Textbook of Atopic Dermatitis

Series in Dermatological Treatment
Published in association with the *Journal of Dermatological Treatment*

Already available

1   Robert Baran, Roderick Hay, Eckhart Haneke, Antonella Tosti, *Onychomycosis*, second edition
    ISBN 9780415385794

2   Ronald Marks, *Facial Skin Disorders*
    ISBN 9781841842103

Of related interest

Steven R Feldman, Kathy C Phelps, Kelly C Verzino, *Handbook of Dermatologic Drug Therapy*
ISBN 9781842142608

Lionel Fry, *Atlas of Dermatology,* fifth edition
ISBN 9781842142370

Arthur Jackson, Graham Colver, Rodney PR Dawber, *Cutaneous Cryosurgery*, third edition
ISBN 9781841845524

Antonella Tosti, Bianca Maria Piraccini, *Diagnosis and Treatment of Hair Disorders*
ISBN 9781841843407

Michael D Zanolli, Steven R Feldman, *Phototherapy Treatment Protocols for Psoriasis and Other Phototherapy-Responsive Dermatoses*, second edition
ISBN 9781842142523

Textbook of Atopic Dermatitis

Edited by

SAKARI REITAMO MD
Hospital for Skin and Allergic Diseases
Helsinki University Central Hospital
Finland

THOMAS A LUGER MD
Clinic for Skin Diseases
and Boltzmann Institute for Immunobiology of the Skin
University of Münster
Germany

MARTIN STEINHOFF MD PhD
Clinic for Skin Diseases
and Boltzmann Institute for Immunobiology of the Skin
University of Münster
Germany

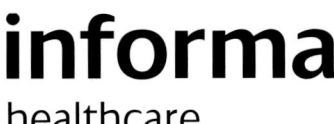

informa
healthcare

First published in the United Kingdom in 2008 by Informa Healthcare, Telephone House, 69–77 Paul Street, London EC2A 4 LQ. Informa Healthcare is a trading division of Informa UK Ltd. Registered Office: 37/41 Mortimer Street, London W1T 3JH. Registered in England and Wales number 1072954.

Tel: +44 (0)20 7017 5000
Fax: +44 (0)20 7017 6699
Website: www.informahealthcare.com

A CIP record for this book is available from the British Library.

Library of Congress Cataloging-in-Publication Data

Data available on application

ISBN-10: 1–84184–246–X
ISBN-13: 978–1–84184–246–2

Distributed in North and South America by
Taylor & Francis
6000 Broken Sound Parkway, NW, (Suite 300)
Boca Raton, FL 33487, USA
Within Continental USA
Tel: 1 (800) 272 7737; Fax: 1 (800) 374 3401
Outside Continental USA
Tel: (561) 994 0555; Fax: (561) 361 6018
Email: orders@crcpress.com

Distributed in the rest of the world by
Cengage Learning Services Limited
Cheriton House
North Way
Andover, Hampshire SP10 5BE, UK
Tel: +44 (0)1264 332424
Email: tps.tandfsalesorder@thomson.com

Composition by C&M Digitals (P) Ltd, Chennai, India
Printed and bound in India by Replika Press Pvt Ltd

Contents

Contributors

Harri Alenius
Finnish Institute of Occupational Health
Helsinki
Finland

Khusru Asadullah
Global Drug Discovery
Bayer Schering Pharma AG
Berlin
Germany

Matthias Augustin MD
Department of Dermatology and Venerology
University Hospital of Hamburg
Hamburg
Germany

Stefan Beissert MD
Department of Dermatology
University of Münster
Münster
Germany

John Berth-Jones
Department of Dermatology
Walsgrave Hospital
Coventry
United Kingdom

Thomas Bieber MD PhD
Department of Dermatology
Rheinische-Friedrich-Wilhelms University of Bonn
Bonn
Germany

Mark Boguniewicz MD
Professor
Division of Pediatric Allergy-Immunology
Department of Pediatrics
National Jewish Medical and Research Center
and University of Colorado School of Medicine
Denver, CO
USA

Randolf MS Brehler MD
Department of Dermatology
University of Münster
Münster
Germany

Michael J Cork PhD MRCP
University Department of Dermatology
Division of Molecular and Genetic Medicine
The Royal Hallamshire Hospital
Sheffield
United Kingdom

Simon Danby
School of Medicine and Biomedical Sciences
University of Sheffield
Sheffield
United Kingdom

Gordon W Duff
School of Medicine and Biomedical Sciences
University of Sheffield
Sheffield
United Kingdom

Sonja A Grundmann
Department of Dermatology
University of Münster
Münster
Germany

Rita Haapakoski
Finnish Institute of Occupational Health
Helsinki
Finland

Ralf G Heine MD FRACP
Department of Allergy
Royal Children's Hospital
Parkville
Victoria
Australia

Gereon Heuft MD
Professor
Department of Psychosomatics and Psychotherapy
University Hospital Münster
Münster
Germany

David J Hill FRACP
Director
Department of Allergy
Royal Children's Hospital
Parkville Victoria
Australia

Clifford S Hosking MD FRACP
Department of Allergy
Royal Children's Hospital
Parkville
Victoria
Australia

Stefanie Kamann
Department of Dermatology
Ludwig-Maximilian-University
Munich
Germany

Antti Lauerma
Finnish Institute of Occupational Health
Helsinki
Finland

Young-Ae Lee
Professor
Pediatric Pneumology and Immunology
Charité University
Campus Virchow-Klinikum
Berlin
Germany

Maili Lehto
Finnish Institute of Occupational Health
Helsinki
Finland

Donald YM Leung MD PhD
National Jewish Medical and Research Center
Denver, CO
USA

Thomas A Luger MD
Clinic for Skin Diseases
and Boltzmann Institute for Immunobiology of the Skin
University of Münster
Münster
Germany

Alice MacGowan
Division of Genomic Medicine
University of Sheffield
Sheffield
United Kingdom

Marcus Maurer MD
Department of Dermatology and Allergy
Allergie-Centrum-Charité
Charité – Universitätsmedizin Berlin
Berlin
Germany

Ekkehard May
Global Drug Discovery
Bayer Schering Pharma AG
Berlin
Germany

Melanic Mertens
Department of Dermatology
University of Münster
Münster
Germany

Manar Moustafa
Division of Genomic Medicine
University of Sheffield
Sheffield
United Kingdom

Salima Mrabet-Dahbi
Department of Clinical Chemistry
and Molecular Diagnostics
Central Laboratory
Hospital of the Philipps-University Marburg
Marburg
Germany

Noreen Nicol MS RN FNP
Clinical Senior Instructor
University of Colorado School of Nursing
Chief Clinical Officer
National Jewish Medical and Research Center
Denver, CO
USA

Natalija Novak MD
Department of Dermatology
Rheinische-Friedrich-Wilhelms University of Bonn
Bonn
Germany

Marc A Radtke MD
Department of Dermatology and Venerology
University Hospital of Hamburg
Hamburg
Germany

Hartmut Rehwinkel
Global Drug Discovery
Bayer Schering Pharma AG
Berlin
Germany

Sakari Reitamo MD
Hospital for Skin and Allergic Diseases
Helsinki University
Central Hospital
Finland

Anita Remitz
Department of Dermatology
Skin and Allergy Hospital
Helsinki
Finland

Harald Renz
Department of Clinical Chemistry
and Molecular Diagnostics
Central Laboratory
Hospital of the Philipps-University Marburg
Marburg
Germany

Heike Schäcke
Global Drug Discovery
Bayer Schering Pharma AG
Berlin
Germany

Gudrun Schneider MD
Department of Psychosomatics and Psychotherapy
University Hospital Münster
Münster
Germany

Stefanie Schoepe
Global Drug Discovery
Bayer Schering Pharma AG
Berlin
Germany

Sonja Ständer MD
Department of Dermatology
University Hospital Münster
Münster
Germany

Martin Steinhoff MD PhD
Clinic for Skin Diseases
and Boltzmann Institute for Immunobiology of the Skin
University of Münster
Münster
Germany

Wolfram Sterry
Department of Dermatology and Allergology
University Hospital
Charité
Berlin
Germany

Rachid Tazi-Ahnini
School of Medicine and Biomedical Sciences
University of Sheffield
Sheffield
United Kingdom

Kristian Thestrup-Pedersen MD PhD
Professor of Dermatology
University of Aarhus
Aarhus
Denmark

Jibu Varghese
School of Medicine and Biomedical Sciences
University of Sheffield
Sheffield
United Kingdom

Yiannis Vasilpoulos
School of Medicine and Biomedical Sciences
University of Sheffield
Sheffield
United Kingdom

Hannele Virtanen
Department of Dermatology
Skin and Allergy Hospital
Helsinki
Finland

Simon Ward
Pediatric Dermatology Clinic
Children's Hospital
Sheffield
United Kingdom

Ulrich Wahn
Pediatric Pneumology and Immunology
Charité University
Campus Virchow-Klinikum
Berlin
Germany

Andreas Wollenberg
Department of Dermatology
Ludwig-Maximilian-University
Munich
Germany

Margitta Worm
Department of Dermatology and Allergy
Allergie-Centrum-Charité
Charité – Universitätsmedizin Berlin
Berlin
Germany

Thomas Zollner
Global Drug Discovery
Bayer Schering Pharma AG
Berlin
Germany

Torsten Zuberbier
Department of Dermatology and Allergy
Allergie-Centrum-Charité
Charité – Universitätsmedizin Berlin
Berlin
Germany

Preface

Atopic dermatitis (AD) is a common disorder which affects infants, children and adults throughout the world with a high socio-economical impact and a broad relevence on the quality of life of these patients. Typical for AD is eczema, a superficial inflammation of the skin. For dermatologists, AD is primarily a clinical diagnosis, which is based on the features suggested by Hanifin and Rajka. In this classification, patients who have no signs of sensitization for environmental antigens, and hence normal immunoglobulin E levels in the serum, are included. New studies suggest that these patients may include up to 50% of the patients with AD, when population-based studies are performed. In contrast, classification by allergologists suggest that AD as a disease where sensitization and hence raised IgE levels plays a central role.

Recent knowledge on common mutations of proteins, especially those of the outer layer of the skin, such as filaggrin, suggest that the skin barrier function in AD can be impaired by both genetic defects in the structure of the skin and the immunological inflammation of AD. Studies both in mouse and man suggest that that a proper barrier function is important not only for the skin but also for the airways. Moreover, the function and regulation of the peripheral as well as central nervous system has been demonstrated to be altered in patients with AD. Thus, this book aims at highlighting our recent advances in understanding the complex interactions between the tissue barrier, the immune and the nervous system.

Treatment of AD remains a challenge. While treatment with topical corticosteroids still forms the primary treatment, long-term data of this treatment is still not sufficient. Ultraviolet therapy and oral immunosuppressive treatment are needed especially in the more severe cases of AD. These treatments are capable of reducing but not replacing corticosteroid treatment. Topical calcineurin inhibitors represent a new treatment alternative which in many cases can totally substitute treatment with topical corticosteroids.

This book gives a broad and intense overview about the clinical manifestations, the pathogenesis as well as present and future treatment modalities of AD. It is aimed to teach both the academic as well as practising dermatologist. We want to thank the publisher for their contribution in putting this book together. The central role of Robert Peden is gratefully acknowledged. We are also grateful for the expertise of all authors who contributed to make this work possible.

Sakari Reitamo, Thomas Luger
and Martin Steinhoff

1

The clinical manifestations of atopic dermatitis

Anita Remitz and Sakari Reitamo

INTRODUCTION

Atopic dermatitis (AD) is a chronic, relapsing, inflammatory skin disease related to other atopic symptoms like allergic rhinitis, allergic conjunctivitis, and asthma. AD usually starts before the age of 2 years and is the first of the atopic symptoms that shows clinical signs. Patients with AD have an increased risk of developing other atopic symptoms later in life. Both endogenous and exogenous factors interact in the development of clinical signs of the disease. Hereditary factors are important, but exogenous causes like the cold climate, stress and pollen are usually necessary to develop clinical symptoms.

The term atopic dermatitis was introduced by Wise and Sulzberger in 1933 as a skin disease characterized by dry skin, pruritus, and chronic relapsing erythematous lesions.[1] The name 'atopy' comes from the Greek meaning 'wrongly placed'. Coca et al had introduced the term atopy to describe a hereditary disorder different from anaphylaxis which was clinically characterized by hay fever and bronchial asthma. The disorder was further characterised by a tendency different from normal subjects, i.e. to become sensitized to environmental factors.[2] In 1967 Ishizaka et al[3] and Johansson[4] showed that IgE antibodies were characteristic of the atopic condition.

The diagnosis of AD is purely clinical; there is no specific clinical symptom or laboratory test. Itch is the main symptom of this disease and the localization of the eczema is often typical (face, jugular, bend of the elbow, hollow of the knee). However, the localization varies with age.

THE LOCALIZATION OF AD AT DIFFERENT AGES

Infancy (0 to 1 year)

The disease often starts around the third month of age and is located on the cheeks and scalp (Figure 1.1). The skin is pruritic and erythematous patches can be seen covered with crusts, which are often secondarily infected (Figure 1.2). Because the rash is scaly and crusted and resembles burnt milk the disease has also been called milk scale. The rash can also develop on the extensor surfaces of the extremities and on the trunk (Figure 1.3). Children with AD often have troubles with sleeping due to pruritus (Figure 1.4). Food allergies are rather common (Figure 1.5).

Childhood (1 to 4 years)

In young children from 1 to 4 years the eczema can still be located on the extensor sites of the extremities (Figure 1.6), but also on the flexural areas (Figure 1.7). It can also be located around the mouth, on the eyelids,

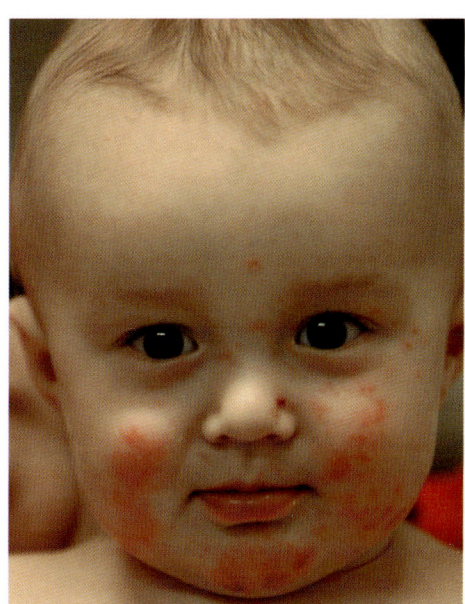

Figure 1.1   AD in an infant.

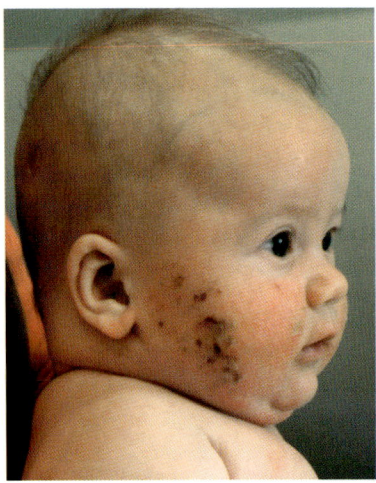

Figure 1.2   Typical milkscale, also called prurigo Besnier.

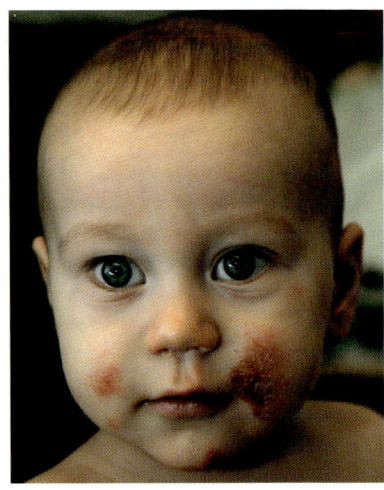

Figure 1.5   AD exacerbated by insensitivity to milk and eggs in a 19-month-old-boy.

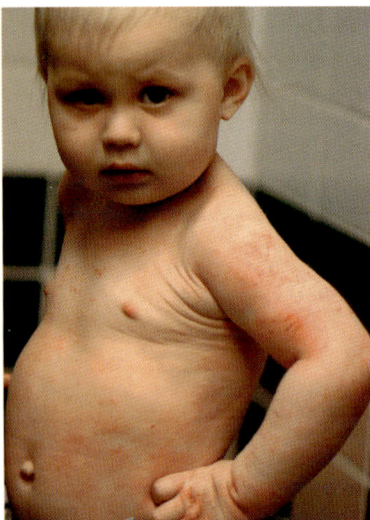

Figure 1.3   AD of the extensor surfaces and trunk in a 1-year-old boy.

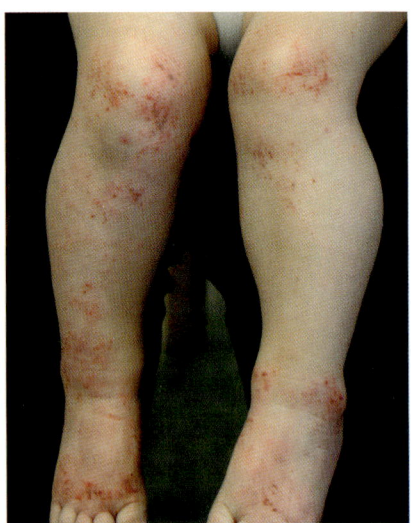

Figure 1.6   AD on extensor surfaces of the lower extremities.

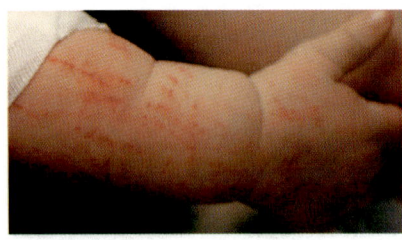

Figure 1.4   Results of intensive pruritus and scratching in a 1-year-old infant.

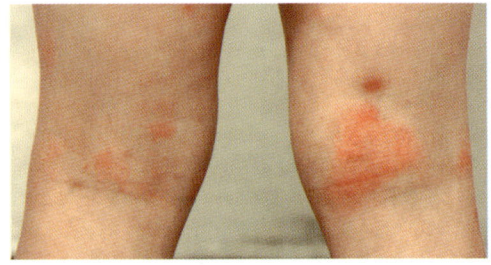

Figure 1.7   AD of the flexures.

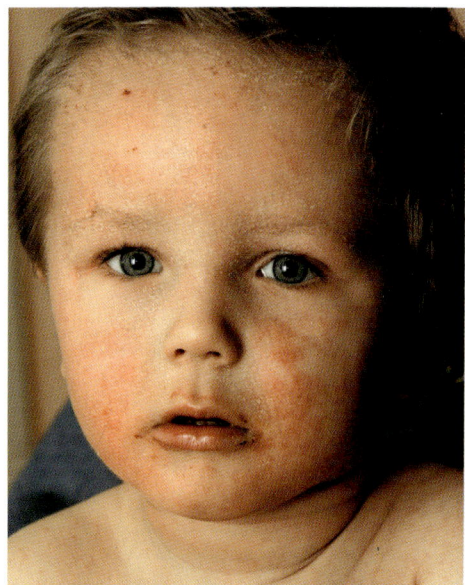

Figure 1.8   Widespread AD with mild scales in a small child.

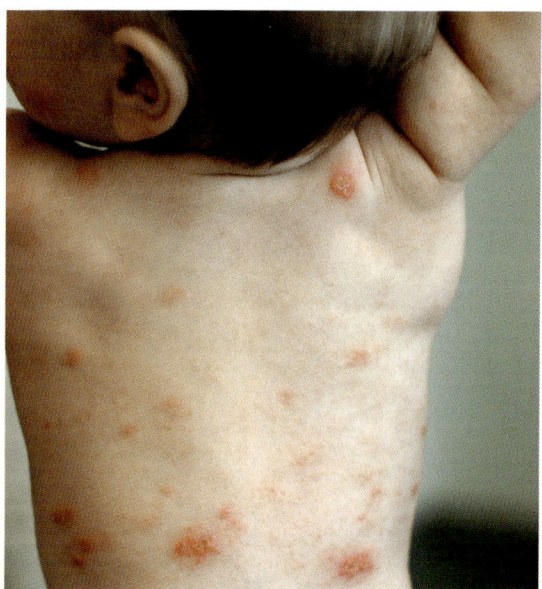

Figure 1.9   Nummular AD in a small child.

neck, and hands (Figure 1.8). The lips can be dry and scaly. The lesions are usually symmetric erythematous papules with excoriations, small crusts, and lichenification (Figure 1.9). Food allergies are less common than in infants.

Adolescents (4 to 16 years)

Children from 4 to 16 years usually develop symmetric eczema on the flexural areas (Figure 1.10), on the hands (Figure 1.11), and feet. The so-called horseback area on the back of the thighs can also be affected (Figures 1.12–13). During the winter months the children can develop eczema on their hands and feet (atopic winter feet) due to wet gloves or socks after playing outside. When the child comes closer to puberty eczema can also be seen on the upper body and face (Figures 1.14–15). Food allergies are unusual.

Adults (over 16 years)

In adults the eczema lesions are typically on the face (Figures 1.16–19), upper body (Figure 1.20), flexural areas (Figures 1.21–22), and hands (Figure 1.23). Sometimes the disease can develop into erythrodermia (Figure 1.24). Stress and climate are important triggering factors.

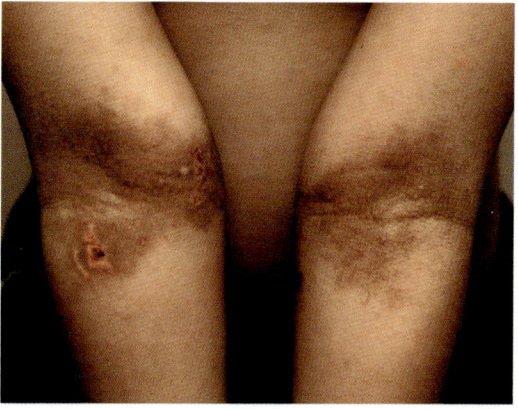

Figure 1.10   Lichenified AD of the elbows in a child of African origin.

DIAGNOSTIC CRITERIA OF AD

Although the diagnosis of AD is purely clinical, it is not always easy to define the disease and therefore several authors have suggested guidelines to help in making the diagnosis. The diagnosis is based on medical history (personal and/or family history) and typical signs and symptoms. However, none of these clinical features is diagnostic for AD. Hanifin et al[5] based their

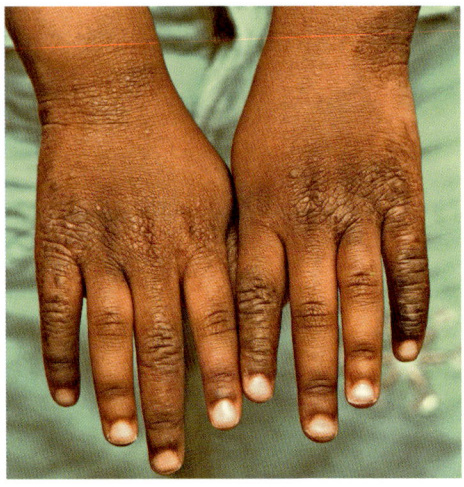

Figure 1.11   Lichenified AD of the hand in a child of African origin.

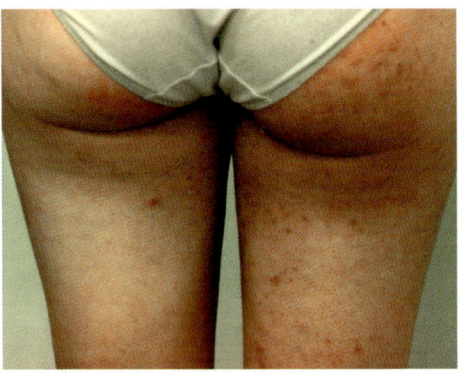

Figure 1.12   AD in the horse-back area in a white young female.

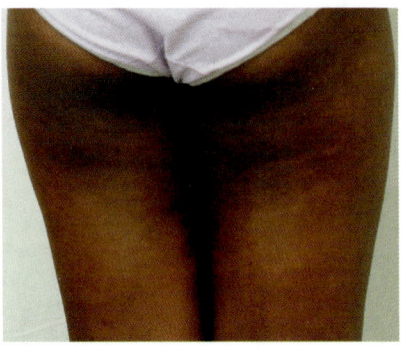

Figure 1.13   AD in the horse-back area in a black young female.

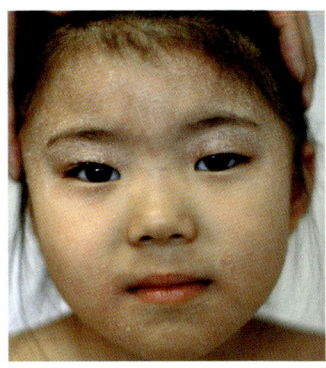

Figure 1.14   AD of the face with scales in a girl of Japanese origin.

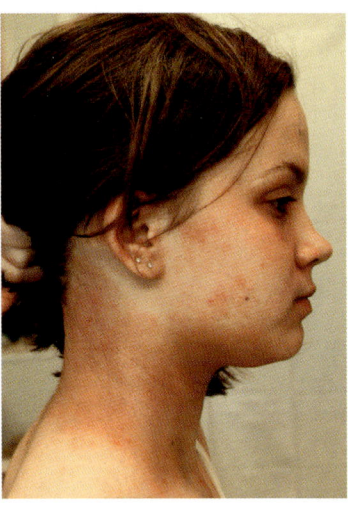

Figure 1.15   Severe AD of the face in a white girl.

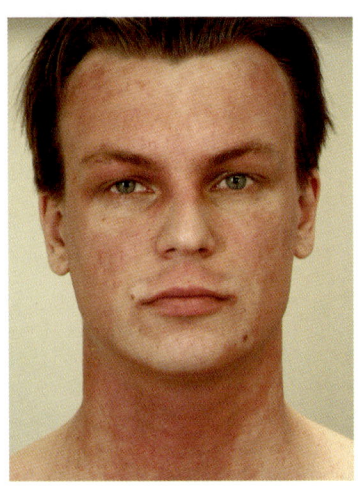

Figure 1.16   AD with widespread erythema in a 25-year-old man.

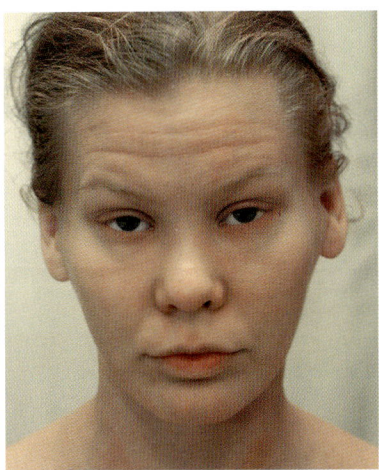

Figure 1.17   Severe AD with oedema but little erythema of the face in a 19-year-old female.

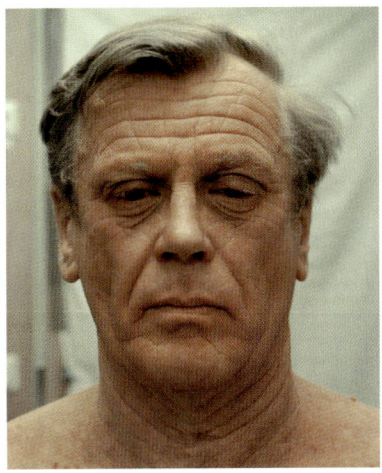

Figure 1.18   Severe AD with profound oedema and erythema of the face in a 56-year-old man.

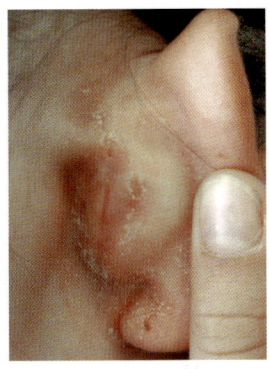

Figure 1.19   Retroauricular eczema in a 20-year-old woman with AD.

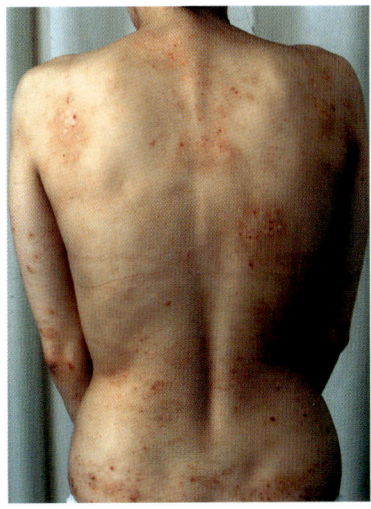

Figure 1.20   Nummular eczema with scars from scratching in a 18-year-old female.

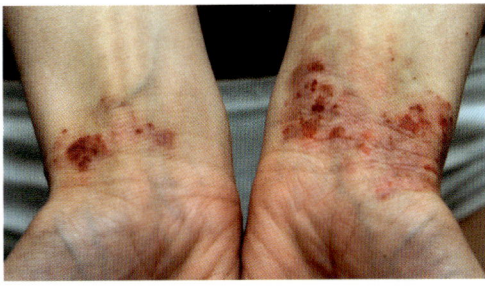

Figure 1.21   Lichenified eczema of the wrist with signs of intense scratching in a 16-year-old female.

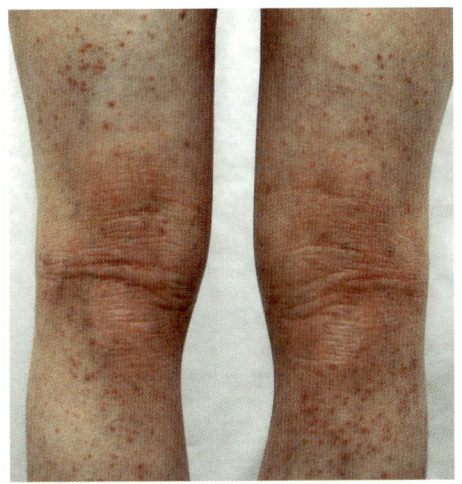

Figure 1.22   Severe lichenified eczema of the knees in a 17-year-old male.

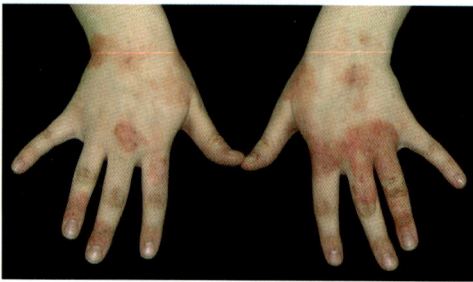

Figure 1.23   Typical irritant eczema of the hands in AD in a 22-year-old female.

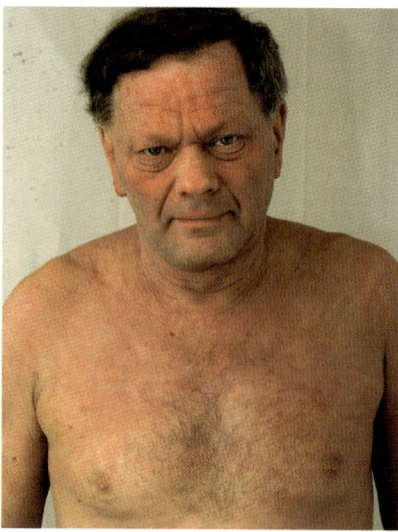

Figure 1.24   Severe erythrodermia in a 51-year-old male with long-standing AD resistant to therapy.

diagnosis on 4 major criteria and several minor criteria (Table 1.1). Williams et al[6] applied and simplified Hanifin and Rajka's criteria and suggested that the patient must have itchy skin (obligatory) and then at least three of the additional features (Table 1.2).

Several investigators have looked at the prevalence of the minor criteria of Hanifin et al in atopic patients. Böhme et al[7] studied 221 children 24 months of age or younger, who were re-examined after 2 years. A control group of 99 children of the same age, with no history of eczema were examined in the same way. They found 7 minor criteria that were met more in atopic children: namely, xerosis (100%), course influenced by environmental factors (87%), facial erythema (54%), skin reactions provoked by ingested food (39%), itch when sweating (34%), positive skin prick tests (29%),

Table 1.1   Hanifin et al: diagnostic criteria. The patient must have at least 3 of the major characteristics and 3 of the minor characteristics to have AD. (Hanifin JM, Rajka G. Diagnostic features of atopic dermititis. Acta Derm Venereol Suppl (Stockh) 1980; 92: 44–7.)

Major characteristics
Pruritus (excoriations can often be seen, Figure 1.25)
Lichenification (flexural lichenification in adults and older children, facial and extensor involvement in infants, Figure 1.26)
Chronic or chronically relapsing course
Personal or family history of atopy (asthma, allergic rhinoconjunctitis, atopic dermatitis, contact urticaria Figure 1.27)

Minor characteristics
Xerosis (dryness of skin)
Ichthyosis (especially with palmar hyperlinearity or keratosis pilaris, Figure 1.28)
Immediate type I reactions to skin test allergens (positive prick test reactions, Figure 1.29)
Elevated serum IgE (about 20% of atopic patients have normal IgE levels)
Early age of onset
Cutaneous infections by *Staphylococus aureus* (Figure 1.30), herpes simplex (Figure 1.31) and other viral infections, warts (Figures 1.32–33), or molluscum contagiosum (Figure 1.34)
Non-specific hand (and/or foot) dermatitis (Figure 1.35)
Nipple eczema (Figure 1.36)
Cheilitis (Figure 1.37)
Recurrent conjunctivitis (Figure 1.38)
Dennie-Morgan infraorbital fold (Figures 1.39–40)
Keratoconus
Anterior subcapsular cataracts
Orbital darkening (Figure 1.41)
Facial pallor/erythema (Figures 1.42–43)
Anterior neck folds
Itch when sweating
Food intolerance
Course influenced by environmental or emotional factors
Intolerance to wool and lipid solvents or any course fabric or non-absorptive occlusive garment, and wet working conditions
Perifollicular accentuation
White dermographism/delayed blanch (Figures 1.44–45)

and hand eczema (28%). Early age of onset was an inclusion criteria for the study. Approximately half of

Table 1.2   Williams et al: diagnostic criteria.
Williams et al suggested that the patients must
have itchy skin and then at least 3 of the additional
features. (Williams HC, Burney PG, Pembroke AC.
Br J Dermatol 1994; 131: 406–16.)

Basic feature (obligatory)
Itchy skin

Additional features (at least 3 of the following)
Skin symptoms in flexural regions such as knee and
    elbow flexures, in front of the wrists
    and neck (in cheeks in children under 10 years)
Asthma or allergic rhinitis (or atopic diseases in close
    relatives in children under 4 years)
Dry skin during the last year
Visible eczema in flexural areas (or on cheeks and/or
    forehead in children under 4 years)
Eczema starting before the age of 2

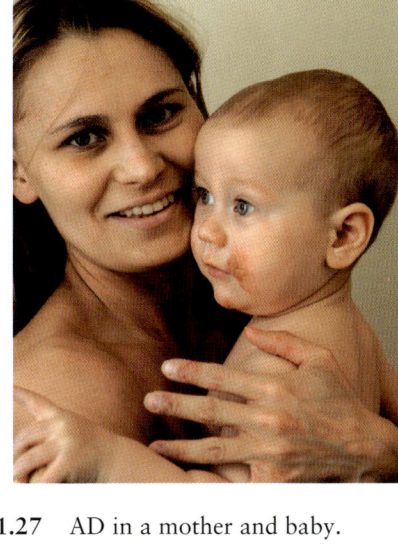

Figure 1.27   AD in a mother and baby.

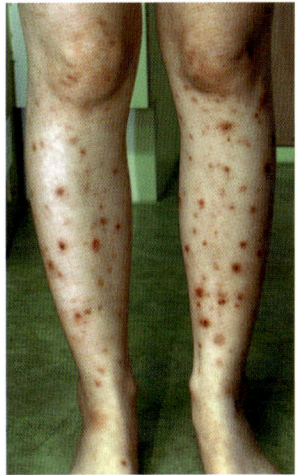

Figure 1.25   Lower extremities with signs of chronic scratching due to intense pruritus in a 16-year-old female patient with AD.

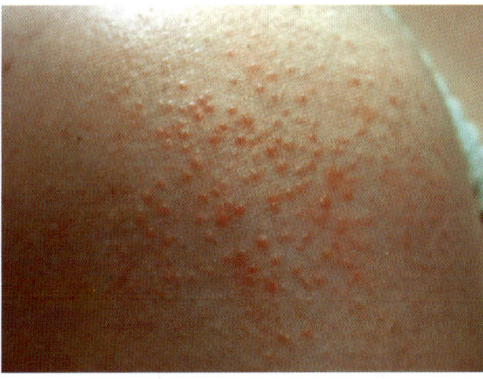

Figure 1.28   Keratosis pilaris is a sign not restricted to AD.

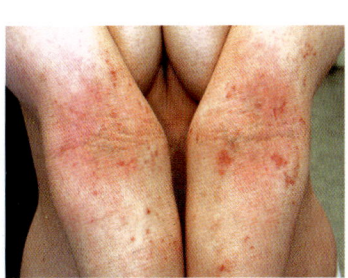

Figure 1.26   Flexural lichenification in a 20-year-old female with AD.

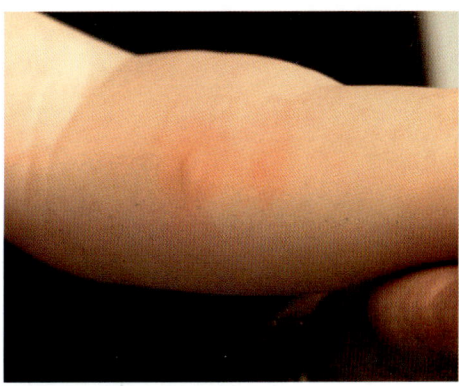

Figure 1.29   Positive prick test reactions to milk and egg-white in a 17-month-old child with food allergy.

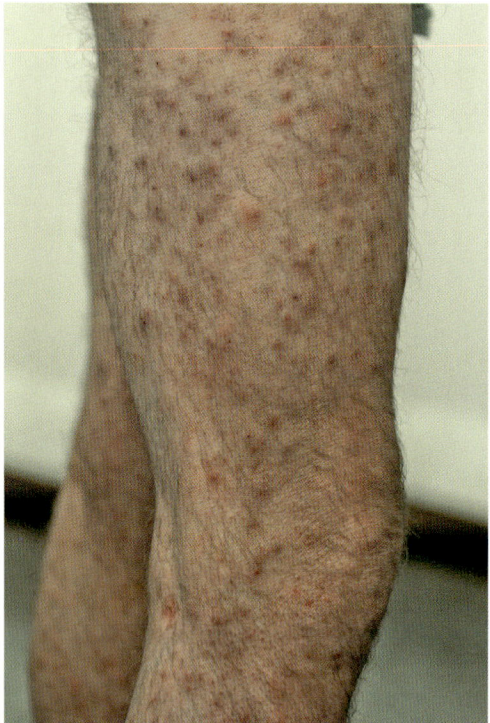

Figure 1.30   Folliculitis caused by *Staphylococcus aureus* in a 54-year-old male with severe AD.

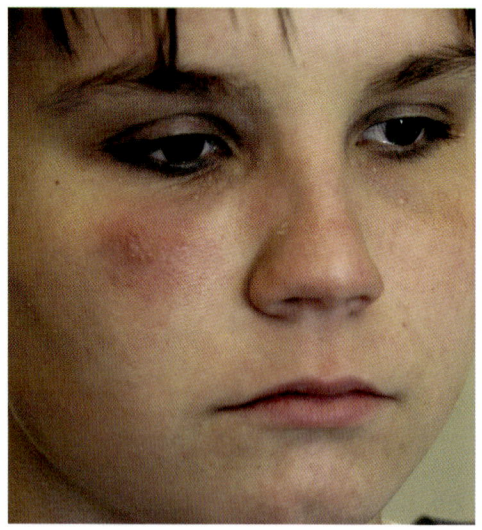

Figure 1.31   Herpes simplex infection at an unusual site in a 15-year-old female with AD.

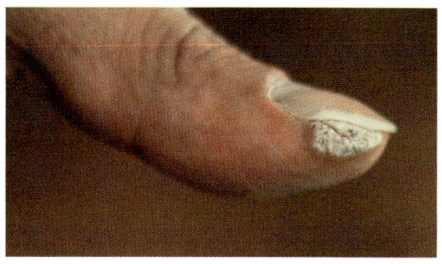

Figure 1.32   Long-standing viral warts in a 36-year-old male with severe AD.

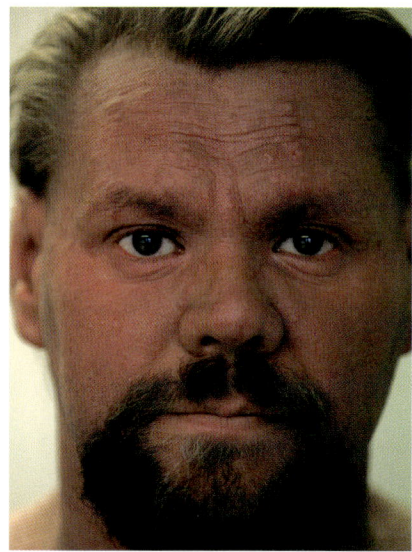

Figure 1.33   Viral warts of the face in the same male as in Figure 1.33.

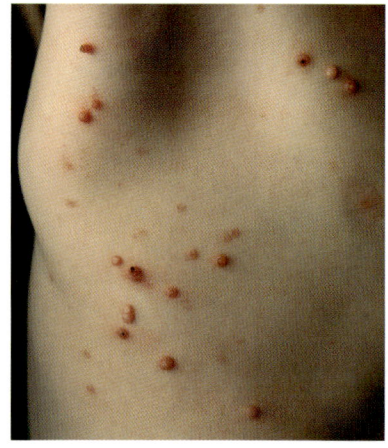

Figure 1.34   Molluscae in a 4-year-old girl.

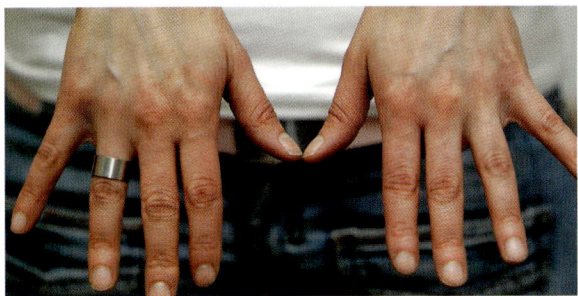

Figure 1.35   Irritant hand eczema in a 25-year-old female with AD.

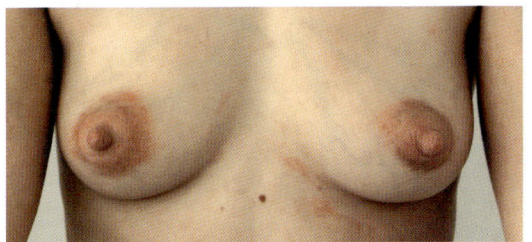

Figure 1.36   Nipple eczema in 24-year-old female with AD.

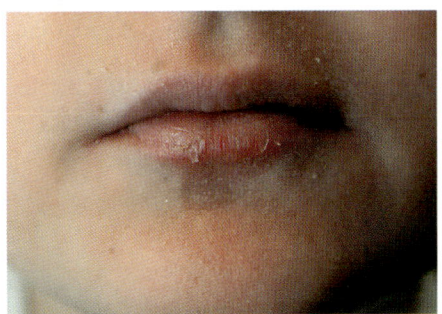

Figure 1.37   Cheilitis in a 17-year-old female with AD.

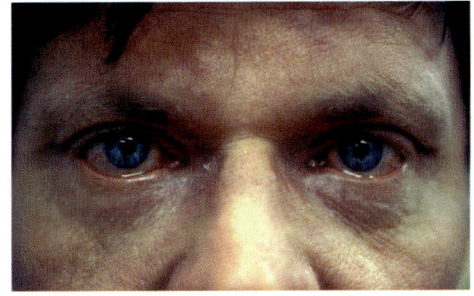

Figure 1.38   Chronic conjunctivitis in a 41-year-old male with severe AD.

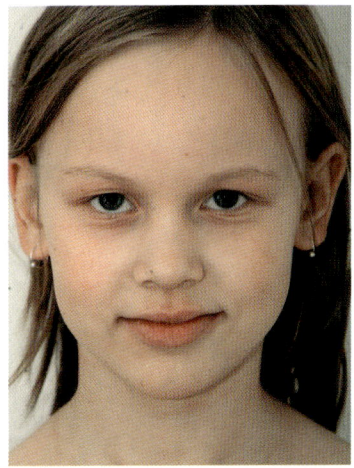

Figure 1.39   Dennie-Morgan infraorbital fold in a young girl.

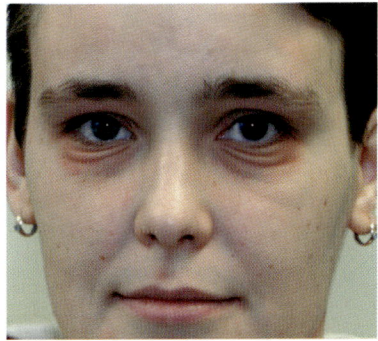

Figure 1.40   Dennie-Morgan fold in a young woman.

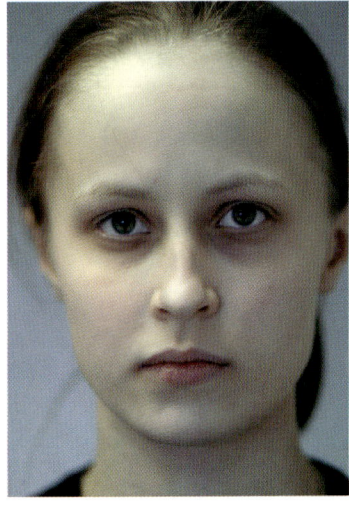

Figure 1.41   Orbital darkening in a 20-year-old female with mild AD.

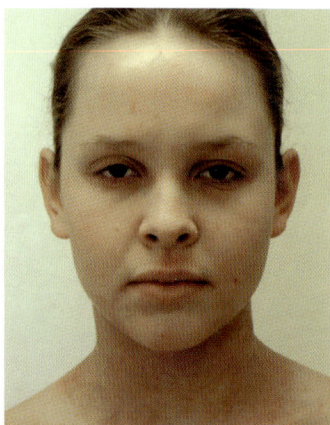

Figure 1.42   Facial pallor in a 20-year-old female with AD.

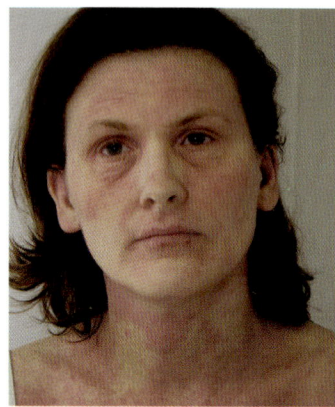

Figure 1.43   Facial erythema in a 45-year-old female with AD and a long-term use of corticosteroids.

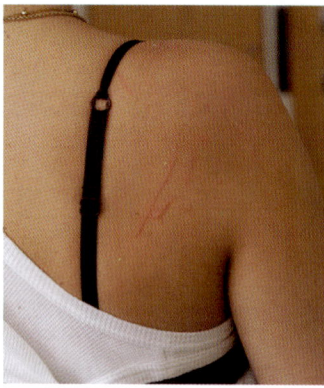

Figure 1.44   White dermographism caused by scratching in 22-year-old female with AD.

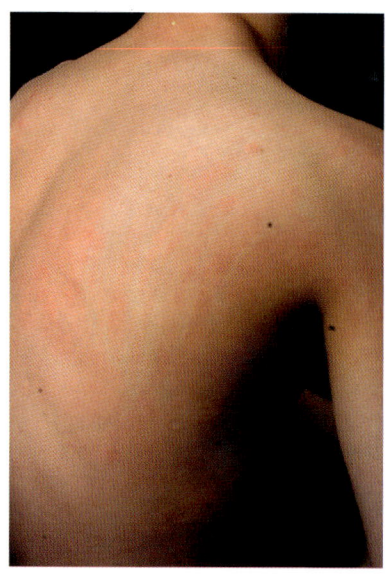

Figure 1.45   Delayed blanch in a 17-year-old male with widespread AD.

the criteria occurred in 3% or fewer of the studied patients and may be of minimal use in this age group.

In addition to age the clinical condition of the patient seems to be of importance on several minor characteristics. Therefore, effective treatment will have an effect on the expression of several signs. The occurrence of the Dennie-Morgan infraorbital fold was low in the infant study by Böhme, but when Diepgen et al[8] studied the age group of 10 to 55 years, it had a prevalence of 69%. As with many symptoms and signs of AD, the Dennie-Morgan sign is clearly dependent on the clinical condition of the patients (Figure 1.46). This applies also to the anterior neck folds (Figure 1.47). The infra-auricular fissure has often been proposed to be a diagnostic feature of AD. Kim et al[9] showed a prevalence of 55% and Tada et al[10] of 82% in atopic patients up to 52 years.

As a conclusion, there are no specific criteria that would occur only in atopic patients. They can, however, help in the diagnosis of AD. The age of the atopic patients seems to be of great importance in the occurrence of the different minor criteria, and racial differences can also be seen. Pruritus seems to be a symptom which is quite resistant to treatment, and can also be provoked by other diseases in patients with AD (Figure 1.48).

Firooz et al[11] studied the frequency of the main criteria (Table 1.3). The most common symptoms were itch, which was seen in 70%, and history of dry skin in 40% of patients.

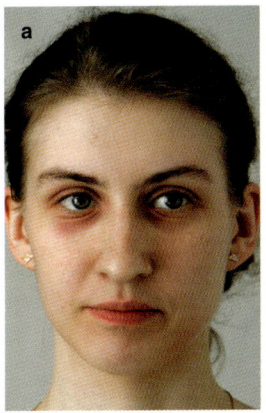
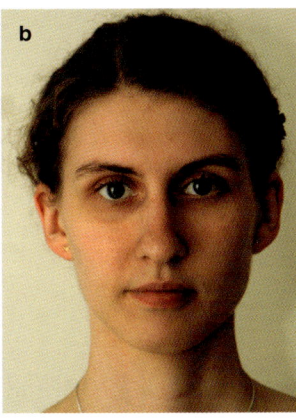

Figure 1.46   Dennie-Morgan infraorbital fold before (a) and after (b) treatment with topical tacrolimus ointment.

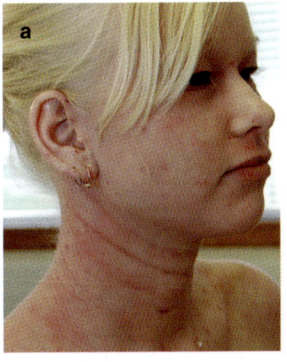
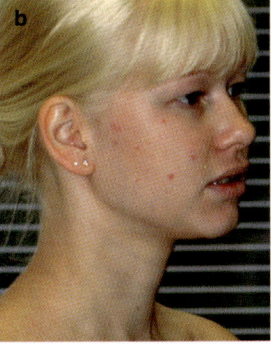

Figure 1.47   Anterior neck folds before (a) and after (b) treatment with topical tacrolimus ointment.

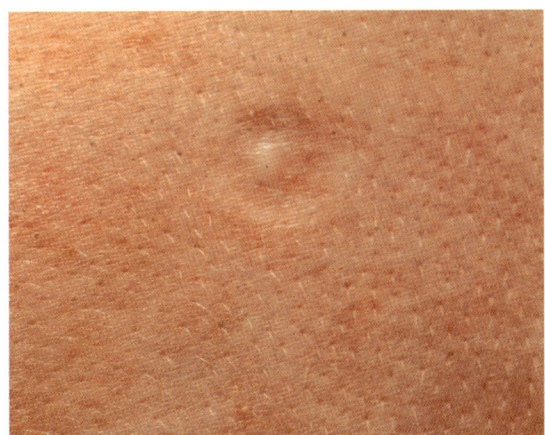

Figure 1.48   Scars caused by intense pruritus and scratching scratching during varicella infection.

Table 1.3   Frequency of the proposed diagnostic criteria for AD in patients and controls. (Firooz A, Davoudi SM, Farahmand AN et al. Validation of the diagnostic criteria for atopic dermititis. Arch Dermatol 1999; 135: 514–16.)

Criteria	No. (%) patients with AD	Controls
Itch	42 (70.0)	128 (36.0)
History of involvement of skin diseases	20 (33.3)	40 (11.2)
History of asthma or hay fever	11 (18.3)	51 (13.3)
History of general dry skin	24 (40.0)	35 (9.8)
Visible flexural eczema	8 (13.3)	9 (2.5)
Onset <2 years	3 (5.0)	0

DIFFERENTIAL DIAGNOSIS

In infancy AD can be mixed with seborrhoeic dermatitis, which also can occur on the face and scalp. These infants often suffer from diaper dermatitis and do not have a family history of atopic diseases. Seborrhoeic disease also subsides after a few weeks when the stimulatory effect of maternal hormones disappears. Ichthyosis vulgaris can be suspected in children with very dry skin and with positive family history of ichthyosis. The typical scaling is seen especially on the extensor surfaces of the extremities after 2 months of age. Scabies can be seen with severe itch and dermatitis. Usually other family members also have symptoms, and the finding of burrows, usually on the hands, and the isolation of mites provide the diagnosis. Psoriasis also sometimes starts in infancy although it is rare. Then the lesions are more defined and can be present with the typical white scale.

In childhood and adolescence the localization of AD is usually on flexural areas and the disease has usually started earlier in infancy. However, the atopic winter foot can sometimes be misdiagnosed to tinea pedis. Impetigo of the face can also sometimes be misdiagnosed as AD. Psoriasis can also start in childhood, usually after streptococcal infections in the form of psoriasis guttata. Pityriasis rosea usually starts with

Table 1.4	Diseases associated with AD
Elevated IgE Immunodeficiency	Hyper-IgE syndrome
	Wiskott-Aldrich syndrome
	Ataxia-telangiectasia
	Selective IgA deficiency
Genodermatoses	Phenylketonuria
	Hypohidrotic ectodermal dysplasia
	Biotin deficiency
	Hartnup disease
	Acrodermatitis enteropathica
	Langerhans cell histiocytosis

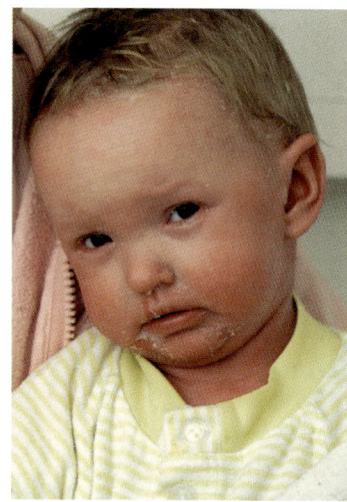

Figure 1.49 A girl with Netherton syndrome

a larger primary lesion which is followed by smaller scaly lesions on the trunk. The lesions subside in approximately 6 weeks.

In adults hand eczema can be a sign of AD, but possible contact allergies have to be excluded if the eczema continues for several months in spite of treatment.

There are also rare conditions where AD has been described as a feature. However, the dermatitis which has been described in these patients rarely fulfils the criteria for AD. AD is also a common disease, so it is possible that these patients have two diseases. The diseases are listed in Table 4. The rare Netherton syndrome is also associated with AD (Figure 1.49).

REFERENCES

1. Wise F, Sulzberger MB. Footnote on problem of eczema, neurodermatitis and lichenification. In: Wise F, Sulzberger MB, eds. Year Book of Dermatology and Syphilogy. Chicago: Year Book Publishers, 1933: 38–9.
2. Coca AF, Cooke RA. On the classification on the phenomenon of hypersensitivities. J Immunol 1923; 8: 163–82.
3. Ishizaka K, Ishizaka T. Identification of xE antibodies as carrier of reaginic activity. J Immunol 1967; 99: 1187–98.
4. Johansson SGO. Raised levels of of a new immunoglobulin (IgND) in asthma. Lancet 1967; 2: 951–53.
5. Hanifin JM, Rajka G. Diagnostic features of atopic dermatitis. Acta Derm Venereol Suppl (Stockh) 1980; 92: 44–7.
6. Williams HC, Burney PG, Pembroke AC. The UK working parties & diagnostic criteria for atopic dermatitis III. Br J Dermatol 1994; 131: 406–16.
7. Böhme M, Svensson Å, Kull I, Wahlgren C-F. Hanifin's and Rajka's minor criteria for atopic dermatitis: Which do 2-year-olds exhibit? J Am Acad Dermatol 2000; 43: 785–92.
8. Diepgen TL, Sauerbrei W, Fartasch M. Development and validation of diagnostic scores for atopic dermatitis incorporating criteria of data quality and practical usefulness. J Clin Epidemiol 1996: 1031–8.
9. Kim KH, Chung JH, Park KC. Clinical evaluation of minor clinical features of atopic dermatitis. Ann Dermatol 1993; 5: 9–12.
10. Tada J, Toi Y, Akiyama H, Arata J. Infra-auricular fissures in atopic dermatitis. Acta Derm Venereol 1994; 74: 129–31.
11. Firooz A, Davoudi SM, Farahmand AN et al. Validation of the diagnostic criteria for atopic dermatitis. Arch Dermatol 1999; 135: 514–16.

2

Genetic dissection of eczema

Young-Ae Lee and Ulrich Wahn

INTRODUCTION

Eczema is a chronic inflammatory skin disease that is characterized by intense pruritus. In the industrialized countries the prevalence of eczema is approximately 15% with a steady increase over the last decades.[1,2] Along with asthma and allergic rhinitis, eczema is commonly associated with the state of atopy which is characterized by the formation of allergy antibodies (IgE) to environmental allergens.

Eczema is commonly the first clinical manifestation of allergic disease. Onset of disease is observed during the first year of life in 57% and during the first 5 years in 87% of patients.[3] For the majority of affected children eczema heralds a lifetime of allergic disease. The development of atopic disease often follows an age-dependent pattern that is known as the 'atopic march'.[4] A susceptible child commonly passes a characteristic sequence of transient or persistent disease stages that begins with eczema and food allergy in the young infant and continues with the development of respiratory airways disease later in childhood and adulthood. The close familial and intra-individual association of these disease entities strongly suggests shared genetic determinants. However, additional epidemiological studies show that parental eczema confers a higher risk of eczema to offspring than parental asthma or allergic rhinitis,[5] indicating the presence of eczema-specific genes.

A strong genetic component in atopy was recognized almost a century ago. Cooke et al first reported that the relatives of patients are at significantly increased risk of developing allergic disease.[6] The initial report already included the observation of non-Mendelian inheritance of allergic disease and the positive correlation of genetic risk with an earlier age of onset. The strongest evidence for the importance of genetic factors in atopic disease stems from twin studies. The concordance rate for eczema among monozygotic twins of about 80%

far exceeds the concordance rate of 20% observed among dizygotic twins.[7,8] These data clearly indicate that the genetic contribution to the expression of eczema is substantial. In addition, studies on the vertical transmission of eczema and atopic disease show that children are more likely to inherit these disorders if the mother is affected (parent-of-origin effect).[9] The predominance of maternal inheritance may be due to environmental factors such as uterine milieu or breast feeding, but may also arise due to genetic mechanisms such as parent-specific gene expression (genomic imprinting).[10] Parent-of-origin effects should therefore be taken into account in the search for eczema genes.

Eczema and atopic disorders are regarded as multifactorial conditions, the onset and severity of which are influenced by both genetic and environmental factors. The data are consistent with an immune etiology shared by all atopic diseases and a congenital target organ defect, the penetrance of which is modified by multiple environmental factors during early childhood. Genetic investigations of atopic disease may prove important in dissecting the clinical entities of atopic disorders that we currently recognize thus providing novel guidelines for their classification. Identification of genes underlying eczema and atopy has the capacity to define primary physiological mechanisms, thereby clarifying disease pathogenesis, identifying pathways and targets for therapeutic intervention, providing opportunity for preclinical diagnosis, and allowing treatment tailored to underlying abnormalities in individual patients.

APPROACHES TO THE GENETIC ANALYSIS OF ECZEMA

Genetic complexity is present when there is no simple correlation between genotype and phenotype. The expression of the disease phenotype cannot be predicted using Mendel's laws of segregation.[11] Typically, there is

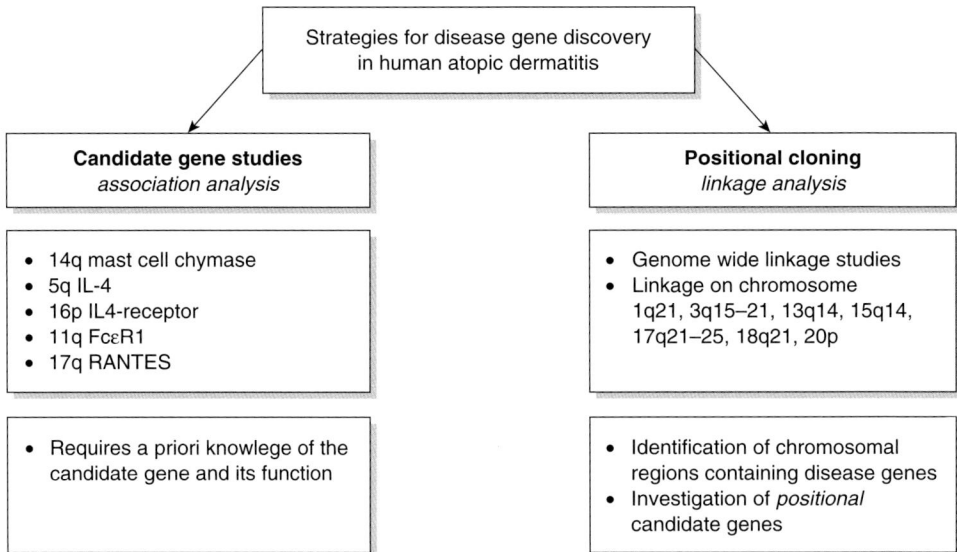

Figure 2.1   Strategies for disease gene discovery in human eczema.

wide temporal and quantitative variability in the disease expression with respect to age of onset, disease duration, and severity. Moreover, disease allele carriers may themselves remain unaffected by disease (incomplete penetrance) because manifestation of the disease may require or be facilitated by the interaction with other genetic or environmental factors. The heritable component of eczema can be regarded as the cumulative effect of multiple disease alleles. The number of genes that influence the trait and the magnitude of the effect imparted by any single locus remains a matter of conjecture. Furthermore, the combination of disease-causing alleles is likely to vary among and even within different ethnic groups (genetic heterogeneity). To identify disease genes for complex traits such as eczema by genetic approaches, the investigation of hundreds to thousands of affected families is required. Major strategies of disease gene identification for eczema in man are summarised in Figure 2.1.

CANDIDATE GENE STUDIES

Several candidate gene studies for eczema have been reported. In this approach candidate genes are selected based on their known function in the pathophysiology of eczema. Based on the hypothesis that variants in these genes alter gene function or expression and may confer susceptibility to the disease, the gene is then screened for sequence variants and the frequency of these variants is compared between groups of patients and controls. Most of the candidate genes explored were initially investigated for asthma and atopy.

Overall, there is substantial variance in the study design, phenotype definition, and size of the study population. As case-control studies may result in false positive findings due to population substructure, some authors have used family-based association tests, such as the transmission disequilibrium test (TDT). The classical TDT requires family triads consisting of a patient and the parents. The transmission of a putative disease from heterozygous parents to an affected offspring is observed. At a locus that is unrelated to the disease the marker alleles will be transmitted with equal probability, whereas a true disease allele would be expected to be transmitted more frequently to an affected child. Modifications of this test for different family structures and certain modes of inheritance have been developed.[12] A number of candidate genes for eczema have been investigated. Those that have been explored in at least 2 independent studies have been summarised in Table 2.1.

Mast cell chymase

Mast cell chymase is a proinflammatory serine protease that is abundantly expressed by dermal mast cells. The expression of mast cell chymase is decreased in non-lesional skin of eczema patients and further decreased in lesional skin suggesting a role of mast cell chymase in suppressing skin inflammation.[13] The gene encoding mast cell chymase (chromosome 14q11) was investigated as a candidate gene for eczema. Two non-coding polymorphisms were studied in 4 Japanese patient groups with eczema, atopic asthma, non-atopic asthma, and allergic rhinitis, each comprising 100 individuals, as well

Table 2.1   Results of association studies for eczema and associated phenotypes

Gene	Chromosomal location	Polymorphism	Population	Study sample	Phenotype	Refs.
Mast cell chymase	14q11	−1903A/G	Japanese	100 cases, 100 controls	AD	(14)
		−1903A/G	Japanese	107 cases, 507 controls	AD with IgE < 500 IU/L	(15)
		−1903A/G	Japanese	169 cases, 100 controls	AD with IgE < 500 IU/L	(16)
		−1903A/G	Japanese	100 cases, 101 controls	no association	(17)
		−1903A/G	Italian	70 cases, 100 controls	no association	(18)
		−1903A/G	Swedish	107 ASP families	no association	(19)
IL4	5q31	−589C/T	Japanese	88 ASP families	AD	(21)
		−589C/T	Japanese	302 cases, 120 controls	no association	(22)
		−589C/T	Swedish	308 individuals	no association	(23)
		−589C/−34C haplotype	Australian	101 families	AD	(24)
αIL4R, IL4 receptor	16p11	Q576R	USA	30 cases, 30 controls	atopy	(25)
		Q551R	Japanese	27 cases, 29 controls	AD	(26)
		Q551R	Japanese	302 cases, 120 controls	no association	(22)
		−327A, −326C, −186A, −184A	Japanese	101 cases, 75 controls	AD	(27)
IL13	5q31	G4257A	German	187 cases, 98 controls	AD	(32)
		G4257A	Japanese	185 cases, 102 controls	AD	(33)
		C1103T			no association	
		G4257A	Canadian	29 cases	AD	(34)
		C1103T			no association	
FcεRI	11q13	Rsal_in2, Rsal_ex7	British	60 families, 88 families	AD	(35)
		FcεRI microsatellite	Swedish	361 ASP families	AD	(19)
RANTES	17	−401G/A	German	188 cases, 98 controls	AD	(37)
		−401G/A, −28G, −2518G	Hungarian	128 cases, 303 controls	no association	(38)

as a group of 100 healthy controls. One of the polymorphisms (−1903A/G) was associated with eczema, and not allergic asthma or allergic rhinitis.[14] In a pediatric cohort, Mao et al divided the probands according to total serum IgE levels. They reported that among children with total IgE serum levels < 500 IU/L, heterozygotes for the −1903 polymorphism were significantly more frequent among patients with eczema compared to unaffected controls.[15] The same polymorphism was evaluated comparing Japanese patients with eczema alone, and those with eczema and allergic airways disease. The association was confirmed in a small subgroup of 47 patients with eczema alone and serum IgE levels of < 500 IU/L.[16] It was suggested that this variant may predispose to non-atopic eczema. However, further investigations failed to replicate the association in other Japanese,[17] Italian,[18] and Swedish[19] populations.

The cytokine gene cluster and cytokine receptors

The chromosomal region 5q31-33 has repeatedly shown evidence for linkage and association with atopic disorders. This region contains a number of interesting functional candidate genes for eczema and atopy including the cytokine gene cluster with the interleukin (IL)-4, IL-13, IL-9, and IL-5 genes, as well as the genes encoding IL-12B, CD14, hepatitis A virus cellular receptor 1, and GM-CSF.

The gene encoding IL-4 was one of the first candidate genes investigated. Evidence for linkage of total serum IgE levels to a marker close to the IL-4 gene was first demonstrated in 170 affected sib pairs originating from 11 Amish families.[20] The cytokine IL-4 plays a key role in the regulation of humoral and allergic responses. IL-4 controls the differentiation of naïve T helper cells into T helper 2 (Th2) effector cells. It induces the expression of Th2 cytokines like IL-5, IL-6, and IL-9, and class switching to IgE.

Suggestive evidence for linkage of genetic markers flanking the IL-4 gene was detected in 88 Japanese affected sib pair families with atopic dermatitis. The promoter polymorphism in the IL-4 gene, −589C/T, was investigated for association using the TDT. Significant overtransmission of the T allele to affected children (0.001) was observed.[21] This association, however, was not confirmed in a larger Japanese study comprising 302 eczema patients and 120 controls.[22] The IL-4 gene was subsequently investigated for linkage and association in a Swedish sample: 308 genotyped individuals were available for a family-based association test of the 589C/T promoter polymorphism. Two discrete phenotypes, eczema per se and specific sensitization as well as the semiquantitative trait 'severity score of eczema' were studied. No linkage or association with the two discrete

phenotypes was observed; however, positive evidence for linkage to the 589C/T promoter polymorphism was detected (P < 0.005). The authors concluded that this chromosomal region influences the severity of eczema.[23] Finally, promoter polymorphisms within the IL-4 gene were investigated for association with childhood eczema in an Australian cohort of 76 nuclear families and 25 trios. In addition to the − 590C/T polymorphism (identical to − 589C/T), a newly identified promoter polymorphism, − 34C/T, was studied. In the initial analysis of each single polymorphism no association was observed; however, combined to form haplotypes, an association of the − 590C/− 34C haplotype with eczema was detected. The authors point out that the association became non-significant after correction for multiple testing. The results remain difficult to interpret, as the suggestive association in this study was reported with the haplotype containing the − 590C allele rather than the T allele which was associated in the initial Japanese report.[24]

The effects of IL-4 are mediated by the IL-4 receptor, a heterodimer consisting of an α-subunit (αIL4R) and either a γc subunit (type 1 receptor) or an IL-13Ra1 unit (type 2 receptor). The gene encoding the α-subunit of the IL-4 receptor (αIL4R) is located on chromosome 16p. Linkage studies in this region were reported for a Swedish and a Danish study group. Söderhäll et al typed two microsatellite markers closely flanking the αIL4R gene in 406 families with at least 2 children with eczema. Linkage analysis was conducted for the phenotypes eczema and specific sensitisation and yielded negative results for both traits. In fact, linkage to this chromosomal region was excluded for a locus-specific effect of $\lambda s = 2$ for eczema and $\lambda s = 3$ for specific sensitisation.[23] Similarly, linkage analysis in 100 nuclear families of the Danish ITA cohort (Inheritance of Type I Allergy) excluded the region of the αIL4R gene with $\lambda s = 2$ for atopy and eczema.

The cDNA of αIL4R was screened for sequence variants in 10 patients with severe eczema or hyper-IgE syndrome and a mutation was identified in position 1902 of the gene leading to an amino acid exchange (Q576R) in the cytoplasmic domain of the αIL4R protein. This mutation was associated with enhanced expression of the low affinity IgE receptor (CD 23) in vitro and a change in the binding specificity of the adjacent tyrosine residue at position 575 to signal-transducing molecules. A significant association of this variant with atopy was detected in a small case control study comprising 30 atopic individuals and 30 controls.[25] Oiso et al genotyped 6 known polymorphisms in the αIL4R gene in a very small sample of 27 patients with eczema and 29 non-atopic controls and reported a positive association of the Gln551Arg polymorphism with eczema (P = 0.01).[26] However, this association was not confirmed in a larger study group of the same ethnic origin.[22] Recently, an association study with promoter polymorphisms of the αIL4R gene was performed. Six promoter polymorphisms were characterized, 5 of which were found to be associated with eczema. The 4 proximal variants formed three common haplotypes named α, β, and γ. The α haplotype was significantly more frequent among 101 eczema patients compared to 75 controls. Promoter assays revealed no significant difference in promoter activity of the α and β haplotypes at baseline and after stimulation in vitro. Therefore, the functional significance of the association remains to be explored.[27]

The IL-13 gene is located in the cytokine gene cluster on chromosome 5q. Several previous investigations support an important role of IL-13 in the pathogenesis of eczema. Increased expression of IL-13 mRNA was observed in acute eczema skin lesions.[28] IL-13 gene expression was also significantly increased in peripheral blood mononuclear cells (PBMCs) of patients with eczema than in controls[29] and was shown to correlate with the severity of eczema.[30] Heinzmann et al characterized a mutation in Exon 4 of the IL-13 gene at position 4257 bp. The A allele of this variant results in an amino acid change with a predicted enhanced receptor binding and increased IL-13 signalling.[31] Liu et al performed an association study of this variant for eczema in 187 affected children and 98 unaffected controls from the German MAS-90 cohort. The presence of the A allele was significantly associated with eczema and elevated serum IgE.[32] Tsunemi et al studied three polymorphisms (A704C, C1103T, G4257A) in 185 adult patients with eczema and 102 controls. They confirmed the association of the A allele of the G4257A variant with eczema[33] as did a Canadian study in a small sample of 29 affected children.[34]

The high affinity IgE receptor (FcεRI)

The high affinity IgE receptor (FcεRI) is expressed on mast cells, basophils, and antigen-presenting cells and mediates allergic reactions by crosslinking with IgE. In humans, FcεRI is expressed either as a trimer or a tetramer. The β subunit functions as a amplifier of FcεRI surface expression and signalling. The gene encoding the β subunit of FcεRI was investigated as a candidate gene for eczema, as polymorphisms within the gene had previously been shown to be linked and associated with asthma and atopy.

Two non-coding sequence variants in Intron 2 and Exon 7, and a coding polymorphism in Exon 7 (E237G) of the FcεRI gene were examined in two independent family cohorts of 60 and 88 families, respectively. Using a family-based association test, a significant overtransmission of the maternal allele was observed. This result was confirmed in the second family set.[35] The functional significance of these polymorphisms is under investigation. In a study of 12 extended pedigrees from Germany, positive evidence for linkage of eczema with an intragenic microsatellite marker was reported.[36] Studying a large sample of 361 nuclear families with siblings affected with eczema, linkage on chromosome 11q was not confirmed, but a positive association of one of the most common alleles of the FcεRI microsatellite marker was found.[19]

RANTES

RANTES is a CC chemokine with chemoattractant properties for eosinophils, lymphocytes, monocytes, and basophils. In view of its role in the mediation of allergic inflammation, the RANTES gene was explored as a candidate gene for eczema. A functional variant in the promoter region (−401G/A) of the RANTES gene was shown to result in an additional consensus site for the GATA transcription factor family and in increased transcriptional activity of the promoter. This variant was associated with eczema in a case control study of 188 children with eczema and 98 controls from Germany.[37] Association of 2 promoter polymorphisms, −401A and −28G, with asthma was detected in an English[37] and a Chinese[37] study group, respectively. In an attempt to replicate the association with eczema in a paediatric population from Hungary, these two and an additional promoter polymorphism in position −2518G were investigated in 128 children with eczema, 102 allergic children without eczema, and 303 age-matched children without allergic disorders. No association of RANTES promoter polymorphisms with eczema, total IgE levels, white blood cell count, or eosinophil cell count was detected.[38]

The results of candidate gene studies have been highly variable. As summarised in Table 2.1, the study populations are often quite small and it is difficult to assess whether positive associations represent true findings or type I errors. The risk of a type I error increases as the number of tests with marker alleles and phenotypes increases. Only few studies address this problem and correct for multiple testing. Commonly, associations found in one study are often not replicated in others. In many cases, direct comparisons of results are not possible due to different study designs, disease definitions, patient recruitment strategies, ethnic background, and environment. Furthermore, the conflicting results of the IL-4 promoter polymorphism make it difficult to draw conclusions about the significance of the findings. The following standards have been proposed for a good association study:

1. Positive associations should be based on large sample sizes and small P values.
2. The study design should include an initial study as well as an independent replication, as well as both family-based and population-based studies.
3. The putative disease allele should affect gene function in a disease-relevant way.[39]

Since the evaluation of strong functional candidate genes for a complex disease across the whole genome may include as many as 5000 tests, a nominal P value of 10^{-5} (0.05/5000) was proposed to provide a low type I error rate. Even more stringent parameters were suggested for genome-wide tests in the absence of convincing functional candidacy or prior evidence of linkage.[40]

INVESTIGATION OF GENE–ENVIRONMENT INTERACTIONS

Eczema and atopy arise in susceptible individuals after interaction with environmental factors. The importance of the environment in the development of allergic disease is clearly reflected by their increase in prevalence over recent decades.[1,2] The investigation of gene–environment interactions in eczema remains a challenge for the near future. Epidemiological studies have documented a correlation of a decline of childhood infections,[41] as associated with a 'western' lifestyle,[42] small family size,[43] and improved hygiene with the emergence of allergic disease. To address a possible influence of childhood infection on the expression of eczema in carriers of the IL-4 receptor (αIL4R) polymorphism Q551R, Callard et al studied 992 children from the ALSPAC cohort. The documented use of antibiotics was used as a surrogate marker for infection. This study revealed a positive association of the 551R allele with eczema during the first 6 months of life (P = 0.02) only in the group of children that had not received antibiotics. In contrast, no difference in the allelic distribution of this marker was observed among children who had used antibiotics. This association was not present at the age of 60 months. The authors conclude that the influence of infection on the immune system of a genetically susceptible individual may be limited to a critical time interval during the first few months of life. The study demonstrates that some genetic determinants may only be detectable if environmental factors are taken into account.[41] The results also demonstrate that studies of gene–environment interaction in humans require much larger study populations in which clinical and environmental data are available.

MENDELIAN DISEASES

An alternative candidate gene approach has been the investigation of rare Mendelian forms of atopic disease in which mutations in single genes impart large effects on phenotype expression. This approach may be particularly well suited to eczema and atopy, as the functional consequences of single gene disorders are easier

to explore and may define fundamental pathways which, when altered, also affect more common forms of atopic disease.

The first Mendelian disorder investigated was the hyper-IgE syndrome. This disorder is characterized by extremely high serum IgE levels, eosinophilia, chronic eczema, recurrent staphylococcal and fungal infections, as well as pneumonia. Additional features may include coarse facial features, osteoporosis, hyperextensible joints, and delayed shedding of primary teeth. Segregation analysis suggests an autosomal dominant mode of inheritance with variable expression of the phenotype. Linkage analysis in 19 affected families revealed significant evidence for linkage on chromosome 4q21.[44] This region also showed linkage to specific sensitization against house dust mites in 66 affected sib pairs from Germany.[45]

The chromosomal region containing the gene mutated in Wiskott-Aldrich syndrome (WAS) was investigated as a candidate gene for eczema. WAS is a rare X-linked recessive immunodeficiency disorder characterized by severe eczema, thrombocytopenia, recurrent infections, and susceptibility to autoimmune disease and lymphoreticular malignancies. The eczema observed in WAS usually presents within the first few months of life and is clinically indistinguishable from eczema. Mutations in the gene encoding Wiskott-Aldrich syndrome protein (WASp) on chromosome Xp23 have been shown to cause WAS.[46] Four polymorphic microsatellite markers flanking the WAS gene were typed in a Swedish study group comprising 406 affected sib pair families with eczema. Three phenotypic traits were investigated: eczema, severity score of eczema, and atopy defined as raised allergen-specific IgE. Modest evidence for linkage was reported at marker MAOB with a maximum lod score of 1.68 (P < 0.05) to the severity score of eczema. Association of genetic markers in this region could not be seen with eczema nor with elevated allergen-specific serum IgE antibodies. These results provide some evidence that either the WAS gene or another gene in the area contributes to the severity of eczema.[47]

Recently, the gene underlying the Mendelian disorder Netherton syndrome has been explored for atopic disorders.[48] Netherton syndrome is a rare autosomal recessive disease characterized by congenital erythroderma and ichthyosis, sparse brittle hair with a specific hair shaft defect (trichorrhexis invaginata), and atopic manifestations, including high levels of serum IgE, eczematous rashes, asthma, hay fever, angioedema, and eosinophilia. Netherton syndrome was mapped to chromosome 5q32 distal of the cytokine gene cluster.[49] The underlying disease gene was identified to be SPINK5. The coding sequence consisting of 33 exons was resequenced and six coding polymorphisms were identified, four of which were genotyped in a panel of 148 families recruited through a child with eczema. Using the TDT test significant overtransmission of the maternal allele of two polymorphisms, Asn368Ser in Exon 13 and Glu420Lys in Exon 14, was observed for the phenotypes eczema, specific sensitisation, and elevated total serum IgE. The association with the Glu420Lys polymorphism was replicated for the phenotypes eczema, specific sensitisation, elevated total serum IgE, and asthma in a second group of 73 families. An independent replication was attempted in a Japanese study of 124 patients with eczema and 110 healthy controls. Two polymorphisms in Intron 12, three polymorphisms in Exons 13, and one polymorphism in Exon 14 were genotyped. Association analysis of the Asn368Ser and Glu420Lys polymorphisms did not show an association with the putative disease allele suggested by the original study. For the two intronic polymorphisms a weak association with eczema was detected. The disparate results of the studies may reflect differences of the study populations in terms of ethnic origin, age, and the study design. Parent-of-origin effects could not be investigated in the Japanese study. The authors concluded that they may not represent general susceptibility factors for eczema in caucasian populations.[9]

A third study was conducted in a Caucasian population from Germany. Association of the coding variants Asn368Ser, Asp386Asn, and Glu420Lys with eczema was tested for using both a case control study including 201 patients and 368 controls and a family-based study on 308 patient-parents trios. The latter approach allowed the authors to investigate maternal overtransmission. Both studies showed no association of the polymorphisms with eczema. The authors concluded that they may not represent general susceptibility factors for eczema in Caucasian populations.[9] The recent finding of a major eczema susceptibility gene originated from the investigation of families with autosomal dominant ichthyosis vulgaris (IV). IV is a disorder of keratinisation that is characterized by hyperlinearity of the palms and fine scaling of the skin. Loss-of-function mutations in the gene encoding filaggrin (*FLG*) have been identified as a common genetic causes.[51] *FLG* is located within the epidermal differentiation complex (EDC) on human chromosome 1q21. Filaggrin is a key protein of the epidermis which plays a key role in the formation of the protective skin barrier. In the outer granular layer of the epidermis, filaggrin is associated with keratin intermediate filaments and aids their packing into bundles. In terminally differentiated keratinocytes, filaggrin is crosslinked to the cornified cell envelope which constitutes an insoluble barrier in the stratum corneum, protecting the organism against environmental agents and preventing epidermal water-loss.[52] Palmer et al reported that the same loss-of-function mutations in *FLG* predispose to eczema and

asthma that occurs in association with eczema.[53] This study demonstrated that a primary defect in the skin barrier plays an important role in the etiology of eczema and provided a molecular link with the epidermal barrier dysfunction that is clinically observed in eczema patients. Unlike most of the previously reported genetic associations, a strong association of *FLG* null mutations with eczema has repeatedly been replicated. Subsequent studies have demonstrated a reduced penetrance of 42% and have estimated that *FLG* mutations account for about 11% of eczema cases in a population based cohort from Germany.[54]

GENOME-WIDE LINKAGE STUDIES AND POSITIONAL CLONING

Positional cloning of eczema genes relies on chromosomal mapping/localisation by linkage analysis, subsequent narrowing of the candidate region by linkage disequilibrium mapping, and finally characterization of sequence variants and their effect on gene function and disease pathogenesis. Genome-wide linkage studies are the first step in the attempt to identify disease genes by positional cloning. This approach exploits the inheritance of the disease in multiply-affected families and identifies chromosomal regions that have been inherited by affected individuals. It therefore allows the identification of disease genes without prior knowledge of putative disease mechanisms and carries the potential to unravel novel genes and molecular pathways that are important in the disease pathogenesis.

In a genetic linkage study, many families, usually hundreds, are investigated in which the phenotype of interest, eczema, segregates. To scan the genome, every proband is genotyped using several hundred genetic markers evenly spaced along all chromosomes. Usually, highly informative genetic markers are used that allow one to trace the inheritance of each chromosomal segment from parents to offspring. One would expect a chromosomal segment containing an eczema gene to be shared among affected family members more often than regions that have no effect on disease susceptibility. The significance of the excess sharing can be expressed in lod scores.[50]

Ten previous genome scans focussing on asthma and elevated IgE levels have been conducted in different ethnic groups and have revealed numerous linkage findings in different chromosomal regions throughout the genome. The major overlapping linkage findings on asthma, were located on chromosomes 1p, 4q, 5p, 5q near the cytokine gene cluster, 6p near the major histocompatibility complex, 7p, 11q near the β chain of the high affinity IgE receptor, 12q, 13q, and 16q.[50]

The localisation and identification of susceptibility genes of complex diseases has been facilitated by including families with an early age of onset in the analysis. This approach has been successful in disease gene identification in breast cancer[50] and chronic inflammatory bowel disease.[50] The first genome scan for eczema was designed to enhance the contribution of genetic factors in the family set. Therefore, only families with at least two children with eczema with an early age of onset (before the second birthday) and severe disease expression were included: 199 complete nuclear families from Germany, Italy, Sweden, and the Netherlands, were included in the study.[51] Highly significant evidence for linkage was detected in a single chromosomal region on chromosome 3q21. This locus was distinct from any previous linkage reports for asthma or atopy phenotypes. The finding therefore suggested that distinct genetic factors predispose to eczema. Further analysis on chromosome 3q21 revealed that a large estimated proportion of 40% of the families contributed to the linkage score. As epidemiological studies suggested an increased risk of allergic disease transmitted by the mother rather than the father, an additional analysis was conducted to assess whether there was an excess of maternal allele sharing (parent-of-origin effect). This investigation revealed significant evidence for a maternal effect at this locus. Subsequently, the underlying disease causing gene has been identified as a novel epidermal collagen gene, collagen 29A1 (COL29A1).[57] Collagens are the most abundant extracelluar matrix (ECM) proteins in vertebrates and play a crucial role in maintaining tissue integrity. Their importance for tissue function has been highlighted by the wide spectrum of human diseases caused by mutations in collagen genes.[58] COL29A1 was located in a two-staged investigation consisting of systematic linkage and association. Scanning of the candidate region and subsequent confirmation of the association in a large independent replication data set. An association with a maternal transmission pattern was detected within a subregion of 1.70 kilobase, which included a single gene, COL29A1. Involvement of COL29A1 in eczema was further supported by its tissue-and cell-specific expression pattern. Highest COL29A1 expression was observed in the epidermis, but also in other epithelial tissues including the lung, small intestine, and colon which are the main manifestation sites of allergic disorders, including asthma and food allergy. This gene expression pattern indicated a potential role of collagen XXIX in a wider spectrum of allergic diseases and suggested a molecular link between eczema, respiratory airways disease, and food allergies which are epidermiologically closely associated.[59,60] Comparative expression analysis if COL29A1 in skin biopsies if eczema,

patients revealed a distinct lack of COL29A1 mRNA and protein in the outer viable layers of the epidermis. This finding indicated that a defective ECM may give rise to the disease, proposing a new disease mechanism in the etiology of eczema.[57]

The second genome-wide scan was conducted in the UK and included 148 families recruited through a child with active eczema.[53] The linkage result on chromosome 3q was not replicated. Instead, additional linkages for eczema on chromosomes 1q21 and 17q25, and for eczema with asthma on chromosome 20p were reported. Notably, all three loci as well as the one previously described on chromosome 3q closely overlap with linkage findings for another chronic inflammatory skin disease, psoriasis. This finding further supported the notion that skin-specific susceptibility factors exist. While eczema and psoriasis are distinct clinical entities that show no epidemiological association, the newly identified candidate regions may contain genetic variants specific to skin barrier function and immunity and may thus facilitate the identification of the underlying disease genes. The candidate region on chromosome 1q21 contains the epidermal differentiation complex and that on chromosome 17q the keratin type I gene cluster. Mutations in a number of genes located in either region have been demonstrated to cause different monogenic disorders of epidermal differentiation and function.[54]

A third genome-wide linkage study for eczema susceptibility genes was conducted in a Swedish study group. Of a total of 406 affected sib pair families, 109 were selected for the genome scan.[55] Similar to the previous studies, 367 microsatellite markers were used and linkage analysis was carried out for three qualitative phenotypes, eczema, extrinsic eczema, and severe eczema, as well as one semi-quantitative phenotype, severity of eczema. Suggestive evidence for linkage was reported for eczema on chromosome 3p24-22, and for eczema combined with elevated allergen-specific IgE levels (atopic eczema) as well as for severe eczema on chromosome 18q21. For the semi-quantitative phenotype severity score of eczema, suggestive evidence for linkage was found in an additional four regions on chromosomes 3q14, 13q14, 15q14-15, and 17q21. The results of the published genome scans are summarised in Table 2.2. Taken together, two chromosomal regions on chromosomes 3q and 17q emerge which are supported by replication and confirmation in the third study. All three studies demonstrate that multiple disease genes predispose to eczema. There is only partial overlap with linkage findings for asthma confirming epidemiological data that suggested the existence of shared genetic susceptibility for all atopic diseases and organ-specific genetic susceptibility.

Table 2.2   Results of genome screens for eczema and related phenotypes

Population	Number of families	1q21	3p22–24	3q15–21	13q14	15q14	17q25	18q21	20p	Refs.
Germany, Sweden, Italy, the Netherlands	199			3q21 AD atopy						(49)
UK	148	1q21AD					17q25 AD		20p AD with asthma	(51)
Sweden	109		3p22–24 AD	3q15 severity of AD	13q14 severity of AD	15q14 severity of AD	17q21 severity of AD	18q21 extrinsic AD		(53)

MOUSE MODELS

Gene mapping by linkage analysis in animal models offers several advantages over the human setting such as reduced genetic heterogeneity in inbred strains and the possibility to generate large numbers of offspring in short generation times. This is particularly useful in the process of disease gene identification in a linked chromosomal segment as key recombinants in a candidate region can more easily be generated by breeding. In addition, the mouse offers a different approach to disease gene identification based on gene targeting by knockout and transgenic techniques. Furthermore, inbred animal strains provide an ideal setting for the investigation of gene–environment interactions as animal experiments can be conducted under conditions of tight environmental control.

Inbred mouse models with susceptibility to eczema like disease and atopy have been used in backcrosses with disease-resistant strains for gene mapping. The NOA (Naruto Research Institute Otsuka Atrichia) shows an ulcerating dermatitis with accumulation of mast cells and increased serum IgE. A susceptibility locus for dermatitis was mapped to a region on mouse chromosome 14[56] that is syntenic to human chromosome 13q14 where linkage of total serum IgE levels and asthma has been reported.[57,58] Two additional modifier loci on mouse chromosomes 7 and 13 have been identified.[59] The respective syntenic regions on human chromosomes 11q13 and 5q13 have repeatedly been linked to atopic phenotypes.[50] Using a positional cloning approach in human populations, the underlying disease gene on chromosome 13q14 has been identified as PHF11. Variants in this gene were found to be associated with specific sensitization and severe asthma,[59] as well as eczema.[59] While the function of PHF11 remains to be elucidated, its expression in cells of the immune system and domain architecture suggest a role in transcriptional regulation.

Another inbred model, the NC/Nga mouse (NC) has been investigated. This mouse is characterized by severe dermatitis with epidermal hyperplasia and increased numbers of mast cells and eosinophils, as well as elevated serum IgE. A locus for the eczema skin-like lesions was located on mouse chromosome 9 in a region syntenic to human chromosomes 11q22-23 and 15q21-25.[60] The latter region has shown linkage to the severity score of eczema in Swedish families.[55] Fine mapping of the proposed eczema loci in the mouse and disease gene identification is pending. Gene discovery by positional cloning in mouse models is facilitated by the availability of breeding strategies such as congenic substitution mapping.[61] The orthologues of genes within a defined mouse chromosome interval are strong candidates for human disease loci and are expected to reveal disease-relevant pathways that can be explored further in human populations. Likewise genes identified in man can be analysed functionally using mouse models.

SUMMARY

Eczema and atopy are multifactorial disorders with a strong genetic basis. Improved methods of genetic analysis and the availability of the sequence of the human genome have led to remarkable progress in identifying chromosomal regions and candidate genes linked to eczema. Recent genetic findings highlight the importance of the epidermis and its role in maintaining the physical and immunological barrier in the pathogenesis of eczema and allergic disease. Functional evaluation of novel disease variants including their predictive value in human populations and possible interactions with environmental factors will require the examination of large numbers of clinically well-characterized patients and families.

The genetic constitution provides the basis for immune responses to environmental stimuli and autoantigens. It is possible that many gene variants that predispose to eczema and atopy have evolved as determinants of natural host resistance to infectious disease. The overlapping linkage findings for eczema and other chronic inflammatory skin conditions favor genes that determine skin-specific disease mechanisms. Future analysis of complex diseases like eczema will benefit from the development and application of analytical methods that have the ability to systematically evaluate the contribution of genes operating in heterogeneous environments. Comprehensive analysis of the genetic components of different pathway(s) that are essential for the development of eczema will be an important tool, since it seems very likely from our current knowledge that many molecular variants acting in concert may be required to induce and maintain expression of the disease.

REFERENCES

1. Kay J, Gawkrodger DJ, Mortimer MJ, Jaron AG. The prevalence of childhood atopic eczema in a general population. J Am Acad Dermatol 1994; 30: 35–9.
2. Taylor B, Wadsworth J, Wadsworth M, Peckham C. Changes in the reported prevalence of childhood eczema since the 1939–45 war. Lancet 1984; 2: 1255–57.
3. Rajka G. Prurigo Besnier (atopic dermatitis) with special reference to the role of allergic factors. The influence of atopic hereditary actors. Acta Derm Venereol (Stockh) 1960; 40: 285–306.
4. Wahn U. What drives the allergic march? Allergy 2000; 55: 591–99.
5. Dold S, Wjst M, von Mutius E, Reitmeir P, Stiepel E. Genetic risk for asthma, allergic rhinitis, and atopic dermatitis. Arch Dis Child 1992; 67: 1018–22.
6. Cooke RA, Van der Veer A. Human sensitization. J Immunol 1916; 1: 201–305.
7. Larsen FS, Holm NV, Henningsen K. Atopic dermatitis. A genetic-epidemiologic study in a population-based twin sample. J Am Acad Dermatol 1986; 15: 487–94.

8. Schultz LF. Atopic dermatitis: a genetic-epidemiologic study in a population-based twin sample. J Am Acad Dermatol 1993; 28: 719–23.

9. Chavanas S, Bodemer C, Rochat A, Hamel-Teillac D, Ali M et al. Mutations in SPINK5, encoding a serine protease inhibitor, cause Netherton syndrome. Nat Genet 2000; 25: 141–2.

10. Wilkins JF, Haig D. What good is genomic imprinting: the function of parent-specific gene expression. Nat Rev Genet 2003; 4: 359–68.

11. Mendel GJ. Versuche über Pflanzen-Hybriden. Verhandlungen des naturforschenden Vereines in Brünn, Abhandlungen, Brünn 1866; 4: 3–47.

12. Spielman RS, Ewens WJ. The TDT and other family-based tests for linkage disequilibrium and association. Am J Hum Genet 1996; 59: 983–89.

13. Li-Weber M, Krammer PH. Regulation of IL4 gene expression by T cells and therapeutic perspectives. Nat Rev Immunol 2003; 3: 534–43.

14. Mao XQ, Shirakawa T, Yoshikawa T, Yoshikawa K, Kawai M et al. Association between genetic variants of mast-cell chymase and eczema. Lancet 1996; 348: 581–3.

15. Mao XQ, Shirakawa T, Enomoto T, Shimazu S, Dake Y et al. Association between variants of mast cell chymase gene and serum IgE levels in eczema. Hum Hered 1998; 48: 38–41.

16. Tanaka K, Sugiura H, Uehara M, Sato H, Hashimoto-Tamaoki T et al. Association between mast cell chymase genotype and atopic eczema: comparison between patients with atopic eczema alone and those with atopic eczema and atopic respiratory disease. Clin Exp Allergy 1999; 29: 800–3.

17. Kawashima T, Noguchi E, Arinami T, Kobayashi K, Otsuka F et al. No evidence for an association between a variant of the mast cell chymase gene and atopic dermatitis based on case-control and haplotype-relative-risk analyses. Hum Hered 1998; 48: 271–4.

18. Pascale E, Tarani L, Meglio P, Businco L, Battiloro E et al. Absence of association between a variant of the mast cell chymase gene and atopic dermatitis in an Italian population. Hum Hered 2001; 51: 177–9.

19. Soderhall C, Bradley M, Kockum I, Wahlgren CF, Luthman H et al. Linkage and association to candidate regions in Swedish atopic dermatitis families. Hum Genet 2001; 109: 129–35.

20. Marsh DG, Neely JD, Breazeale DR, Ghosh B, Freidhoff LR et al. Linkage analysis of IL4 and other chromosome 5q31.1 markers and total serum immunoglobulin E concentrations. Science 1994; 264: 1152–6.

21. Kawashima T, Noguchi E, Arinami T, Yamakawa-Kobayashi K, Nakagawa H et al. Linkage and association of an interleukin 4 gene polymorphism with atopic dermatitis in Japanese families. J Med Genet 1998; 35: 502–4.

22. Tanaka K, Sugiura H, Uehara M, Hashimoto Y, Donnelly C et al. Lack of association between atopic eczema and the genetic variants of interleukin-4 and the interleukin-4 receptor alpha chain gene: heterogeneity of genetic backgrounds on immunoglobulin E production in atopic eczema patients. Clin Exp Allergy 2001; 31: 1522–7.

23. Söderhäll C, Bradley M, Kockum I, Luthman H, Wahlgren CF et al. Analysis of association and linkage for the interleukin-4 and interleukin-4 receptor b;alpha; regions in Swedish atopic dermatitis families. Clin Exp Allergy 2002; 32: 1199–202.

24. Elliott K, Fitzpatrick E, Hill D, Brown J, Adams S et al. The −590C/T and −34C/T interleukin-4 promoter polymorphisms are not associated with atopic eczema in childhood. J Allergy Clin Immunol 2001; 108: 285–7.

25. Hershey GK, Friedrich MF, Esswein LA, Thomas ML, Chatila TA et al. The association of atopy with a gain-of-function mutation in the alpha subunit of the interleukin-4 receptor. N Engl J Med 1997; 337: 1720–5.

26. Oiso N, Fukai K, Ishii M. Interleukin 4 receptor alpha chain polymorphism Gln551Arg is associated with adult atopic dermatitis in Japan. Br J Dermatol 2000; 142: 1003–6.

27. Hosomi N, Fukai K, Oiso N, Kato A, Ishii M et al. Polymorphisms in the promoter of the interleukin-4 receptor alpha chain gene are associated with atopic dermatitis in Japan. J Invest Dermatol 2004; 122: 843–5.

28. Hamid Q, Naseer T, Minshall EM, Song YL, Boguniewicz M et al. In vivo expression of IL-12 and IL-13 in atopic dermatitis. J Allergy Clin Immunol 1996; 98: 225–31.

29. Katagiri K, Itami S, Hatano Y, Takayasu S. Increased levels of IL-13 mRNA, but not IL-4 mRNA, are found in vivo in peripheral blood mononuclear cells (PBMC) of patients with atopic dermatitis (eczema). Clin Exp Immunol 1997; 108: 289–94.

30. Koning H, Neijens HJ, Baert MR, Oranje AP, Savelkoul HF. T cell subsets and cytokines in allergic and non-allergic children. I. Analysis of IL-4, IFN-gamma and IL-13 mRNA expression and protein production. Cytokine 1997; 9: 416–26.

31. Heinzmann A, Mao XQ, Akaiwa M, Kreomer RT, Gao PS et al. Genetic variants of IL-13 signalling and human asthma and atopy. Hum Mol Genet 2000; 9: 549–59.

32. Liu X, Nickel R, Beyer K, Wahn U, Ehrlich E et al. An IL13 coding region variant is associated with a high total serum IgE level and atopic dermatitis in the German multicenter atopy study (MAS-90). J Allergy Clin Immunol 2000; 106: 167–70.

33. Tsunemi Y, Saeki H, Nakamura K, Sekiya T, Hirai K et al. Interleukin-13 gene polymorphism G4257A is associated with atopic dermatitis in Japanese patients. J Dermatol Sci 2002; 30: 100–7.

34. He JQ, Chan-Yeung M, Becker AB, Dimich-Ward H, Ferguson AC et al. Genetic variants of the IL13 and IL4 genes and atopic diseases in at-risk children. Genes Immun 2003; 4: 385–9.

35. Cox HE, Moffatt MF, Faux JA, Walley AJ, Coleman R et al. Association of atopic dermatitis to the beta subunit of the high affinity immunoglobulin E receptor. Br J Dermatol 1998; 138: 182–7.

36. Folster-Holst R, Moises HW, Yang L, Fritsch W, Weissenbach J et al. Linkage between atopy and the IgE high-affinity receptor gene at 11q13 in atopic dermatitis families. Hum Genet 1998; 102: 236–9.

37. Nickel RG, Casolaro V, Wahn U, Beyer K, Barnes KC et al. Atopic dermatitis is associated with a functional mutation in the promoter of the C-C chemokine RANTES. J Immunol 2000; 164: 1612–16.

38. Kozma GT, Falus A, Bojszko A, Krikovszky D, Szabo T et al. Lack of association between atopic eczema/dermatitis syndrome and polymorphisms in the promoter region of RANTES and regulatory region of MCP-1. Allergy 2002; 57: 160–3.

39. Anonymous. Freely associating. Nat Genet 1999; 22: 1–2.

40. Dahlman I, Eaves IA, Kosoy R, Morrison VA, Heward J et al. Parameters for reliable results in genetic association studies in common disease. Nat Genet 2002; 30: 149–50.

41. Yazdanbakhsh M, Kremsner PG, van Ree R. Allergy, parasites, and the hygiene hypothesis. Science 2002; 296: 490–4.

42. Yemaneberhan H, Bekele Z, Venn A, Lewis S, Parry E et al. Prevalence of wheeze and asthma and relation to atopy in urban and rural Ethiopia. Lancet 1997; 350: 85–90.

43. Strachan DP. Hay fever, hygiene, and household size. BMJ 1989; 299: 1259–60.

44. Grimbacher B, Schaffer AA, Holland SM, Davis J, Gallin JI et al. Genetic linkage of hyper-IgE syndrome to chromosome 4. Am J Hum Genet 1999; 65: 735–44.

45. Kurz T, Strauch K, Heinzmann A, Braun S, Jung M et al. A European study on the genetics of mite sensitization. J Allergy Clin Immunol 2000; 106: 925–32.

46. Derry JM, Ochs HD, Francke U. Isolation of a novel gene mutated in Wiskott-Aldrich syndrome. Cell 1994; 78: 635–44.

47. Bradley M, Soderhall C, Wahlgren CF, Luthman H, Nordenskjold M et al. The Wiskott-Aldrich syndrome gene as a candidate gene for atopic dermatitis. Acta Derm Venereol 2001; 81: 340–2.

48. Walley AJ, Chavanas S, Moffatt MF, Esnouf RM, Ubhi B et al. Gene polymorphism in Netherton and common atopic disease. Nat Genet 2001; 29: 175–8.

49. Chavanas S, Garner C, Bodemer C, Ali M, Teillac DH et al. Localization of the Netherton syndrome gene to chromosome

5q32, by linkage analysis and homozygosity mapping. Am J Hum Genet 2000; 66: 914–21.

50. Descargues P, Deraison C, Bonnart C, Kreft M, Kishibe M et al. Spink5-deficient mice mimic Netherton syndrome through degradation of desmoglein 1 by epidermal protease hyperactivity. Nat Genet 2005; 37: 56–65.

51. Smith FJ, Irvine AD, Terron-Kwiatkowski A, Sandilands A, Clampbell LE et al. Loss-of-function mutations in the gene encoding filaggrin cause ichthyosis vulgaris. Nat Genet 2006; 38: 337–42.

52. Candi E, Schmidt R, Melino G. The cornified envelope: a model of cell death in the skin. Nat Rev Mol Cell Biol 2005; 6: 328–40.

53. Palmer CN, Irvine AD, Terron-Kwiatkowski A, Zhao Y, Liao H et al. Common loss-of-function variants of the epidermal barrier protein filaggrin are a major predisposing factor for eczema. Nat Genet 2006; 38: 441–6.

54. Marenholz I, Nickel R, Ruschendorf F, Schulz F, Esparza-Gordillo J et al. Filaggrin loss-of-function mutations predispose to phenotypes involved in the atopic march. J Allergy Clin Immunol 2006; 118: 866–71.

55. Hoffjan S, Ober C. Present status on the genetic studies of asthma. Curr Opin Immunol 2002; 14: 709–17.

56. Lee YA, Wahn U, Kehrt R, Tarani L, Businco L et al. A major susceptibility locus for eczema maps to chromosomes 3q21. Nat Genet 2000; 26: 470–73.

57. Soderhall C, Marenholz I, Kerscher T, Gruber C, Worm M et al. Variants in a novel epidermal collagen gene (COL29A1) are associated with eczema. PLOS Biology 2007; 5: 1952–61.

58. Myllyharju J, Kivirikko KI. Collagens, modifying enzymes and their mutations in humans, files and worms. Trends Genet 2004; 20: 33–43.

59. Spergel JM, Paller AS. Eczema and the atopic march. J Allergy Clin Immunol 2003; 112: S118–S127.

60. Sicherer SH, Sampson HA. Food hypersensitivity and eczema: pathophysiology, epidemiology, diagnosis, and management. J Allergy Clin Immunol 1999; 104: S114–A122.

61. Cookson WO, Ubhi B, Lawrence R, Abecasis GR, Walley Aj et al. Genetic linkage of childhood eczema to psoriasis susceptibility loci. Nat Genet 2001; 27: 372–3.

62. Irvine AD, McLean WH. The molecular genetics of the genodermatoses: progress to date and future directions. Br J Dermatol 2003; 148: 1–13.

63. Bradley M, Soderhall C, Luthman H, Wahlgren CF, Kockum I et al. Susceptibility loci for eczema on chromosomes 3, 13, 15, 17 and 18 in a Swedish population. Hum Mol Genet 2002; 11: 1539–48.

64. Natori K, Tamari M, Watanabe O, Onouchi Y, Shiomoto Y et al. Mapping of a gene responsible for dermatitis in NOA (Naruto Research Institute Otsuka Atrichia) mice, an animal model of allergic dermatitis. J Hum Genet 1999; 44: 372–6.

65. Daniels SE, Bhattacharrya S, James A, Leaves NI, Young A et al. A genome-wide search for quantitative trait loci underlying asthma. Nature 1996; 383: 247–50.

66. Kimura K, Noguchi E, Shibasaki M, Arinami T, Yokouchi Y et al. Linkage and association of atopic asthma to markers on chromosome 13 in the Japanese population. Hum Mol Genet 1999; 8: 1487–90.

67. Watanabe O, Tamari M, Natori K, Onouchi Y, Shiomoto Y et al. Loci on murine chromosomes 7 and 13 that modify the phenotype of the NOA mouse, an animal model of eczema. J Hum Genet 2001; 46: 221–4.

68. Kohara Y, Tanabe K, Matsuoko K, Kanda N, Matsuda H et al. A major determinant quantitative-trait locus responsible for eczema-like skin lesions in NC/Nga mice is located on Chromosome 9. Immunogenetics 2001; 53: 15–21.

69. Rogner UC, Avner P. Congenic mice: cutting tools for complex immune disorders. Nat Rev Immunol 2003; 3: 243–52.

3

The pathogenesis of atopic dermatitis

Natalija Novak and Thomas Bieber

INTRODUCTION

The skin is much more than just a protective coat and encounters a high number of antigens at the interface between the body and the surrounding environment.[1,2] Atopic dermatitis (AD) is a chronic inflammatory skin disease, clinically and histologically very similar to contact dermatitis. AD can occur at any age and has a high prevalence in children. In past years, the rising interest in this disease has been forced by its increasing prevalence in Western societies and its contribution to the worsening of health care costs.[3] AD offers a wide clinical spectrum ranging from minor forms presented by a few dry eczematous patches to major forms with erythematous rash.[4] Cardinal features of AD are erythematous eczematous skin lesions, flexural lichenifications or papules which go along with an intense pruritus and cutaneous hyperreactivity.[5,6] Various names, such as atopic eczema, neurodermitis constitutionalis, endogenous eczema, eczema flexurarum, Besnier's prurigo, asthma eczema, or hay fever eczema have been created for this disease and indicate that still no precise clinical definition of AD exists.[7] Additionally, the exact pathophysiological mechanisms leading to AD are still elusive and various studies have tried to unravel the key factors leading to this disease.[8]

Since Prausnitz et al described the existence of a human serum factor that reacts with allergens in 1921, much effort has been made to characterize the effector molecules of human immunity in depth. Today we know that the antibody called immunoglobulin E (IgE) which was discovered in 1967 by Ishizaka[9] is composed of 2 identical heavy and 2 identical light chains. These chains form the antigen-binding and the constant Fc domain, through which the IgE molecule binds to its cell surface receptors. Most individuals react with an increase of serum IgE levels as a defensive response to parasitic infections. IgE-mediated hypersensitivity reactions are largely regulated by T lymphocytes and it

is generally accepted that the increased prevalence of atopic diseases in recent years is due to a disturbed balance of Th1 cells and Th2 cells with a clear predominance of Th2 cells.[10] The latter preferentially produce interleukin (IL)-4, IL-5, IL-10, and IL-13, which induce IgE production and activation of eosinophils, thereby facilitating the typical features of allergic diseases. The exact reasons for this disturbance are unknown but are generally attributed to the Western lifestyle.[11]

In regard to AD, two types have been identified: the allergic form, which affects about 70–80% of the patients and occurs in the context of sensitizations towards environmental allergens and elevated serum IgE level, and the intrinsic, non-allergic form, affecting a minority of 20–30% of the patients, occurring with low IgE serum levels and the absence of any detectable sensitizations.[12] This suggests that elevated allergen specific IgE levels are not a prerequisite in the pathogenesis of AD. In recent times the concept of a 'pure' type of AD without any previous or actual associated respiratory diseases is distinguished from the 'mixed' counterpart associated with sensitizations against aero-allergens or food allergens, implying that elevated IgE serum levels can be associated with this disease but are not an obligate parameter for defining the disease.

PREDISPOSING FACTORS

The hygiene hypothesis

The generally held belief is that human foetal lymphocytes are skewed towards a Th2 profile as a consequence of intrauterine priming by placental cytokines, hormones, and possibly by transplacental allergen exposure.[13] During the postnatal period, in non-atopic individuals the Th2 profile switches into a Th1 profile, probably in consequence of stimulation by different infectious agents. In contrast, in atopic individuals this reversal does not take place during the first month of life and gives rise to immunological reactions of the Th2 type. Additionally, factors of the modern lifestyle, such as the use of antibiotics, the reduction of the family size, and the increase of hygienic strategies, lead to a reduction of bacterial stimulations and support this development.[14]

Other risk factors include low birth weight, maternal smoking, early infection with respiratory syncytial virus, vaccination against *Bordetella pertussis,* and early allergen contacts.[15]

Recently, an effective prevention of early atopic diseases in children at risk from *Lactobacillus GG* has been described.[16] In this study, perinatal administration of probiotics halved the development of AD during the first 2 years of life.

Other primary prevention strategies constitute in main part of the avoidance of early allergen exposures, i.e. food and inhalation or breast-feeding, which is considered as the first choice for atopic infants. As another strategy, it has been found that the administration of antihistamines over a time period of 12–24 months was able to delay/prevent the development of asthma in AD children later in their lives.[17]

Genetic mechanisms

The early age of onset, the familial occurrence of the disease and the high concordance rate of 77% in monozygotic twins and 15% in dizygotic twins suggest that AD represents a genetically complex disease, which develops against a background of gene–gene and gene–environment interactions.[18] A number of candidate genes have been proposed by several research groups and have sometimes provided contradictory results about numerous linkages to various chromosomal regions. The genetic studies on AD may be classified into two different approaches: linkage gene analysis studies and the studies of candidate genes. The first strategy is aimed at detecting an association of the AD phenotype with any of the chromosome regions. Meanwhile candidate gene studies investigate the association of polymorphisms of a specific gene with the atopic phenotype and are restricted to a single, already known gene locus.

Several chromosomes contain candidate genes, especially on chromosome 5q31-33 containing the Th2 cytokine genes IL-3, IL-4, IL-5, IL-13 and GM-CSF.[19] In 1998, linkage analysis showed a gene encoded at 16p11.2-12 to be linked to the total serum IgE level.[20] This gene region is the location of the IL-4 receptor alpha gene (IL-4Rα). It was suspected that mutations leading to an increased IL-4 receptor reactivity such as Q576R could be responsible for elevated IgE secretion.[21] Further on, polymorphisms affecting at least 4 different amino acids in the cytoplasmic domain of

IL-4Rα may significantly influence the outcome of IL-4 receptor signalling and consequently IgE secretion.[12]

Additionally, a linkage of high total IgE with 12q21-1q24.1, where the genes for interferon-γ (IFN-γ) and stem cells factor (KIT-ligand/mast-cell growth factor) are located, was detected.[22]

Cookson et al found that the gene locus 11q13, which represents the region for the β-chain of the high affinity receptor for IgE, has been linked to the AD phenotype and provided the first evidence for an effect of maternal imprinting on atopy,[23] as he revealed a significant sharing of maternally inherited alleles in region 11q13 in sib pairs with atopic IgE responsiveness.[22] AD has also been associated with a low-producer transforming-growth factor phenotype.[24] Similarly, variants of the IL-13 coding region,[25] functional mutations of the proximal promoter of the RANTES gene and the linkage of AD to chromosome 3q21, a region encoding the costimulatory molecules CD80 and CD86, have been identified as susceptible loci for AD.[26]

The disturbance of skin function

Intense pruritus and scratching in combination with a cutaneous hyperreactivity and reduced threshold for pruritus underlie the vicious circle of the continuous mechanical stimulation and the dysregulated cytokine release by keratinocytes.

As a basic defect of AD, the altered lipid composition of the stratum corneum is responsible for the xerotic aspect of the skin and determines a higher permeability to allergens and irritants, which could be typically found in AD patients.[27] Ceramides serve as the major water-holding molecules in the extracellular space of the cornified envelope, and the barrier function of these complex structures is provided by a matrix of structural proteins bound to ceramides.[28] A reduced content of ceramides has been reported in the cornified envelope of healthy and diseased epidermis in AD patients. This abnormal expression of ceramides leads to an abnormal expression of sphingomyelin deacylase-like enzymes. Even non-involved skin of AD patients is characterized by an severe dryness and an impairment of the barrier function of the stratum corneum, indicated by an increased transepidermal water loss. As an additional factor, ceramidase, which breaks down ceramide into sphingosine and fatty acid, is secreted significantly more from the bacterial flora obtained from lesional and non-lesional skin of AD patients. In the active phase of the disease, pH values shift towards alkalinity at both eczematous and uninvolved skin sites.[29] Altogether the susceptibility to irritants in AD can be described as a primary, continuous defect of epidermal differentiation and functions in the presence of subclinical inflammation-induced skin damage in

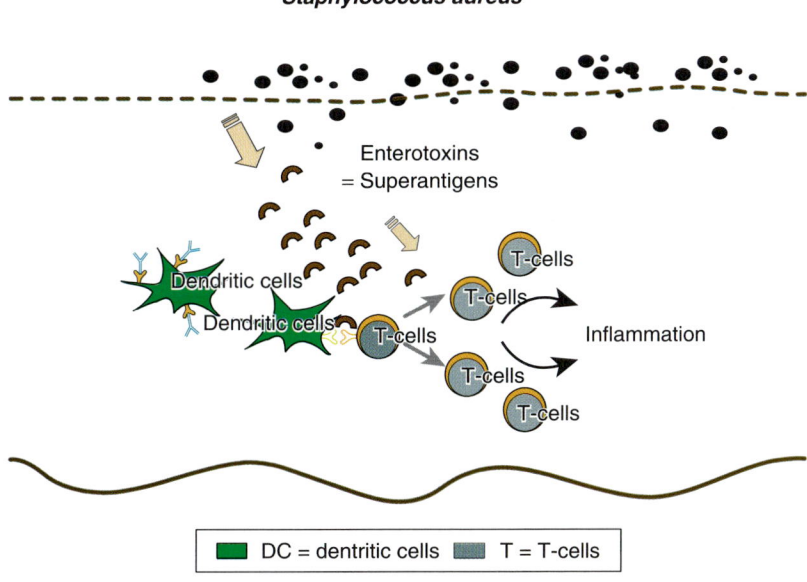

Figure 3.1 *Staphylococcus aureus*-derived enterotoxins (SEA/SEB) amplify the proliferation of T cells and trigger the proinflammatory immune response in AD in this way.

combination with a further impairment of the skin barrier during the active phase of the disease.

PROVOCATION FACTORS

Food and aeroallergens

Food allergies have a pathogenetic role in a subset of AD patients, particularly in infants, and contribute to the severity of the disease by the induction of skin lesions. In most of the cases, these food allergens are derived from egg, wheat, milk, soy, and peanut. Food-allergen specific T cells have been cloned from the lesional and non-lesional skin of AD patients.[30]

Intranasal or bronchial inhalation challenge with aeroallergens such as house dust mite or animal dander can lead to the development or worsening of AD skin lesions and the degree of IgE sensitizations to aeroallergens is directly associated with the severity of the disease, while the reduction of exposures to some common allergens such as house dust mite is associated with a significant improvement of AD in some cases.[31]

As a proof of concept the successful application of aeroallergens such as cat dander in the atopy patch test (APT) shows that it is possible to elicit eczematous skin lesions solely by external application of aeroallergens to the skin.[32] The APT is assumed to evaluate the clinical relevance of IgE-mediated sensitization in AD patients. The intermittent or continuous flow of aeroallergens and autoantigens in the process of facilitated antigen presentation may define the pathophysiological basis of the recurrent and self-perpetuating course of AD.[33]

Microbes

Pityrosporum ovale is a lipophilic yeast commonly found on the head and neck area and is thought to elicit immediate and late-phase reactions in these patients. In over 60% of the AD patients even IgE to *Pityrosporum ovale* can be detected in the peripheral blood supporting the hypothesis of the importance of this organisms in AD.[34]

Staphylococcus aureus is found in over 90% of patients with chronic AD skin lesions, reaching a density of approximately 1 million per cm^2.[35] Acute exudative skin lesions can contain over 10 million of this organism per cm^2 and increased numbers have been found even in normal skin and the nasal vestibula or intertriginous areas of AD patients.[36] In contrast, only 5% of normal subjects harbour this organism on their skin surface.

Scratching is an important factor, enhancing the binding of the bacteria by disturbing the skin barrier and exposing extracellular matrix molecules known to act as adhesions to *Staphylococcus aureus* (such as fibronectin, collagens, fibrinogen, elastin, laminin). In addition, bacterial binding seems to be higher at skin sites with Th2-mediated inflammation by the induction of an enhanced production of these adhesins. *S. aureus* is capable of secreting toxins, such as enterotoxin A (SEA) and B (SEB) or toxic shock syndrome toxin-1 at the skin surface, which serve as so-called 'superantigens'[37] (Figure 3.1).

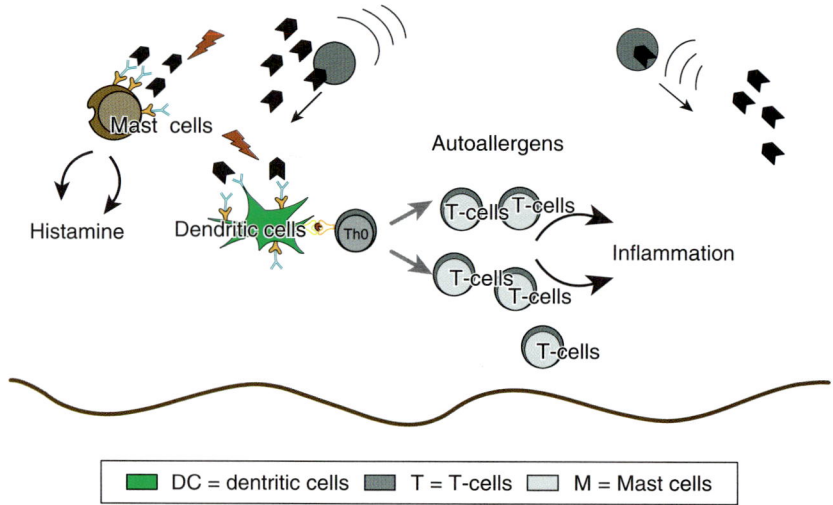

Figure 3.2   As an additional factor, autoallergens amplify the immunologic reactions in AD patients.

S. aureus superantigens are presented as 'ordinary' antigens in the peptide-presenting groove of the major histocompatibility complex MHC to the respective antigen-specific T cell. On the other hand, the intact proteins are capable of bridging the MHC complex to all T cells with the same β-chain family, irrespective of their antigen specificity.

An analysis of the peripheral blood skin homing CLA+ T cells from these patients and T cells in their skin lesions shows that they have undergone a T-cell receptor Vb expansion consistent with superantigenic stimulation.[38] Superantigens augment the synthesis of allergen-specific IgE and induce glucocorticoid resistance in these patients.[39] In most of the AD patients specific IgE antibodies against staphylococcal superantigens could be found, which correlate with disease severity. AD skin is also deficient in antimicrobial peptides needed for host defence against bacteria, fungi and viruses. Together, the higher colonisation with microbial hosts in combination with an inadequate host defence might perpetuate the course of disease.

Autoallergens

Immunoglobulin E autoreactivity has been implicated as an immunopathogenetic factor in AD. In addition, molecular analysis of allergens has revealed striking similarities between environmental allergens and human proteins, leading to the hypothesis that autoimmune reactions might also play a role.[40] Recently, IgE-reactive autoantigens directed against human proteins have been cloned from human epithelial copy DNA (cDNA) expression libraries and have been found to represent primarily intracellular proteins.[41] Autoantigens characterized for

AD are *Hom s 1-5* and *DSF70*.[42] These autoantigens seem to act as adjuvants to the immunological mechanisms in AD patients with elevated IgE levels, as they have been detected in IgE-immune complexes of AD sera and the release of autoallergens from the damaged tissue, putatively triggered by mechanical factors such as scratching, could trigger responses mediated by mast cells, T cells, and IgE (Figure 3.2). This notion is supported by the observation that IgE autoallergen levels decrease in consequence of successful treatment. Together these finding imply that immune responses initiated by environmental allergens might be maintained by human endogenous antigens.

Contact allergens

Possible contact allergens, which can penetrate the epidermal skin barrier in AD patients more easily due to its impairment, include nickel, latex, vehicle of external preparations, and fragrances. Furthermore, irritative agents such as wool or disinfectants might lead to some exacerbation of the disease. Therefore, avoidance or even reduction of these factors in the environment should be one of the basic principles in the management of the disease.[18]

Neuroimmunological factors

One important provocation factor of AD, which can lead to the exacerbation of the disease, is stress. Even though the exact mechanisms of the interaction of the skin immune system and the nervous system have not yet been identified, it is believed that this phenomenon might be mediated by neuroimmunological factors such as neuropeptides, which can be found within the epidermal nerve fibres in close association with epidermal Langerhans cells (LCs).[43] Some of these neuroimmunological mediators, such as calcitonin gene-related peptide (CGRP), are able to exert an inhibitory effect on the antigen presenting capacity of LCs. In addition, activated keratinocytes are able to produce the neuropeptide proopiomelanocortin-derived hormones (α-MSH), which in turn seem to promote IL-10 secretion in order to induce negative feedback signals for the downregulation of the inflammatory reactions in the skin.[44] Mast cell tryptase and proteinase-activated receptor-2 as well as IL-31 have been observed to be up-regulated in patients with AD, mediators which may not only be involved in inflammation but also pruritus. Thus, various neuroimmunological mechanism in the skin of AD patients may contribute to new therapeutical intervention strategies in the future.[45]

IMMUNOPATHOGENIC FACTORS

Monocytes

Increased cyclic adenosine monophosphate (cAMP) hydrolysis by genetically determined overactive phosphodiesterase in monocytes leads to an increased production of mediators such as prostaglandin E and IL-10.[46] This mechanism turns to inhibit Th2 responses and accentuates IL-4 secretion by Th2 cells and it appears that in addition to prostaglandin E2, IL-10 acts to regulate the balance between Th1 and Th2 functional responses, accounting for many atopic features, including IL-4, IL-5, and IL-6 production by T cells, increased IgE synthesis, decreased interferon-γ production and impaired cell-mediated immune responses.[47] The question of a defect at the level of monocytes has been an issue for a long time. It has been suggested that monocytes from atopic individuals display enhanced survival and release distinct soluble mediators. Monocytes of patients with allergic AD display enhanced surface expression of the high and low affinity receptor for IgE (FcεRI and FcεRII) and the IL-4Rα chain and in this way can be distinguished from monocytes in patients with non-allergic AD, in which the expression of these surface markers is low.[12] Additionally, the composition of different monocyte subsets,[48] which have been identified in the peripheral blood recently, is distinct in the acute phase of the disease.

Eosinophils

The common presence of peripheral blood eosinophilia and elevated serum levels of eosinophil granule proteins suggests that eosinophil degranulation plays a major role in AD. Increased serum levels of eosinophils with enhanced survival have been detected and especially on eosinophils from allergic AD patients, the functional CD137 receptor,[49] which stimulates T-cell activation and differentiation, could be detected. The granular protein elevations found in the peripheral blood correlate with the disease activity. In the skin, Th2 cytokines, together with chemokines such as eotaxin and monocyte chemoattractant protein 4, promote the influx of activated eosinophils into the skin of AD patients.[50] Extensive eosinophil major basic protein deposition has been demonstrated in the lesional skin.[51]

Keratinocytes

Dysregulated signal transduction in epithelial cells could favour an exaggerated response to inflammatory stimuli. Altered cytokine synthesis by skin cells is proposed to increase the expression of TNF-α, IL-1β, and IL-12 mRNA in the skin of AD patients after contact with detergents or aeroallergens.[52] An intrinsic defect of keratinocytes found in AD leads to an enhanced secretion of GM-CSF, IL-1 and TNF-α and might result in main part from the altered transcriptional control or activation of the signal transduction cascade.

T cells

One of the most prominent features of AD is the pronounced skin infiltration with activated CD4+ T cells in skin lesions. Immunohistological investigations have shown that the dermal infiltrate in the skin lesions is mainly composed of CD4+ and CD8+ cells with a CD4:CD8 ratio similar to that found in the peripheral blood. It is well known that the human immune system harbours a powerful army of cutaneous T cells, which seem to be highly activated and bear the cutaneous lymphocyte antigen (CLA) on their surface, which enables them to be immediately recruited into the skin on invasion of foreign antigens.[53] Homing of T cells to the skin is determined by the interaction of CLA with vascular cell surface antigens expressed on dermal blood vessels, such as E-selectin. Other important co-factors in this homing process are alpha-6 integrin, VCAM-1, ICAM-1, and IL-8 which are found in higher levels in the peripheral blood of AD patients.[54] Following antigen presentation by DC, Th0 precursors are triggered to differentiate into Th1 or Th2 cells. While the Th1 response is associated with delayed-type hypersensitivity reactions (DTH) and the predominance of interferon-γ and IL-2 secretion, the Th2 pattern is associated with an increased secretion of IgE and IgE-mediated reactions as even as the predominance of IL-4, IL-5, and IL-13.[55] In this regard, AD has a particular status, since it is clinically a cell-mediated hypersensitivity reaction. Analyses of biopsy samples from unaffected skin of AD patients have an increased number of Th2 cells expressing mRNA of IL-4 and IL-13. While acute AD lesions do not contain significant numbers of cells expressing mRNA of IL-5, IL-12, GM-CSF, or IL-12, the mRNA amount of these cytokines increases in the chronic phase while the mRNA level of IL-4 and IL-13 expressing cells decreases. Together with kinetic studies from lesional skin of APT reactions a biphasic course of AD is suggested, in which the initial phase is characterized by a Th2 pattern. This phase switches into the chronic phase, predominated by a clear Th1 profile.[56] This switch is probably started by local production of IL-12 from infiltrating eosinophils or inflammatory dendritic epidermal cells, or both.

Inflammatory cytokines and chemokines in the skin

The paradoxical reduction in cell-mediated immunity in AD is a result of the increased production of immunosuppressive cytokines such as IL-10 and TGF-β that have been observed in AD. Further on, the chemoattractant for CD4+ T cells, as even as the chemokines T cells expressed and secreted (RANTES), macophage-derived chemokine (MDC) and thymus and activation-regulated chemokine (TARC) could be found in AD.[57]

Persistent skin inflammation in chronic skin lesions could be induced by mediators which enhance the survival of eosinophils, monocytes/macrophages and DC such as IL-5 or GM-CSF, which can be found in high numbers in chronic AD skin.[58]

CONCLUSIONS AND FUTURE PERSPECTIVES

The pathophysiology of AD is rather heterogeneous. First, antigen-presenting cells are located at the interface between the environment and the skin. DC in tissues are highly specialised for capturing and processing foreign or autologous antigens or haptens. Uptake of high-molecular-weight antigens by DC may occur through macropinocytosis or more specifically through a number of membrane receptors such as FcεRII or FcεRI, the high affinity receptor for IgE.[59] Inflammatory dendritic epidermal cells (IDEC)[60] have been reported as FcεRI bearing DC.

Thus, epidermal LC and IDEC in the skin lesions of AD patients express the high affinity receptor for IgE (FcεRI), indicating a crucial role in antigen presentation as well as hyperreactivity.

Furthermore, DCs expressing high receptor densities probably induce the synthesis and release of mediators, which help to enhance the subsequent antigen presentation. Hence antigen uptake and aggregation of FcεRI on DC may lead to the de novo synthesis and release of mediators capable of directing T cells towards a defined phenotype and function of Th1 or Th2 cells.

In general various cells such as LCs, IDEC, macrophages, T cells, B cells, keratinocytes, endothelial cells, eosinophils, and mast cells orchestrate the pathophyiology of AD with different dominance at various stages. These cells communicate with each other in cylokines, predominantly Th2-dominated, as well as chemokines, prostanoid, proteases, and reactive oxygen species products. Undoubtedly, the high affinity IgE receptor plays a crucial role in this context. Dissecting these interactions at the cellular and molecular level will lead to a deeper understanding of the pathophysiology of AD.

Hyperstimulatory cells of the DCc lineage.[61] However, it was the combination of immunomorphological and ultrastructural characterizations which led to the delineation of two different epidermal DC populations in this disease: Langerhans cells (LC) and inflammatory dendritic epidermal cells (IDEC).[62–64] Classical epidermal LC are characterized by their tennis racket shaped cytoplasmic Birbeck granules and their CD1a+, Langerin (CD207)+[65] phenotype. In contrast, IDEC lack the typical Birbeck granules but express the mannose receptor (CD206), which mediates the uptake of bacterial components by endocytotic processes.[62,66–72] A hallmark of both epidermal LC and IDEC in the skin lesions of AD patients is the elevated expression of the high affinity receptor for IgE (FcεRI) and their putative role in antigen focusing.[73]

Indeed the receptor is not constitutively expressed on DC but seems to be regulated by signals of the inflammatory surrounding micromilieu such as local IgE, a reducing microenvironment or TGF-β levels. The highest expression of FcεRI is displayed on LC and IDEC from lesional skin of AD and correlated positively with the IgE serum level. Recent concepts support the hypothesis that IDEC, which are assumed to be of a rather monocytic origin, are recruited in the acute phase of AD into the epidermis by signals mediated from cells of the inflammatory micromilieu. Interestingly, after successful topical treatment of the AD lesions, the number of IDEC in the epidermis decreases below the detecting level, indicating that this cell type is strongly related to the state of inflammation of the skin.

FcεRI-bearing DC play a crucial role in the pathophysiology of AD, since they may represent the missing link between aeroallergens penetrating the epidermis due to the reduced skin barrier and antigen-specific cells infiltrating the skin lesions. This concept is strongly supported by the observation that the presence of FcεRI-expressing, LC-bearing IgE molecules is a prerequisite for producing eczematous skin lesions by the

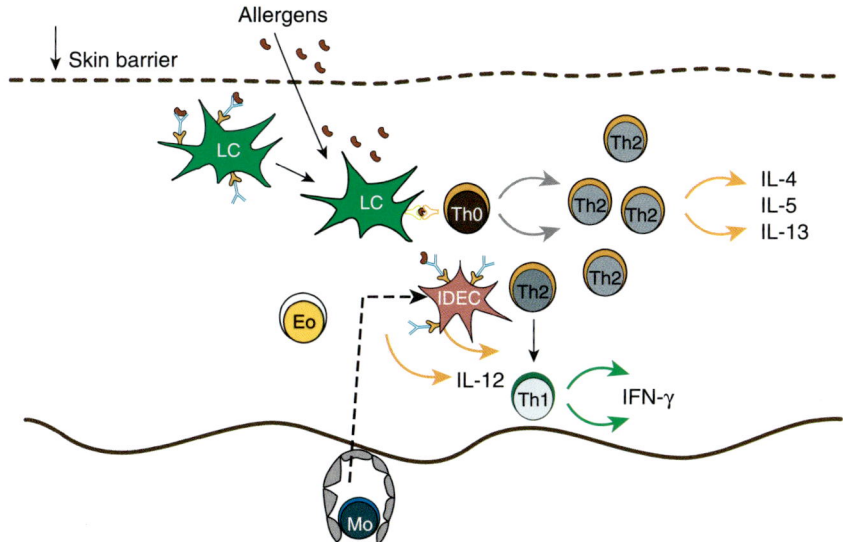

Figure 3.3 Allergens invading the epidermis due to the reduced skin barrier in AD patients are taken up by FcεRI-bearing dendritic cells such as Langerhans cells (LC), processed and presented to allergen-specific T cells. This leads to an increased proliferation of allergen-specific T cells of the Th2 type. In addition, keratinocytes (KC) release proinflammatory cytokines which contribute to the inflammation of the skin. Inflammatory dendritic epidermal cells (IDEC), which are recruited from monocytes of the peripheral blood (Mo) and eosinophils (Eo) might release IL-12 and promote the switch into an immune response of the Th1 type in which IFN-γ producing T cells predominate.

application of aeroallergens to the skin of AD patients in the atopy patch test.

Multimeric ligands, which have been shown to be taken up by FcεRI-mediated endocytosis are channelled into MHC class II compartments and peptide loading of newly synthesized MHC class II molecules leads to an optimal antigen presentation to CD4+ T cells. DC expressing high receptor densities will display full activation upon FcεRI receptor ligation, most probably inducing the synthesis and release of mediators, which might help to enhance the subsequent antigen presentation (Figure 3.3).

It is possible, that FcεRI-expressing DC armed with specific IgE can boost the secondary immune response and further trigger the IgE synthesis by recruiting and activating more antigen-specific Th2 cells or IDEC from the peripheral blood into the skin. DC are the most potent stimulators of naïve T cells, i.e. they are committed to initiate primary immune responses. It cannot be excluded that even complex allergenic structures efficiently captured via FcεRI on DC are processed by these cells in a way leading to the unmasking and presentation of cryptic peptides/epitopes, the T cell never met before. This would initiate a primary reaction against these unhidden antigens, thereby helping to increase the variety of the IgE specificities. Antigen uptake and aggregation of FcεRI on DC could lead to the de novo

synthesis and release of mediators capable of directing T cells toward a defined phenotype and function of Th1 or Th2 cells.

REFERENCES

1. Bos JD. The skin as an organ of immunity. Clin Exp Immunol 1997; 107: 3–5.
2. Bos JD, Zonneveld I, Das PK et al. The skin immune system (SIS): distribution and immunophenotype of lymphocyte subpopulations in normal human skin. J Invest Dermatol 1987; 88: 569–73.
3. Taylor B, Wadsworth J, Wadsworth M, Peckham C. Changes in the reported prevalence of childhood eczema since the 1939–45 war. Lancet 1984; 2: 1255–7.
4. Leung DY, Bieber T. Atopic dermatitis. Lancet 2003; 361: 151–60.
5. Kay AB. Allergy and allergic diseases. Second of two parts. N Engl J Med 2001; 344: 109–13.
6. Kay AB, Allergy and allergic diseases. First of two parts. N Engl J Med 2001; 344: 30–7.
7. Johansson SG, Hourihane JO, Bousquet J et al. A revised nomenclature for allergy. An EAACI position statement from the EAACI nomenclature task force. Allergy 2001; 56: 813–24.
8. Cooper KD, Atopic dermatitis: recent trends in pathogenesis and therapy. J Invest Dermatol 1994; 102: 128–37.
9. Ishizaka K, Tomioka H, Ishizaka T, Mechanisms of passive sensitization. I. Presence of IgE and IgG molecules on human leukocytes. J Immunol 1970; 105: 1459–67.

10. Bukantz SC, Clemens von Pirquet and the concept of allergie. J Allergy Clin Immunol 2002; 109: 724–6.

11. Schafer T, Dockery D, Kramer U, Behrendt H et al. Experiences with the severity scoring of atopic dermatitis in a population of German pre-school children. Br J Dermatol 1997; 137: 558–62.

12. Novak N, Kruse S, Kraft et al. Dichotomic nature of atopic dermatitis reflected by combined analysis of monocyte immunophenotyping and single nucleotide polymorphisms of the interleukin-4/interleukin-13 receptor gene: the dichotomy of extrinsic and intrinsic atopic dermatitis. J Invest Dermatol 2002; 119: 870–5.

13. Van Bever HP, Early events in atopy. Eur J Pediatr 2002; 161: 542–6.

14. Prescott SL, Holt PG, Abnormalities in cord blood mononuclear cytokine production as a predictor of later atopic disease in childhood. Clin Exp Allergy 1998; 28: 1313–16.

15. Lau S, Illi S, Sommerfeld C, Niggemann B et al. Early exposure to house-dust mite and cat allergens and development of childhood asthma: a cohort study, Multicentre Allergy Study Group. Lancet 2000; 356: 1392–7.

16. Kalliomaki M, Salminen S, Arvilommi H et al. Probiotics in primary prevention of atopic disease: a randomised placebo-controlled trial. Lancet 2001; 357: 1076–9.

17. Allergic factors associated with the development of asthma and the influence of cetirizine in a double-blind, randomised, placebo-controlled trial: first results of ETAC, Early Treatment of the Atopic Child. Pediatr Allergy Immunol 1998; 9: 116–24.

18. Meagher LJ, Wines NY, Cooper AJ, Atopic dermatitis: review of immunopathogenesis and advances in immunosuppressive therapy. Australas J Dermatol 2002; 43: 247–54.

19. Forrest S, Dunn K, Elliott K, Fitzpatrick E et al. Identifying genes predisposing to atopic eczema. J Allergy Clin Immunol 1999; 104: 1066–70.

20. Deichmann KA, Heinzmann A, Forster J et al. Linkage and allelic association of atopy and markers flanking the IL4-receptor gene. Clin Exp Allergy 1998; 28: 151–5.

21. Hershey GK, Friedrich MF, Esswein LA et al. The association of atopy with a gain-of-function mutation in the alpha subunit of the interleukin-4 receptor. N Engl J Med 1997; 337: 1720–5.

22. Cookson W. The genetics of atopy. J Allergy Clin Immunol 1994; 94: 643–4.

23. Cookson WO, Young RP, Sandford AJ et al. Maternal inheritance of atopic IgE responsiveness on chromosome 11q. Lancet 1992; 340: 381–4.

24. Arkwright PD, Chase JM, Babbage S et al. Atopic dermatitis is associated with a low-producer transforming growth factor beta(1) cytokine genotype. J Allergy Clin Immunol 2001; 108: 281–4.

25. Cox HE, Moffatt MF, Faux JA et al. Association of atopic dermatitis to the beta subunit of the high affinity immunoglobulin E receptor. Br J Dermatol 1998; 138: 182–7.

26. Cookson WO. Genetic aspects of atopic allergy. Allergy 1998; 53: 9–14.

27. Fartasch M. Epidermal barrier in disorders of the skin. Microsc Res Tech 1997; 38: 361–72.

28. Gfesser M, Abeck D, Rugemer J et al. The early phase of epidermal barrier regeneration is faster in patients with atopic eczema. Dermatology 1997; 195: 332–6.

29. Gfesser M, Rakoski J, Ring J, The disturbance of epidermal barrier function in atopy patch test reactions in atopic eczema. Br J Dermatol 1996; 135: 560–5.

30. van Reijsen FC, Felius A, Wauters EA et al. T-cell reactivity for a peanut-derived epitope in the skin of a young infant with atopic dermatitis. J Allergy Clin Immunol 1998; 101: 207–9.

31. Tan BB, Weald D, Strickland I, Friedmann PS, Double-blind controlled trial of effect of housedust-mite allergen avoidance on atopic dermatitis. Lancet 1996; 347: 15–18.

32. Ring J, Darsow U, Behrendt H, Role of aeroallergens in atopic eczema: proof of concept with the atopy patch test. J Am Acad Dermatol 2001; 45: S49–52.

33. Darsow U, Vieluf D, Ring J. Evaluating the relevance of aeroallergen sensitization in atopic eczema with the atopy patch test: a randomized, double-blind multicenter study, Atopy Patch Test Study Group. J Am Acad Dermatol 1999; 40: 187–93.

34. Devos SA, van der Valk PG. The relevance of skin prick tests for Pityrosporum ovale in patients with head and neck dermatitis. Allergy 2000; 55: 1056–8.

35. Leung DY, Atopic dermatitis and the immune system: the role of superantigens and bacteria. J Am Acad Dermatol 2001; 45: S13–16.

36. Capoluongo E, Giglio AA, Lavieri MM et al. Genotypic and phenotypic characterization of Staphylococcus aureus strains isolated in subjects with atopic dermatitis. Higher prevalence of exfoliative B toxin production in lesional strains and correlation between the markers of disease intensity and colonization density. J Dermatol Sci 2001; 26: 145–55.

37. Cho SH, Strickland I, Boguniewicz M et al. Fibronectin and fibrinogen contribute to the enhanced binding of Staphylococcus aureus to atopic skin. J Allergy Clin Immunol 2001; 108: 269–74.

38. Strickland I, Hauk PJ, Trumble AE et al. Evidence for superantigen involvement in skin homing of T cells in atopic dermatitis. J Invest Dermatol 1999; 112: 249–53.

39. Hauk PJ, Hamid QA, Chrousos GP et al. Induction of corticosteroid insensitivity in human PBMCs by microbial superantigens. J Allergy Clin Immunol 2000; 105: 782–7.

40. Valenta R, Natter S, Seiberler S et al. Autoallergy: a pathogenetic factor in atopic dermatitis? Curr Probl Dermatol 1999; 28: 45–50.

41. Seiberler S, Bugajska-Schretter A, Hufnagl P et al. Characterization of IgE-reactive autoantigens in atopic dermatitis. 1. Subcellular distribution and tissue-specific expression. Int Arch Allergy Immunol 1999; 120: 108–16.

42. Ochs RL, Muro Y, Si Y et al. Autoantibodies to DFS 70 kd/transcription coactivator p75 in atopic dermatitis and other conditions. J Allergy Clin Immunol 2000; 105: 1211–20.

43. Asahina A, Hosoi J, Murphy GF, Granstein RD. Calcitonin gene-related peptide modulates Langerhans cell antigen-presenting function. Proc Assoc Am Physicians 1995; 107: 242–4.

44. Luger TA, Schauer E, Trautinger F et al. Production of immunosuppressing melanotropins by human keratinocytes. Ann N Y Acad Sci 1993; 680: 567–70.

45. Wollenberg A, Bieber T, Atopic dermatitis: from the genes to skin lesions. Allergy 2000; 55: 205–13.

46. Gantner F, Gotz C, Gekeler V et al. Phosphodiesterase profile of human B lymphocytes from normal and atopic donors and the effects of PDE inhibition on B cell proliferation. Br J Pharmacol 1998; 123: 1031–8.

47. Hanifin JM, Chan SC. Monocyte phosphodiesterase abnormalities and dysregulation of lymphocyte function in atopic dermatitis. J Invest Dermatol 1995; 105: 84S–8S.

48. Novak N, Allam P, Geiger E et al. Characterization of monocyte subtypes in the allergic form of atopic eczema/dermatitis syndrome. Allergy 2002; 57: 931–5.

49. Heinisch IV, Bizer C, Volgger W et al. Functional CD137 receptors are expressed by eosinophils from patients with IgE-mediated allergic responses but not by eosinophils from patients with non-IgE-mediated eosinophilic disorders. J Allergy Clin Immunol 2001; 108: 21–8.

50. Taha RA, Minshall EM, Leung DY et al. Evidence for increased expression of eotaxin and monocyte chemotactic protein-4 in atopic dermatitis. J Allergy Clin Immunol 2000; 105: 1002–7.

51. Kay AB, Barata L, Meng Q et al. Eosinophils and eosinophil-associated cytokines in allergic inflammation. Int Arch Allergy Immunol 1997; 113: 196–9.

52. Pastore S, Mascia F, Giustizieri ML et al. Pathogenetic mechanisms of atopic dermatitis. Arch Immunol Ther Exp (Warsz) 2000; 48: 497–504.

53. Trautmann A, Akdis M, Brocker EB et al. New insights into the role of T cells in atopic dermatitis and allergic contact dermatitis. Trends Immunol 2001; 22: 530–2.

54. Hwang ST. Mechanisms of T-cell homing to skin. Adv Dermatol 2001; 17: 211–41.

55. Wistokat-Wulfing A, Schmidt P, Darsow U et al. Atopy patch test reactions are associated with T lymphocyte-mediated allergen-specific immune responses in atopic dermatitis. Clin Exp Allergy 1999; 29: 513–21.

56. Grewe M, Gyufko K, Schopf E et al. Lesional expression of interferon-gamma in atopic eczema. Lancet 1994; 343: 25–6.

57. Yawalkar N, Uguccioni M, Scharer J et al. Enhanced expression of eotaxin and CCR3 in atopic dermatitis. J Invest Dermatol 1999; 113: 43–8.

58. Bratton DL, Hamid Q, Boguniewicz M et al. Granulocyte macrophage colony-stimulating factor contributes to enhanced monocyte survival in chronic atopic dermatitis. J Clin Invest 1995; 95: 211–18.

59. Sallusto F, Cella M, Danieli C et al. Dendritic cells use macropinocytosis and the mannose receptor to concentrate macromolecules in the major histocompatibility complex class II compartment: downregulation by cytokines and bacterial products. J Exp Med 1995; 182: 389–400.

60. Novak N, Kraft S, Haberstok J et al. A reducing microenvironment leads to the generation of FcepsilonRIhigh inflammatory dendritic epidermal cells (IDEC). J Invest Dermatol 2002; 119: 842–9.

61. Bieber T, Dannenberg B, Prinz JC et al. Occurrence of ige-bearing epidermal Langerhans cells in atopic eczema: a study of the time course of the lesions and with regard to the IgE serum level. J Invest Dermatol 1989; 93: 215–19.

62. Wollenberg A, Kraft S, Hanau D et al. Immunomorphological and ultrastructural characterization of Langerhans cells and a novel, inflammatory dendritic epidermal cell (IDEC) population in lesional skin of atopic eczema. J Invest Dermatol 1996; 106: 446–53.

63. Wollenberg A, Bieber T. Two populations of cd1a+ epidermal dendritic cells expressing B7 molecules in human skin. Br J Dermatol 1998; 138: 358–9.

64. Taylor RS, Baadsgaard O, Hammerberg C et al. Hyperstimulatory CD1a+CD1b+CD36+ Langerhans cells are responsible for increased autologous T lymphocyte reactivity to lesional epidermal cells of patients with atopic dermatitis. J Immunol 1991; 147: 3794–802.

65. Birbeck MS, Breathnach AS, Everall JD. An electron microscope study of basal melanocytes and high-level clear cells (Langerhans cells) in vitiligo. J Invest Dermatol 1961; 37: 51–64.

66. Stahl PD, Ezekowitz RA. The mannose receptor is a pattern recognition receptor involved in host defense. Curr Opin Immunol 1998; 10: 50–5.

67. Wollenberg A, Wen S, Bieber T. Langerhans cell phenotyping: a new tool for differential diagnosis of inflammatory skin diseases. Lancet 1995; 346: 1626–7.

68. Yin ET, Galanos C, Kinsky S et al. Picogram-sensitive assay for endotoxin: gelation of limulus polyphemus blood cell lysate induced by purified lipopolysaccharides and lipid a from gram-negative bacteria. Biochim Biophys Acta 1972; 261: 284–9.

69. Miller L, Blank U, Metzger H et al. Expression of high-affinity binding of human immunoglobulin E by transfected cells. Science 1989; 244: 334–7.

70. Letourneur O, Sechi S, Willette-Brown J et al. Glycosylation of human truncated Fc epsilon RI alpha chain is necessary for efficient folding in the endoplasmic reticulum. J Biol Chem 1995; 270: 8249–56.

71. Turner H, Kinet JP, Signalling through the high-affinity IgE receptor Fc epsilonRI. Nature 1999; 402: B24–30.

72. Engering AJ, Cella M, Fluitsma D et al. The mannose receptor functions as a high capacity and broad specificity antigen receptor in human dendritic cells. Eur J Immunol 1997; 27: 2417–25.

73. Novak N, Kraft S, Bieber T. IgE receptors. Curr Opin Immunol 2001; 13: 721–6.

4

Epidermal barrier dysfunction in atopic dermatitis

Michael J Cork, Simon Danby, Yiannis Vasilopoulos, Manar Moustafa, Alice MacGowan, Jibu Varghese, Gordon W Duff, Rachid Tazi-Ahnini and Simon J Ward

INTRODUCTION

Atopic dermatitis (AD) is a chronic inflammatory skin disease associated with cutaneous hyper-reactivity to environmental triggers that are innocuous to normal, non-atopic individuals.[1] Major contributors to this hyperactivity are the many changes in the cutaneous and systemic immune responses in individuals with AD.[2] One example is the production of raised levels of total serum immunoglobulin IgE and specific IgE to common allergens.[3] However, the link between AD and allergen-specific IgE remains hotly debated.[4] A recent systematic review revealed that the association with raised IgE was much lower in children with mild to moderate AD than in children with severe disease.[3] It has been postulated that the non-allergic, intrinsic dermatitis could be a pure, transitional form of AD.[5] This raises the question: is there a genetic and environmental basis for primary intrinsic, non-allergic dermatitis? A logical place to look is the skin barrier, given its role in protecting against environmental stimuli.

Another area of AD research that points us to the skin barrier and the influence of the environment is the rising prevalence of AD and concomitant rise in exposure to environmental agents. The prevalence of AD has been rising progressively in developed countries since the 1940s.[6–12] How can the prevalence of AD have increased so dramatically if it is only determined genetically? This rise in prevalence suggests that environmental factors must be crucial in the expression of the disease.[9]

AD is a multifactorial, heterogenous genetic disease arising as a result of the interaction of many genes with environmental factors. The most likely model for the development of AD is a gene dosage and environmental dosage effect. For example, if an individual has a mutation in 5 major genes for AD, then the environmental factors required to develop the disease may be minimal. If the mutations are only present in 2 of the genes, then a much greater environmental exposure may be required to develop the disease.[13]

Several environmental factors have been associated with AD, including washing with soap and detergents, washing with hard water, and exposure to house dust mites.[14–22] However, there are few formal longitudinal studies that indicate how the home environment has changed over the past 50 years. We have reviewed data regarding exposure to soap and detergents, frequency of washing, and exposure to house dust mites.[23] An example of these changes is the increased use of soap and detergent personal wash products between 1981 and 2001 in the United Kingdom, where the sales rose (inflation adjusted) from £76 million to £453 million, while the population only rose from 56.3 million to 59.1 million.[23] The frequency of personal washing has also changed over the past 40 years. In 1961 the average use of water for personal washing was 11 litres per person per day, rising to 51 litres per person per day in 1997/98.[23] In the United Kingdom, there have also been changes in the heating, ventilation, insulation, and floor coverings of houses over the past 40 years, which have created an increasingly optimal environment for the house dust mite.[23] All these environmental agents damage the skin barrier directly, and, coupled with the increasing prevalence of AD, also suggest that breakdown of the skin barrier may be a very important event in the development of the disease.

From an immunological perspective it has been suggested that barrier breakdown in AD is a secondary consequence of the inflammatory response to irritants and allergens, the 'inside-outside hypothesis'.[24] Alternatively, it has been hypothesized that the xerosis,[25] the permeability barrier abnormality,[26,27] or both, could drive the activity of AD, the 'outside-inside hypothesis'.[27,28] Which is the correct hypothesis? Barrier function appears to fluctuate in relation to disease activity, suggesting that changes in barrier function may drive disease activity.[28] In addition, barrier damage induced, for example, by surfactants (sodium lauryl sulphate) or skin stripping causes the release and production of cytokines such as interleukin (IL)-1α, IL-β, tumor necrosis factor (TNF)-α and granulocyte–macrophage colony–stimulating factor,[29,30] indicating that barrier disruption alone leads to cytokine production, inflammation, and a flare of dermatitis.[27] AD has a very wide spectrum of disease severity. At the mild end, the dermatitis is usually intrinsic, with no elevation of specific or non-specific IgE, and this immunological state may be maintained for the duration of the disease. This can usually be controlled for most of the time with a complete emollient regimen and intermittent use of calcineurin inhibitors and mild to moderate topical corticosteroids.[31,32] At the other end of the disease severity spectrum, in very severe AD, the total IgE level may be > 10 000 units and multiple specific IgEs are above the top of the scale. This very severe dermatitis may only be controlled with systemic agents such as cyclosporin and mycophenolate.[33] Are mild AD and very severe AD the same disease? Are the contributions of the 'inside-outside' and 'outside-inside' hypothesis mechanisms different in AD of different severities?

If a disturbance in epidermal barrier function represents one of the primary events in the development of AD, the genes that regulate barrier function are a logical place to look for changes/variants that predispose to the disease. This is not a new idea: in 1999 Alain Taieb proposed that a genetic predisposition to a defective skin barrier was a primary event in the development of AD allowing allergen penetration and enhanced T_H2 responses.[34] Three groups[35–38] have identified variants/changes in genes regulating the integrity of the epidermal barrier and have shown that they are strongly associated or linked with AD. The likely functional consequence of these genetic changes is a premature breakdown of the skin barrier, resulting in a thin skin barrier. A thin, defective epidermal barrier could enhance the penetration of irritants and allergens into and through the skin barrier. This could activate the immune response by facilitating interaction between antigens and the immune effector cells present in the skin (Figure 4.1).[2] Increased penetration of allergens through the epidermis could also promote the initiation of an inflammatory response within the stratum corneum/stratum granulosum by inducing the release of pro-inflammatory cytokines from keratinocytes.[27]

Intra-individual variations in epidermal barrier structure and function

Although AD can affect any area of the body, it preferentially affects the flexures and the face. In babies aged less than 6 months, the face and scalp are the most common sites affected.[39] In older children, the most common sites affected are the antecubital and popliteal fossae.[40,41] In addition to the classical patterns of AD, there are several site-specific variants.[42] Eyelid eczema is common in adolescents, affecting up to 21% of these individuals,[40] and has been associated with hay fever and exposure to other aeroallergens such as house dust mites.[43] The infra-auricular and retro-auricular sites are particularly prone to fissuring, probably as a reaction to repeated minor trauma.[40,44,45]

Many factors could explain the areas of predisposition to AD, including the thickness of the stratum corneum and the variation in exposure to irritants and allergens at different body sites. Hanifin[46] commented that the stratum corneum over the eyelids is extremely thin and that these areas are vulnerable to the irritants and allergens entering in contact with the periorbital areas because these zones are rubbed and scratched unconsciously. Only three studies[47–49] have evaluated epidermal thickness in multiple body sites and have shown that it is thinnest in the eyelid[47] and genitals.[49] The next thinnest sites are the flexor forearm and posterior auricular areas[49] (Figure 4.2). Interestingly, these are two of the areas of predisposition to AD indicated above. The thickness of the epidermis in the antecubital fossae was not recorded.

The epidermal barrier to the penetration of exogenous substances, such as irritants, allergens, and drugs, is located in the deeper part of the stratum corneum.[50,51] It is, therefore, expected that the percutaneous penetration of exogenous substances varies in different body areas according to differences in the thickness of the stratum corneum. The most detailed studies on the regional variation of the percutaneous penetration of an exogenous substance have been made using topical corticosteroids. In some studies, where the percutaneous penetration of corticosteroids was measured in vitro using cadaver skin from different body sites,[52] the greatest percutaneous penetration was observed for scrotal and posterior auricular skin and the lowest for plantar skin. The definitive study on in vivo regional variation in percutaneous penetration of topical corticosteroids was performed in human male volunteers with normal skin.[53] Feldman et al applied [14]carbon-labelled hydrocortisone to different body areas and measured the penetration of hydrocortisone by recording[14] carbon activity in the urine over the subsequent 5 days. They observed the greatest

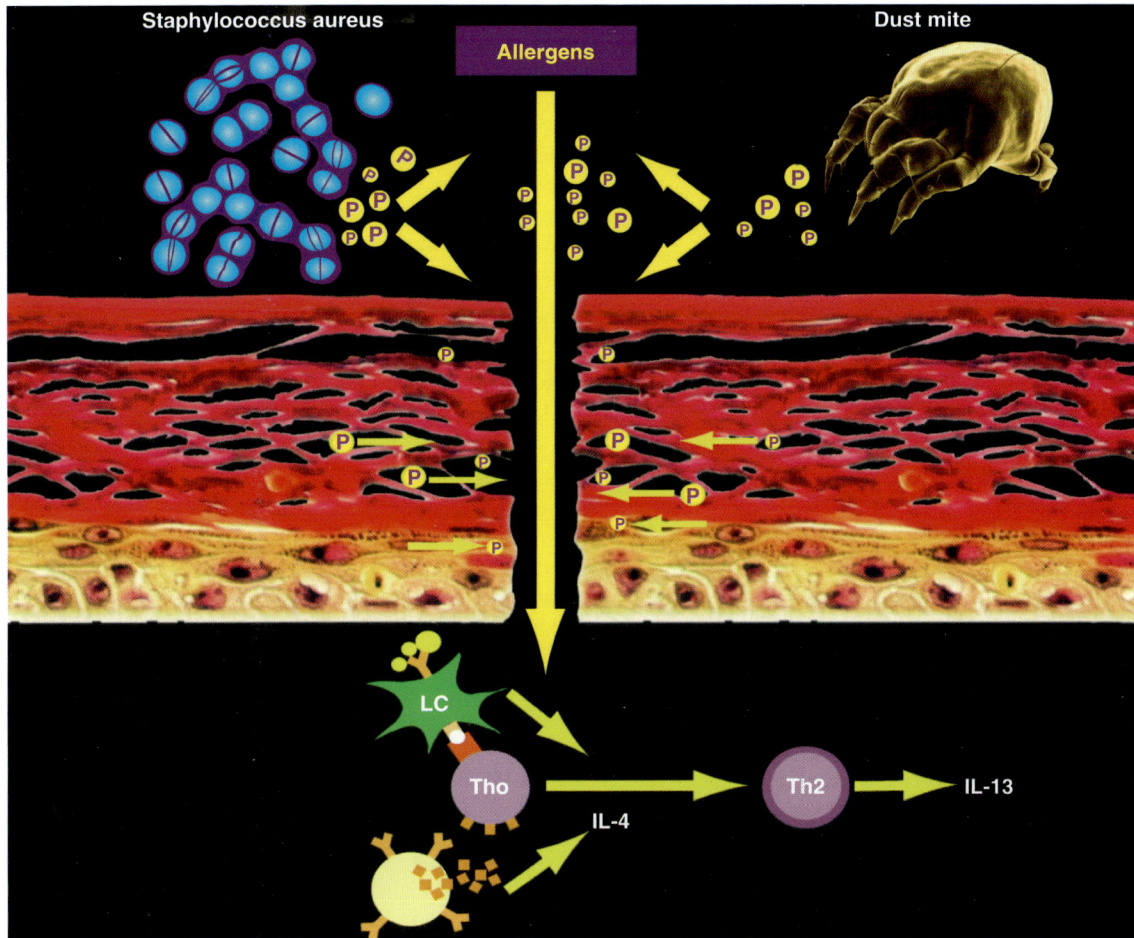

Figure 4.1   There is a defective skin barrier in the stratum corneum in individuals with AD. This arises due to changes in several protease, protease inhibitor and filaggrin genes. The result of these changes is to increase the protease activity within the stratum corneum, which leads to the premature breakdown of the skin barrier. Proteases are also produced by environmental agents such as house dust mites and *Staphylococcus aureus*, and these further damage the skin barrier. The damaged skin barrier then permits the penetration of allergens, which can then induce T_H1 to T_H2 switching. The defective skin barrier is therefore the initial event in the development of AD.

percutaneous penetration of hydrocortisone in the skin of the face, eyelid, and scrotum, and the lowest penetration in plantar skin. There was a 300–fold greater penetration of hydrocortisone through the eyelid compared to plantar skin. These differences cannot be explained by differences in blood flow.[54,55]

The percutaneous penetration of topically applied drugs in different body areas shows the same pattern of variation as the thickness of the stratum corneum,

with the highest penetration through the thinnest stratum corneum.[49] Although regional differences in the percutaneous penetration of irritants and allergens have not been investigated, it seems reasonable to speculate that the pattern might be similar to that observed for the penetration of a topically applied drug, such as hydrocortisone.

Regional variations in epidermal thickness and drug penetration[49,53] indicate that the eyelids, posterior

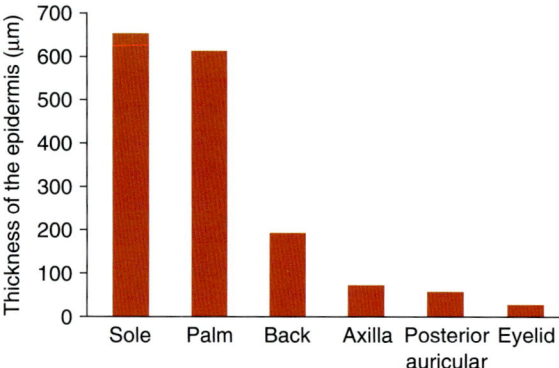

Figure 4.2 The thickness of the epidermis in skin samples from different body sites (Lee & Huang, 2002[49]). The epidermis is thinnest in skin from the plantar aspect of the foot.

auricular areas, other parts of the face, and flexures have a thin epidermal barrier with decreased barrier function (Figure 4.2). These skin sites can be visualized as having 'low epidermal barrier reserve', that is, they are more vulnerable to any exogenous agent that could further decrease the thickness and functional integrity of the epidermal barrier.

Although AD can involve any body site, the eyelids, posterior auricular areas, and flexures are the earliest sites of involvement in infants, the sites where the disease persists longer[39] and with 'low epidermal barrier reserve'. It is probable that these body sites are the most vulnerable to penetration of irritants and allergens[46] and, therefore, represent the first and most persistent sites of disease involvement.

INTER-INDIVIDUAL VARIATION IN SKIN BARRIER FUNCTION

Although there are intra-individual variations in skin barrier thickness and function, which correlate with the earliest and most persistent sites of AD, not all children develop the disease. In addition to intra-individual variations in epidermal barrier function, there are also inter-individual variations.[56] The variability between different measurements at the same site and for the same individual has been estimated to be 8% by site and 21% by day-to-day. The variation between individuals is larger, ranging from 35 to 48%.[57,58] On the basis of the trans-epidermal water loss (TEWL) measurements, there appears to be a 20–40% difference in the skin barrier function at a given regional site between individuals.[57] There is also a wide range for the percutaneous absorption of topically applied drugs,

which may vary by up to 30–fold between individuals on the forearm.[59] Between–subject differences in the absorption of drugs in different body sites are not completely explainable by variations in the thickness of the stratum corneum and corneocyte size. In certain individuals, a defect in epidermal barrier function may only become apparent when the skin is stressed. An example is the skin of aged people in which baseline TEWL measurements are similar to younger adults. However, if the barrier is damaged, recovery to normal is much slower than in a younger adult.[60] It has been suggested that this decreased ability to repair the epidermal barrier after an environmental insult may not only explain inter-individual variation in barrier function but also the increased susceptibility of some individuals to irritant contact dermatitis.[61] The inter-individual variation in skin permeability to drugs in the 'normal population' suggests that there could be genetic variants associated with increased barrier permeability to drugs in some individuals. The 'normal population', from which adult 'normal' skin samples are obtained, may include individuals who had AD as a child or those who may have suffered previously from irritant contact dermatitis or sensitive skin but are apparently 'normal' at the time of testing. These individuals could be those who show increased skin permeability to topically applied drugs. In support of this hypothesis there are data indicating that epidermal barrier function in non-lesional skin from patients with AD is different from that of subjects who never suffered from this disease.[62–64] In one study,[62] the average thickness of the stratum corneum was 12.2 µm in non-lesional skin from individuals with AD and 19.7 µm in controls who had not had AD. In other studies,[63,64] TEWL measurements were also much higher in non-lesional skin from individuals with AD than in the skin of those with no history of AD.

HOW ATOPIC IS ATOPIC DERMATITIS?

Two types of AD have been defined.[65,66] The extrinsic form of the disease is associated with increased levels of total serum IgE and increased levels of specific IgE to environmental allergens,[65] while the intrinsic form is associated with total serum IgE within the age-adjusted normal range and no elevation of specific IgEs to environmental allergens.[66] The link between AD and allergen-specific IgE remains, however, uncertain and controversial.[3,66–70] A recent systematic review[3] asked the question, 'how atopic is AD?'. This is the first work that compared results of population-based studies with those of hospital-based studies. The comparison is important because hospital-based studies include a large proportion of patients with severe dermatitis while the majority of patients included in population-based studies have mild or moderate disease. It was found that in hospital-based studies the percentage of children with extrinsic, 'atopic' dermatitis ranged between 47 and 75%. In contrast, in population-based studies the percentage of children with extrinsic, 'atopic' dermatitis ranged from 7.4 to 78%.[3] Up to 66% of patients with dermatitis did not have measurable allergen-specific IgE in the serum at the time of measurement. The same work also showed that high levels of specific IgE antibodies and/or total serum IgE levels were significantly associated with the severity of dermatitis.

A major gap in the literature is the absence of longitudinal studies on IgE measurements.[3] These studies could help determine if, in some subjects, elevation of total serum IgE and allergen-specific IgE occurs transiently and may remain undetected when measurements are performed only on one occasion. In a study where children with AD were followed during the development of respiratory allergic disease,[71] subjects who were initially negative to the skin prick test became positive over the next 10 years. It has been postulated that non-allergic, intrinsic dermatitis might be considered as the pure, primary, transitional form of AD.[71,72] Could the genetic basis of the pure, primary, intrinsic, transitional form of AD[72] be represented by genetic variants that predispose to a defective epidermal barrier?

THE SKIN BARRIER

The epithelium serves as a first line of defence between the body and the environment (Figure 4.3). Disturbance of the epidermal barrier can favour the penetration of microbes and allergens. Enhanced penetration of agents with antigenic properties increases the risk of sensitization because it allows interaction between allergens and allergen-presenting cells in the skin, and triggers the onset of inflammation once sensitization has occurred (Figure 4.1). Increased penetration of irritants through the skin facilitates the occurrence of non-allergic inflammatory reactions. The skin barrier is, therefore, an important shield against environmental injury.

The barrier to the penetration of irritants and allergens is located in the lower part of the stratum corneum (Figures 4.3, 4.4). The structural integrity of the stratum corneum is maintained by the presence of modified desmosomes, called corneodesmosomes. Corneodesmosomes lock the corneocytes together and provide tensile strength for the stratum corneum to resist shearing forces (Figures 4.3, 4.4). Elias[73] visualized the stratum corneum as being similar to a brick wall, with the corneocytes analogous to bricks and the lipid lamellae acting as cement. Extending this model, the corneodesmosomes may be thought of as analogous to

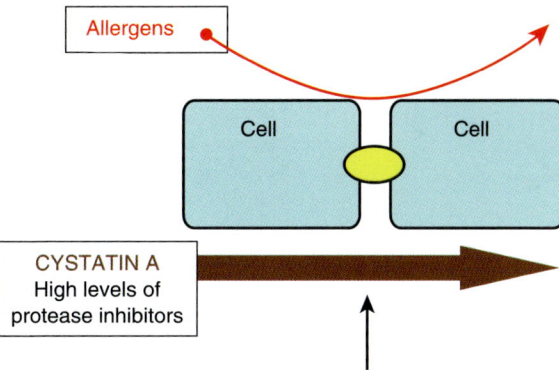

Figure 4.3   In normal skin, there are low levels of proteases such as stratum corneum chymotryptic enzyme (SCCE) and high levels of protease inhibitors such as cystatin A and LEKTI. This results in breakdown of the corneodesmosomes (yellow oval) only in the uppermost layers of the stratum corneum. Thereby, the thickness of the stratum corneum is maintained at a constant. This provides a resilient skin barrier that prevents the penetration of allergens through the stratum corneum.

iron rods that pass down though holes in the bricks to give the wall its tensile strength.[74]

Corneocytes are flattened cells that represent the final differentiation stages of the outermost keratinocytes of the granular layer, when these cells lose their subcellular organelles and nuclei and become densely packed with keratin fibres.[75] In humans, the stratum corneum has an average of 20 corneocyte layers, each corneocyte being approximately 30 μm in diameter.[76] The thickness of the stratum corneum can vary in different body regions to increase the level of protection to areas that experience greater friction, such as the soles of the feet, and palms of the hands.[49] During the formation of corneocytes, the granular cells spill out their lamellar granule contents into the extracellular space to form the lipid lamellae matrix, which encases the corneocytes like cement.[77] The lipid lamellae help prevent internal water loss and penetration of water-soluble materials (Figure 4.4). They also give flexibility to the barrier and ensure that it is as tight as possible. The lipid lamellae matrix is a crystalline substance composed of ceramides, cholesterol, fatty acids, and cholesterol esters,[78] and is believed to exist as a single and coherent lamellar gel.[79]

Disturbed maturation of the lamellar bodies has been demonstrated in atopic skin,[79] consisting of a decreased release of the acid, lipid, and enzyme constituents of the stratum corneum, leading to a defective barrier function.

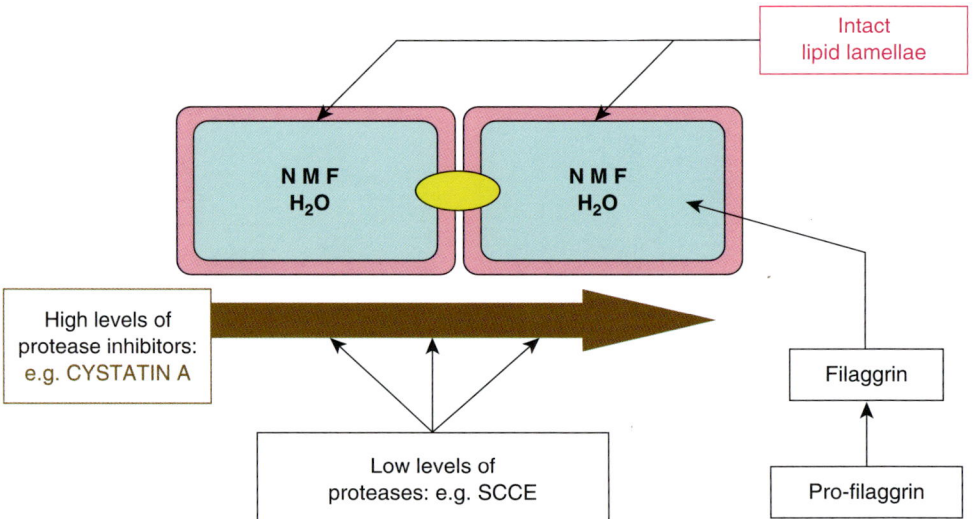

Figure 4.4   The integrity of the skin barrier involves several components, including the regulation of proteolysis of corneodesmosomes (see Figure 4.3), the lipid lamellae, and generation of natural moisturising factor (NMF).

The lipid lamellae provide a water resistant layer around the corneocytes, which helps prevent water loss from the corneocytes. NMF is generated from the breakdown products of the structural protein: filaggrin. NMF attracts water and retains it within the corneocytes causing them to swell. The swollen corneocytes prevent gaps/cracks from developing between them and therefore help to make the stratum corneum resistant to the penetration of allergens.

A disturbance in the extruding mechanism of lamellar lipids, resulting in decreased lipid contents of the stratum corneum, has also been described in eczematous skin.[18] Other reported alterations in AD have included a considerable deficiency in the main barrier lipid components[80] and an increase in sphingomyelin deacylase activity, resulting in decreased ceramide production.[81]

Corneodesmosomes are specialised desmosomes, which bind the corneocytes together in the stratum corneum[82] and are incorporated into the corneocyte envelope. They consist of the cadherin family of extracellular transmembrane glycoproteins, desmoglein and desmocollin (reviewed by Rawlings).[78] Within the corneocytes, desmoglein and desmocollin are linked to keratin filaments via corneodesmosomal plaque proteins, including plakoglobin, desmoplakin, and plakophillin. Desmoglein and desmocollin pass from the corneocyte envelope into the lipid lamellae between the corneocytes and bind to the same proteins on adjacent cells.[83] Corneodesmosin is a 52kDa protein specifically expressed in keratinizing epithelia.[82,84,85] Following secretion into the extracellular space, corneodesmosin is translocated to the transition zone between the stratum granulosum and the stratum corneum[86] and incorporated into the desmosomes. This marks the transition from desmosome to corneodesmosome.

Desquamation is the process by which the epidermal barrier is maintained at a constant thickness. The corneocytes that are shed from the skin surface are continually replaced from underneath by keratinocytes undergoing terminal differentiation. Thus, there is a fine balance between basal cell proliferation and corneocyte desquamation involved in maintaining an epithelium of constant thickness.[87] Desquamation also treads a fine balance between breaking the barrier down enough to allow a continual renewal of epidermal cells, and leaving it intact enough to prevent allergens and irritants from penetrating through to the deeper layers of the skin. The current model of the processes involved in desquamation has been provided by Caubet et al.[88] The model describes a network of degradatory proteases, regulated by protease inhibitors, which breaks down the extracellular corneodesmosomal adhesion proteins that bind the corneocytes together, and in doing so allows the corneocytes to shed from the skin surface (Figures 4.3, 4.4). A cocktail of serine, cysteine, and aspartic proteases are secreted into the extracellular spaces of the stratum corneum during desquamation to facilitate the breakdown of the corneodesmosomes.[89–91] According to the model of desquamation proposed by Caubet et al,[88] inactive protease precursors are activated by tryptic cleavage, and regulated by a complementary cocktail of protease inhibitors. Cleavage of the extracellular corneodesmosomal proteins by the proteases leads to a weakening of the bonds between the corneocytes and a reduction in corneocyte cohesion.

Among the proteases involved in the process of desquamation are the stratum corneum chymotryptic enzyme (SCCE) and the stratum corneum tryptic enzyme (SCTE) [87,92–95] (Figures 4.3, 4.4). These are serine proteases that are expressed in granular keratinocytes and present within the extracellular spaces of the stratum corneum.[95,96] SCCE has been shown to hydrolyze corneodesmosin and desmocollin 1, whilst SCTE is also capable of cleaving desmoglein1.[88] Both SCCE and SCTE are produced as inactive precursors. Removal of pro-peptides by trypsin digestion leads to the formation of the proteolytically active enzymes.[92,94] Studies have shown that SCTE is capable of activating SCCE,[88] in addition to itself,[87,94,95] suggesting that SCTE may serve as a regulator of SCCE activity. Other enzymes capable of degrading corneodesmosomal adhesion proteins include the cysteine proteases cathepsin L2/stratum corneum thiol protease and stratum corneum L-like enzyme; [91,97] the aspartic protease cathepsin D;[98] and several glycosidases.[78]

The activities of the proteases involved in desquamation are regulated by several protease inhibitors coexpressed to balance the rate of corneodesmosome cleavage. SCCE activity is inhibited by the serine leukoprotease inhibitor (SLPI),[99] which can itself be inactivated by members of the cathepsin family.[100] SCCE is also inhibited by elafin, also known as skin-derived antileukoprotease (SKALP), which has been shown to covalently bind to corneocytes.[101] Lymphoepithelial Kazal-type 5 serine protease inhibitor (LEKTI), encoded by the *SPINK5* gene, may also have anti-SCCE activity. It is expressed in similar areas to SCCE and has been linked to Netherton syndrome,[102] a skin condition involving severe barrier dysfunction. Human epidermis also expresses the cystatin protease inhibitors α and M/E, which are specific for cysteine proteases (Figures 4.3, 4.4).[103]

GENETIC REGULATION OF SKIN BARRIER FUNCTION

There is an increasing body of evidence that a genetically determined primary defect in the skin barrier may be central to the development of AD. It has been demonstrated that transgenic mice over-expressing human SCCE develop changes in their skin similar to those seen in chronic AD.[92] Over-expression of SCCE in those mice might have led to a premature breakdown

of the corneodesmosomes, with increasing corneocyte desquamation and thinning of the skin barrier. The resulting impairment of skin barrier function may have favoured the penetration of irritants and allergens and consequent development of dermatitis (Table 4.1).

In order to evaluate the possibility that genetic variations within the SCCE gene are indeed associated with dysregulation of SCCE activity in humans, leading to a thin skin barrier, the SCCE gene was screened for variations, and an associations study was performed in children with AD and in normal controls.[36] A 4 base-pair insertion was identified in the 3'-untranslated region of the kallikrein 7 gene, encoding SCCE (Figure 4.5). The common allele was AACC and the rare allele was AACCAACC. A significant genetic association was found between the rare AACCAACC variant of the SCCE gene and AD. The patients with AD were then stratified into those who did not have high levels of serum IgE (intrinsic AD) and those who did (extrinsic AD). The highest association between the rare variant of the SCCE gene and AD was observed in the subgroup of patients who did not have elevated IgE levels (odds ratio: 4.47; 95% confidence interval: 1.49–13.38; $P = 0.0039$). The association was not significant in the subgroup of patients with high levels of serum IgE.

It is known that determinants of mRNA stability are frequently positioned in the 3'-untranslated region of the genes and that any mutation in this region can alter expression levels of the encoded protein.[104–106] Thus, the AACC insertion could increase the half life of SCCE mRNA, leading to an increased production of the enzyme in the skin of individuals with intrinsic AD. The over-expression of SCCE would cause a premature lysis of the corneodesmosomal proteins. The consequent enhancement in corneocyte desquamation would produce a thin defective epidermal barrier that would allow penetration of irritants, thereby favouring the development of an inflammatory response (Figure 4.5).

Genetic mutations have also been identified in genes encoding members of the protease inhibitors involved in desquamation. Mutations in the *SPINK5* gene, which encodes LEKTI, have been linked to Netherton syndrome.[35,102,107,108] Individuals with this disorder display marked barrier dysfunction, involving altered desquamation and impaired keratinization.[109] Ultrastructural analyses of skin from patients with Netherton syndrome show that there is a marked increase in corneodesmosome cleavage and a reduction in inter-corneocyte cohesion.[109] Transgenic studies using *SPINK5* (–/–) mice have demonstrated that LEKTI deficiency results in abnormal desmosome cleavage in the upper granular layer of the epidermis, which is caused by increased SCCE and SCTE activity.[110] Increased protease activity in the skin of *SPINK5* (–/–) mice leads to increased

Table 4.1 Genetic dysfunction of epidermal integrity and effects of endogenous and exogenous proteases

Protein	Gene	Abbreviation	Dysfunction	Reference
Stratum corneum chymotryptic enzyme	KLK7	SCCE	Genetic association between a mutation in the SCCE gene and AD. Results suggested that altered SCCE expression might lead to an increased rate of desmosome breakdown and a weakening of the skin barrier.	36
			Transgenic mice over-expressing SCCE. The mice displayed epidermal hyperproliferation and decreased skin barrier function. Their phenotype was similar to that seen in chronic itchy dermatitis.	92
Stratum corneum tryptic enzyme	KLK5	SCTE	Shown to degrade corneodesmosomal proteins. Altered function may lead to similar changes to those associated with abnormal SCCE expression.	88
Stratum corneum thiol protease		SCTP	Responsible for the degradation of extracellular structural proteins. Can function in acidic environments like the stratum corneum. Altered function may lead to similar changes to those associated with abnormal SCCE expression.	91
Desmoglein		DSG	The distribution of different isoforms of desmoglein affects the structure and function of the stratum corneum. Transgenic mice abnormally expressing DSG3 within the stratum corneum developed scaling and altered lipid lamellae. The ultrastructure of the stratum corneum showed premature loss of cohesion of corneocytes.	Elias PM et al. J Cell Biol 2001; 153: 243–9
			Targeted disruption of the DSG3 gene in mice led to a loss of keratinocytes cell adhesion. The mice developed a phenotype similar to that seen in pemphigus vulgaris.	120
			Abnormal DSG3 expression in the epidermis of transgenic mice resulted in epidermal hyperproliferation and abnormal differentiation.	Merritt AJ et al. Mol Cell Biol 2002; 22: 5846-58
Desmocollin		DSC	Transgenic mice lacking desmocollin 1 develop a very weak epidermis, and display barrier defects and abnormal differentiation.	121

(Continued)

Table 4.1   (Continued)

Protein	Gene	Abbreviation	Dysfunction	Reference
Corneodesmosin		CDSN		
Desmoplakin		DP	Transgenic null mice die in utero. Analysis of the embryos revealed a critical role for desmoplakin in anchoring intermediate filaments to desmosomes, and in desmosome assembly and/or stabilization. Mutation in the gene encoding desmoplakin led to a null allele that was associated with the inherited skin disorder, striate palmoplantar keratoderma.	122,123
Serine leukoprotease inhibitor		SLPI		
Skin derived antileukoprotease		SKALP		99; Alkemade JA et al. J Cell Sci 1994; 107: 2335–42; Wiedow O et al. J Invest Dermatol 1993; 101: 305–9
Lymphoepithelial kazal type 5 serine protease inhibitor	SPINK5	LEKTI	SPINK5 deficient mice develop the key features of Netherton syndrome. The barrier defects were attributed to increased epidermal protease activity and an increased rate of desmoglein 1 cleavage.	110
			SPINK5 mutant mice develop a fragile stratum corneum and die due to dehydration through increased TEWL. Data suggested that the fragility of the corneodesmosomes was being caused by increased proteolysis of corneodesmosin.	111
House dust mite protease		Der p1/p2	Purified Der p1 and p2 were shown to elicit an allergic reaction and to have proteolytic activity.	134
Cathepsin L			The lysosomal protease cathepsin L is an important regulator of keratinocyte and melanocyte differentiation during hair follicle morphogenesis and cycling	Tobin D et al. Am J Pathol 2002; 160: 1807–21; Roth W et al. FASEB J 2000; 14: 2075–86
Cathepsin D			Cathepsin D is involved in the regulation of transglutaminase I and epidermal differentiation	Egberts F et al. J Cell Sci 2004; 117:2295-2307
Cystatin M/E				Zeeuwen PL et al. Hum Mol Genet 2004; 13: 1069–79

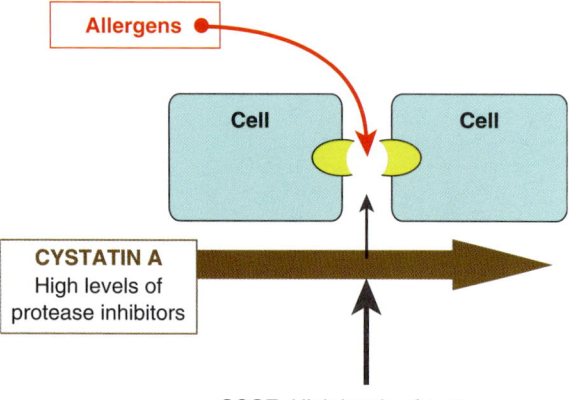

Figure 4.5 In children with AD, who have the AACC3'UTR repeat variant in their KLK7 (SCCE) gene, increased levels of proteases are produced,[36] which results in excessive breakdown of the corneodesmosomes (yellow ovals) and causes a defective skin barrier. This then allows the penetration of allergens that can trigger a flare of AD. This occurs in the presence of normal levels of protease inhibitors such as cystatin A and LEKTI.

breakdown of desmoglein 1[110] and corneodesmosin,[111] which is consistent with the premature cleavage of corneodesmosomes observed in the skin of patients with Netherton syndrome. Several studies have also linked mutations in the *SPINK5* gene with AD.[35,112,113]

Cystatins are cysteine protease inhibitors expressed within the epidermis. Several studies have shown that the cystatins might afford protection from proteolysis by bacterial and viral proteases.[114] Transgenic mice carrying a null mutation in the gene encoding cystatin M/E display severe barrier abnormalities and die shortly after birth.[103] Mice lacking cystatin M/E have abnormalities in cornification and desquamation with hyperkeratosis[103] (Table 4.1).

Cystatin A is a protease inhibitor that is expressed in the stratum corneum and stratum granulosum. Decreased expression of cystatin A has been found in the skin of patients with AD.[115] The cystatin A gene maps to chromosome 3q21, which has been identified as a major susceptibility locus for AD.[116] Normally there are high levels of the cystatin A protease inhibitor within the stratum corneum, which, with other protease inhibitors such as LEKTI, inhibit the activity of endogenous proteases produced within the skin (Figures 4.3, 4.4). Cystatin A is also secreted in sweat and forms a layer over the surface of the skin that protects the skin from exogenous proteases such as those produced by house dust mites and *Staphylococcus* aureus[117] (Figure 4.6).

We have identified a +344c variant in the Cystatin A gene and found a significant association with AD.[38] This variant results in decreased mRNA stability and therefore decreased levels of the cystatin A protease inhibitor, both within the skin and in the sweat[38] (Figures 4.7, 4.8, 4.9). The decreased levels of cystatin A in sweat are not able to inhibit the activity of exogenous proteases, such as those from house dust mites (Figure 4.8). This results in increased deterioration of the corneodesmosomes, breaking down of the stratum corneum and allows the penetration of allergens (Figure 4.9).[38] The integrity of the epidermal barrier is maintained by a balance between the levels of both endogenous and exogenous proteases and protease inhibitors. Cystatin A is a potent inhibitor of the endogenous cathepsins (B, H and L) within the epidermis, and exogenous (Der p1 and Der f1) proteases from house dust mites. The Der p1 and Der f1 proteases can also induce T_H1/T_H2 switching.[118,119] The cystatin A +344c variant may therefore represent an important contribution to both the defective epidermal barrier and T_H2 switching.[38]

Transgenic knockout mice studies have revealed the importance of several adhesion proteins for the assembly of functional desmosomes and maintenance of a functional skin barrier (Table 4.1). Desmoglein $3^{-/-}$ mice develop traumatized skin that displays a marked separation of desmosomes under electron microscopy.[120] Mice lacking desmocollin 1 have been shown to have flaky and fragile epidermis, with acanthyosis in the granular layer.[121] Desmoplakin is also important in epidermal sheet formation[122] (Table 4.1). Mice lacking desmoplakin have few desmosomes and a marked reduction in barrier integrity.[123] It could be hypothesized that mutations within genes encoding adhesion proteins, which alter the ability of these proteins to preserve skin barrier integrity, might also play a role in the development of AD.

Changes in both protease and protease inhibitor genes could be combined in some patients to produce even more severe breakdown of the skin barrier (Figure 4.10).

Filaggrin is a structural protein incorporated into the cornified cell envelope. The majority of filaggrin does not persist beyond the two deepest layers of stratum corneum.[124,125] Filaggrin is extensively deaminated through the actions of the enzyme peptidyl-deiminase. It is subsequently degraded into small peptides and then free amino acids. The free amino acids are then catabolised into the constituents of natural moisturizing factor (NMF) such as pyrolidine carboxylic acid and urolaic acid.[125]

NMF is essential for the retention of water within corneocytes, and results in their optimal hydration and swelling. This prevents the development of gaps between

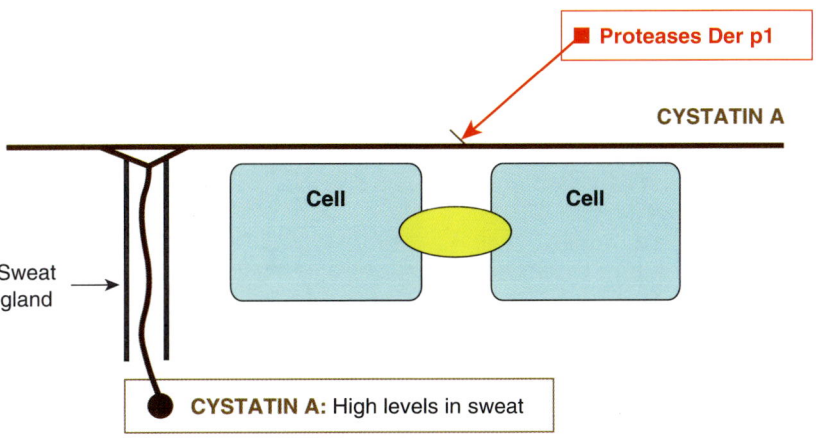

Figure 4.6   In normal skin, the protease inhibitor, cystatin A, is secreted in sweat and flows out onto the surface of the stratum corneum forming a protective layer. Exogenous proteases from, for example, house dust mites (Der p1) are inhibited by the protective layer of the cystatin A protease inhibitor and, as a result, cannot break down the corneodesmosomes. The protective layer of protease inhibitor on the surface of normal skin provides another mechanism to maintain a resilient skin barrier.

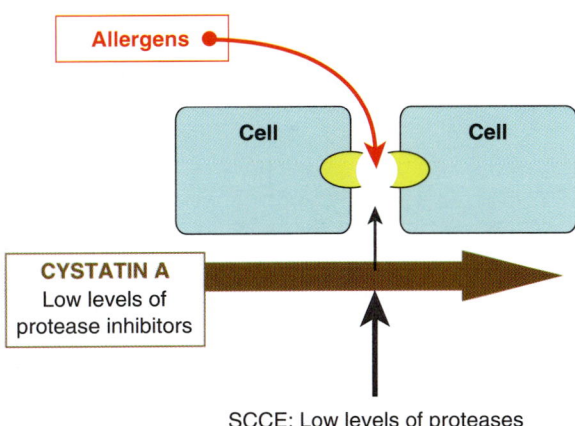

Figure 4.7   In children with AD who have the +344 cystatin A variant,[36] the messenger RNA for cystatin A is less stable, consequently there is less cystatin A protein within the stratum corneum. This change means that even with a normal quantity of proteases within the stratum corneum, its activity is increased and produces excessive breakdown of the corneodesmosomes. This allows the penetration of allergens that can then trigger flares of AD.

the corneocytes, enhancing the integrity of the stratum corneum and making it resistant to the penetration of irritants and allergens (Figure 4.4).

There are decreased levels of both filaggrin and NMF in the skin of patients with AD.[115,125] Loss of function variants in the filaggrin gene have been shown to be linked with AD.[37] This provides an explanation for both the decreased levels of filaggrin and NMF within the stratum corneum of patients with AD. This may, in turn, lead to a decreased ability of the corneocytes to retain water, resulting in their shrinkage. As corneocytes shrink, this results in gaps developing between them, creating a defective epidermal barrier, which is then vulnerable to the penetration of irritants and allergens.

The different genetic variants that contribute to a defective epidermal barrier are illustrated in Figure 4.11. These include increased levels of proteases such as SCCE,[36] and decreased levels of protease inhibitors such as LEKTI[110] and cystatin A.[38] Loss of function variants in the filaggrin gene may result in decreased generation of NMF and a decreased ability of the corneocytes to hold water. These genetic variants may occur on their own but could also be combined to produce more severe breakdown of the epidermal barrier.

SECONDARY PROTEASES

When endogenous proteases, such as SCCE, are produced in excessive quantities, the corneocytes desquamate prematurely, producing a thin skin barrier. This then facilitates the penetration of irritants and allergens, which can trigger a flare of the AD. Cells within the inflammatory infiltrate can produce proteases that further damage the skin barrier. These proteases can be considered as a product of the inflammatory response

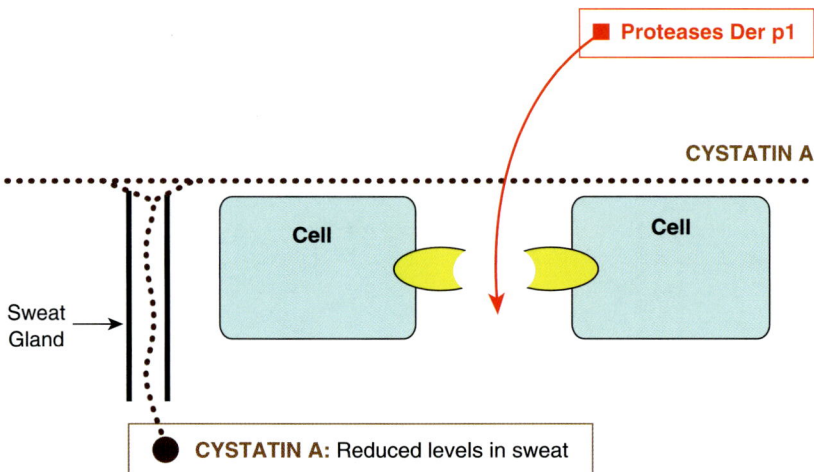

Figure 4.8   In a child with AD who has the +344 cystatin A variant,[38] there is less cystatin A protease inhibitor secreted in the sweat. Therefore, the layer of cystatin A protease inhibitor over the surface of the skin can be visualised as incomplete and is insufficient to provide protection against exogenous proteases such as Der p1. The exogenous proteases can, therefore, break down the corneodesmosomes, leading to a defective skin barrier.

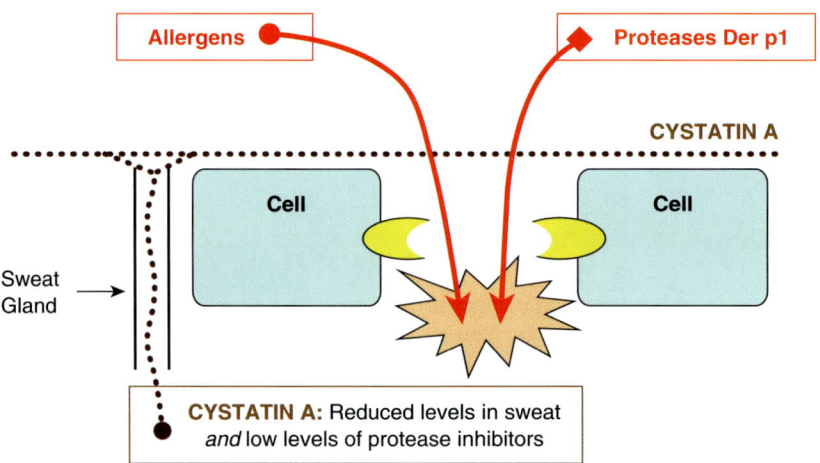

Figure 4.9   In a child with AD, with the +344 cystatin A variant,[38] the incomplete protective layer of protease inhibitor on the surface of the skin allows exogenous proteases (i.e. Der p1) to break down the corneodesmosomes. This results in a reduced integrity of the stratum corneum barrier and allergens can penetrate through to trigger a flare of AD. The proteases from house dust mites (Der p1, Der f1) not only break down the skin barrier, but can also act as allergens themselves, triggering a flare of AD.

(secondary proteases), and their levels will be proportional to the severity of a flare of AD. Mast cell chymase (MCC) is a chymotrypsin-like serine protease primarily stored in secretory mast cell granules. In one study,[126] the number of MCC–positive cells was significantly increased in the lesional skin of patients with AD, in comparison with non-lesional skin. However, there was no significant difference in the number of MCC–positive cells between the non-lesional skin of patients with AD and the skin of normal controls, suggesting that increased MCC activity may be associated with active dermatitis. In another study in mice,[127] injection of MCC into the normal skin induced an inflammatory response similar to that observed in AD.

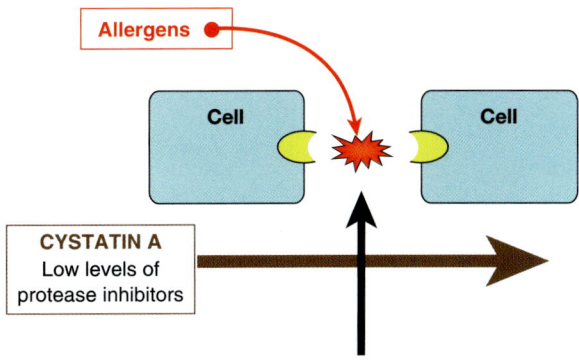

Figure 4.10   Genetic variants that determine a defective skin barrier can occur in isolation, as illustrated for the protease KLK7 (SCCE) in Figure 4.5 and for the protease inhibitor, cystatin A, in Figures 4.7 & 4.8.

It is also possible that genetic variants could be combined in some individuals with AD: for example, a change in the protease gene, KLK7 & (SCCE),[36] might be combined with a change in the protease inhibitor gene, cystatin A.[38] This would result in both an increased level of proteases (SCCE), and decreased levels of protease inhibitor (cystatin A), resulting in a more severe breakdown of the skin barrier than if the individual changes were present on their own.

There is also evidence that MCC may participate in the development of chronic dermatitis by inducing eosinophil infiltration.[128] Variants within the MCC gene have been associated with AD in children.[129] The association was strongest in individuals with low levels of total serum IgE.[129] Instead, in adults with AD, a polymorphism in the promoter region of the MCC gene has been associated with high levels of total serum IgE.[130]

EXOGENOUS PROTEASES

House dust mites are a source of over 30 different proteins that can induce IgE–mediated responses.[131] Some of these proteins are cysteine and serine proteases.[132] Some of these proteins have been shown to cleave adhesion proteins and to increase the permeability of lung epithelium.[133] Patch tests have demonstrated that two proteins with proteolytic activity derived from house dust mites, Der p1 and Der p2, can elicit irritative or immune reactions that are not linked to raised levels of IgE against house dust mites, suggesting that these proteins cause skin irritation or immune activation through a direct proteolytic activity.[134]

As reviewed by Storck,[135] *Staphylococcus aureus* has been implicated as an environmental factor in the pathogenesis of AD since the nineteenth century. *Staphylococcus*

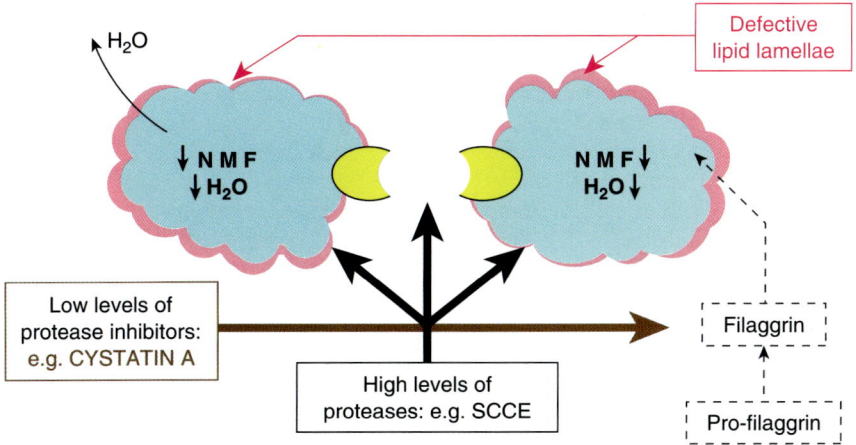

Figure 4.11   The changes in protease and protease inhibitor genes may also be combined with changes in the lipid lamellae and NMF levels. Changes in the lipid lamellae may result from primary changes in genes that regulate their synthesis and/or be secondary to increased protease activity.[167]

Changes in the filaggrin gene[37] may result in decreased levels of NMF and a raising of the pH within the stratum corneum. The decreased levels of NMF would result in a decreased ability to retain water within the corneocytes. This would allow gaps/cracks to open between the corneocytes, further exacerbating the defective skin barrier. A rise in the pH within the stratum corneum could result in enhanced protease activity[167] further contributing to a defective skin barrier in AD.

aureus is not a member of the normal microflora colonizing the skin, apart from carriage in the nasal and perineal areas. In contrast, in the skin of patients with AD, up to 14×10^6 organisms per cm^2 are present in eczematous lesions.[136] *Staphylococcus aureus* may play a role in the chronicity and severity of AD through its release of superantigenic exotoxins.[137] In addition to their immunological effects, these toxins may also directly damage the skin barrier. *Staphylococci* produce proteinases that could break down corneodesmosomes by a mechanism similar to that described above for SCCE.[138] In addition, *Staphylococcus aureus* secretes sphingosine deacylase and glycerophospholipids that may interfere with the formation of the lipid lamellae.[139] Thus, exogenous proteases and lipases produced by house dust mites and *Staphylococcus aureus* may contribute to the breakdown of the skin barrier in AD (Figure 4.1).

GENE–ENVIRONMENT INTERACTIONS: pH AND DETERGENTS

The skin has long been known to have an acidic pH (the acid mantle) that contributes to the optimal barrier function of this tissue.[140] The average surface pH of the forearm of a healthy male is around 5.4 to 5.9.[141] In humans, the skin surface pH at birth is near–neutral (pH 6.5) compared with children and adults.[142–144] In newborn rats, the stratum corneum reaches adult pH levels during the first few days after birth,[145,146] whereas similar changes take a few weeks to occur in human newborns.[144,147]

Although the acid mantle of the stratum corneum was initially thought to originate from exogenous sources (microbial metabolites, free fatty acids of pilo–sebaceous origin, and eccrine gland-derived products, such as amino and lactic acids),[148–150] recent studies have demonstrated that endogenous pathways (generation of by-products of keratinization, synthesis of free fatty acids from phospholipid hydrolysis by the secretory phospholipase A2, and the non-energy-dependent sodium–proton exchanger) are additional sources.[151–153] The acid mantle has multiple effects on the skin. Firstly, it has a strong antimicrobial effect,[154,155] decreases skin colonization by pathogenic bacteria,[149,154,156] and favours the adhesion of non-pathogenic bacteria to the stratum corneum.[157] Secondly, several lines of evidence indicate a role for skin surface pH on desquamation, permeability barrier homeostasis, and stratum corneum integrity/cohesion. A delay in epidermal barrier recovery occurs when the skin is immersed in neutral pH buffers.[158] Moreover, epidermal barrier abnormalities are noticed when the skin pH is increased by blocking either the secretory phospholipase A2 or the non-energy dependent sodium–proton exchanger, and these abnormalities are corrected by co-exposure of inhibitor-treated areas to an acidic buffer.[153,159]

Skin pH variations have been clearly documented in some skin diseases. Anderson[160] found a total body pH elevation in seborrheic dermatitis, AD, and xeroderma. Others[161] demonstrated a significantly higher skin surface pH in a group of school children with AD compared to controls. In AD patients, skin pH was reported to be 0.5 units higher than in control subjects.[162] Similar studies[161,163] documented that skin pH is higher in AD patients than in healthy controls even on uninvolved skin. Seidenari et al[163] also demonstrated that skin pH values are higher in patients with active lesions than in asymptomatic patients.

Many enzymes involved in skin barrier homeostasis and restoration have been shown to be pH-dependent.[164] The skin protease SCCE exhibits a neutral pH optimum.[90] A change in pH from 7.5 to 5.5 reduces SCCE activity by 50%.[90,165] The thiol cystein protein (cathepsin LZ) and the aspartate protease (cathepsin D) have an acid pH optimum and probably mediate desquamation in the upper layers of normal skin.[89,97,166] The SCCE/SCTE proteases could initiate the degradation of corneodesmosomes in the lower layers of the stratum corneum in normal skin and in all layers of the stratum corneum in diseased skin, where the neutral pH (pH 7.0) predominates.[166] The importance of pH to the activity of skin proteases was demonstrated in hairless mice treated with 'superbases' that neutralize skin surface pH.[167] This caused rapid activation of serine proteases, with consequent degradation of corneodesmosomes. The resulting decrease in skin barrier cohesion/integrity was detectable with the skin stripping/TEWL assay.

Stratum corneum pH is also important for the generation and degradation of the lipid lamellae. The lipid-generating enzymes, β-glucocerebrosidase and sphingomyelinase, also exhibit low acid pH optimum.[164,168–170] Application of 'superbases' to hairless mouse skin has been demonstrated to decrease glucocerebrosidase activity, which has been shown to generate incompletely processed lipid lamellae membranes, as assessed by electron microscopy.[167] Raising the pH of the stratum corneum surface can, therefore, cause enhanced desquamation of corneocytes by increasing the activity of serine proteases such as SCCE and also by interfering with the normal lipid processing required for the formation of the lipid lamellae.

In an individual with a genetic predisposition to increased skin protease activity, for example due to the rare AACCAACC variant of the SCCE gene,[36] there will be constantly high levels of SCCE protein in the stratum corneum. If the pH of the skin is then raised from the pH of normal skin (5.5) to 7.0 or higher, the SCCE protease activity will be further increased, with further enhancement of corneocyte desquamation and thinning of the stratum corneum (Figure 4.12). The most common environmental agents that can raise the

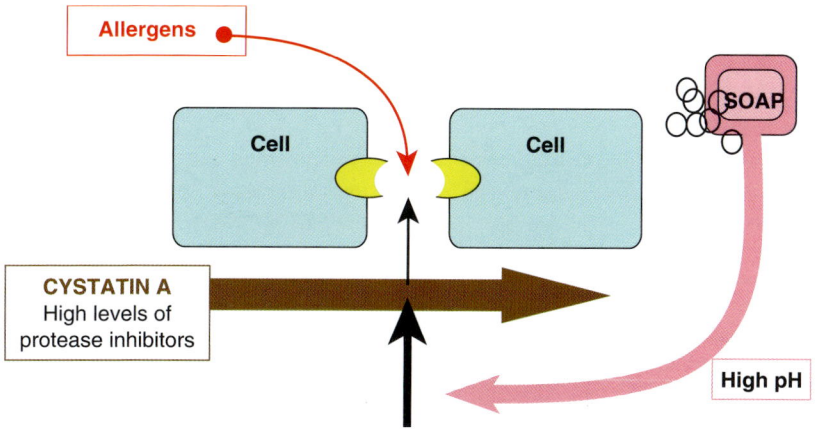

SCCE: High levels of proteases

Figure 4.12   Soap and detergents are very important environmental triggers in AD. The use of soap and detergents raises the pH of the skin from the normal of 5.5, up to 7.5, and sometimes higher, to 10.[62]

Proteases, such as SCCE, are pH sensitive and they have enhanced activity at neutral pH.[167] Washing with soap and detergents provides an important environmental trigger that directly interacts with changes in protease genes (e.g. SCCE), leading to exacerbated skin barrier breakdown in AD.

pH of the skin surface are soap and other detergents. Washing the skin with soap causes an increase of the pH on the palms by 3 units for more than 90 minutes.[171] White et al[62] measured the thickness of the stratum corneum in normal skin and in non-lesional eczematous skin before and after washing with soap. Prior to washing, the stratum corneum was thicker in normal skin (19.7 μm) than in non-lesional eczematous skin (13.7 μm). Washing with soap caused further thinning of the stratum corneum in both the normal and the non-lesional eczematous skin, which is consistent with an increased activity of skin proteases such as SCCE, resulting in premature breakdown of the corneodesmosomes. The observed differences between normal skin and non-lesional eczematous skin could be explained by differences in the level of SCCE expression in the skin determined by genetic variants in the SCCE gene.[40] This is an excellent example of a gene–environment interaction, producing the AD clinical phenotype (Figure 4.12).[172]

Detergents are widely used in cleaning human skin. They work by emulsifying the skin surface lipids (both foreign and natural), which can then be washed off by water. Surfactants can damage the skin, provoking scaling, dryness, tightness and roughness, erythema and swelling.[173–176] The use of soap and detergents is one of the most common causes of irritant contact dermatitis of the hands and can trigger flares of AD.[177]

The detergent sodium lauryl sulphate is used as the standard test of skin susceptibility to irritation. The negative effects of surfactants on skin barrier function are demonstrated by an increased TEWL, which is more severe in subjects with AD than in normal controls.[178] Surfactants can solubilize lipids, and it has been postulated that this could be the mechanism by which they increase TEWL.[178,179] However, measurements of lipid solubilization by sodium lauryl sulphate suggest that, at concentrations ranging between 0.1% and 2%, it removes very small amounts of free fatty acids, cholesterol, and esters.[175] The acute irritant effects of soap and detergents could be partially explained by the release of pro-inflammatory cytokines from corneocytes.[29,30] However, enhanced desquamation and thinning of the stratum corneum associated with changes in skin pH may probably explain the negative effects of many detergents on skin barrier function. The potential negative effects of surfactants on the skin barrier of people with AD should be taken into account when choosing topical products. For example, aqueous cream is a generic emollient soap substitute, designed to be used instead of soap in people with AD and related disease and contains sodium lauryl sulphate at 1% concentration. The use of aqueous cream as a leave-on emollient rather than as a wash-off soap substitute has been associated with irritant reactions and exacerbations of AD,[31] probably occurring as a result of the irritative effects of sodium lauryl sulphate described above. This illustrates the importance of understanding that topical pharmaceutical and cosmetic products can have both positive and negative effects on the skin barrier. If used incorrectly, these products can damage the skin barrier and as a result exacerbate, rather than improve, the control of AD.

GENE–ENVIRONMENT INTERACTIONS: TOPICAL CORTICOSTEROIDS

The positive anti-inflammatory effects of topical corticosteroids have to be balanced with their potential to induce cutaneous atrophy as a result of the inhibition of the synthesis of collagen and glycosaminoglycans,[180–182] and also against their effects on the integrity of the epidermal barrier.[183-185] A significant increase in TEWL has been observed in patients following the long-term application of topical corticosteroids.[186,187] Short-term application of topical corticosteroids (3 weeks) has also been associated with a significant increase in TEWL from normal skin.[184] It appears, therefore, that within 3 weeks, topical corticosteroids can cause significant disruption of the epidermal barrier. These findings should not surprise, considering that even a single supra-physiological dose of endogenous glucocorticoids induced by stress has been shown to impair epidermal barrier homeostasis.[25,188]

Sheu et al[183] performed biopsies on the facial skin of patients previously treated with topical corticosteroids on their faces for 4 months to 4 years. The skin of patients treated with topical corticosteroids differed from that of control subjects in that it showed up to a 70% reduction in the thickness of the stratum corneum by light microscopy, a marked decrease in the number of intercellular lipid lamellae, and a marked reduction in the number of membrane-coated granules at the stratum granulosum/stratum corneum interface by electron microscopy. The reduction in the number of cell layers in the stratum corneum and reduced lipid lamellae was reflected in an increased TEWL in the topical corticosteroid-treated patients (21.3 ± 11.8 g/m^2 per hour) compared with normal controls (6.7 ± 1.29 g/m^2 per hour).[183,187]

Kao et al[185] investigated the effects of short-term (3 days) application of very potent topical corticosteroids (clobetasol propionate 0.05%) in normal human volunteers. The baseline TEWL was not changed after this treatment compared to controls. However, when the skin was tape-stripped, the TEWL was much higher from the clobetasol-treated skin than from that treated with vehicle. Similar results were obtained in murine skin treated with clobetasol propionate 0.05%.[185] Measurements of the amount of proteins on the tape strips removed from the mouse skin revealed larger quantities from the clobetasol-treated site than from sites treated with vehicle.[185] This indicates that tape stripping removed more corneocytes from the skin treated with clobetasol than from the skin treated with vehicle. The ability of the stratum corneum to resist tape stripping is imparted by the corneodesmosomes, which lock the corneocytes together. As increasing numbers of corneodesmosomes are cleaved, more corneocytes will be removed with successive tape strips. The more corneocytes that are removed per tape strip the greater the disruption to the skin barrier and the higher the TEWL. In the study by Kao et al,[185] the number of corneocytes lost by tape stripping and the TEWL increased in a dose-dependent manner. Electron micrographs of the skin of these mice revealed a 35% reduction in the number of corneodesmosomes in the lower part of the stratum corneum in mice treated with clobetasol compared with those treated with vehicle, which explains why tape stripping removed significantly more corneocytes from clobetasol-treated skin than from vehicle-treated skin. Kao et al[185] also found changes in the lipid lamellae similar to those reported by Sheu et al.[183,188] Thus, short-term treatment (3 days) with very potent topical corticosteroids appears to cause disruption of both the corneodesmosomes and lipid lamellae, resulting in a decrease in the functional integrity of the epidermal barrier.

Corticosteroids bind to glucocorticoid nuclear receptors, which in turn bind to corticosteroid-responsible elements in the promoter region of multiple genes.[189] At concentrations as low as 10^{-10} molar, corticosteroids have been shown to up-regulate SCCE gene expression in vitro.[190] An increased production of SCCE protein following topical application of corticosteroids would help explain the degradation of corneodesmosomes observed after 3 days' application of clobetasol propionate to the skin of mice.[185]

We have shown that application of clobetasol propionate, one finger-tip unit twice daily for 4 days, to normal human skin, induces the expression of the mRNA for SCCE[191] and may, therefore, have a detrimental effect on epidermal barrier function by promoting corneodesmosome breakdown. The application of potent topical corticosteroids for 2 weeks and moderately potent topical corticosteroids (twice per day) for 4 weeks can also lead to significant damage to the stratum corneum;[192,193] however, topical corticosteroids are an extremely effective treatment for severe flares of AD. How is this compatible with the negative effects of topical corticosteroids on the skin barrier as a result of increased SCCE protease production? The most likely explanation is that during a severe flare of AD there are several other sources of proteases, including inflammatory cells (secondary proteases), and *Staphylococcus aureus*. The anti-inflammatory actions of topical corticosteroids can decrease production of all these sources of proteases and the overall effects of topical corticosteroids in the middle of a flare on the skin barrier will, therefore, be positive, improving barrier function. Before development of a severe flare of AD or after resolution of the flare, the main sources of proteases in the stratum corneum are endogenous proteases such as SCCE. The levels of SCCE will be increased in non-lesional eczematous skin as a result of the variation in the SCCE gene associated with AD.[36] Further increase in the levels of SCCE induced by topical corticosteroids will worsen the epidermal barrier dysfunction. The disruption of the stratum corneum barrier observed after even short-term exposure to topical corticosteroids[185] supports this hypothesis. Outside a flare of AD, the overall effects of topical corticosteroids on the skin barrier may, therefore, be negative as these drugs may enhance its breakdown. This helps explain why short-term treatment of a flare of AD with topical corticosteroids is very effective while their long-term use can lead to problems such as flare rebound and steroid addiction.

Rebound flare after the discontinuation of topical corticosteroids is not uncommon. It occurs both in the context of an underlying skin disease, such as AD, and also in normal skin after prolonged application of topical corticosteroids.[194,195] Rebound flare was observed in all of the patients studied by Sheu et al.[183] The rebound flare following discontinuation of topical corticosteroids has similarities to that observed following other forms of barrier disruption. Barrier disruption results in the initiation of cytokine cascade, followed by an inflammatory response.[29,30,196] Several of the cytokines released following barrier disruption can induce transcription from the protease genes and lead to further barrier breakdown.[197] An extreme form of rebound flare following the discontinuation of topical corticosteroids is 'the red burning skin syndrome'.[198] In all the reported cases, patients had used topical corticosteroids for prolonged periods on delicate skin sites, such as the face and genitals. Patients initially developed pruritus followed by burning and erythema. Further application of topical corticosteroids led to an exacerbation of the condition, described as corticosteroid addiction. A possible mechanism is that as the potent TCS cause a thinning of the naturally thin stratum corneum on the face this allows more allergens to penetrate, inducing persistent flares of the AD. As a result the patient uses more TCS to treat the flare, but this causes further thinning of the stratum corneum and, consequently, greater allergen penetration, causing more flares.[183,185] A vicious circle is therefore established. Thus, an understanding of the kinetics of protease production around a flare of AD helps us understand how to use treatments such as topical corticosteroids more safely.

CONCLUSIONS

'Inside-outside'[24] or 'outside-inside'[27] hypothesis: which is correct? We suggest that both may be important at different times in the evolution of AD, in intrinsic and extrinsic AD, and in ADs of different severities. Intrinsic AD, without an elevated level of non-specific or specific IgE, is common (up to 66% of cases) in children with mild or moderate AD recruited from the community.[3] It has been postulated that non-allergenic, intrinsic AD can be considered as a pure, transitional form of the disease.[72] In a proportion of children with intrinsic AD, the disease will remain intrinsic, while in others, the allergic nature of the disease will manifest with time.[71]

In children with intrinsic AD there is a strong association with an insertion in the 3'-untranslated region of the gene encoding the protease SCCE.[36]

In mild, intrinsic AD the use of an irritant such as soap in patients with the genetic predisposition to a skin barrier breakdown related to the variant of the SCCE gene may be sufficient on its own to produce barrier disruption. This stimulates the production of inflammatory cytokines[29,30] and leads to the development and persistence of eczematous lesions. These would be eczematous lesions produced according to the 'outside-inside' hypothesis. AD is an example of a gene dosage and environmental dosage effect disease. At one end of the spectrum, a single change in one skin barrier gene may predispose to AD but require exposure to an environmental agent such as soap and detergents for the disease to be expressed. At the other end of the spectrum a combination of changes in several skin barrier genes could, on their own, lead to severe skin barrier breakdown and development of more severe AD. Environmental factors such as soap, detergents, and exogenous proteases derived from house dust mites and *Staphylococcus aureus* would further exacerbate the barrier breakdown and AD. At the severe end of the spectrum, other genetic changes may also be important, for example, changes in the genes that regulate the production of IgE.

The hypothesis that non-allergenic intrinsic AD might be considered as a pure transitional form of the disease[72] is compatible with the skin barrier genetic data. The SCCE variant is strongly associated with intrinsic but not extrinsic AD.[36] A proportion of the patients with intrinsic AD will never develop increased levels of serum IgE. In some infants, the disease may start as the intrinsic, non-allergenic form of AD, with a defective epidermal barrier. The alterations in epidermal barrier integrity and function allow the penetration of allergens through the skin, facilitating the interaction of these allergens with the local antigen-presenting cells and immune effector cells. During the first 6 months of a baby's life, the T_H1 cells are most vulnerable to switching to T_H2, resulting in increased production of IL-4 and IL-5 and increased production of IgE.[199] By this chain of events, the intrinsic AD of some young children may become extrinsic AD. In very mild, permanently intrinsic AD the 'outside-inside hypothesis'[27] may explain the entire disease process. In AD that starts as intrinsic but then switches to extrinsic, both the 'outside-inside hypothesis' [27] and the 'inside-outside hypothesis'[24] may probably explain different aspects of the disease process at different points in time of the disease development. The genetic predisposition to a defective skin barrier could be considered as a starting point in the atopic march. The number and functional significance of changes in skin barrier genes could help determine the severity of barrier breakdown and allergen penetration. In addition, an understanding of the kinetics of protease production in the skin of AD patients could help treatments such as topical corticosteroids to be used more safely and effectively. The environmental exposure to irritants and allergens would also be very important in unmasking/exacerbating defective skin barrier function. This, in turn, could influence T_H1/T_H2 switching and the change from intrinsic, non-allergic AD to extrinsic, allergic AD.

CLINICAL IMPLICATIONS OF SKIN BARRIER DYSFUNCTION IN ATOPIC DERMATITIS

Our increasing awareness that epidermal barrier dysfunction is an extremely important component of the pathophysiology of AD should focus our attention on everything that comes into contact with the skin. This includes environmental agents such as soap, detergents, bacterial infection and inhalant allergens such as house dust mites, and the topical formulations used to treat AD. Exposure to soap and detergents has been recognized as an exacerbating environmental factor in AD for more than 40 years. The detrimental effects were thought to arise through damage to the lipid lamellae. It now appears that the rise in skin pH produced by soap and detergents is also very important in enhancing the activity of skin proteases. Ensuring that the washing regimen of people with AD is completely free from any type of soap or detergent wash product is, therefore, very important. Soap and detergent wash products can be replaced with emollient wash products.[200] For some products, such as shampoos, it is not possible to eliminate all detergents. However, it is possible to reduce the chance that they will damage the skin barrier by using the mildest surfactants in the lowest concentrations. As shampoos inevitably flow onto the face, the careful selection of these products is important. There are now emollient wash products designed for the shower, bath, and hand washing, such as Aveeno cream and wash; Balneum Plus cream and wash; E45 cream, bath, and wash; Hydromol cream and bath; Lipobase cream; and Oilatum cream and bath. Emollient bath, shower, and wash products should be combined with emollient creams and ointments to improve skin barrier function. In view of the damaging effect of detergents it is important to select appropriately formulated products. Emollient creams containing high concentrations of surfactants have been shown to induce irritant reactions in the majority of children attending a paediatric AD clinic.[201] The ideal approach is to let the patients select which product(s) they find most suitable for their skin.

Environmental agents such as house dust mites produce cysteine proteases that enhance T_H2 responses and the production of specific IgEs.[118,119] However, the same proteases can also break down corneodesmosomes and lead to an increased barrier dysfunction. Measures to reduce exposure to house dust mites may, therefore, be important in all patients with AD.[23] *Staphylococcus aureus* is also a source of exogenous proteases, which could break down the skin barrier. These proteases are probably very important in secondarily infected lesions of AD, but their negative effects on the skin barrier may also be important in non-lesional eczematous skin.

Topical corticosteroids are an important short-term treatment for severe flares of AD. However, if topical corticosteroids are used for prolonged periods and particularly on delicate skin sites, they can cause cutaneous atrophy[183,201–204] and damage the stratum corneum. Prolonged use of topical corticosteroids may damage the skin barrier on delicate skin sites enough to enhance the penetration of irritants and allergens. This may provide the explanation for the phenomenon of post-topical steroid rebound and steroid addiction.[198] One way to reduce the chronic use of topical corticosteroids is to introduce calcineurin inhibitors, such as pimecrolimus and tacrolimus, into treatment regimens. Mild to moderate flares of AD can be treated with pimecrolimus, which does not damage the skin barrier.[32,203–206] In patients with recurrent flares of severe AD who require large quantities of potent topical corticosteroids, tacrolimus can be used as an alternative, or it can be rotated with the potent topical corticosteroid.[207] The key message is to control everything that comes into contact with the skin in order to reduce the damage to the skin barrier and the number of flares of AD. Our new understanding of the breakdown of the skin barrier in AD also provides opportunities to produce new treatments which can more effectively repair the skin barrier than existing emollients.

REFERENCES

1. Leung DYM, Bieber T. Atopic dermatitis. Lancet 2003; 361: 151–60.
2. Leung DYM, Boguniewicz M, Howell MD, Nomura I, Hamid QA. New insights into atopic dermatitis. J Clin Invest 2004; 113: 651–7.
3. Flohr C, Johansson SG, Wahlgren CF, Williams H. How atopic is atopic dermatitis? J Allergy Clin Immunol 2004; 114: 150–8.

4. Pepys J. Atopy. In: Gill PGH, Coombs RRA, Lachman PJ, eds. Clinical aspects of immunology. 3rd ed. Oxford: Blackwell Science 1975: 877–902.

5. Novak N, Allam JP, Bieber T. Allergic hyperreactivity to microbial components – a trigger factor of 'intrinsic' atopic dermatitis? J Allergy Clin Immunol 2003; 112: 215–6.

6. Fergusson DM, Horwood IJ, Beatrais AI, Shannon FT, Taylor B. Eczema and infant diet. Clin Allergy 1981; 11: 325–31.

7. Taylor B, Wadsworth J, Wadsworth M, Peckham C. Changes in the reported prevalence of childhood eczema since the 1939–1945 war. Lancet 1984; 2: 1255–7.

8. Shultz-Larsen F, Holm NV, Hennigsen K. Atopic dermatitis: A geneti-epidemiological study in a population-based twin sample. J Am Acad Dermatol 1986; 15: 487–94.

9. Williams HC. Is the prevalence of atopic dermatitis increasing? Clin Exp Dermatol 1992; 17: 385–91.

10. Neame RI, Berth-Jones J, Kirinczuk JJ, Graham-Brown RAC. Prevalence of atopic dermatitis in Leicester: a study of methodology and examination of possible ethnic variation. Br J Dermatol 1995; 132: 772–7.

11. Thestrup-Pedersen K. The incidence and pathophysiology of atopic dermatitis. J Eur Acad Dermatol Venereol 1996; 7 (suppl 1): 53–7.

12. Yura A, Shimizu T. Trends in the prevalence of atopic dermatitis in school children: longitudinal study in Osaka Prefecture, Japan, from 1985 to 1997. Br J Dermatol 2001; 115: 966–73.

13. Hall IP. Candidate gene approaches: gene-environmental interactions. Clin Exp Allergy 1998; 28 (suppl 1): 74–6.

14. Abe T, Ohkido M, Yamamoto K. Studies on skin surface barrier function: - skin surface lipids and transepidermal water loss in atopic skin during childhood. J Dermatol 1978; 5: 223–9.

15. Al-Jaberi H, Marks R. Studies of the clinically uninvolved skin in patients with dermatitis. Br J Dermatol 1984; 111: 437–43.

16. White FH, Gohari K. Some aspects of desmosomal morphology during differentiation of hamster cheek pouch. J Submicrosc Cytol 1984; 16: 407–22.

17. Hamami I, Marks R. Abnormalities in clinically normal skin: a possible explanation of the 'angry back syndrome'. Clin Exp Dermatol 1988; 13: 328–33.

18. Melnik B, Hollman J, Erler E, Verhoeven B, Plewig G. Microanalytical thin layer chromatography of all major stratum corneum lipids. J Invest Dermatol 1989; 92: 231–4.

19. Colloff MJ. Exposure to house dust mites in houses of people with atopic dermatitis. Br J Dermatol 1992; 127: 322–7.

20. Tan BB, Weald D, Strickland I, Friedmann PS. Double-blind controlled trial of effect of housedust-mite allergen avoidance on atopic dermatitis. Lancet 1996; 347: 15–8.

21. McNally NJ, Williams HC, Phillips DR et al. Atopic eczema and domestic water hardness. Lancet 1998; 352: 527–31.

22. McNally NJ, Williams HC, Phillips DR. Atopic eczema and the home environment. Br J Dermatol 2001; 145: 730–6.

23. Cork MJC, Murphy R, Carr J et al. The rising prevalence of atopic eczema and environmental trauma to the skin. Dermatol Pract 2002; 10: 22–6.

24. Leung DY. Atopic dermatitis: new insights and opportunities for therapeutic intervention. J Allergy Clin Immunol 2000; 105: 860–76.

25. Denda M, Sato J, Tsuchiya T, Elias PM, Feingold KR. Low humidity stimulates epidermal DNA synthesis and amplifies the hyperproliferative response to barrier disruption: implication for seasonal exacerbations of inflammatory dermatoses. J Invest Dermatol 1998; 111: 873–8.

26. Ghadially R, Reed JT, Elias PM. Stratum corneum structure and function correlates with phenotype in psoriasis. J Invest Dermatol 1996; 107: 558–64.

27. Elias PM, Wood LC, Feingold KR. Epidermal pathogenesis of inflammatory dermatoses. Am J Contact Dermatol 1999; 10: 119–26.

28. Chamlin SL, Kao J, Freiden IJ et al. Ceramide-dominant barrier repair lipids alleviate childhood atopic dermatitis: changes in barrier function provide a sensitive indicator of disease activity. J Am Acad Dermatol 2002; 47: 198–208.

29. Wood LC, Elias PM, Calhoun C et al. Barrier disruption stimulates interleukin-1 alpha expression and release from a preformed pool in murine epidermis. J Invest Dermatol 1996; 106: 397–403.

30. Wood LC, Stalder AK, Liou A et al. Barrier disruption increases gene expression of cytokines and the 55kD TNF receptor in murine skin. Exp Dermatol 1997; 6: 98–104.

31. Cork MJ, Britton J, Butler L et al. Comparison of parent knowledge, therapy utilization and severity of atopic eczema before and after explanation and demonstration of topical therapies by a specialist dermatogy nurse. Br J Dermatol 2003; 149: 582–9.

32. Wahn U, Bos JD, Goodfield M et al. Efficacy and safety of pimecrolimus cream in the long-term management of atopic dermatitis in children. Pediatrics 2002; 110(1 pt1): e2.

33. Harper JI, Ahmed I, Barclay G et al. Cyclosporin for severe childhood atopic dermatitis: short course versus continuous therapy. Br J Dermatol 2000; 142: 52–8.

34. Taieb A. Hypothesis: from epidermal barrier dysfunction to atopic disorders. Contact Dermatitis 1999; 41: 177–80.

35. Walley AJ, Chavanas S, Moffatt MF et al. Gene polymorphism in Netherton and common atopic disease. Nat Genet 2001; 29: 175–8.

36. Vasilopoulos Y, Cork MJ, Murphy R et al. Genetic association between an AACC insertion in the 3'UTR of the stratum corneum chymotryptic enzyme gene and atopic dermatitis. J Invest Dermatol 2004; 123: 62–6.

37. Palmer CN, Irvine AD, Terron-Kwiatkowski A et al. Common loss-of-function variants of the epidermal barrier protein filaggrin are a major predisposing factor for atopic dermatitis. Nat Genet 2006; 38: 441–6.

38. Vasilopoulos Y, Cork MJ, Teare D et al. A non-synonymous substitution of cystatin A, a cysteine protease inhibitor of house dust mite protease, leads to decreased mRNA stability and shows a significant association with atopic dermatitis. Allergy 2007; 62: 514–19.

39. Kunz B, Ring J. Clinical features and diagnostic criteria of atopic dermatitis. In: Harper J, Oranje A, Prose N, eds. Textbook of Pediatric Dermatogy. Oxford: Blackwell Science 2002: 199–214.

40. Schudel P, Wüthrich B. Klinische Verlaufsbeobachtungen bei Neurodermitis atopica nach dem Kleinkindesalter. Z Hautkr 1985; 60: 479–86.

41. Dotterud LK, Kvammen B, Lund E, Falk ES. Prevalence and some clinical aspects of atopic dermatitis in the community of Sor-Varanger. Acta Derm Venereol 1995; 75: 50–3.

42. Przybilla B, Ring J, Ruzicka T. Clinical aspects of atopic eczema: synopsis. In: Przybilla B, Ring J, Ruzicka T, eds. Handbook of atopic eczema. Berlin: Springer 1991; 132–8.

43. Wüthrich B. Atopic dermatitis flare provoked by inhalent allergens. Dermatologica 1989; 178: 51–3.

44. Fartasch M, Diepgen TL, Hornstein OP. Atopic dermatitis – ichthyosis vulgaris – hyperlinear palms – an ultrastructural study. Dermatologica 1989; 178: 202–5.

45. Tada J, Toi Y, Akiyama H, Arata J. Infra-auricular fissures in atopic dermatitis. Acta Derm Venereol 1994; 74: 129–31.

46. Hanifin, J.M. Atopic dermatitis. In: Marks R, editor. Eczema. London: Dunitz 1992; 77–101.

47. Barker DE. Skin thickness in the human. Plast Reconstr Surg 1951; 7: 115–6.

48. Southwood WF. The thickness of the skin. Plast Reconstr Surg 1955; 15: 423–9.

49. Lee Y, Hwang K. Skin thickness of Korean adults. Surg Radiol Anat 2002; 24: 183–9.

50. Scheuplein RJ, Blank IH. Permeability of the skin. Physiol Rev 1971; 51: 702–47.

51. Schaefer H, Zesch A, Stuttgen G. Skin permeability. Berlin: Springer; 1982.

52. Marzulli FN. Barrier to skin penetration. J Invest Dermatol 1962; 39: 387–93.

53. Feldman RJ, Maibach HI. Regional variation in percutaneous penetration of ^{14}C cortisol in man. J Invest Dermatol 1967; 48: 181–3.

54. Schaefer KE, Scheer K. Regional differences in CO2 elimination through the skin. Exp Med Surg 1951; 9: 449–57.

55. Cronin E, Staughton RB. Percutaneous absorption: regional variations and the effect of hydration and epidermal stripping. Br J Dermatol 1962; 74: 265–72.

56. Schaefer H, Stutggen G, Zesch A, Schalla W, Gazith J. Quantitative determination of percutaneous absorption of radio-labeled drugs in vitro and in vivo by human skin. Curr Probl Dermatol 1978; 7: 80–94.

57. Blichmann CW, Serup J. Reproducibility and variability of trans-dermal water loss measurements. Acta Derm Venereol 1989; 67: 206–10.

58. Oestmann E, Lavrijsen AP, Hermans J, Ponec M. Skin barrier function in healthy volunteers as assessed by transepidermal water loss and vascular response to hexyl nicotinate: intra- and inter-individual variability. Br J Dermatol 1993; 128: 130–6.

59. Maibach HI. In vivo percutaneous penetration of corticoids in man and unresolved problems in their efficacy. Dermatologica 1976; 152 (suppl 1): 11–25.

60. Ghadially R, Brown B, Sequeira-Martin SM, Feingold KR, Elias PM. The aged permeability barrier: structural, functional, and lipid biochemical abnormalities in humans and a senescent murine model. J Clin Invest 1995; 95: 2281–90.

61. Halkier-Sorenson L, Thestrup-Pedersen K. The efficacy of a moisturizer (locobase) among cleaners and kitchen assistants during everyday exposure to water and detergents. Contact Dermatitis 1993: 29; 1–6.

62. White MI, McEwan Jenkinson D, Lloyd DH. The effect of wash-ing on the thickness of the stratum corneum in normal and atopic individuals. Br J Dermatol 1987; 116: 525–30.

63. Werner Y, Linberg M. Transepidermal water loss in dry and clinically normal skin in patients with atopic dermatitis. Acta Derm Venereol 1985; 65: 102–5.

64. Ogawa H, Yoshiike T. Atopic dermatitis: studies of skin perme-ability and effectiveness of topical PUVA treatment. Pediatr Dermatol 1992; 9: 383–5.

65. Wollenberg A, Bieber T. Allergy Review Series V: The skin as target for IgE-mediated allergic reactions. Atopic dermatitis: from the genes to skin lesions. Allergy 2000; 55: 205–13.

66. Schmid-Grendelmeier P, Simon D, Simon HU, Akdis CA, Wuthrich B. Epidemiology, clinical features, and immunology of the 'intrinsic' (non-IgE-mediated) type of atopic dermatitis (con-stitutional dermatitis). Allergy 2001; 56: 841–9.

67. Johansson SGO, Hourihane JOB, Bousquet J et al. A revised nomenclature for allergy. An EAACI position statement from the EAACI nomenclature task force. Allergy 2001; 56: 813–24.

68. Johansson C, Tengvall Linder M, Aalberse RC, Scheynius A. Elevated levels of IgG and IgG4 to Malassezia allergens in atopic eczema patients with IgE reactivity to Malassezia. Int Arch Allergy Immunol 2004; 135: 93–100.

69. Bos JD. Atopiform dermatitis. Br J Dermatol 2002; 147: 426–9.

70. Hanifin JM. Atopiform dermatitis: do we need another confus-ing name for atopic dermatitis? Br J Dermatol 2002; 147: 430–2.

71. Novembre E, Cianferoni A, Lombardi E et al. Natural history of 'intrinsic' atopic dermatitis. Allergy 2001; 56: 452–3.

72. Novak N, Bieber T. Allergic and nonallergic forms of atopic dis-eases. J Allergy Clin Immunol 2003; 112: 252–62.

73. Elias PM. Epidermal lipids, barrier function and desquamation. J Invest Dermatol 1983; 80: 44–9.

74. Cork MJ, Robinson DA, Vasilopoulos Y et al. New perspectives on epidermal barrier dysfunction in atopic dermatitis: gene-environment interactions. J Allergy Clin Immunol 2006; 118: 3–21.

75. Lavker RM, Matoltsy AG. Formation of horny cells: the fate of organelles and differentiation products in ruminal epithelium. J Cell Biol 1970; 44: 501–12.

76. Menon GK, Feinfold KR, Elias PM. The lamellar secretory response to barrier disruption. J Invest Dermatol 1992; 98: 279–89.

77. Lavker RL. Membrane coating granules: the fate of the dis-charged lamellae. J Ultrastruct Res 1976; 55: 79–86.

78. Rawlings AV. Trends in stratum corneum research and the man-agement of dry skin conditions. Int J Cosmetic Sci 2003; 25: 63–95.

79. Fartasch M, Diepgen TL. The barrier function in atopic dry skin: disturbance of membrane-coating granule exocytosis and forma-tion of epidermal lipids? Acta Derm Venereol 1992; 176: 26–31.

80. Mecheleidt O, Kaiser HW, Sanhoff K. Deficiency of epidermal protein-bound omega-hydroxyceramides in atopic dermatitis. J Invest Dermatol 2002; 119: 166–73.

81. Hara J, Higuchi K, Okamoto R, Kawashima Y, Imokawa G. High-expression of sphingomyelin deacylase is an important determinant of ceramide deficiency leading to barrier disruption in atopic dermatitis. J Invest Dermatol 2000; 115: 406–13.

82. Serre G, Mils V, Haftek M et al. Identification of late differen-tiation antigens of human cornified epithelia, expressed in re-organized desmosomes and bound to cross-linked envelope. J Invest Dermatol 1991; 97: 1061–72.

83. Buxton RS, Cowin P, Franke WW et al. Nomenclature of the desmosomal cadherins. J Cell Biol 1993; 121: 481–3.

84. Guerrin M, Simon M, Montezin M et al. Expression cloning of human corneodesmosin proves its identity with the product of the S gene and allows improved characterization of its processing dur-ing keratinocyte differentiation. J Biol Chem 1998; 273: 22640–7.

85. Lundström A, Serre G, Haftek M, Egelrud T. Evidence for a role of corneodesmosin, a protein which may serve to modify desmo-somes during cornification, in stratum corneum cell cohesion and desquamation. Arch Dermatol Res 1994; 286: 369–75.

86. Haftek M, Serre G, Thivolet J. Immunochemical evidence for a possible role of cross-linked keratinocyte envelopes in stratum corneum cohesion. J Histochem Cytochem 1991; 39: 1531–8.

87. Egelrud T. Purification and preliminary characterization of stra-tum corneum chymotryptic enzyme: a proteinase that may be involved in desquamation. J Invest Dermatol 1993; 101: 200–4.

88. Caubet C, Jonca N, Brattsand M et al. Degradation of cor-neodesmosome protein by two serine proteases of the kallikrein family, SCTE/KLK5/hK5 and SCCE/KLK7/hK7. J Invest Dermatol 2004; 122: 1235–44.

89. Horikoshi T, Igarashi S, Uchiwa H, Brysk H, Brysk MM. Role of endogenous cathepsin D-like and chymotrypsin-like proteolysis in human epidermal desquamation. Br J Dermatol 1999; 141: 453–9.

90. Ekholm IE, Brattsand M, Egelrud T. Stratum corneum tryptic enzyme in normal epidermis: a missing link in the desquamation process? J Invest Dermatol 2000; 114: 56–63.

91. Watkinson A. Stratum corneum thiol protease (SCTP): A novel cysteine protease of late epidermal differentiation. Arch Dermatol Res 1999; 291: 260–8.

92. Hansson L, Backman A, Ny A et al. Epidermal overexpression of stratum corneum chymotryptic enzyme in mice: a model for chronic itchy dermatitis. J Invest Dermatol 2002; 118: 444–9.

93. Suzuki Y, Nomura J, Koyama J, Horii I. The role of proteases in stratum corneum: involvement in stratum corneum desquama-tion. Arch Dermatol Res 1994; 286: 369–75.

94. Egelrud T, Lundström A. A chymotrypsin-like proteinase that may be involved in desquamation in plantar stratum corneum. Arch Dermatol 1991; 283: 108–12.

95. Ekholm IE, Egelrud T. The expression of stratum corneum chymotryptic enzyme in human anagen hair follicles: further evidence for its involvement in desquamation-like process. Br J Dermatol 1998; 139: 585–90.

96. Sondell B, Thornell LE, Stigbrand T, Egelrud T. Immunolocalisation of stratum corneum chymotryptic enzyme in human skin and oral

epithelium with monoclonal antibodies: evidence of a proteinase specifically expressed in keratinizing squamous epithelia. J Histochem Cytochem 1994; 42: 459–65.

97. Bernard D, Mehul B, Thomas-Collignon A et al. Analysis of proteins with caseinolytic activity in a human stratum corneum extract revealed a yet unidentified cystein protease and identified the so-called 'stratum corneum thiol protease' as cathepsin 12. J Invest Dermatol 2003; 120: 592–600.

98. Horikoshi T, Chen S-H, Rajaraman S, Brysk H, Brysk MM. Involvement of cathepsin D in the desquamation of human stratum corneum. J Invest Dermatol 1998; 110: 547.

99. Franzke CW, Baici A, Bartel J, Christophers E, Wiedow O. Antileukoprotease inhibits stratum corneum chymotryptic enzyme. J Biol Chem 1996; 271: 21886–90.

100. Taggart CC, Lowe GJ, Greene CM et al. Cleave and inactivate secretory leukoprotease inhibitor. J Biol Chem 2001; 276: 33345–52.

101. Molhuizen HO, Alkemade HA, Zeeuwen PL et al. SKALP/elafin: an elastase inhibitor from cultured human keratinocytes. Purification, cDNA sequence, and evidence for transglutaminase cross-linking. J Biol Chem 1993; 268: 12028–32.

102. Chavanas S, Bodemer C, Rochat A. Mutations in SPINK5, encoding a serine protease inhibitor, cause Netherton syndrome. Nat Genet 2000; 25: 141–2.

103. Zeeuwen PL, Van Vlijmen-Willems IM, Jensen BJ et al. Cystatin M/E expression is restricted to differentiated epidermal keratinocytes and sweat glands: a new skin-specific proteinase inhibitor that is a target for cross-linking by transglutaminase. J Invest Dermatol 2001; 116: 693–701.

104. Bilenoglu O, Basak AN, Russell JE. A 3'UTR mutation affects beta-globin expression without altering the stability of its fully processed mRNA. Br J Haematol 2002; 119: 1106–14.

105. Frittitta L, Ercolino T, Bozzali M et al. A cluster of three single nucleotide polymorphisms in the 3'-untranslated region of human glycoprotein PC-1 gene stabilizes PC-1 mRNA and is associated with increased PC-1 protein content and insulin resistance-related abnormalities. Diabetes 2001; 50: 1952–5.

106. Di Paola R, Frittitta L, Miscio G et al. A variation in 3' UTR of hPTP1B increases specific gene expression and associates with insulin resistance. Am J Hum Genet 2002; 70: 806–12.

107. Sprecher E, Chavanas S, DiGiovanna JJ et al. The spectrum of pathogenic mutations in SPINK5 in 19 families with Netherton syndrome: implications for mutation detection and first case of prenatal diagnosis. J Invest Dermatol 2001; 117: 179–87.

108. Komatsu N, Takata M, Otsuki N et al. Elevated stratum corneum hydrolytic activity in Netherton syndrome suggests an inhibitory regulation of desquamation by SPINK 5-derived peptides. J Invest Dermatol 2002; 118: 436–43.

109. Comel M. Ichthyosis linearis circumflexa. Dermatologica 1949; 98: 133–6.

110. Descargues P, Deraison C, Bonnart C et al. SPINK5-deficient mice mimic Netherton syndrome through degradation of desmoglein 1 by epidermal protease hyperreactivity. Nat Genet 2005; 37: 56–65.

111. Yang T, Liang D, Koch PJ et al. Epidermal detachment, desmosomal dissociation, and destabilization of corneodesmosin in SPINK5−/− mice. Genes Dev 2004; 18: 2354–8.

112. Kato A, Fukai K, Oiso N et al. Association of SPINK5 gene polymorphisms with atopic dermatitis in the Japanese population. Br J Dermatol 2003; 148: 665–9.

113. Nishio Y, Noguchi E, Shibasaki M et al. Association between polymorphisms in the SPINK5 gene and atopic dermatitis in the Japanese. Genes Immun 2003; 4: 515–7.

114. Dubin G. Proteinaceous cysteine protease inhibitors. Cell Mol Life Sci 2005; 62: 653–69.

115. Seguchi T, Cui CY, Kusuda S et al. Decreased expression of filaggrin in atopic skin. Arch Dermatol Res 1996; 288: 442–6.

116. Lee YA, Wahn U, Kehrt R et al. A major susceptibility locus for atopic dermatitis maps to chromosome 3q21. Nat Genet 2000; 26: 470–3.

117. Kato T, Tahai T, Mitsuishi K, Okumura K, Ogawa H. Cystatin A inhibits IL-8 production by keratinocytes stimulated with Der P1 and DER F1: Biochemical skin barrier against house dust mites. J Allergy Clin Immunol 2005; 116: 169–76.

118. Gough L, Schultz O, Sewell HF, Shakib F. The cysteine protease activity of the major dust mite allergen DER p 1 selectively enhances the immunoglobulin E antibody response. J Exp Med 1999; 190: 1897–902.

119. Comoy EE, Pestel J, Duez C et al. The house dust mite allergen, Dermatophagoides pteryssinus, promotes type 2 responses by modulating the balance between IL-4 and IFN-gamma. J Immunol 1998; 160: 2456–62.

120. Koch PJ, Mahoney MG, Ishikawa H et al. Target disruption of the pemphigus vulgaris antigen (desmoglein 3) gene in mice causes loss of keratinocyte cell adhesion with a phenotype similar to pemphigus vulgaris. J Cell Biol 1997; 137: 1091–102.

121. Chidgey M, Brakebusch C, Gustafsson E et al. Mice lacking desmocollin 1 show epidermal fragility accompanied by barrier defects and abnormal differentiation. J Cell Biol 2001; 155: 821–32.

122. Vasioukhin V, Bowers E, Bauer C, Degenstein L, Fuchs E. Desmoplakin is essential in epidermal sheet formation. Nat Cell Biol 2001; 3: 1076–85.

123. Gallicano GI, Kouklis P, Bauer C et al. Desmoplakin is required early in development for assembly of desmosomes and cytoskeletal linkage. J Cell Biol 1998; 143: 2009–22.

124. Richards S, Scott IR, Harding CR et al. Evidence for filaggrin as a component of the cell envelope of the newborn rat. Biochem J 1988; 253: 153–60.

125. Harding CR, Bartolone J, Rawlings AV. Effects of natural moisturizing factor and lactic isomers on skin function. In: Loden M and Maibach HI edt. Dry Skin & Moisturisers, Chemistry and Function, Dermatology: Clinical & Basic Science Series, Ch 19 pp 229–241. CRC Press 2000.

126. Badertscher K, Bronnimann M, Karlen S, Braathen LR, Yawalkar N. Mast cell chymase is increased in atopic dermatitis but not in psoriasis. Arch Dermatol Res 2005; 296: 503–6.

127. Tomimori Y, Tsuruoka N, Fukami H et al. Role of mast cell chymase in allergen-induced biphasic skin reaction. Biochem Pharmacol 2002; 64: 1187.

128. Tomimori Y, Muto T, Fukami H et al. Chymase participates in chronic dermatitis by inducing eosinophil infiltration. Lab Invest 2002; 82: 789–94.

129. Mao XQ, Shirakawa T, Enomoto T et al. Association between variants of mast cell chymase gene and serum IgE levels in eczema. Hum Hered 1998; 48: 38–41.

130. Iwanaga T, McEuen A, Walls AF et al. Polymorphism of the mast cell chymase gene (CMA1) promoter region: lack of association with asthma but association with serum total immunoglobulin E levels in adult atopic dermatitis. Clin Exp Allergy 2004; 34: 1037–42.

131. Stewart GA, Thompson PJ. The biochemistry of common aeroallergens. Clin Exp Allergy 1996; 26: 1020–44.

132. Yasueda H, Mita H, Akiyama K et al. Allergens from Dermatophagoides mites with chymotryptic activity. Clin Exp Allergy 1993; 23: 384–90.

133. Winton HL, Wan H, Cannell MB et al. Class specific inhibition of house dust mite proteinases which cleave cell adhesion, induce cell death and which increase the permeability of lung epithelium. Br J Pharmacol 1998; 124: 1048–59.

134. Deleuran M, Ellingsen AR, Paludan K, Schou C, Thestrup-Pedersen K. Purified Der p1 and p2 patch tests in patients with atopic dermatitis: evidence for both allergenicity and proteolytic irritancy. Acta Derm Venereol 1998; 78: 241–3.

135. Storck H. Experimentelle Untersuchung zur Frage der Bedeutung von Mikroben in der Ekzemgenese. Dermatogica Helvetica 1948; 96: 177–262.

136. Leyden J, Marples R, Klingman A. Staphylococcus aureus in the lesions of atopic dermatitis. Br J Dermatol 1974; 90: 523–30.

137. Leung DY, Harbeck R, Bina P et al. Presence of IgE antibodies to staphylococcal exotoxins on the skin of patients with atopic dermatitis. Evidence for a new group of allergens. J Clin Invest 1993; 92: 1374–80.

138. Miedzobrodzki J, Kaszycki P, Bialecka A, Kasprowicz A. Proteolytic activity of Staphylococcus aureus strains isolated from the colonized skin of patients with acute-phase atopic dermatitis. Eur J Clin Microbiol Infect Dis 2002; 21: 269–76.

139. Otto M. Virulence factors of the coagulase-negative staphylo-cocci. Front Biosci 2004; 9: 841–63.

140. Schade A, Marchionini A. Der Säuremantel der Haut (nach Gaskettenmessung). Klin Wochensohr 1928; 7: 12–14.

141. Braun-Falco O, Korting HC. Der Normale pH- Wert der Haut. Hautarzt 1986; 3: 126–9.

142. Taddei A. Ricerche, mediante indicatori, sulla relazione attuale della cute nel neonato. Riv Ital Ginecol 1935; 18: 496–501.

143. Behrendt H, Green M. Skin pH pattern in the newborn infant. Am J Dis Child 1958; 95: 35–41.

144. Visscher MO, Chatterjee R, Munson KA, Pickens WL, Hoath SB. Changes in diapered and non diapered infant skin over the first month of life. Pediatr Dermatol 2000; 17: 45–51.

145. Behne MJ, Barry NP, Hanson KM et al. Neonatal development of the stratum corneum pH gradient: localisation and mecha-nisms leading to emergence of optimal barrier function. J Invest Dermatol 2003; 120: 998–1006.

146. Fluhr JW, Mao-Qiang M, Brown BE et al. Functional con-sequences of a neutral pH in neonatal rat stratum corneum. J Invest Dermatol 2004; 123: 140–51.

147. Fox C, Nelson D, Wareham J. The timing of skin acidification in very low birth weight infants. J Perinatol 1998; 18: 272–5.

148. Marchionini A, Hausknecht W. Sauremantel der haut und bakte-rienabwehr. Klin Wochenschr 1938; 17: 663–6.

149. Puhvel SM, Reisner RM, Sakamoto M. Analysis of lipid compo-sition of isolated human sebaceous gland homogenates after incubation with cutaneous bacteria: thin-layer chromatography. J Invest Dermatol 1975; 64: 406–11.

150. Ament W, Huizenga JR, Mook GA, Gips CH, Verkee GJ. Lactate and ammonia concentration in blood and sweat during incremen-tal cycle ergometer exercise. Int J Sports Med 1997; 18: 35–9.

151. Fluhr JW, Elias PM. Stratum corneum pH: formation and func-tion of the 'acid mantle'. Exog Dermatol 2002; 1: 163–75.

152. Rippke F, Schreiner V, Schwanitz HJ. The acidic milieu of the horny layer: new findings on the physiology and pathophysiol-ogy of the skin pH. Am J Clin Dermatol 2002; 3: 261–72.

153. Behne MJ, Meyer JW, Hanson KM et al. NHE1 regulates the stra-tum corneum permeability barrier homeostasis. Microenvironment acidification assessed with fluorescence lifetime imaging. J Biol Chem 2002; 277: 47399–406.

154. Rebell G, Pillsbury DM, de Saint Phalle M, Ginsburg D. Factors affecting the rapid disappearance of bacteria placed on the nor-mal skin. J Invest Dermatol 1950; 14: 247–63.

155. Leyden JJ, Kligman AM. The role of microorganisms in diaper dermatitis. Arch Dermatol 1978; 114: 56–9.

156. Aly R, Maibach HI, Rahman R, Shinefield HR, Mandel AD. Correlation of human in vivo and in vitro cutaneous antimicro-bial factors. J Infect Dis 1975; 131: 579–83.

157. Bibel DJ, Aly R, Lahti L, Shinefield HR, Maibach HI. Microbial adherence to vulvar epithelial cells. J Med Microbiol 1987; 23: 75–82.

158. Mauro T, Holleran WM, Grayson S et al. Barrier recovery is impeded at neutral pH, independent of ionic effects: Implications for extracellular lipid processing. Arch Dermatol 1998; 290: 215–22.

159. Fluhr JW, Kao J, Jain M et al. Generation of free fatty acids from phospholipids regulates stratum corneum acidification and integrity. J Invest Dermatol 2001; 117: 44–51.

160. Anderson DS. The acid-base balance of the skin. Br J Dermatol 1951; 63: 283–96.

161. Eberlein-Konig B, Schafer T, Huss-Marp J et al. Skin surface pH, stratum corneum hydration, trans-epidermal water loss and skin roughness related to atopic eczema and skin dryness in a population of primary school children. Acta Derm Venereol 2000; 80: 188–91.

162. Locker G. Permeabilitätsprüfung der Haut Ekzemkranker und Hautgesunder für den neun Indikator Nitrazingelh 'Geigy', Modifizierung der alkaliresistenzprobe, pH-verlauf in der Tiefe des stratum corneum. Dermatologica 1961; 124: 159–82.

163. Seidenari S, Giusti G. Objective assessment of the skin of chil-dren affected by atopic dermatitis: a study on pH, capacitance and TEWL in eczematous and clinically uninvolved skin. Acta Derm Venereol 1995; 75: 429–33.

164. Schmuth M, Man MQ, Weber F et al. Permeability barrier disor-der in Nieman-Pick disease: sphingomyelin-ceramide processing required for normal barrier homeostasis. J Invest Dermatol 2000; 115: 459–66.

165. Caubet C, Jonca N, Brattsand M et al. Degradation of cor-neodesmosome proteins by two serine proteases of the kallikrein family, SCTE/KLK5/hK5 and SCCE/KLK7/hK7. J Invest Dermatol 2004; 83: 761–73.

166. Elias PM. The epidermal permeability barrier: from the early days at Harvard to emerging concepts. J Invest Dermatol 2004; 122(2): xxxvi–xxxix. doi:10.1046/j.0022–202X.2004.22233.x

167. Hachem JP, Man MQ, Crumrine D et al. Sustained serine pro-teases activity by prolonged increase in pH leads to degradation of lipid processing enzymes and profound alterations of barrier function and stratum corneum integrity. J Invest Dermatol 2005; 125: 510–20.

168. Uchida Y, Hara M, Nishio H et al. Epidermal sphingomyelins are precursors for selected stratum corneum ceramides. J Lipid Res 2000; 41: 2071–82.

169. Holleran WM, Takagi Y, Menon GK et al. Processing of epidermal glycosylceramides is required for optimal mammalian cutaneous permeability barrier function. J Clin Invest 1993; 91: 1656–64.

170. Jensen JM, Schutze S, Forl M, Kronke M, Proksch E. Roles for tumour necrosis factor receptor p55 and sphingomyelinase in repairing the cutaneous permeability barrier. J Clin Invest 1999; 104: 1761–70.

171. Mucke H, Mohr K-T, Rummler A, Wutzler P. Untersuchungen über den haut-pH-wert der hand nach anwendeung von seife. Reinigungs-und Händedesinfektionsmitteln. Pharmazie 1993; 48: 468–9.

172. Hornby SJ, Ward SJ, Gilbert CE et al. Environmental risk factors in congenital malformations of the eye. Ann Trop Paediatr 2002; 22: 67–77.

173. Kligman AM, Wooding WM. A method for the measurement and evaluation of irritants on human skin. J Invest Dermatol 1967; 49: 78–94.

174. Imokawa G. Comparative study on the mechanism of irritation by sulphate and phosphate type of anionic surfactants. J Soc Cosmet Chem 1980; 31: 45–66.

175. Froebe CL, Simion FA, Rhein LD, Cagan RH, Kligman A. Stratum corneum lipid removal by surfactants: relation to in vivo irritation. Dermatologica 1990; 181: 277–83.

176. Ananthapadmanabhan KP, Moore DJ, Subramanyan L, Misra M, Meyer F. Cleansing without compromise: the impact of cleansers on the skin barrier and the technology of mild cleansing. Dermatol Ther 2004; 17 (suppl 1): 16–25.

177. Meding B, Swanbeck G. Prevalence of hand eczema in an indus-trial city. Br J Dermatol 1987; 116: 627–34.

178. Cowley NC, Farr PM. A dose-response study of irritant reactions to sodium lauryl sulphate in patients with seborrhoeic dermatitis and atopic eczema. Acta Derm Venereol 1992; 72: 432–5.

179. Kirk JF. Effect of handwashing on skin lipid removal. Acta Derm Venereol 1966; 57: 24–71.

180. Haapasaari KM, Risteli J, Koivukangas V, Oikarinen A. Comparison of the effect of hydrocortisone, hydrocortisone-17–butyrate and betamethasone on collagen synthesis in human skin in vivo. Acta Derm Venereol 1995; 75: 269–71.

181. Haapasaari KM, Risteli J, Karvonen J, Oikarinen A. Effect of hydrocortisone, methylprednisolone and momethasone furoate on collagen synthesis in human skin in vivo. Skin Pharmacol 1997; 10: 261–4.

182. Oikarinen A, Haapasaari KM, Sutinen M, Tasanen K. The molecular basis of glucocorticoid-induced skin atrophy: topical glucocorticoid apparently decreases both collagen synthesis and the corresponding collagen mRNA level in human skin in vivo. Br J Dermatol 1998; 139: 1106–10.

183. Sheu HM, Lee JYY, Chai CY, Kuo K. Depletion of stratum corneum intercellular lipid lamellae and barrier function abnormalities after long-term topical corticosteroids. Br J Dermatol 1997; 136: 884–90.

184. Kolbe L, Kligman AM, Schreiner V, Stoudemayer T. Corticosteroid-induced atrophy and barrier impairment measured by non-invasive methods in human skin. Skin Res Technol 2001; 7: 73–7.

185. Kao JS, Fluhr JW, Man MQ et al. Short-term glucocorticoid treatment compromises both permeability barrier homeostasis and stratum corneum integrity: inhibition of epidermal lipid synthesis accounts for functional abnormalities. J Invest Dermatol 2003; 120: 456–64.

186. Frosch PJ, Wendt H. Human models for quantification of corticosteroid adverse effects. In: Maibach HI, Lowe NJ, editors. Models in Dermatology. Volume 2. Basel: Karger; 1985: 5–15.

187. Sheu HM, Chang CH. Alterations in water content of the stratum corneum following long-term topical corticosteroids. J Formos Med Assoc 1991; 90: 664–9.

188. Sheu HM, Lee JY, Kuo KW, Tsai JC. Permeability barrier abnormality of hairless mouse epidermis after topical corticosteroid: characterization of stratum corneum lipids by ruthenium tetroxide staining and high-performance thin-layer chromatography. J Dermatol 1998; 25: 281–9.

189. Goulding NJ. The molecular complexity of glucocorticoid actions in inflammation – a four-ring circus. Curr Opin Pharmacol 2004; 4: 629–36.

190. Yousef GM, Scorilas A, Magklara A, Soosaipillai A, Diamandis EP. The KLK7 (PRSS6) gene, encoding for the stratum corneum chymotryptic enzyme is a new member of the human kallikrein gene family – genomic characterization, mapping, tissue expression and hormonal regulation. Gene 2000; 254: 119–28.

191. Cork MJ, Robinson D, Vasilopoulos Y et al. Interaction of topical corticosteroids and pimecrolimus with the skin barrier: Implications for efficacy and safety of treatment for atopic dermatitis. J Am Acad Dermatol 2006; 54 (Suppl S): AB3.

192. Cork M, Robinson D, Vasilopoulos Y, Ferguson A. The effects of topical corticosteroids and pimecrolimus on skin barrier function, gene expression and topical drug penetration in atopic eczema and unaffected controls. J Am Acad Dermatol 2007; 56 (Suppl 2): AB69.

193. Cork MJ, Varghese J, Hadcraft J et al. Differences in the effect of topical corticosteroids and calcineurin inhibitors on the skin barrier – implications for therapy. J Invest Dermatol 2007; 127: S45.

194. Zheng PS, Lavker RM, Lehmann P, Kligman AM. Morphologic investigations on the rebound phenomenon after corticosteroid-induced atrophy in human skin. J Invest Dermatol 1984; 82: 345–52.

195. Björnberg A. Erythema craquele provoked by corticosteroids on normal skin. Acta Derm Venereol 1982; 62: 147–51.

196. Nickoloff BJ, Naidu Y. Perturbation of epidermal barrier function correlates with initiation of cytokine cascade in human skin. J Am Acad Dermatol 1994; 30: 535–46.

197. Esche C, de Benedetto A, Beck LA. Keratinocytes in atopic dermatitis: inflammatory signals. Curr Allergy Asthma Rep 2004; 4: 276–84.

198. Rapaport MJ, Lebwohl M. Corticosteroid addiction and withdrawal in the atopic: the red burning skin syndrome. Clin Dermatol 2003; 21: 201–14.

199. Holt PG. The role of genetic and environmental factors in the development of T-cell mediated allergic disease in early life. Paediatr Respir Rev 2004; 5 (suppl A): S27–30.

200. Cork MJ. The importance of skin barrier function. J Dermatolog Treat 1997; 8: S7–13.

201. Cork MJ, Timmins J, Holden C et al. An audit of adverse drug reactions to aqueous cream in children with atopic eczema. The Pharmaceutical Journal via PJ online 2003; 271: 747–8.

202. Furue M, Terao H, Rikihisa W et al. Clinical dose and adverse effects of topical corticosteroids in daily management of atopic dermatitis. Br J Dermatol 2003; 148: 128–33.

203. Cork MJ. Treatment of atopic dermatitis from a skin barrier perspective. J Invest Dermatol 2005a; 125: 611.

204. Cork MJ. Skin barrier damage: Cause or consequence of atopic dermatitis? J Am Acad Dermatol 2005b; 52 (Suppl 3): 9.

205. Eichenfield LF, Lucky AW, Boguniewicz M et al. Safety and efficacy of pimecrolimus (ASM 981) cream 1% in the treatment of mild and moderate atopic dermatitis in children and adolescents. J Am Acad Dermatol 2002; 46: 495–503.

206. Kapp A, Papp K, Bingham A et al. Long-term management of atopic dermatitis in infants with topical pimecrolimus, a non-steroid, anti-inflammatory drug. J Allergy Clin Immunol 2002; 110: 277–84.

207. Reitamo S, Ortonne JP, Sand C et al. A multicentre, randomized, double-blind, controlled study of long-term treatment with 0.1% tacrolimus ointment in adults with moderate to severe atopic dermatitis. Br J Dermatol 2005; 152; 1282–9.

5

Staphylococcus aureus in atopic dermatitis

Donald YM Leung

INTRODUCTION

Atopic dermatitis (AD) is a chronic inflammatory skin disease commonly seen in patients with a history of asthma or allergic rhinitis.[1] Intensely pruritic skin lesions evolve as the result of complex interactions between IgE bearing antigen-presenting cells, T cell activation, mast cell degranulation, keratinocytes, eosinophils, and a combination of immediate and cellular immune responses (see Chapter 3). A number of factors can trigger this inflammatory skin cascade including irritants, foods, aeroallergens, and infection (see Chapter 13).

The current chapter will examine the role of *Staphylococcus aureus* in the pathogenesis of AD acting not only as a trigger but also having skin disease-sustaining effects resulting from its proinflammatory properties.[2] These effects are, in part, due to the potent toxins, e.g. superantigens, they produce. An understanding of the mechanisms underlying enhanced *S. aureus* colonization and infection in AD and identification of the molecules involved in triggering atopic skin inflammation has important implications in our current approach to the management of AD and the development of new therapies for patients with this common skin condition.

PREVALENCE OF *STAPHYLOCOCCUS AUREUS* IN ATOPIC DERMATITIS

S. aureus colonizes the skin of most patients with active AD.[3] In contrast, the skin of less than 5% of normal subjects is colonized by this bacterium. Furthermore, when present on normal skin, *S. aureus* is usually low in number and is mainly confined to the intertriginous areas. Notably, the presence of *S. aureus* on atopic skin depends on the skin lesion: *S. aureus* can be isolated

from 55–75% of clinically unaffected atopic skin lesions, 85–91% of chronic lichenified lesions and 80–100% of acute exudative skin lesions.[4]

The density of *S. aureus* on acutely inflamed AD lesions is generally more than 1000-fold higher than on nonlesional AD skin. Clinical superinfection with *S. aureus* can reach 10^7 organisms per cm^2 on acute exudative AD skin lesions. Thus, atopic skin provides a favourable environment for the colonization and proliferation of *S. aureus*. These patients can have a sudden exacerbation of skin disease due to *S. aureus* infection. Secondarily infected patients show greater clinical improvement to combined treatment with anti-staphylococcal antibiotics and topical corticosteroids, as compared to topical corticosteroids alone, supporting the concept that *S. aureus* contributes to atopic skin inflammation in AD.[5,6]

MECHANISM(S) FOR ENHANCED *STAPHYLOCOCCUS AUREUS* COLONIZATION

The mechanism(s) leading to increased *S. aureus* colonization in AD are poorly understood. It is likely to result from a combination of processes which include defective skin barrier function, loss of certain innate antibacterial activities from changes in antimicrobial peptide levels, or reduced immune responses necessary for eradication and defence against bacteria, as well as changes in skin surface pH values toward alkalinity.[7] There has also been much interest in the potential role of lipid deficiencies in atopic skin since lipids have antimicrobial effects and reduced lipid content in atopic skin may lead to increased transepidermal water loss contributing to the dryness and cracked, brittle skin which predisposes to *S. aureus* colonization.[8,9] These factors are not mutually exclusive. All are likely to play a role in *S. aureus* colonization of AD skin varying according to the patient's genetic predisposition and environment.

Increased *S. aureus* adherence

The initial step in colonization or infection requires attachment of *S. aureus* to skin surfaces. The skin of patients with AD has been demonstrated to have increased adherence for *S. aureus*.[10] The reason for increased binding of *S. aureus* to AD skin is not completely understood but is thought to be due to the underlying skin inflammation. This concept is supported by the following studies:

1. Acute AD skin lesions are colonized with greater numbers of *S. aureus* than chronic skin lesions, unaffected atopic skin or normal non-atopic.[3,4] Scratching probably enhances *S. aureus* binding by disturbing the skin barrier and releasing proinflammatory cytokines which upregulate extracellular matrix molecules known to act as adhesins for *S. aureus*.[11] Furthermore, cracks in the epidermal layer from scratching or skin dryness can expose underlying extracellular matrix molecules which can serve as an anchor for attachment of *S. aureus* to the skin.
2. It has been found that treatment with anti-inflammatory medications such as topical corticosteroids or tacrolimus significantly reduces the numbers of *S. aureus* found on atopic skin.[12,13] Corticosteroids have no direct antimicrobial effects. Thus, it is very likely that atopic skin inflammation leads to the expression of attachment sites which promote colonization of *S. aureus*. Please see Table 5.1.
3. We have studied *S. aureus* binding to skin lesions in mice undergoing Th1-or Th2-mediated inflammatory responses.[14] Bacterial binding to frozen skin sections was found to be significantly greater at skin sites with Th2-mediated inflammation than skin sites with Th1-mediated inflammation. Importantly this increased bacterial binding did not occur in IL-4 gene knockout mice suggesting that IL-4 plays a critical role in the enhancement of *S. aureus* binding to skin. Conversely when normal mouse skin was incubated in vitro with IL-4, as compared to interferon-gamma, increased *S. aureus* binding occurred only to skin explants treated with IL-4.

Recently, several staphylococcal cell surface molecules, termed 'adhesins' (aside from protein A), have been identified which are responsible for the initial interactions between *S. aureus* and extracellular matrix proteins in the skin. These include fibronectin-binding

---

Table 5.1 Factors contributing to *S. aureus* colonization/infection in atopic dermatitis

- Impaired skin barrier function
- Reduced skin lipid content in atopic dermatitis
- Skin surface pH toward alkalinity
- Increased skin adherence to *S. aureus* due to increased fibronectin and fibrinogen
- Decreased production of endogenous antimicrobial peptides (beta defensins, LL-37) by keratinocytes

---

proteins A and B, clumping factors A and B which are fibrinogen-binding proteins, and collagen adhesins.[11] Relevant to atopic inflammation, IL-4, but not interferon-gamma, is known to induce fibronectin production by skin fibroblasts.[15]

Recently, we found that fibronectin and fibrinogen, but not collagen, are involved in the binding of *S. aureus* to Th2-induced inflammatory skin lesions. This is supported by the following observations:

1. *S. aureus* mutants that were selectively deficient in fibronectin- or fibrinogen-binding proteins, as compared to their corresponding wild-type parent strains, demonstrated reduced binding to allergen-sensitised/challenged Th2, but not Th1, skin reactions in mice.[14] Consistent with these studies, *S. aureus* mutants deficient in fibronectin- or fibrinogen-binding proteins demonstrated reduced binding to human AD skin but not psoriatic skin or normal skin.[16] In contrast, a *S. aureus* collagen adhesin-negative mutant did not show decreased binding to Th2-mediated inflamed skin.
2. When *S. aureus* was pre-incubated with either human serum albumin, fibronectin, collagen, or fibrinogen in an attempt to block the *S. aureus* binding proteins, only fibronectin and fibrinogen significantly reduced the level of *S. aureus* binding to Th2-induced skin inflammation sites. Interestingly, the *S. aureus* binding sites were primarily confined to the stratum corneum.

Overall these data suggest a selective mechanism by which Th2, as compared to Th1, responses can enhance *S. aureus* binding to the skin. Thus, IL-4 induced fibronectin synthesis, in combination with plasma exudation of fibrinogen, could provide a mechanism by which the atopic/inflammatory environment mediates enhanced *S. aureus* attachment to the skin. Interestingly, the *S. aureus* fibronectin-binding MSCRAMM FnbpA is a bifunctional protein that also binds to fibrinogen.[17]

This observation is consistent with our observations suggesting that blocking the binding of *S. aureus* to fibrinogen and fibronectin may be an important therapeutic target for reduction of *S. aureus* colonization in atopic skin.

Decreased innate immune response

Using electron microscopy, Morishita et al[18] found colonies of *S. aureus* distributed on the surface of the epidermis as well as growing between layers of keratinocytes. This study suggests that an exponential increase in *S. aureus* could result from failure of the innate immune response to restrict the growth of microorganisms. Indeed, a direct comparison of AD and psoriasis showed that about 30% of AD patients suffered from infections whereas only 6.7% of psoriasis patients had this complication,[19] despite the fact that both skin diseases have defective skin barrier function.[20] It has been speculated that the reduced prevalence of infections in psoriasis may be associated with the increased production of antimicrobial peptides.[21]

Two major classes of antimicrobial peptides have been found in mammalian skin: beta-defensins[22,23] and cathelicidins.[24,25] They have been shown to have antimicrobial activities against bacterial, fungal, and viral pathogens.[22,25] In the skin, keratinocytes are the primary producer of these peptides. The mechanism of action for these cationic antimicrobial peptides involves disruption of the microbial membrane to interfere with intracellular functions.[27] Expression of some of these peptides is constitutive (e.g. human-beta-defensin 1 (HBD-1)),[21] whereas others (HBD-2 and LL-37, a cathelicidin) are accumulated following skin injury or inflammation. Animal models have shown that the expression of antimicrobial peptides is essential for the ability of skin to resist bacterial infection.[28,29]

Recently, we compared the expression of antimicrobial peptides in these two skin diseases to determine if the increased susceptibility to infection in AD is due to a deficiency in antimicrobial peptides.[30] In this study, we compared the expression of HBD-2 and LL-37 in AD skin lesions to psoriatic lesions and normal skin using immunohistochemical staining, Western and immuno-dot blotting, and quantitative real-time reverse transcriptase-polymerase chain reaction (real-time RT-PCR). By immunohistochemistry and immuno-dot blot, we confirmed that there was abundant LL-37 and HBD-2 in the skin of all patients with psoriasis. Immunostaining of LL-37 and HBD-2, however, was significantly decreased in AD lesions. Real-time RT-PCR showed significantly lower expression of HBD-2 and LL-37 mRNA in AD lesions than in psoriasis lesions.

The importance of expression of both antimicrobial peptides was studied by evaluating the combined antimicrobial effects of LL-37 and HBD-2 on *S. aureus*.[30] The combination of LL-37 and HBD-2 showed synergistic antimicrobial activity by effectively killing *S. aureus* more than either antimicrobial peptide alone. Thus, a deficiency in antimicrobial peptide expression could account for the ability of *S. aureus* to readily colonize and infect skin from patients with AD.

Since acute AD skin lesions are associated with marked overexpression of IL-4 and IL-13, we then studied the effects of IL-4 and IL-13 on TNF-beta induced HBD-2 expression in a human keratinocyte cell line. IL-4 alone or in combination with IL-13 significantly suppressed TNF-beta-induced expression of HBD-2 in keratinocytes. These data suggest that the low expression of antimicrobial peptide expression in atopic dermatitis may be acquired as the result of allergic immune responses.

IMMUNE RESPONSE TO *STAPHYLOCOCCUS AUREUS*

The exact mechanisms by which *S. aureus* induces skin inflammatory responses in AD are unknown. However, a number of staphylococcal products, such as protein A, lipoteichoic acid, and various toxins have been observed to induce activation of cells involved in the pathogenesis of AD including mast cells, T cells, keratinocytes, and macrophages.[4] Unlike hyperimmuno-globulinaemia E syndrome, patients with AD rarely make IgE against constituents of the *S. aureus* cell wall. However, AD has been associated with the production of high level IgE against superantigens.[31] As such there has been a great deal of interest in mechanisms by which superantigens could contribute to the skin inflammation of AD.

Superantigens

An important strategy by which *S. aureus* exacerbates or maintains skin inflammation in AD is by secreting a group of toxins known as superantigens (Figure 5.1). Superantigens bind directly without antigen processing to constitutively expressed HLA-DR molecules on professional antigen-presenting cells such as macrophages or dendritic cells, and to gamma interferon-induced HLA-DR molecules on non-professional antigen-presenting cells such as keratinocytes.[32] This results in the release of proinflammatory cytokines by these HLA-DR+ cells, or via the subsequent activation of T cells. The stimulation of T cells by superantigens results in the activation of lymphocytes expressing specific T cell receptor V-beta

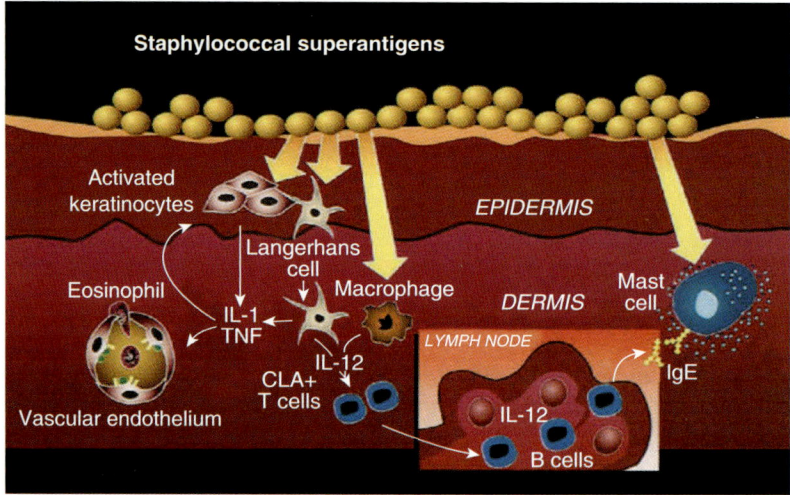

Figure 5.1 Immune actions of staphylococcal superantigens. (Reprinted with permission from Leung DY. Atopic dermatitis: new insights and opportunities for therapeutic intervention. J Allergy Clin Immunol 2000; 105: 860–76.)

regions. While all bacterial superantigens cause marked stimulation of T cells, they frequently cause the expansion of different portions of the T cell repertoire. Identification of specific T cell receptor V-beta expansions can be useful in supporting the concept that tissue inflammation is mediated by superantigens.[33]

A variety of observations support a role for superantigens in the pathogenesis of AD (Table 5.2).

1. The majority of AD patients have *S. aureus* cultured from their skin that secrete superantigens such as enterotoxins A, B, and toxic shock syndrome toxin-1 (TSST-1).[31,34,35] An analysis of the peripheral blood skin homing T cells expressing cutaneous lymphoid antigen (CLA) from these patients as well as their skin lesions reveals that they have undergone a T cell receptor V-beta expansion within both their CD4+ T cells and their CD8+ T cells indicative of superantigen stimulation.[36,37] TCR V-beta skewing was not present within the CLA[+] T cell subsets of patients with plaque psoriasis or normal controls. TCR BV genes from the presumptively superantigen-expanded populations of skin homing T cells were cloned and sequenced from AD subjects, and consistent with a superantigen-driven effect, were found to be polyclonal.
2. Most AD patients make specific IgE antibodies directed against the superantigens found on their skin.[34,35] Basophils from patients with IgE to superantigens release histamine on exposure to the

Table 5.2   Role of staphylococcal superantigens in atopic dermatitis

- AD severity correlates with presence of IgE to superantigens
- Superantigens augment allergen-induced skin inflammation by activating infiltrating mononuclear cells and inducing mast cell degranulation
- Superantigens induce dermatitis on application to skin by patch testing
- Patients recovering from toxic shock syndrome develop chronic eczema
- Superantigens induce the skin homing receptor on T cells
- Peripheral blood mononuclear cells from AD, as compared to normal controls, have higher proliferative responses to superantigens

relevant superantigen, but not in response to superantigens to which they make no specific IgE.[31] These data suggest that superantigens induce specific IgE in AD patients and chronic mast cell degranulation in vivo when the superantigens penetrate their impaired skin barrier. This promotes the itch-scratch cycle, thereby contributing to the evolution of skin rashes in AD.

3. A correlation has been found between the presence of IgE to superantigens and severity of AD.[34,35] Colonization with superantigen-producing *S. aureus* is greatest in patients with IgE to staphylococcal superantigens. Of note, in one study there was no difference in skin severity between patients with or without superantigen-producing *S. aureus* unless patients made an IgE response to the superantigen present on their skin.[35] Patients with superantigen-producing *S. aureus* on their skin have increased IgE levels to specific allergens. This is consistent with in vitro studies demonstrating superantigens augment allergen-specific IgE synthesis by binding to HLA-DR on B cells.[38] Utilizing a human-SCID mouse model of skin inflammation, *S. aureus* superantigens have been reported to enhance allergen-induced skin inflammation.[39] Skin homing peripheral blood T cells have also been shown to respond to superantigen and contribute to eosinophilia and IgE production in AD.[40,41]

4. Epicutaneous application of SEB to normal skin or unaffected AD skin induces skin erythema and induration.[42] In one study, half of the AD patients experienced a flare of their skin disease in the elbow flexure ipsilaterally to where the SEB was applied. These observations provide direct evidence that superantigens can exacerbate and sustain skin inflammation with AD. It has also been found that the T cells infiltrating into skin patch test sites stimulated with SEB are selectively expanded with a T cell repertoire (increased expression of T cell receptor V-beta 3, 12, and 17) consistent with SEB stimulation.[43] Furthermore, in a prospective study, 14 of 68 patients recovering from toxic shock syndrome (TSS) developed chronic eczematoid dermatitis, whereas no patients recovering from gram-negative sepsis developed eczema.[44] These investigators concluded that superantigens may induce an atopic eczematoid process in the skin. Kawasaki syndrome, a multi-system vasculitis thought to be caused by superantigens, has also been associated with a 10–fold higher prevalence of AD than disease controls.[45,46]

A number of factors probably contribute to skin inflammation induced by superantigens. In vitro, superantigens can cause marked activation of Th2 cells. Mouse Th2 cells expanded by superantigen induce IL-4 dependent skin inflammation when injected into the skin of mice.[47] Saloga et al[48,49] also found that epicutaneous application and intracutaneous injection of SEB elicits a strong inflammatory skin response in wild-type BALB/c mice, but not T cell deficient SCID mice suggesting that superantigen-induced skin inflammation is T cell dependent.

Importantly, superantigens have been demonstrated to induce T cell expression of the CLA skin homing receptor via stimulation of IL-12 production.[50] As shown in Figure 5.1, staphylococcal superantigens secreted at the skin surface can penetrate the skin to stimulate epidermal macrophages or Langerhans cells (LCs) to produce IL-1 and tumour necrosis factor-alpha. Local production of IL-1 and TNF induces the expression of E-selectin on vascular endothelium,[51] allowing an initial influx of CLA+ Th2 memory/effector cells. IL-12 secreted by superantigen-stimulated LCs which migrate to skin-associated lymph nodes can upregulate the expression of CLA on T cells. These actions result in the formation of additional skin-homing memory T cells which can promote skin inflammation.

Chronic AD is frequently associated with colonization by superantigen-producing *S. aureus* and increased infiltration of monocyte/macrophages.[1] To examine a potential role for microbial superantigens in the prolongation of monocyte-macrophage survival, Bratton et al[52] incubated peripheral blood monocytes from AD subjects with TSS toxin-1 (TSST-1), a superantigen, and examined its effects on monocyte apoptosis. TSST-1, in a concentration dependent manner, significantly inhibited monocyte apoptosis and stimulated production of the prosurvival cytokines GM-CSF, IL-1, and tumour necrosis factor-alpha. Their data also showed that GM-CSF production was the primary cytokine responsible for inhibition of apoptosis creating conditions favouring persistent tissue inflammation and skin colonization with *S. aureus*.

Alpha toxin

Aside from superantigens, staphylococci can express other toxins which contribute to skin inflammation. Ezepchuk et al[53] found that AD *S. aureus* isolates which failed to secrete superantigens, produced alpha toxin. All of these staphylococcal strains also expressed staphylococcal protein A. The superantigens, TSST-1, SEA, SEB, and exfoliative toxin as well as protein A did not induce significant cytotoxic damage on keratinocytes. In contrast, alpha toxin induced profound keratinocyte cytotoxicity that was time and dose dependent. Additionally, alpha toxin induced the release of tumour necrosis factor-alpha from keratinocytes rapidly after addition to cultures. In contrast, protein A and staphylococcal superantigens stimulated tumour necrosis factor-alpha secretion from keratinocytes over an extended period of time.

Alpha toxin exerts its effects by forming a transmembrane pore that behaves like a calcium ionophore. Because cellular membrane disruption with resultant intracellular calcium mobilization is a potent stimulus for the synthesis of the lipid mediator platelet-activating factor, the ability of beta toxin to induce platelet-activating factor production was recently studied by Travers et al.[54] Treatment of a human keratinocyte cell line with alpha toxin resulted in significant levels of platelet-activating factor. Alpha toxin also stimulated arachidonic acid release in keratinocytes. Pretreatment of keratinocytes with platelet-activating factor receptor antagonists blunted alpha toxin-induced arachidonic acid release, suggesting a role for alpha toxin-produced platelet-activating factor in this process. Of note, retroviral-mediated expression of the platelet-activating factor receptor into the platelet-activating factor receptor–negative epithelial cell line KB resulted in an augmentation of alpha toxin-mediated intracellular calcium mobilization and arachidonic acid release. These studies suggest that alpha toxin-mediated signalling can be augmented via the epidermal platelet-activating factor receptor providing a novel mechanism by which alpha toxin can augment the skin inflammatory response.

MANAGEMENT OF *STAPHYLOCOCCUS AUREUS* IN ATOPIC DERMATITIS

Antibiotic/steroid combinations

Extensive serous weeping, folliculitis, and pyoderma indicate bacterial infection usually secondary to *S. aureus* in patients with AD. The concept that infection with *S. aureus* can exacerbate acute AD, and colonization promotes chronic skin inflammation, provides a rationale for use of anti-staphylococcal therapy in patients with poorly controlled AD. Systemic anti-staphylococcal antibiotics are particularly helpful in the treatment of acute exacerbations of AD due to diffuse *S. aureus* infection.[55–57] Erythromycin and the newer macrolide antibiotics (azithromycin and clarithromycin) are usually beneficial for patients who are not infected with a macrolide-resistant *S. aureus* strain. However, for macrolide-resistant *S. aureus*, a penicillinase-resistant penicillin (e.g. dicloxacillin) should be used. First-generation cephalosporins also offer effective coverage for *S. aureus*. Topical mupirocin is useful in the treatment of localized impetiginized skin lesions.[5]

Owing to the increased risk of bacterial resistance that may occur with frequent use of antibiotics, it is important to combine antimicrobial therapy with effective skin care since it is well established that the excoriated inflamed skin of AD predisposes to *S. aureus* colonization and infection. Use of antibiotic therapy must be carried out with good skin hydration to restore skin barrier function and effective anti-inflammatory therapy to reduce overall skin inflammation. Exacerbating factors such as food allergens, inhalant allergens, irritants, and emotional triggers should be identified and eliminated as they can alter response to therapy. Since the major reservoir for *S. aureus* is in the nose, intranasal antibiotics may be needed to reduce overall skin carriage of *S. aureus*.[58]

Several studies have demonstrated that the combination of topical corticosteroids with an antibiotic is significantly more effective in reducing skin inflammation due to AD than using the topical corticosteroid or topical antibiotic alone.[59–61] The observation that combined treatment of AD with antibiotics and corticosteroids is more effective than corticosteroids alone suggests that *S. aureus* secretes products that can induce steroid resistance. This may contribute to the spectrum of corticosteroid responsiveness that exists in AD.[62] Recently, we reported that when T cells are stimulated with superantigens, as compared to other stimuli, they become resistant to the immunosuppressive effects of corticosteroids.[63] This is consistent with the observation that antibiotics, even at concentrations that do not suppress their growth, are known to reduce superantigen production by *S. aureus*.[64]

At a cellular level, corticosteroids exert their biological effects by binding to a specific intracellular receptor, i.e. the glucocorticoid receptor (GR). Cloning of the human GR gene has revealed that alternative splicing of the GR pre-mRNA generates two homologous isoforms, termed GRbeta and GRbeta.[65,66] GRbeta is the steroid-activated transcription factor which, in the hormone-bound state, modulates the expression of steroid-sensitive genes. GRbeta differs from GRbeta only in its COOH terminus with replacement of the last 50 amino acids of the latter with a unique 15 amino acid sequence. This difference renders GRbeta unable to bind corticosteroids, and antagonises the activity of GRbeta. Interestingly, superantigens are a potent inducer of GRbeta expression in T cells and may account for their ability to induce corticosteroid resistance.[63]

Non-antibiotic approaches for control of *Staphylococcus aureus*

Antiseptics

In patients who cannot be weaned off antibiotic therapy, alternative approaches should be considered for control of *S. aureus*. This would include topical antibacterial cleansers which have been shown to be effective in reducing bacterial skin flora.[67] The antiseptic gentian violet has been shown to significantly decrease *S. aureus* on AD skin accompanied by a reduction in the clinical severity of skin disease.[68,69] Use of 10% povidone-iodine solution has been reported to result in a 10–100-fold decrease in the density of *S. aureus* on AD skin.[70] Finally,

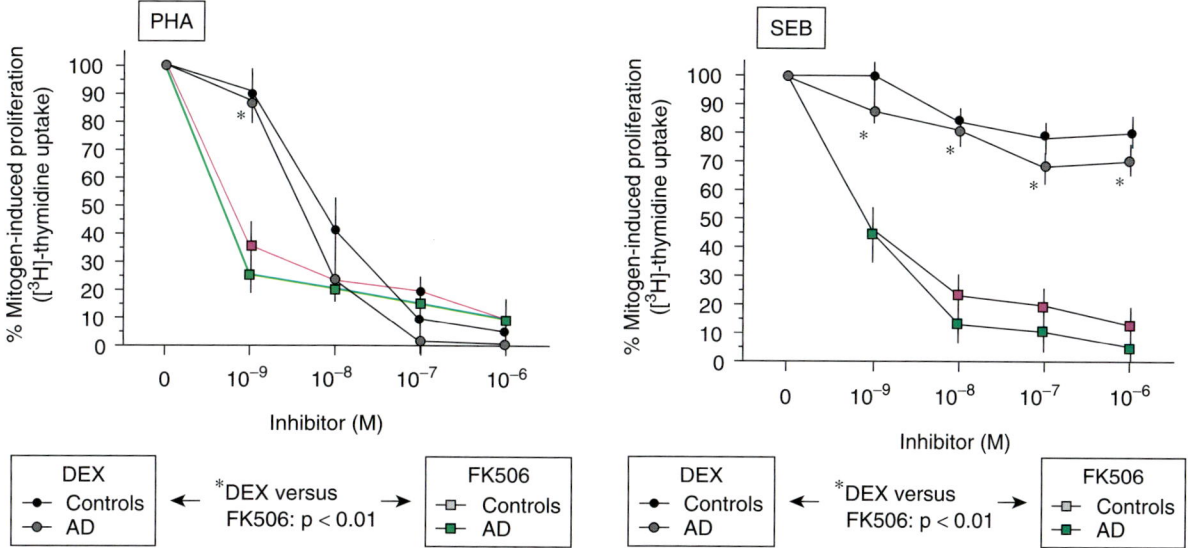

Figure 5.2 Effect of dexamethasone (DEX) and FK506 on PHA vs SEB stimulated T cell proliferation response to superantigens vs PHA. (Reprinted with permission from Hauk PJ, Leung DY. Tacrolimus (FK 506): a new treatment approach in superantigen-associated diseases like atopic dermatitis? J Allergy Clin Immunol 2000; 107: 391–2.)

daily bathing with an antibacterial soap has been found to significantly reduce the number of S. aureus on the skin and result in clinical improvement of AD.[71] It should be noted that all these anti-infective strategies may be limiting as they can be too irritating for the inflamed skin of some patients with AD.

Phototherapy

Phototherapy or photochemotherapy is effective in the treatment of AD. Although its mechanisms of action are not completely understood, it is thought that these may be due to immunosuppressive and anti-inflammatory effects. It has also been shown that UV irradiation or psoralen plus UVA (PUVA) inhibits growth of S. aureus via a direct bactericidal effect.[72] Treatment of S. aureus with UV irradiation or PUVA has also been found to inhibit superantigen production in a dose-dependent manner.[73] These bacteriostatic effects of UV radiation along with its suppressive effects on superantigen production may contribute to the therapeutic efficacy of phototherapy in AD.

Topical tacrolimus

Several multicentre, controlled studies have demonstrated that FK506 in ointment form (tacrolimus) can effectively reduce the clinical symptoms of AD within 3–5 days of initiating therapy.[74–77] Tacrolimus acts by binding to a cyclophilin-like cytoplasmic protein, FK506

binding protein, and this complex in turn inhibits calcineurin, which is a phosphatase needed for activation of NF-AT, a critical transcription factor needed for gene transcription of multiple Th1- and Th2-like cytokines including IL-2, IL-4, and IL-5.[78] Remitz et al[13] found that application of 0.1% tacrolimus ointment significantly decreased the number of S. aureus on the skin of AD patients within the first week of treatment. Since tacrolimus has no direct inhibitory effect on bacterial growth, the reduction in number of S. aureus following the clinical improvement of AD by tacrolimus treatment is probably due to its anti-inflammatory actions. As shown in Figure 5.2, superantigen-induced T cell activation is resistant to the anti-proliferation effects of dexamethasone, a prototypic corticosteroid. However, FK506 was highly effective at inhibiting superantigen-induced T cell activation.[79] Thus, tacrolimus ointment may be an effective treatment option for steroid-insensitive AD patients colonized with S. aureus-secreting superantigens.

CONCLUSIONS

Colonization and infection with S. aureus contributes to the severity of AD. The inflamed skin of atopic patients avidly binds S. aureus. Once attached to the skin, staphylococcal superantigens can augment allergic

Table 5.3 **Therapeutic approach to reduce *S. aureus***	

- Restore skin barrier function
- Antibiotics for acute treatment
- Topical anti-inflammatory agents:
  - corticosteroids
  - macrolide immunomodulators
- Antiseptics
- Phototherapy

skin inflammation and reduce corticosteroid sensitivity (Table 5.3). Reduction in *S. aureus* colonization requires effective skin care to control skin inflammation which predisposes to *S. aureus* colonization/infection. These observations suggest a role for antibiotic/corticosteroid combinations or non-steroidal topical macrolide immuno-suppressive ointments in the treatment of AD.

REFERENCES

1. Leung DY. Atopic dermatitis: new insights and opportunities for therapeutic intervention. J Allergy Clin Immunol 2000; 105: 860–76.
2. Leung DYM. Role of Staphylococcus aureus in atopic dermatitis. In: Bieber T, Leung DYM, eds. Atopic Dermatitis. New York: Marcel Dekker, Inc, 2002: 401–18.
3. Leyden JJ, Marples RR, Kligman AM. Staphylococcus aureus in the lesions of atopic dermatitis. Br J Dermatol 1974; 90: 525–30.
4. Hauser C, Prins C, Lacour M. The role of infectious agents in atopic dermatitis. In: Leung DYM, ed. Atopic Dermatitis: from Pathogenesis to Treatment. New York: Chapman & Hall, 1996: 67–112.
5. Lever R, Hadley K, Downey D et al. Staphylococcal colonization in atopic dermatitis and the effect of topical mupirocin therapy. Br J Dermatol 1988; 119: 189–98.
6. Nilsson EJ, Henning CG, Magnusson J. Topical corticosteroids and Staphylococcus aureus in atopic dermatitis. J Am Acad Dermatol 1992; 27: 29–34.
7. Mempel M, Schmidt T, Weidinger S et al. Role of Staphylococcus aureus surface-associated proteins in the attachment to cultured HaCaT keratinocytes in a new adhesion assay. J Invest Dermatol 1998; 111: 452–6.
8. Miller SJ, Aly R, Shinefeld HR et al. In vitro and in vivo anti-staphylococcal activity of human stratum corneum lipids. Arch Dermatol 1988; 124: 209–15.
9. Imokawa G, Abe A, Jin K et al. Decreased level of ceramides in stratum corneum of atopic dermatitis: an etiologic factor in atopic dry skin? J Invest Dermatol 1991; 96: 523–6.
10. Cole GW, Silverberg NL. The adherence of Staphylococcus aureus to human corneocytes. Arch Dermatol 1986; 122: 166–9.
11. Foster TJ, Höök M. Surface protein adhesins of Staphylococcus aureus. Trends Microbiol 1998; 6: 484–8.
12. Stalder JF, Fleury M, Sourisse M et al. Local steroid therapy and bacterial skin flora in atopic dermatitis. Br J Dermatol 1994; 131: 536–40.
13. Remitz A, Kyllonen H, Granlund H et al. Tacrolimus ointment reduces staphylococcal colonization of atopic dermatitis lesions. J Allergy Clin Immunol 2001; 107: 196–7.
14. Cho SH, Strickland I, Tomkinson A et al. Preferential binding of Staphylococcus aureus to skin sites of Th2-mediated inflammation in a murine model. J Invest Dermatol 2001; 116: 658–63.
15. Postlethwaite AE, Holness MA, Katai H et al. Human fibroblasts synthesize elevated levels of extracellular matrix proteins in response to interleukin 4. J Clin Invest 1992; 90: 1479–85.
16. Cho SH, Strickland I, Boguniewicz M et al. Fibronectin and fibrinogen contribute to the enhanced binding of Staphylococcus aureus to atopic skin. J Allergy Clin Immunol 2001; 108: 269–74.
17. Wann ER, Gurusiddappa S, Höök M. The fibronectin-binding MSCRAMM FnbpA of Staphylococcus aureus is a bifunctional protein that also binds to fibrinogen. J Biol Chem 2000; 275: 13863–71.
18. Morishita Y, Tada J, Sato A et al. Possible influences of Staphylococcus aureus on atopic dermatitis – the colonizing features and the effects of staphylococcal enterotoxins. Clin Exp Allergy 1999; 29: 1110–17.
19. Christophers E, Henseler T. Contrasting disease patterns in psoriasis and atopic dermatitis. Arch Dermatol Res 1987; 279(Suppl): S48–51.
20. Grice K, Sattar H, Baker H, Sharratt M. The relationship of transepidermal water loss to skin temperature in psoriasis and eczema. J Invest Dermatol 1975; 64: 313–15.
21. Fulton C, Anderson GM, Zasloff M et al. Expression of natural peptide antibiotics in human skin. Lancet 1997; 350: 1750–1.
22. Harder J, Bartels J, Christophers E et al. A peptide antibiotic from human skin. Nature 1997; 387: 861.
23. Stolzenberg ED, Anderson GM, Ackermann MR et al. Epithelial antibiotic induced in states of disease. Proc Natl Acad Sci U S A 1997; 94: 8686–90.
24. Gallo RL, Ono M, Povsic T et al. Syndecans, cell surface heparan sulfate proteoglycans, are induced by a proline-rich antimicrobial peptide from wounds. Proc Natl Acad Sci U S A 1994; 91: 11035–39.
25. Frohm M, Agerberth B, Ahangari G et al. The expression of the gene coding for the antibacterial peptide LL-37 is induced in human keratinocytes during inflammatory disorders. J Biol Chem 1997; 272: 15258–63.
26. Gropp R, Frye M, Wagner TO et al. Epithelial defensins impair adenoviral infection: implication for adenovirus-mediated gene therapy. Hum Gene Ther 1999; 10: 957–64.
27. Gallo RL, Murakami M, Ohtake T et al. Biology and clinical relevance of naturally occurring antimicrobial peptides. J Allergy Clin Immunol 2002; 110: 823–31.
28. Nizet V, Ohtake T, Lauth X et al. Innate antimicrobial peptide protects the skin from invasive bacterial infection. Nature 2001; 414: 454–7.
29. Panyutich A, Shi J, Boutz PL et al. Porcine polymorphonuclear leukocytes generate extracellular microbicidal activity by elastase-mediated activation of secreted proprotegrins. Infect Immun 1997; 65: 978–85.
30. Ong PY, Ohtake T, Brandt C et al. Endogenous antimicrobial peptides and skin infections in atopic dermatitis. N Engl J Med 2002; 347: 1151–60.
31. Leung DY, Harbeck R, Bina P et al. Presence of IgE antibodies to staphylococcal exotoxins on the skin of patients with atopic dermatitis. Evidence for a new group of allergens. J Clin Invest 1993; 92: 1374–80.
32. Kotzin BL, Leung DY, Kappler J et al. Superantigens and their potential role in human disease. Adv Immunol 1993; 54: 99–166.
33. Leung DYM, Schlievert PM. Superantigens in human disease: Future directions in therapy and elucidation of disease pathogenesis. In: Leung DYM, Huber B, Schleivert PM, eds. Superantigens: Molecular Biology, Immunology and Relevance to Human Disease. New York: Marcel Dekker, Inc, 1997: 581–602.
34. Bunikowski R, Mielke M, Skarabis H et al. Prevalence and role of serum IgE antibodies to the Staphylococcus aureus-derived

superantigens SEA and SEB in children with atopic dermatitis. J Allergy Clin Immunol 1999; 103: 119–24.

35. Nomura I, Tanaka K, Tomita H et al. Evaluation of the staphylococcal exotoxins and their specific IgE in childhood atopic dermatitis. J Allergy Clin Immunol 1999; 104: 441–6.

36. Strickland I, Hauk PJ, Trumble AE et al. Evidence for superantigen involvement in skin homing of T cells in atopic dermatitis. J Invest Dermatol 1999; 112: 249–53.

37. Bunikowski R, Mielke ME, Skarabis H et al. Evidence for a disease-promoting effect of Staphylococcus aureus-derived exotoxins in atopic dermatitis. J Allergy Clin Immunol 2000; 105: 814–19.

38. Hofer MF, Harbeck RJ, Schlievert PM. Staphylococcal toxins augment specific IgE responses by atopic patients exposed to allergen. J Invest Dermatol 1999; 112: 171–6.

39. Herz U, Schnoy N, Borelli S et al. A human-SCID mouse model for allergic immune response bacterial superantigen enhances skin inflammation and suppresses IgE production. J Invest Dermatol 1998; 110: 224–31.

40. Akdis M, Akdis CA, Weigl L et al. Skin-homing, CLA+ memory T cells are activated in atopic dermatitis and regulate IgE by an IL-13-dominated cytokine pattern: IgG4 counter-regulation by CLA- memory T cells. J Immunol 1997; 159: 4611–19.

41. Akdis M, Simon HU, Weigl L et al. Skin homing (cutaneous lymphocyte-associated antigen-positive) CD8+ T cells respond to superantigen and contribute to eosinophilia and IgE production in atopic dermatitis. J Immunol 1999; 163: 466–75.

42. Strange P, Skov L, Lisby S et al. Staphylococcal enterotoxin B applied on intact normal and intact atopic skin induces dermatitis. Arch Dermatol 1996; 132: 27–33.

43. Skov L, Olsen JV, Giorno R et al. Application of Staphylococcal enterotoxin B on normal and atopic skin induces up-regulation of T cells by a superantigen-mediated mechanism. J Allergy Clin Immunol 2000; 105: 820–6.

44. Michie CA, Davis T. Atopic dermatitis and staphylococcal superantigens. Lancet 1996; 347: 324.

45. Brosius CL, Newburger JW, Burns JC et al. Increased prevalence of atopic dermatitis in Kawasaki disease. Pediatr Infect Dis J 1988; 7: 863–6.

46. Leung DY, Meissner HC, Shulman ST et al. Prevalence of superantigen-secreting bacteria in patients with Kawasaki disease. J Pediatr 2002; 140: 742–6.

47. Müller KM, Jaunin F, Masouye I et al. Th2 cells mediate IL-4-dependent local tissue inflammation. J Immunol 1993; 150: 5576–84.

48. Saloga J, Enk AH, Becker D et al. Modulation of contact sensitivity responses by bacterial superantigen. J Invest Dermatol 1995; 105: 220–4.

49. Saloga J, Leung DY, Reardon C et al. Cutaneous exposure to the superantigen staphylococcal enterotoxin B elicits a T-cell-dependent inflammatory response. J Invest Dermatol 1996; 106: 982–8.

50. Leung DY, Gately M, Trumble A et al. Bacterial superantigens induce T cell expression of the skin-selective homing receptor, the cutaneous lymphocyte-associated antigen, via stimulation of interleukin 12 production. J Exp Med 1995; 181: 747–53.

51. de Vries IJ, Langeveld-Wildschut EG, van Reijsen FC et al. Adhesion molecule expression on skin endothelia in atopic dermatitis: effects of TNF-alpha and IL-4. J Allergy Clin Immunol 1998; 102: 461–8.

52. Bratton DL, Hamid Q, Boguniewicz M et al. Granulocyte macrophage colony-stimulating factor contributes to enhanced monocyte survival in chronic atopic dermatitis. J Clin Invest 1995; 95: 211–18.

53. Ezepchuk YV, Leung DY, Middleton MH et al. Staphylococcal toxins and protein A differentially induce cytotoxicity and release of tumour necrosis factor-alpha from human keratinocytes. J Invest Dermatol 1996; 107: 603–9.

54. Travers JB, Leung DYM, Johnson C et al. Augmentation of staphylococcal alpha-toxin signaling by the epidermal platelet-activating factor receptor. J Invest Dermatol 2003; 120: 789–94.

55. Abeck D, Mempel M. Staphylococcus aureus colonization in atopic dermatitis and its therapeutic implications. Br J Dermatol 1998; 139(Suppl 53): 13–16.

56. Boguniewicz M, Sampson H, Leung SB et al. Effects of cefuroxime axetil on Staphylococcus aureus colonization and superantigen production in atopic dermatitis. J Allergy Clin Immunol 2001; 108: 651–2.

57. Skov L, Baadsgaard O. Role of infection in atopic dermatitis. In: Leung DYM, Greaves MW, eds. Allergic Skin Diseases: A Multidisciplinary Approach. New York: Marcel Dekker, Inc, 2000: 449–62.

58. Doebbeling BN, Reagan DR, Pfaller MA et al. Long-term efficacy of intranasal mupirocin ointment. A prospective cohort study of Staphylococcus aureus carriage. Arch Intern Med 1994; 154: 1505–8.

59. Ramsay CA, Savoie LM, Gilbert M. The treatment of atopic dermatitis with topical fusidic acid and hydrocortisone acetate. J Eur Acad Dermatol Venereol 1996; 7: S15–22.

60. Wachs GN, Maibach HI. Co-operative double-blind trial of an antibiotic/corticoid combination in impetiginized atopic dermatitis. Br J Dermatol 1976; 95: 323–8.

61. Leyden JJ, Kligman AM. The case for steroid–antibiotic combinations. Br J Dermatol 1977; 96: 179–87.

62. Clayton MH, Leung DY, Surs W et al. Altered glucocorticoid receptor binding in atopic dermatitis. J Allergy Clin Immunol 1995; 96: 421–3.

63. Hauk PJ, Leung DY. Tacrolimus (FK506): new treatment approach in superantigen-associated diseases like atopic dermatitis? J Allergy Clin Immunol 2001; 107: 391–2.

64. Herbert S, Barry P, Novick RP. Subinhibitory clindamycin differentially inhibits transcription of exoprotein genes in Staphylococcus aureus. Infect Immun 2001; 69: 2996–3003.

65. Bamberger CM, Bamberger AM, de Castro M et al. Glucocorticoid receptor beta, a potential endogenous inhibitor of glucocorticoid action in humans. J Clin Invest 1995; 95: 2435–41.

66. Leung DYM, Bloom JW. Update on glucocorticoid action and resistance. J Allergy Clin Immunol 2003; 111: 1–20.

67. Stalder JF, Fleury M, Sourisse M et al. Comparative effects of two topical antiseptics (chlorhexidine vs $KMnO_4$) on bacterial skin flora in atopic dermatitis. Acta Derm Venereol Suppl (Stockh) 1992; 176: 132–4.

68. Brockow K, Grabenhorst P, Abeck D et al. Effect of gentian violet, corticosteroid and tar preparations in Staphylococcus aureus-colonized atopic eczema. Dermatology 1999; 199: 231–6.

69. Brockow K, Grabenhorst P, Traupe B. Gentian violet for the treatment of atopic eczema antibacterial and clinical efficacy. J Invest Dermatol 1997; 109: 463.

70. Akiyama H, Tada J, Toi JH et al. Changes in Staphylococcus aureus density and lesion severity after topical application of povidone-iodine in cases of atopic dermatitis. J Dermatol Sci 1997; 16: 23–30.

71. Breneman DL, Hanifin JM, Berge CA et al. The effect of antibacterial soap with 1.5% triclocarban on Staphylococcus aureus in patients with atopic dermatitis. Cutis 2000; 66: 296–300.

72. Yoshimura M, Namura S, Akamatsu H et al. Antimicrobial effects of phototherapy and photochemotherapy in vivo and in vitro. Br J Dermatol 1996; 135: 528–32.

73. Yoshimura-Mishima M, Akamatsu H, Namura S et al. Suppressive effect of ultraviolet (UVB and PUVA) radiation on superantigen production by Staphylococcus aureus. J Dermatol Sci 1999; 19: 31–6.

74. Rfuzicka T, Bieber T, Schopf E et al. A short-term trial of tacrolimus ointment for atopic dermatitis. European Tacrolimus Multicenter Atopic Dermatitis Study Group. N Engl J Med 1997; 337: 816–21.

75. Boguniewicz M, Fiedler VC, Raimer S et al. A randomized, vehicle-controlled trial of tacrolimus ointment for treatment of atopic dermatitis in children. Pediatric Tacrolimus Study Group. J Allergy Clin Immunol 1998; 102: 637–44.

76. Reitamo S, Van Leent EJ, Ho V et al. Efficacy and safety of tacrolimus ointment compared with that of hydrocortisone acetate ointment in children with atopic dermatitis. J Allergy Clin Immunol 2002; 109: 539–46.

77. Reitamo S, Rustin M, Ruzicka T et al. Efficacy and safety of tacrolimus ointment compared with that of hydrocortisone butyrate ointment in adult patients with atopic dermatitis. J Allergy Clin Immunol 2002; 109: 547–55.

78. Allen BR. Tacrolimus ointment: its place in the therapy of atopic dermatitis. J Allergy Clin Immunol 2002; 109: 401–3.

79. Hauk PJ, Leung DY, Tacrolimus (FK506): a new treatment approach in superantigen-associated diseases like atopic dermatitis? J Allergy Clin Immunol 2001; 107: 391–2.

6

Role of viruses

Andreas Wollenberg and Stefanie Kamann

INTRODUCTION

Patients affected by atopic dermatitis (AD) tend to develop common viral infections such as herpes simplex, molluscum contagiosum or verruca vulgaris more frequently than non-atopics. These infections do not exhibit other clinical features in atopics than in non-atopics, are treated similarly in both patient groups, and will not be discussed in this chapter. In addition, widespread disseminated viral infections occur in the skin lesions of AD. These infections have been described according to the causative virus as eczema molluscatum (EM), eczema vaccinatum (EV) or eczema herpeticum (EH). Though all these diseases are relatively rare and little is known about their specific pathogenesis, some of them are among the true medical emergencies in dermatology. EV and EH represent the probably most feared complications of AD. Here, we touch EM, which is more annoying than dangerous, but difficult to treat, briefly cover the most severe but nowadays only exceptionally occurring EV, and handle in depth the clinically most important aspects of diagnosis and treatment of EH.

ECZEMA MOLLUSCATUM

Disseminated eruption of molluscum contagiosum virus (MCV) in an AD patient is known as EM. It is mostly a disease of children. The relatively small, skin-coloured frequently umbilicated papules vary in size (Figure 6.1). Though most papules are confined to the eczematous lesions of the underlying AD, autoinoculation of the virus may cause aberrant papules in other body regions. There is no fever, no malaise, and no general symptoms associated with EM.

MCV was found to have unique genes not found in variola virus, that encode proteins which help the virus avoid immune detection, and 59 MCV genes are

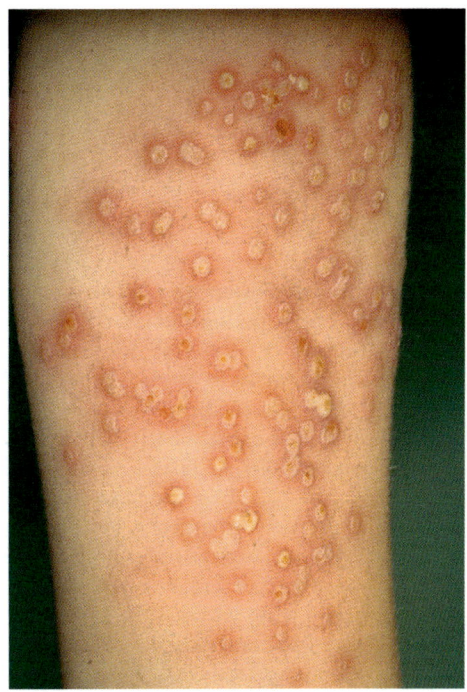

Figure 6.1 Eczema molluscatum. A disseminated eruption of whitish, umbilicated papules on eczematous skin which show considerable variation in size.

predicted to encode previously uncharacterized proteins, including MHC class I, chemokine, and glutathione peroxidase homologues, which may be linked with MCV pathogenesis and provide considerable insights into how viruses can evade antiviral defence mechanisms.[1]

The soluble interleukin (IL)-18 binding protein (IL-18BP) of poxviruses represents a new immune escape strategy. As IL-18 is a proinflammatory cytokine that can enhance both the innate and acquired immunity, the poxvirus-encoded IL-18BPs binding to IL-18 with high affinity and inhibiting IL-18 mediated IFN-γ induction interrupts the normal immune response to MCV antigens.[2]

Treatment of EM greatly depends on the physician's personal opinion and experience. Patients pretreated with topical steroids or topical immunomodulators are usually taken off these drugs for a few weeks to allow mounting of a natural immune response against the virus.[3] In addition, a smaller number of lesions may be expressed with a suitably shaped forceps. Half an hour's pretreatment with a cream containing a eutectic mixture of local anaesthetics will both reduce pain and soften the lesion for easier removal. Topical application of imiquimod or other topical immunostimulatory drugs shows promising results and may become a future treatment option.[4] As the virus is easily spread by a scratching hand, we recommend the application of gauze dressings to cover the affected areas.

ECZEMA VACCINATUM

Disseminated eruption of vaccinia in an AD patient is known as eczema vaccinatum (EV). Vaccination with vaccinia virus has been performed for about two hundred years to prevent or attenuate smallpox infection caused by the variola virus in humans.[5] Following the declaration of smallpox eradication by the WHO in 1980, all countries have subsequently stopped vaccination of the general public. As of this writing, vaccination is essentially restricted to special forces, military personnel and specialized laboratory workers, but heteroinoculation of vaccinia virus may cause infection in contact persons.[6] In case of a release of variola virus as a biological weapon, ring vaccination of first and second contacts with vaccinia virus is recommended by the health authorities and may lead to EV.[7]

Along with its legacy of enormous success, the live virus smallpox vaccine has the dubious distinction of having one of the highest rates of vaccine-associated adverse events seen among all vaccines currently in routine use.[6] As AD is a contraindication to smallpox vaccination, accidental contact vaccination accounted for more cases of EV (65%) than did intentional primary vaccination.[8] The incidence of EV in the USA was 123 per million primary vaccinees, with case fatality rates of approximately 1–5%.[9,10]

A disseminated eruption of blisters and pustules, predominantly scattered throughout the lesional skin, together with fever and severe illness, describes the clinical picture of EV. Seemingly contradictory are published data, that two-thirds of EV patients did not have active disease at the time of vaccinia virus exposure.[8] This may in part be explained by a lack of AD patients

to upregulate the antimicrobial cathelicidin peptide LL-37 in response to vaccinia virus exposure.[11] As most dermatologists have not seen EV patients during their residency, the Centres for Disease Control has set up a highly useful smallpox related internet training module with a number of excellent clinical pictures including EV (http://www.bt.cdc.gov/Agent/Smallpox/Smallpox.asp. The diagnosis of EV is easily made on clinical grounds, and may be confirmed by electron microscopic demonstration of poxvirus structures from the blister fluid.

Vaccinia immune globulin (VIG) may be administered to patients with EV in a dose of 0.6 ml/kg if available, given intramuscularly in divided doses over a 24–36 hour period. This may be repeated in 2 to 3 days if improvement does not occur.[12] The VIG quantities are limited at present, but the pharmaceutical industry is currently producing larger quantities of VIG which will be suitable for intravenous use in a yet to be defined dosage regimen.

ECZEMA HERPETICUM

The first description of EH dates back to 1887, when the Austrian dermatologist Moritz Kaposi described 10 children with eczema larvare infantum complicated by a vesicopustular eruption.[13] Today, the term Kaposi's varicelliform eruption is used for any disseminated cutaneous infection with the herpes simplex virus (HSV) type 1 or 2, which may include AD, eczema, Darier disease,[14] pemphigus foliaceus,[15] mycosis fungoides,[16] Sézary syndrome,[17] ichthyosis vulgaris,[18] Hailey-Hailey disease,[19] and burn patients.[20] In contrast, EH should be restricted to disseminated HSV infection as a complication of an eczematous skin disease.[21]

Patients with EH frequently present with a disseminated, distinctly monomorphic eruption of dome-shaped vesicles (Figures 6.2–6.3), accompanied by fever, malaise, and lymphadenopathy. Within 2 weeks, the blisters usually dry out, forming crusts that fill eroded pits (Figure 6.4). Atypical variants with characteristic, disseminated 'slits' in tense erythematous plaques may also occur. Head, neck, and upper body are most frequently affected. Lesions generally heal over 2 to 6 weeks. Mortality of disseminated HSV infection, such as EH, was up to 80% prior to effective antiviral treatment and may be associated with systemic viramia leading to a multiple organ involvement and encephalitis.[22,23]

Disseminated HSV infections such as EH can be complicated by keratoconjunctivitis, encephalitis, meningitis, and neonatal herpes. The nature and severity of disease depends on several factors, including site of

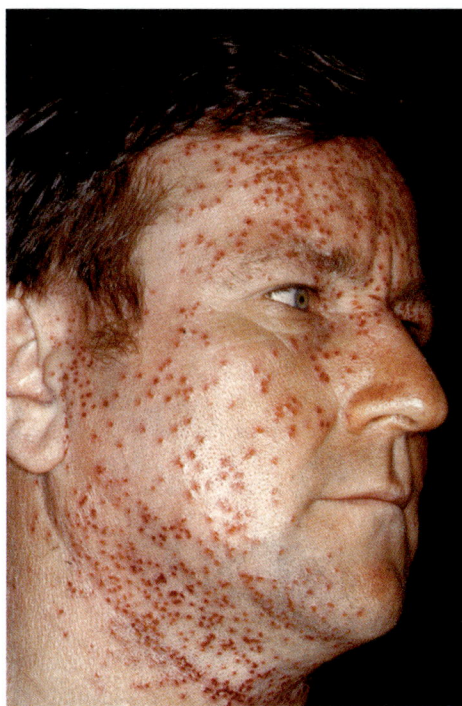

Figure 6.2 Eczema herpeticum, vesiculo-pustular stage. A disseminated eruption of distinctly monomorphic, dome-shaped blisters and secondary pustules on eczematous skin is suggestive of eczema herpeticum.

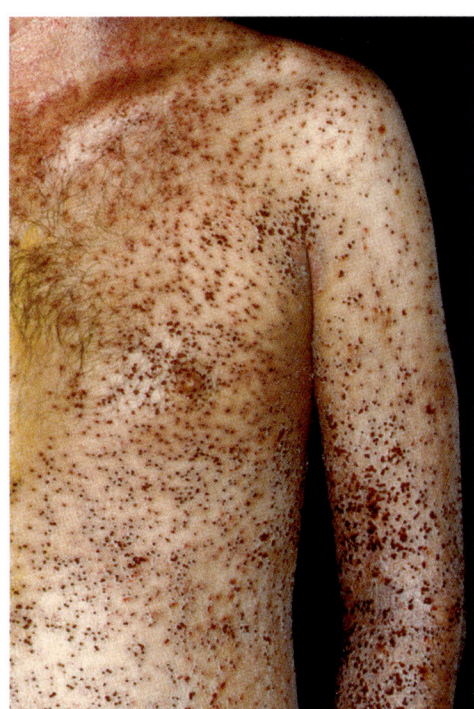

Figure 6.4 Eczema herpeticum, crust stage. After a few days, the blisters are drying out and form crusts that fill eroded pits.

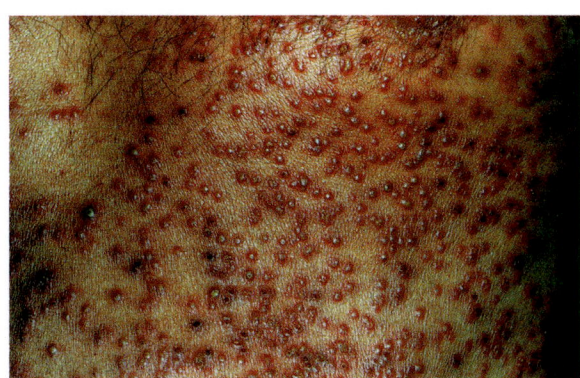

Figure 6.3 Eczema herpeticum, vesiculo-pustular stage. A disseminated eruption of distinctly monomorphic, dome-shaped blisters and secondary pustules on eczematous skin is suggestive of eczema herpeticum.

Population-based epidemiological data on EH are difficult to obtain because of its rarity. The number of patients treated in university hospitals for this disease is said to have increased over the years.[24] Whether this is due to the increased incidence of AD, to the increased mobility of patients allowing them to reach a dermatology unit more easily, or to an increase of EH as such remains unclear. Only a few studies have investigated a larger number of patients with EH,[24,25] and the predisposing factors are essentially those associated with severe manifestations of AD as such: an early onset of the underlying AD and a high total serum IgE level.[25] More than 75% of the patients with EH had not received corticosteroid treatment in the 4 weeks prior to onset of EH, arguing against a role for topical corticosteroids in the development of EH.[25]

Diagnostic procedures in eczema herpeticum

In most cases, the typical clinical features of EH allow the differential diagnosis to widespread impetigo or other disseminated infections, contact dermatitis, or

virus inoculation, age, immune status of the host, and genetic variations in virus strains or infected persons.

chickenpox. The clinical diagnosis can be confirmed by polymerase chain reaction (PCR) for viral DNA, by electron microscopic detection of herpes group virus from blister fluid, or by commercial immunofluorescence tests for cells affected by HSV. The diagnosis is supported by demonstration of large multinucleated cells in the blister fluid and conventional light microscopy (Tzanck test). A less sensitive method is viral culture, and less specific methods are serologic tests. The choice of the optimal test depends on the clinical manifestation of the disease.[25]

In all EH cases, the patient's personal history and family history of concomitant atopic diseases, such as allergic rhinoconjunctivitis and bronchial asthma, as well as personal and environmental history of herpes labialis, should be well documented to allow further information about predisposing factors for EH. Serum IgE levels usually correlate with the severerity of AD.[25]

Differential blood count, erythrocyte sedimentation rate (ESR), and body temperature may exhibit signs of viramia, while serum creatinine levels should be measured before starting systemic aciclovir therapy. Bacterial swabs will show bacterial colonization or infection with *Staphylococcus aureus* or other bacteria.

Patients with EH should be seen by an ophthalmologist to monitor for herpetic keratitis. A neurologist should examine the patient if meningeal involvement is suspected. Clinical features of CNS infection with HSV may be headache, confusion, and fever. Areas with decreased attenuation in the temporal lobes in the CT scan of the head, abnormalities in the EEG, and pleocytosis and increased protein levels in the cerebrospinal fluid will only be found if the herpes encephalitis is suspected and the tests are ordered.[26]

Pathogenesis of eczema herpeticum

Infection of epithelial cells with HSV is initiated by contact of the virus with mucosa or abraded skin.[27] Replication of HSV in epidermal and dermal cells follows, and HSV can even be spread via the lymphatics to regional lymph nodes.[28] This may explain the severity and large affected area during primary infection. During this initial infection, HSV gains access to sensory neurons to establish latent infection. Reactivation and replication of latent HSV can be induced by stimuli such as light, trauma, or immunosuppression. Patients with a compromised cell-mediated immunity, as present in AD, are at risk of developing recurrent and severe HSV infections.

Primary infection with HSV may not be apparent but may also cause herpetic gingivostomatitis. Herpes labialis is typically caused by HSV reactivation, the well-known herpes simplex recidivans in loco. EH may be caused by primary or secondary HSV infection.[25]

The impaired skin barrier of patients with severe AD, together with the spongiosis, makes it easier for the virus to invade the skin and bind to its cellular receptors. A desmosomal protein, nectin-1, has recently been identified as one of the relevant HSV receptors in man.[29] In AD, there is a Th2 cell predominance with increased production of the Th2 cytokines IL-4 and IL-13.[30] IL-4 induces IgE production and prevents differentiation of interferon (IFN)-γ producing Th1 cells. The lower levels of IFN-γ in the skin of patients with AD may allow the viruses to overgrow.[6]

A patient's ability to defend himself against HSV infection may critically depend on the production of antiviral type-I interferons. Plasmocytoid dendritic cells (PDC) are a novel dendritic cell subset that circulate in the blood and make up 0.1% of peripheral blood mononuclear cells.[31] As PDCs produce a large amounts of antiviral type I interferon (IFN)-α and IFN-β upon viral infection and are capable of inducing both Th1 and Th2 responses, their presence seems most important for the susceptibility of patients to viral skin infections. We demonstrated recently that AD patients have an impaired recruitment of PDC into their skin lesions as compared with other inflammatory skin diseases such as psoriasis or contact dermatitis, which provides a rationale why patients with AD show a predisposition to viral skin infections.[32]

The induction of antimicrobial peptides such as the antiviral cathelicidin LL-37 is an important mechanism of innate immune defence and may be induced by proinflammatory stimuli.[11] Physiological concentrations of the cathelicidin LL-37 induce antiviral activity and significant killing of HSV in antiviral assays,[11] but a defective upregulation of LL-37 has been demonstrated in skin lesions of AD patients.[33] Moreover, skin of EH patients exhibits significantly lower levels of LL-37 protein expression compared with skin of AD patients.[11] Human cathelicidin expression is inversely correlated to the serum IgE level.[11]

Therapy of eczema herpeticum

Optimal therapy of EH is a combination of topical and systemic actions, and should be started at the earliest possible time. Systemic antiviral chemotherapy is the mainstay of EH treatment, supported by topical antiviral chemotherapy in case of eye involvement (herpetic keratitis). Oral antibiotics are frequently given to control bacterial superinfection, and oral cephalosporine preparations (e.g. cefadroxil, 2×1 g/day) are our treatment of first choice. Topical administration of antiseptic lotions may improve the clinical course of EH by drying out the vesicles and preventing bacterial superinfection.

The role of anti-inflammatory therapy in acute EH stages, including glucocorticosteroids, is controversial, because the wanted anti-inflammatory activity of gluco-corticosteroids and topical immunomodulators is inevitably associated with an unwanted attenuation of the antiviral immune defence of the skin immune system. Despite lacking evidence, many clinicians tend to avoid glucocorticosteroids in the acute phase of EH. In our own institution, topical and systemic steroids are freely given once systemic antiviral therapy has been started.

Antiviral chemotherapy of eczema herpeticum

Systemic antiviral chemotherapy must be given to avoid complications of a disseminated HSV infection such as HSV encephalitis or herpetic keratitis. Currently, the most potent drugs used for HSV therapy are nucleoside analogues which interfere with viral DNA replication. Before the introduction of aciclovir treatment, the mortality rate of EH leading to multiple organ involvement and encephalitis was about 70%.[22]

Aciclovir
Aciclovir is a nucleoside analogue that is converted by herpes virus-encoded kinases to its monophosphate metabolites. This metabolization step can only occur in HSV-infected cells. After conversion to monophosphate, further activation to di- and triphosphate is catalysed by cellular enzymes. The nucleoside triphosphate interacts with the herpes virus DNA polymerase, resulting in inhibition of viral DNA synthesis. Aciclovir has repeatedly been shown to be highly efficient and safe with systemic administration. Shortening of disease duration by oral aciclovir has been demonstrated in a multicentre, double-blind placebo-controlled study with EH patients.[34]

The currently recommended regimen for EH and other severe HSV infections, such as neonatal herpes, HSV encephalitis, or HSV infection in HIV patients, is a 7-day course of intravenous aciclovir (3×5–10 mg/kg/day), which may be prolonged according to the clinical course of the disease. For children less than 12 years old with EH, more accurate dosage can be achieved by using surface area calculations. The recommended dose is then 3×750 mg/m^2/day for 7 days. Oral aciclovir has a lower bioavailibility (15–30%) than intravenously given aciclovir, and should therefore be restricted to the treatment of mild EH (5×400 mg/day).

Prophylactic treatment of recurrent genital HSV infections with low-dose long-term oral aciclovir in a dosage of 2×200 mg/day[35,36] or 2×400 mg/day[37,38] was shown to reduce the number of recurrent episodes. Although there are no studies about aciclovir prophylaxis in patients who tend to develop EH, oral aciclovir in a dosage of 2×200 mg/day may be a therapeutic option in cases with severe recurrent EH.

Aciclovir has a nephrotoxic potential when systemically given, but slow infusion reduces the incidence of renal disturbances. Dose reduction is mandatory in renal insufficient patients and calculated according to creatinine levels. Aciclovir resistance, which appears in 4.7%[39] to 17%[40] of immunocompromised patients, is rarely seen in EH patients.

Although there is no evidence of a teratogenic effect of aciclovir, it is still a matter of discussion if aciclovir should be given during pregnancy. On the other hand, EH during pregnancy may lead to intrauterine infection of the foetus in about 50% by transplacental transmission. Intrauterine infection mostly occurs during the first 20 weeks of pregnancy and leads to an increased rate of abort, death, and birth defects.[41] Although it has never been the subject of larger, well-controlled studies, an individual risk-benefit evaluation is made for each patient, usually resulting in intravenous treatment with aciclovir.[42] A randomized, placebo-controlled study in 46 pregnant women with first episodes of genital herpes, who were treated with either 3×400 mg/day oral aciclovir from 36 weeks' gestation until delivery or with placebo, showed no birth defects in the aciclovir-treated women.[43] Moreover, no HSV could be isolated at time of birth in the 21 aciclovir-treated women, permitting a vaginal delivery, while 9 from 25 placebo-treated woman had to undergo a Caesarean section due to a current HSV infection.[43] According to the manufacturer, 1246 pregnancy outcomes with prenatal exposure to aciclovir collected from 1984 to 1999 showed no increase in the number of birth defects. Thus, a disseminated HSV infection such as EH during pregnancy should be treated with intravenous aciclovir (3×5–10 mg/kg/day) for at least 7 days to avoid HSV-induced abort, death, and birth defects.

Valaciclovir
Valaciclovir is the L-valyl ester prodrug of aciclovir. During first pass metabolism, valaciclovir is almost completely converted to aciclovir. It has an increased oral bioavailibility. Orally given valaciclovir has been compared to oral aciclovir in genital HSV infection, demonstrating the advantage of a more convenient dosing regimen with a potential for improved compliance. There are no studies about the efficacy of valaciclovir in the treatment of EH. We recommend a 7 day course of oral valaciclovir (3×500 mg/day) for EH treatment, which should be prolonged according to the clinical course of the disease.[40]

Herpes prophylaxis with valaciclovir has been studied in a randomized, double-blind trial in a dosing regimen of 1×1000 mg/day, 500 mg/day and 250 mg/day valaciclovir which produced a statistically significant suppression of genital herpes recurrence, as did 2×400 mg/day aciclovir.[38,40] Although there are no data about prophylaxis of recurrent episodes of EH with valaciclovir, we would recommend valaciclovir in a dosage of 2×20 mg/day.

Penciclovir

Penciclovir is a nucleoside deoxyguanosine analogue that inhibits the DNA synthesis of HSV. The safety profile and antiviral activity spectrum of penciclovir is largely identical to aciclovir. After entering the virus-infected cells, penciclovir is phosphorylated to its triphosphate state and is inserted in the viral DNA in place of the nucleotide guanine, thus inhibiting replication of the virus. While aciclovir has a 100-fold higher inhibitory activity, this is compensated by the longer intracellular half-life of penciclovir.

Penciclovir can be used either intravenously or topically. Intravenous penciclovir is not currently licenced as treatment for HSV infections, but doses of 2×5 mg/kg/day were as effective as aciclovir in clinical trials.[44] In topical formulations, penciclovir was found to have a stronger effect in mucocutaneous HSV-induced lesions than aciclovir.[45] Penciclovir has not been studied in EH patients.

Famciclovir

Famciclovir, the diacetate ester derivative of 6-deoxypenciclovir, is the oral prodrug of penciclovir. During bowel passage, it is almost completely converted to penciclovir. In immunocompetent patients, famciclovir provides comparable benefits to aciclovir in genital HSV infection.[46] Famciclovir has not been studied in EH, but a treatment regimen of famciclovir 3×250 mg/day for at least 7 days has been recommended for mild clinical courses of EH.[47]

Foscarnet

Foscarnet is a phosphonate and acts as a substrate analogue of pyrophosphate formed during viral DNA synthesis. Phosphonates inhibit the viral DNA polymerase independent of thymidine kinases and thus are the treatment of choice for patients with aciclovir resistance. Intravenous foscarnet was shown to be highly effective in HIV patients with aciclovir-resistant HSV infection.[48] Though data about administration in EH are lacking, it can be considered as an alternative therapy in rare cases of aciclovir resistance. The currently recommended dosage in HSV infections is intravenous foscarnet 3×40 mg/kg/day for at least 10 days.[48] There is no oral formulation of this drug available. Slow infusion, extensive prehydration, and dose adjustment based on creatinine clearance is recommended because foscarnet is highly nephrotoxic.

Topical treatment of eczema herpeticum

There is no evidence that the additional use of topical antiviral agents on the skin may improve the clinical course of EH in comparison to systemic antiviral chemotherapy alone. Yet, it makes sense to combine systemic antiviral chemotherapy with topical antiviral agents in HSV keratitis and in mucocutaneous lesions.

Ophthalmic therapy

Fortunately, patients with EH rarely suffer from herpetic eye disease. However, in cases exhibiting herpetic lid lesions and reduced corneal sensitivity, local prophylactic treatment should be instituted to prevent ocular complications such as epithelial and stromal keratitis, uveitis, and secondary glaucoma.

Besides ophthalmic topical antiviral agents such as trifluridine, idoxuridine, or brivudin, which belong to the group of 5-substituted 2′-desoxyuridines, topical formulas of the nucleoside analogue aciclovir have been developed for the treatment of HSV-induced epithelial keratitis. In HSV stromal keratitis and uveitis, topical and systemic antivirals must be combined with corticosteroids to suppress the associated immune-mediated inflammation.

Trifluorothymidine 1% eyedrops as well as 3% aciclovir ointment are typically instituted prophylactically as well as in established epithelial keratitis. Trifluorothymidine has been approved since 1962 and shown to be highly effective in the treatment of herpetic keratitis.[49,50] However, to reach therapeutic levels frequent application ($7-9$ x/d) is necessary. Aciclovir ointment $3-5$ x/d has also shown excellent efficacy with resolution of typical dendritic corneal lesions within one day of treatment.[51] Moreover, good intraocular penetration of topically administered aciclovir is advantageous over trifluorothymidine.[52] Application of topical idoxuridine (Ophthal®) also demonstrates good activity in the treatment of ocular HSV infection but is less effective than trifluorothymidine and aciclovir. Due to its systemic toxicity it is strongly limited to topical usage.[53]

Topical brivudin is not licenced yet, but its worldwide approval is in progress. Studies showed a superior efficacy of brivudin in the topical treatment of herpetic keratitis with a more pronounced therapeutic effect than idoxuridine or aciclovir.[54]

Mucocutaneous lesions

Several studies have also shown an influence of topical aciclovir in mucocutaneous HSV lesions.[45] These ambiguous data, and the potency for contact sensitization, possibly resulting in drug eruptions following oral administration in sensitized individuals,[55] is why we do not use aciclovir cream on the skin of EH patients.

Topical penciclovir could also be shown to be as convenient and as effective as 3% aciclovir ointment for the treatment of mucocutaneous HSV lesions, with even a tendency towards a shorter time of resolution of all symptoms in patients treated with 1% penciclovir.[45]

Topical foscarnet was found to be a good alternative in the treatment of HSV-induced mucocutaneous lesions in HIV patients resistant to aciclovir, or with genital herpes.[56,57]

The study results of topical interferon in HSV keratitis or mucocutaneous lesions are promising but its topical formula is not licenced yet.[58]

Due to the lack of data about treatment of EH with topical aciclovir, penciclovir, or foscarnet, and the potency of contact sensitization, we do not add topical antiviral agents to antiviral chemotherapy in EH except in herpetic keratitis.

Vaccination techniques for EH prevention

A small percentage of EH patients tends to develop recurrent episodes of EH. At present, the only way to control this HSV reactivation is prophylactic antiviral chemotherapy, usually with low-dose oral aciclovir.

New therapeutic approaches are currently being developed to enhance the immune response against HSV. In guinea pig models, immunization with HSV-2 glycoprotein or a mixture of the recombinant HSV-1 glycoproteins B and D has been shown to reduce number and duration of recurrent genital HSV-2 infections or HSV-1 induced herpetic keratitis.[59] Human trials conducted with immunization alone or immune response modifiers such as imiquimod or resiquimod alone or a combination also showed promising results for genital HSV infections.[60–62] Further investigations are needed to evaluate if immunotherapy may become an effective method to prevent HSV infections and EH recurrences in patients with AD.

Interferon therapy for eczema herpeticum

Many studies on interferons for the treatment of HSV have been performed during recent years. Two main types of IFN, type I and type II, are known: type I or 'viral' IFNs are secreted by PDC upon viral infection and include IFN-α and IFN-β; type II IFN is IFN-γ. IFNs exhibit potent antiviral properties by the expression of IFN-stimulated genes (ISG) which inhibit virus replication, and the production of virion progeny.[63] In clinical trials, IFNs were found to control HSV-1 spread and shedding in recurrent herpetic lesions and could even inhibit HSV replication almost as well as high-dose aciclovir.[64,65] Moreover, topical administration of a plasmid DNA encoding IFN-α1 onto mouse corneas prior to HSV infection suggests a possible beneficial effect of IFN in HSV infection.[58] Although these studies show promising results, more have to be performed to evaluate the efficacy and risks of interferon therapy in disseminated HSV infection. Especially, it is not clear how interferon may act in patients with AD as it exhibits strong immunostimulatory effects.

REFERENCES

1. Senkevich T, Bugert J, Sisler J, Koonin E, Darai G et al. Genome sequence of a human tumorigenic poxvirus: prediction of specific host response-evasion genes. Science 1996; 273: 813–16.
2. Xiang Y, Moss B. IL-18 binding and inhibition of interferon gamma induction by human poxvirus-encoded proteins. Proc Natl Acad Sci USA 1999; 96: 11537–42.
3. Wetzel S, Wollenberg A. Eczema molluscatum in tacrolimus treated atopic dermatitis. Eur J Dermatol 2004; 14: 73–4.
4. Syed TA, Goswami J, Ahmadpour OA, Ahmad SA. Treatment of molluscum contagiosum in males with an analog of imiquimod 1% in cream: a placebo-controlled, double-blind study. J Dermatol 1998; 25: 309–13.
5. Fenner F, Henderson DA, Arita I, Jezek Z, Ladnyi ID. Smallpox and its eradication. In: The pathogenesis, immunology and pathology of smallpox and vaccinia. Geneva: World Health Organization, 1988: 122–67.
6. Engler RJM, Kenner J, Leung DY. Smallpox vaccination: risk considerations for patients with atopic dermatitis. J Allergy Clin Immunol 2002; 110: 357–65.
7. Wollenberg A, Engler R. Vaccination and adverse reactions to smallpox vaccine. Curr Opin Allergy Clin Immunol 2004; 4: 271–5.
8. Copeman PWM, Wallace HJ. Eczema vaccinatum. Br Med J 1964; 2: 906–8.
9. Highet AS, Kurst J. Viral infections. In: Champion RH, Burton JL, Edling FJG eds. Textbook of Dermatology. London: Blackwell, 1992: 872–3.
10. Lane JM, Millar JD. Risk of smallpox vaccination complications in the United States. Am J Epidemiol 1971; 93: 238–40.
11. Howell M, Wollenberg A, Gallo R, Flaig M, Streib J et al. Cathelicidin deficiency predisposes to eczema herpeticum. J Allergy Clin Immunol 2006; 117: 836–41.
12. Henderson DA, Inglesby TV, Bartlett JG, Ascher MS, Eitzen E et al. Smallpox as a biological weapon. JAMA 1999; 281: 2127–37.
13. Kaposi M. Pathologie und Therapie der Hautkrankheiten. 1887; 3: 483.
14. Higgins CR, Schofield JK, Tatnall FM, Leigh IM. Natural history, management and complications of herpes labialis. J Med Virol 1993; 1: 22–6.
15. Martins-Castro R, Proenca N, de Salles-Gomes LF. On the association of some dermatoses with South American pemphigus foliaceus. Int J Dermatol 1974; 13: 271–5.
16. Masessa JM, Grossman ME, Knobler EH, Bank DE. Kaposi's varicelliform eruption in cutaneous T cell lymphoma. J Am Acad Dermatol 1989; 21: 133–5.
17. Brion N, Guillaume JC, Dubertret L, Touraine R. [Disseminated cutaneous herpes of the adult and Sezary syndrome (author's transl)]. Ann Dermatol Venereol 1981; 108: 517–21.
18. Verbov J. Fixed drug eruption due to phenazone in a hypnotic. Br J Dermatol 1972; 86: 438.
19. Schirren H, Schirren C, Schlupen E, Volkenandt M, Kind P. Exacerbation of Hailey-Hailey disease by infection with herpes simplex virus. Detection with polymerase chain reaction. Hautarzt 1995; 46: 494–7.
20. Nishimura M, Maekawa M, Hino Y, Mihara K, Kohda H. Kaposi's varicelliform eruption. Development in a patient with a healing second-degree burn. Arch Dermatol 1984; 120: 799–800.
21. Wollenberg A, Wetzel S, Burgdorf W, Haas J. Viral infections in atopic dermatitis: pathogenic aspects and clinical management. J Allergy Clin Immunol 2003; 112: 667–74.
22. Sanderson IR, Brueton LA, Savage MO, Harper JI. Eczema herpeticum: a potentially fatal disease. Br Med J (Clin Res Ed) 1987; 294: 693–4.
23. Wheeler CE, Jr., Abele DC. Eczema herpeticum, primary and recurrent. Arch Dermatol 1966; 93: 162–73.

24 Bork K, Brauninger W. Increasing incidence of eczema herpeticum: analysis of seventy-five cases. J Am Acad Dermatol 1988; 19: 1024–9.

25 Wollenberg A, Zoch C, Wetzel S, Plewig G, Przybilla B. Predisposing factors and clinical features of eczema herpeticum - a retrospective analysis of 100 cases. J Am Acad Dermatol 2003; 49: 198–205.

26 McGrath N, Anderson N, Croxson M, Powell K. Herpes simple encephalitis treated with acyclovir: diagnosis and long term outcome. J Neurol Neurosurg Psychiatry 1997; 63: 321–6.

27 Corey L, Spear PG, Fong IW, Ho J, Toy C et al. Infections with herpes simplex viruses (1). N Engl J Med 1986; 314: 686–91.

28 Whitley RJ. Herpes simplex virus infection. Semin Pediatr Infect Dis 2002; 13: 6–11.

29 Yoon M, Spear PG. Disruption of adherens junctions liberates nectin-1 to serve as receptor for herpes simplex virus and pseudorabies virus entry. J Virol 2002; 76: 7203–8.

30 Leung D, Bieber T. Atopic dermatitis. Lancet 2003; 361: 151–60.

31 Cella M, Jarrossay D, Facchetti F, Alebardi O, Nakajima H et al. Plasmacytoid monocytes migrate to inflamed lymph nodes and produce large amounts of type I interferon. Nat Med 1999; 5: 919–23.

32 Wollenberg A, Wagner M, Günther S, Towarowski A, Tuma E et al. Plasmacytoid dendritic cells: a new cutaneous dendritic cell subset with distinct role in inflammatory skin diseases. J Invest Dermatol 2002; 119: 1096–102.

33 Ong PY, Ohtake T, Brandt C, Strickland I, Boguniewicz M et al. Endogenous antimicrobial peptides and skin infections in atopic dermatitis. N Engl J Med 2002; 347: 1151–60.

34 Niimura M, Nishikawa T, Martin A, Booth A, Brocklehurst P et al. Treatment of eczema herpeticum with oral acyclovir. Am J Med 1988; 85: 49–52.

35 Fong IW, Ho J, Toy C, Lo B, Fong MW. Value of long-term administration of acyclovir and similar agents for protecting against AIDS-related lymphoma: case-control and historical cohort studies. Clin Infect Dis 2000; 30: 757–61.

36 Wood M. Antivirals in the context of HIV disease. J Antimicrob Chemother 1996; 37: 97–112.

37 Carlton S, Evans T, Tyring S. New antiviral agents for dermatologic disease. Semin Cutan Med Surg 1998; 17: 243–55.

38 Ormrod D, Scott L, Perry C. Valaciclovir: a review of its long term utility in the management of genital herpes simplex virus and cytomegalovirus infections. Drugs 2000; 59: 839–63.

39 Modiano P, Salloum E, Gillet-Terver MN, Barbaud A, Georges JC et al. Acyclovir-resistant chronic cutaneous herpes simplex in Wiskott-Aldrich syndrome. Br J Dermatol 1995; 133: 475–8.

40 Perry CM, Faulds D. Valaciclovir. A review of its antiviral activity, pharmacokinetic properties and therapeutic efficacy in herpesvirus infections. Drugs 1996; 52: 754–72.

41 Rappersberger K. Infektionen mit Herpes-simplex und Varizella-Zoster-Viren in der Schwangerschaft. Klinische Manifestationen bei Mutter, Fötus und Neugeborenen- therapeutische Optionen. Hautarzt 1999; 50: 706–14.

42 Wollenberg A, Degitz K. Herpetic eczema in pregnancy. Dtsch Med Wochenscr 1995; 120(41): 1395–8.

43 Scott L, Sanchez P, Jackson G, Zeray F, Wendel G. Acyclovir suppression to prevent cesarean delivery after first-episode genital herpes. Obstet Gynecol 1996; 87: 69–73.

44 Lazarus HM, Belanger R, Candoni A, Aoun M, Jurewicz R et al. Intravenous penciclovir for treatment of herpes simplex infections in immunocompromised patients: results of a multicenter, acyclovir-controlled trial. The Penciclovir Immunocompromised Study Group. Antimicrob Agents Chemother 1999; 43: 1192–7.

45 Lin L, Chen XS, Cui PG, Wang JB, Guo ZP et al. Topical application of penciclovir cream for the treatment of herpes simplex facialis/labialis: a randomized, double-blind, multicentre, aciclovir-controlled trial. J Dermatolog Treat 2002; 13: 67–72.

46 Mertz GJ, Loveless MO, Levin MJ, Kraus SJ, Fowler SL et al. Oral famciclovir for suppression of recurrent genital herpes simplex virus infection in women. A multicenter, double-blind, placebo-controlled trial. Collaborative Famciclovir Genital Herpes Research Group. Arch Intern Med 1997; 157: 343–9.

47 Perry CM, Wagstaff AJ. Famciclovir. A review of its pharmacological properties and therapeutic efficacy in herpesvirus infections. Drugs 1995; 50: 396–415.

48 Safrin S, Crumpacker C, Chatis P, Davis R, Hafner R et al. A controlled trial comparing foscarnet with vidarabine for acyclovir-resistant mucocutaneous herpes simplex in the acquired immunodeficiency syndrome. The AIDS Clinical Trials Group. N Engl J Med 1991; 325: 551–5.

49 Kaufman HE, Varnell ED, Thompson HW. Trifluridine, cidofovir, and penciclovir in the treatment of experimental herpetic keratitis. Arch Ophthalmol 1998; 116: 777–80.

50 Kessler HA, Hurwitz S, Farthing C, Benson CA, Feinberg J et al. Pilot study of topical trifluridine for the treatment of acyclovir-resistant mucocutaneous herpes simplex disease in patients with AIDS (ACTG 172). AIDS Clinical Trials Group. J Acquir Immune Defic Syndr Hum Retrovirol 1996; 12: 147–52.

51 Tabery HM. Healing of recurrent herpes simplex corneal epithelial lesions treated with topical acyclovir A non-contact photomicrographic in vivo study in the human cornea. Acta Ophthalmol Scand 2001; 79: 256–61.

52 Poirier RH, Kingham JD, de Miranda P, Annel M. Intraocular antiviral penetration. Arch Ophthalmol 1982; 100: 1964–7.

53 Wilhelmus K. The treatment of herpes simplex virus epithelial keratitis. Trans Am Ophthalmol Soc 2000; 98: 505–32.

54 Panda A, Das GK, Khokhar S, Rao V, Nevin T et al. Efficacy of four antiviral agents in the treatment of uncomplicated herpetic keratitis. Can J Ophthalmol 1995; 30: 256–8.

55 Wollenberg A, Baldauf C, Ruëff F, Przybilla B. Allergische Kontaktdermatitis und Arzneiexanthem auf Aciclovir – Kreuzreaktion auf Ganciclovir. Allergo J 2000; 9: 96–9.

56 Pechere M, Wunderli W, Trellu-Toutous L, Harms M, Saura JH et al. Treatment of acyclovir-resistant herpetic ulceration with topical foscarnet and antiviral sensitivity analysis. Dermatology 1998; 197: 278–80.

57 Snoeck R, Gerard M, Sadzot-Delvaux C, Andrei G, Balzarini J et al. Meningoradiculoneuritis due to acyclovir-resistant varicella zoster virus in an acquired immune deficiency syndrome patient. J Med Virol 1994; 42: 338–47.

58 Noisakran SJ, Carr DJ. Therapeutic efficacy of DNA encoding IFN-alpha1 against corneal HSV-1 infection. Curr Eye Res 2000; 20: 405–12.

59 Stanberry LR, Burke R, Myers MG. Herpes simplex virus glycoprotein treatment of recurrent genital herpes. J Infect Dis 1988; 157: 156–63.

60 Harrison CJ, Miller RL, Bernstein DI. Reduction of recurrent HSV disease using imiquimod alone or combined with a glycoprotein vaccine. Vaccine 2001; 19: 1820–6.

61 Koelle D. Vaccines for herpes simplex virus infections. Curr Opin Investig Drugs 2006; 7: 136–41.

62 Straus SE, Corey L, Burke RL, Savarese B, Barnum G et al. Placebo-controlled trial of vaccination with recombinant glycoprotein D of herpes simplex virus type 2 for immunotherapy of genital herpes. Lancet 1994; 343: 1460–3.

63 Katze M, He Y, Gale M. Viruses and interferon: a fight for supremacy. Immunology 2002; 2: 675–87.

64 Mikloska Z, Cunningham AL. Alpha and gamma interferons inhibit herpes simplex virus type 1 infection and spread in epidermal cells after axonal transmission. J Virol 2001; 75: 11821–6.

65 Sainz B, Jr., Halford WP. Alpha/Beta interferon and gamma interferon synergize to inhibit the replication of herpes simplex virus type 1. J Virol 2002; 76: 11541–50.

7

Atopic dermatitis: the role of fungi

Randolf BS Brehler, Melanie Mertens, and Thomas A Luger

INTRODUCTION

Atopic dermatitis (AD) is a chronic, itching, inflammatory skin disease with increasing incidence especially in countries with a Western lifestyle. Genetic factors, immunodeviation, skin barrier defects and exposure to allergens, air pollution, and other environmental factors are postulated to be relevant for the pathogenesis of this skin disease. Nevertheless so far we do not have one consistent pathogenetic concept of AD. There is increasing evidence that AD is not only one entity; in this context an extrinsic form of AD has been defined, which is characterised by elevated serum IgE levels and immediate-type sensitization against environmental allergens. In contrast to extrinsic AD, which can be triggered by exposure to allergens and various other environmental factors, the intrinsic form is characterized by normal serum IgE levels and absent sensitization to aero-allergens. But also in patients with the intrinsic form of AE IgE- and T-cell-mediated reactivity against *Malassezia sympodialis* was found.

Staphylococcus aureus superantigens can trigger IgE production and can induce skin inflammation. There is increasing evidence that other microorganisms may also be involved in the pathogenesis of AD. Significant differences in the colonisation of the skin have been observed between normal skin and the eczematous skin of patients with AD.

The relevance of the skin flora for AD is indicated by:

- The efficacy of a topical treatment with antiseptics such as clioquinol and triclosan.
- The efficacy of topically applied antibiotics such as sulphonamides, gentamicin, and mupirocin.
- The efficacy of topically applied gammaglobulins.
- The efficacy of oral antibiotics and antimycotics in controlled studies.

In this chapter we give an overview about the relevance of fungi in the pathogenetic concepts of AD.

FUNGI WITH RELEVANCE FOR ATOPIC DERMATITIS

In recent years evidence has grown that yeasts, especially of the genera *Malassezia* and *Candida* can be relevant for the pathogenesis of AD.[1-4]

Many clinical studies demonstrate that the colonisation of the skin and subsequent sensitization to *Malassezia* yeasts can trigger skin inflammation and play a role in the pathogenesis of AD. *Malassezia* yeasts are members of the normal human cutaneous flora but on the other hand these fungi are associated with different skin diseases such as pityriasis versicolor, *Malassezia folliculitis* and seborrhoeic dermatitis.

The concentration of yeasts on the skin must not necessarily be increased in yeast-associated diseases; therefore individual immunological or skin barrier alterations may be primarily relevant for the development of the above-mentioned diseases. Several studies demonstrate that exclusively patients with AD are sensitized to these yeasts. Sensitization was shown by skin tests with *Malassezia* extracts and by the analysis of *Malassezia*-specific IgE antibodies. Patients with head and neck AD (HNAD) are especially sensitized to these microorganisms.

While the skin colonisation with *Malassezia* species should be a trigger for AD, the gastrointestinal colonisation with *Candida albicans* may also be of relevance. Like *Malassezia* from the skin, *C. albicans* can frequently be cultivated from faeces of healthy individuals and sensitization also to *C. albicans* was observed mostly in patients with AD.

Information about the skin colonisation with *Candida* yeasts is rare but there is evidence that this yeast can also be isolated in a higher percentage from the skin of patients with AD than from the skin of healthy controls.

MALASSEZIA INFECTION IN ATOPIC DERMATITIS

Nomenclature of *Malassezia* yeasts

Malassezia yeasts were first identified in the late 1800s and in later studies different names have been used. Because of two main forms of the yeasts, an oval and a round form, their old names are *Pityrosporum ovale* and *Pityrosporum orbiculare*. In the current nomenclature the term *Malassezia* is favoured.

There are 7 different species of *Malassezia (M. furfur, M. pachydermatis, M. sympodialis, M. globosa, M. slooffiae, M. restricta, M. obtusa)* characterized by biochemical and molecular methods, but the clinical significance of each of these species is not clearly understood. Epidemiological studies gave evidence that the prevalence of the different *Malassezia* species vary between healthy individuals and patients with various skin diseases. On the other hand there was also a variation of the most commonly isolated species in different countries.

Skin colonization with *Malassezia*

A great variation in the density and presence in various skin locations has been reported. Highest concentrations were found on the scalp and the upper trunk, lowest on the hands.[5] The density of *Malassezia* yeasts decreases with increasing age; on the other hand the number of yeast cells is larger in adults compared to children.[6,7]

The colonization of the skin with *Malassezia* was analysed in 112 individuals suffering from seborrhoeic dermatitis (20 of 39 were HIV-positive patients), pityriasis versicolor (18 patients), AD (18 patients), and 37 control patients without dermatological lesions. *M. globosa* was the most common species, isolated from 37.5% of the investigated individuals, followed by *M. sympodialis* in 31.3%, and *M. furfur* in 31.3%. In patients with pityriasis versicolor and in HIV-positive patients *M. globosa* was predominant in 67% and 85% of the cases. In non-HIV patients with AD or seborrhoeic dermatitis, *M. furfur* and *M. restricta* were isolated in 72% and 26% of the cases, respectively. It has been concluded that *Malassezia* species were present on the skin of patients with and without dermatological diseases. *Malassezia globosa* especially was found in a high frequency on the skin of patients with dermatological disorders suggesting a higher pathogenicity of this species.[8]

Specific IgE antibodies to *Malassezia*

Specific IgE antibodies to *Malassezia* have been analysed in several clinical trials and were found in 20–100% of the analysed serum samples. The prevalence was highest in adults with HNAD, lower in adults with AD in other

Table 7.1 Specific IgE antibodies to *Malassezia* in different populations. (Modified from Bayrou O, Pecquet C, Flahault A et al. Head and neck atopic dermatitis and Malassezia-furfur-specific IgE antibodies. Dermatology 2005; 211: 107–13.)

Author	Population	Positive %
Johansson et al[9]	AD children	19
Wessels et al[10]	AD	49
	Atopy, no AD	3.7
Jensen-Jarolim et al[11]	HNAD	35
Broberg et al[12]	AD, patients 0–21 years old	14
	Atopy but no AD	3
Lindgren et al[13]	AD, children 4–16 years old	21.8
Back et al[14]	AD	44
Kawano et al[15]	AD	77
Nissen et al[16]	AD	93
Scalabrin et al[17]	AD adults	65
	AD children	13
Kim et al[18]	HNAD	68
Devos et al[19]	HNAD	100
	Non-HNAD	13.6
Mayser et al[20]	HNAD	55
	Generalised AD	34
	AD of the extremities	10
Johansson et al[21]	HNAD	55
	Non-HNAD	19
Arzumanyan et al[22]	AD	28
Bayrou et al[4]	HNAD	100
	Non-HNAD	28
	Contact eczema	0
	Seborrheic dermatis	6.25

localisations and lowest in children (Table 7.1). The localisation of AD was included only in a few studies, but all of these trials reported a high prevalence of sensitization to *Malassezia*, especially in HNAD.

Patients with other skin diseases were sensitized to *Malassezia* species only in single cases.

In the study from Bayrou specific IgE to *Malassezia* was found in all 106 serum samples of patients with HNAD, in 7 of the 25 patients with AD in other localisations, in 1 of 16 patients with seborrhoeic dermatitis and in none of the patients with contact dermatitis. A strong correlation was found between the severity of HNAD and specific IgE levels. Specific IgE antibodies to *Malassezia* were a very good and specific marker of HNAD in this study.[4]

Table 7.2   Skin prick tests to *Malassezia* in different populations. (Modified from Bayrou O, Pecquet C, Flahault A et al. Head and neck atopic dermatitis and Malassezia-furfur-specific IgE antibodies. Dermatology 2005; 211: 107–13.)

Author	Population	Positive %
Clemmensen et al[23]	HNAD	32
Waersted et al[24]	HNAD	28
	Non-HNAD	6
Young et al[25]	AD	59
	Atopy, no AD	0
Kieffer et al[26]	HNAD	79
	Non-HNAD	45
	Seborrheic dermatitis	0
Rokugo et al[27]	AD < 10 years	39
	AD > 10 years	64
Broberg et al[12]	AD 0–21 years	23
	Atopy, no AD	0
Broberg et al[28]	HNAD 14–53 years	55
	Non-HNAD	15
Tanaka et al[29]	AD	40
Nissen et al[16]	AD	60
Kim et al[18]	HNAD	45
Devos et al[19]	HNAD	13.5
	Non-HNAD	86.5
Johansson et al[21]	HNAD	56
	Non-HNAD	36
	Seborrhoeic dermatitis	0
	Healthy controls	0
Khosravi et al[54]	AD	49.6
	Healthy controls	6.7

Table 7.3   Patch tests with *Malassezia* allergens in different populations

Author	Population	Positive %
Tengvall-Linder et al[30]	AD	53.3
	Seborrhoeic dermatitis	0
	Healthy controls	0
Rokugo et al[27]	AD	64
	Healthy controls	3
Kieffer et al[26]	AD	13
	Seborrhoeic dermatitis	0
	Healthy controls	0
Johansson et al[21]	AD	37.8
	HNAD	41
	Seborrhoeic dermatitis	7.1
	Healthy controls	0

Skin prick tests with *Malassezia*

Positive skin prick tests with *Malassezia* extracts were found in a range between 13.5–79% of patients with AD (Table 7.2). Only a minority of patients without AD, including patients with *Malassezia*-related skin diseases like seborrhoeic dermatitis, were sensitized.

Immediate-type sensitization to *Malassezia* species is therefore almost exclusively found in patients with AD. Nevertheless the concentration of these yeasts was found to be higher on the skin of healthy volunteers and patients with skin diseases other than AD. This indicates that *Malassezia* itself is not a pathogen in AD, but the interaction of microorganisms with the immune system of patients with AD may be altered. Barrier destruction may be a primary defect of the AD skin and thus may enhance the penetration of yeast allergens

through the skin. Therefore a skin barrier defect may be responsible for sensitization to this species of microorganisms which belongs to the normal skin flora.

Atopy patch test with *Malassezia*

Atopy patch testing with aero-allergens is an established diagnostic procedure and a positive test demonstrates that AD can be aggravated due to exposure to aero-allergens. In this context house the dust mite, especially, is a frequent trigger factor for AD in previously sensitized patients.

Malassezia allergens were used in atopy patch tests (APT) in a few clinical studies (Table 7.3). Positive test results were observed in patients with AD. These patients had significantly higher *Pityrosporum orbiculare*-specific IgE serum levels.[30] All healthy controls were negative in patch tests with *Malassezia* extracts in this study.

In a second study recombinant *Malassezia* allergens (Mal s 1, Mal s 5, and Mal s 6) were used in addition to *M. furfur* extract:[21] 67% of 132 patients with mild to severe AD were positive, while 13 of 14 patients with seborrhoeic dermatitis and all 33 healthy controls were negative.

In conclusion there is evidence that *Malassezia* can induce eczematous reactions in already sensitized patients with AD and can play therefore a role as a trigger in eliciting and maintaining eczema. It may be advisable to add *Malassezia* allergens to the APT panel.

Other immunological responses to *Malassezia*

Malassezia can stimulate keratinocytes to produce inflammatory cytokines such as TNF-α, IL-6, and IL-8.[31] The maturation of dendritic cells can be induced by *Malassezia* and can therefore induce an increased production of

TNF-α, IL-1β, and IL18 in these cells.[32,33] Aspres et al summarized the mechanisms of *Malassezia* yeasts in the pathogenesis of AD. *Malassezia* yeasts trigger a variety of immunological mechanisms by the stimulation of specific IgE antibodies and the stimulation of allergen specific T cells. IgE-associated activation of allergen-specific T cells stimulates cell-mediated immune responses, mainly involving TH$_2$ cytokine expression. This could be augmented by immediate-type hypersensitivity responses from direct stimulation of IgE-bearing cells and additionally through *Malassezia*-induced complement activation and the release of cytokines by keratinocytes. These mechanisms could cause itch; scratching leads to further skin barrier dysfunction and skin inflammation. A continuous exposure to *Malassezia* allergens could then be responsible for repeated triggering of the host immune system.[34]

CANDIDA INFECTION IN ATOPIC DERMATITIS

More than 50 different *Candida* species have been characterized and many of these species can be isolated from human sources but only a few are dominant. *Candida* can be isolated from normal skin but is more frequently present in the gastrointestinal tract and on mucous membranes. *Candida* colonisation does not imply illness; *Candida* is present in up to 65% of asymptomatic individuals.[35] Skin diseases like immune deficiency, diabetes mellitus, hormonal dysfunction, and the use of drugs like oral antibiotics and corticosteroids predispose to infections with *Candida* yeasts.

Candida colonization and atopic dermatitis

It has been reported that *Candida* species especially *Candida albicans* can be cultivated more frequently from normal and lesional skin of patients with AD than from healthy controls.[35,36] More important is the colonization of the gastrointestinal system with *Candida* yeasts, which has been demonstrated in 70% of patients with AD and in 54% of healthy controls.[37]

Sensitisation to *Candida albicans*

Skin prick tests with *C. albicans* extract have been performed in several clinical studies and were found to be positive in 22 to 94% of patients with AD. Furthermore the number of positive patients correlated with the severity of the skin disease (Table 7.4).

Specific IgE to *Candida*

Specific IgE antibodies to *C. albicans* extracts were found in the range between 25–88% of patients

Table 7.4 Skin prick tests with *Candida* extracts in different populations

Author	Population	Positive %
Savolainen et al[38]	AD	52
	Allergic rhinitis	22
	Healthy controls	5
Kortekangas-Savolainen et al[39]	Severe AD	94
	Moderate AD	76
	Mild AD	25
	Allergic rhinitis	8
	Healthy controls	2
Tanaka et al[29]	AD	30
	Healthy controls	10
Nissen et al[16]	AD	27

Table 7.5 Patch tests with *Candida* allergens in different populations

Author	Population	Positive %
Tanaka et al[29]	Healthy controls	86
	AD	49
Matsumura et al[42]	Healthy controls	84
	Respiratory disease	90
	AD	34

with AD.[14,16,17,29,38,40,41–46] A cross-reactivity between allergens from *C. albicans* and *Malassezia* was described by Doeckes et al.[40] As a result of inhibition tests they postulated a primary sensitization to *Malassezia* and a secondary IgE reactivity to *C. albicans* allergens due to cross-reactive IgE antibodies.

Delayed-type hypersensitivity to *Candida albicans*

Patch tests or scarification patch tests with *C. albicans* were performed in some clinical studies. Positive results were observed in fewer patients with AD compared to healthy controls and patients with respiratory diseases but without AD (Table 7.5). In lymphocyte stimulation/ transformation tests (LTT) the stimulation of PBMC from donors with AD to *C. albicans* allergens was significant lower compared to cells from healthy controls.[29]

Table 7.6 Treatment of AD patients with antifungal drugs. (Modified from Faergemann J. Atopic dermatitis and funghi. Clin Microbiol Rev 2002; 15: 545–63.)

Author	Duration	Treatment	Design	Results
Ikezawa et al[47]	8 weeks	Oral itraconazole/probiotics	Crossover study	Active > probiotics
Svejgaard et al[48]	1 week	Oral itraconazole	Double blind	Active > placebo
Bäck et al[49]	3 months	Oral itraconazole	Double blind	Active = placebo
Clemmensen et al[23]	4 weeks	Oral ketoconazole	Double-blind crossover	Active > placebo
Bäck et al[14]	4 months	Oral ketoconazole	Open	Active > placebo
Morita et al[45]	3 months	Oral ketoconazole or oral fluconazole	Open	Ketoconazole = fluconazole
Lintu et al[50]	30 days	Oral ketoconazole	Double blind	Active > placebo
White et al[51]		Topical hydrocortisone + miconazole	Open	Active > placebo
Broberg et al[52]	4 weeks	Topical hydrocortisone + miconazole	Double blind	Active = placebo
Mayser et al[55]	28 days	Topical ciclopiroxolamine	Double blind	Active > placebo

Both test systems demonstrate that the *C. albicans*-specific T cell does not seem to play a role in the pathogenesis of AD.

It was concluded that persistent exposure to *C. albicans* leads to the development of immediate-type hypersensitivity and a decrease or loss of delayed-type hypersensitivity to this allergen.

ANTIFUNGAL TREATMENT OF PATIENTS WITH ATOPIC DERMATITIS

The yeast colonization of the skin can be reduced by a topical antifungal treatment; a systemic therapy also reduces yeast on mucous membranes. The efficacy of an antifungal treatment in AD patients was studied in a few clinical trials which are summarised in Table 7.6.

In most clinical trials a systemic antifungal treatment was effective and reduced the severity of AD. Unspecific anti-inflammatory effects of the drugs used are quite possible and the efficacy of antifungal treatment in AD may not be related to the reduction of yeasts.

CONCLUSION

There are conflicting data in the literature about the role of fungi in AD. The colonization of the skin with *Malassezia* species, the subsequent sensitization to this yeast, and positive patch tests with *Malassezia* extracts in patients with AD are not convincing proofs for the relevance of this yeast in the pathogenesis of AD; it could be a result of the skin barrier defect in these patients. On the other hand phylogenetically conserved allergen structures such as manganese superoxide dismutase (MnSOD) are present in fungi and in human cells. Interestingly, IgE- and T-cell-mediated reactivity against *Malassezia* was found in patients with extrinsic as in patients with intrinsic AE and occurs specifically in AE patients.[56] In a subset of patients with AD sensitization to *Malassezia*, MnSOD should result in enhancing skin inflammation due to a molecular mimicry and cross-reactivity between fungal and human proteins.[53] Therefore fungi are not causative for the development of AD but may aggravate the skin disease in some patients. New double-blind, placebo-controlled clinical trials with sufficient numbers of patients with well-characterized AD must clarify which patients with AD have a significant benefit from an antifungal therapy.

REFERENCES

1. Faergemann J. Atopic dermatitis and funghi. Clin Microbiol Rev 2002; 15: 545–63.
2. Allam J-P, Bieber T. Review of recent journal highlights focusing on atopic dermatitis. Clin Exp Dermatol 2003; 28: 577–8.
3. Roll A, Cozzio A, Fischer B, Schmid-Grendelmeier P. Microbial colonization and atopic dermatitis. Curr Opin Allergy Clin Immunol 2004; 4: 373–8.

4. Bayrou O, Pecquet C, Flahault A et al. Head and neck atopic dermatitis and Malassezia-furfur-specific IgE antibodies. Dermatology 2005; 211: 107–13.

5. Leeming JP, Notman FH, Holland KT. The distribution and ecology of Malassezia furfur and cutaneous bacteria on human skin. J Appl Bacteriol 1989; 67: 47–52.

6. Bergbrant IM, Faergemann J. Variations of Pityrosporum orbiculare in middle-aged and elderly individuals. Acta Derm Venereol 1988; 68: 537–40.

7. Bergbrant IM, Broberg A. Pityrosporum ovale culture from the forehead of healthy children. Acta Derm Venerol 1994; 74: 260–1.

8. Rincon S, Celis A, Sopo L, Motta A, Cepero de Garcia MC. Malassezia yeast species isolated from patients with dermatologic lesions. Biomedica 2005; 25: 189–95.

9. Johansson S, Karlstrom K. IgE-binding components in Pityrosporum orbiculare identified by an immunoblotting technique. Acta Derm Venereol 1991; 71: 11–16.

10. Wessels MW, Doekes G, Van Ieperen-Van Dijk AG, Koers WJ, Young E. IgE antibodies to Pityrosporum ovale in atopic dermatitis. Br J Dermatol 1991; 125: 227–32.

11. Jensen-Jarolim E, Poulsen LK, With H et al. Atopic dermatitis of the face, scalp, and neck: type I reaction to the yeast Pityrosporum ovale? J Allergy Clin Immunol 1992; 89: 44–51.

12. Broberg A, Faergemann J, Johansson S et al. Pityrosporum ovale and atopic dermatitis in children and young adults. Acta Derm Venereol 1992; 72: 187–92.

13. Lindgren L, Wahlgren CF, Johansson SG, Wiklund I, Nordvall SL. Occurrence and clinical features of sensitization to Pityrosporum orbiculare and other allergens in children with atopic dermatitis. Acta Derm Venereol 1995; 75: 300–4.

14. Back O, Scheynius A, Johansson SG. Ketoconazole in atopic dermatitis. Therapeutic response is correlated with decrease in serum IgE. Arch Dermatol Res 1995; 287: 448–51.

15. Kawano S, Nakagawa H. The correlation between the levels of anti-Malassezia furfur IgE antibodies and severities of face and neck dermatitis of patients with atopic dermatitis. Arerugi 1995; 44: 128–33.

16. Nissen D, Petersen LJ, Esch R et al. IgE-sensitization to cellular and culture filtrates of fungal extracts in patients with atopic dermatitis. Ann Allergy Asthma Immunol 1998; 81: 247–55.

17. Scalabrin DM, Bavbek S, Perzanowski MS et al. Use of specific IgE in assessing the relevance of fungal and dust mite allergens to atopic dermatitis: a comparison with asthmatic and nonasthmatic control subjects. J Allergy Clin Immunol 1999; 104: 1273–9.

18. Kim TY, Jang IG, Park YM, Kim HO, Kim CW. Head and neck dermatitis: the role of Malassezia furfur, topical steroid use and environmental factor in its causation. Clin Exp Dermatol 1999; 24: 226–31.

19. Devos SA, van der Valk PGM. The relevance of skin prick tests for Pityrosporum orbiculare in patients with head and neck dermatitis. Allergy 2000; 55: 1056–8.

20. Mayser P, Gross A. IgE antibodies to Malassezia furfur, M. sympodialis and Pityrosporum orbiculare in patients with atopic dermatitis, seborrheic eczema or pityriasis versicolor, and identification of respective allergens. Acta Derm Venereol 2000; 80: 357–61.

21. Johansson C, Sandstrom MH, Bartosik J et al. Atopy patch test reactions to Malassezia allergens differentiate subgroups of atopic dermatitis patients. Br J Dermatol 2003; 148: 479–88.

22. Arzumanyan VG, Serdyuk OA, Kozlova NN et al. IgE and IgG antibodies to Malassezia spp. yeast extract in patients with atopic dermatitis. Bull Exp Biol Med 2003; 135: 460–3.

23. Clemmensen OJ, Hjorth N. Treatment of dermatitis of the head and neck with ketoconazole in patients with type I sensitivity to Pityrosporum orbiculare. Semin Dermatol 1983; 2: 26–9.

24. Waersted A, Hjorth N. Pityrosporum orbiculare – a pathogenic factor in atopic dermatitis of the face, scalp and neck? Acta Derm Venereol 1985; 114: 146–8.

25. Young E, Koers WJ, Berrens L. Intracutaneous tests with Pityrosporon extract in atopic dermatitis. Acta Derm Venereol Suppl (Stockh) 1989; 144: 122–4.

26. Kieffer M, Bergbrant IM, Faergemann J et al. Immune reactions to Pityrosporum ovale in adult patients with atopic and seborrheic dermatitis. J Am Acad Dermatol 1990; 22: 739–42.

27. Rokugo M, Tagami H, Usuba Y, Tomita Y. Contact sensitivity to Pityrosporum ovale in patients with atopic dermatitis. Arch Dermatol 1990; 126: 627–32.

28. Broberg A, Faergemann J, Johansson S et al. Pityrosporum ovale and atopic dermatitis in children and young adults. Acta Derm Venereol 1992; 72: 187–92.

29. Tanaka M, Aiba S, Matsumura N, Aoyama H et al. IgE-mediated hypersensitivity and contact sensitivity to multiple environmental allergens in atopic dermatitis. Arch Dermatol 1994; 130: 1393–401.

30. Tengvall-Linder M, Johansson C, Scheynius A, Wahlgren CF. Positive patch test reactions to Pityrosporim orbiculare in atopic dermatitis patients. Clin Exp Allergy 2000; 30: 122–31.

31. Watanabe S, Kano R, Sato H, Nakamura Y, Hasegawa A. The effects of Malassezia yeasts on cytokine production by human keratinocytes. J Invest Dermatol 2001; 116: 769–73.

32. Buentke E, Zargari A, Heffler LC et al. Uptake of the yeast Malassezia furfur and its allergenic components by human immature CD1a+ dendritic cells. Clin Exp Allergy 2000; 30: 1759–70.

33. Buentke E, Heffler LC, Wallin RP et al. The allergenic yeast Malassezia furfur induces maturation of human dendritic cells. Clin Exp Allergy 2001; 31: 1583–93.

34. Aspres N, Anderson C. Malassezia yeasts in the pathogenesis of atopic dermatitis. Australas J Dermatol 2004; 45: 199–205.

35. Odds FC, ed. Candida and Candidosis, 2nd edn. Baltimore: WB Saunders, 1988.

36. Arzumanyan VG, Magarshak OO, Semenov BF. Yeast fungi in patients with allergic diseases: species variety and sensitivity to antifungal drugs. Biull Eksp Biol Med 2000; 129: 601–4.

37. Buslau M, Menzel I, Holzmann H. Fungal flora of human faeces in psoriasis and atopic dermatitis. Mycoses 1988; 33: 90–4.

38. Savolainen J, Lammintausta K, Kalimo K, Viander M. Candida albicans and atopic dermatitis. Clin Exp Allergy 1993; 23: 332–9.

39. Kortekangas-Savolainen O, Kalimo K, Lammintausta K, Savolainen J. IgE-binding components of baker's yeast (Saccharomyces cerevisiae) recognized by immunoblotting analysis. Simultaneous IgE binding to mannan and 46-48 kD allergens of Saccharomyces cerevisiae and Candida albicans. Clin Exp Allergy 1993; 23: 179–84.

40. Doekes GMJ, Kaal MJH, van Leperen-van Dijk AG. Allergens of Pityrosporum ovale and Candida albicans. II. Physicochemical characterization. Allergy 1993; 48: 401–8.

41. Nermes M, Falth-Magnusson K, Savolainen J, Viander M, Bjorksten B. A comparison of the development of antibody responses to the polysaccharide antigen (Candida albicans mannan) in atopic and healthy infants and children. Clin Exp Allergy 1996; 26: 164–70.

42. Matsumura N, Aiba S, Tanaka M et al. Comparison of immune reactivity profiles against various environmental allergens between adult patients with atopic dermatitis and patients with allergic respiratory diseases. Acta Derm Venereol 1997; 77: 388–91.

43. Kawamura MS, Aiba S, Tagami H. The importance of CD54 and CD86 costimulation in T cells stimulated with Candida albicans and Dermatophagoides farinae antigens in patients with atopic dermatitis. Arch Dermatol Res 1998; 290: 603–9.

44. Savolainen J, Kortekangas-Savolainen O, Nermes M et al. IgE, IgA, and IgG responses to common yeasts in atopic patients. Allergy 1998; 53: 506–12.

45. Morita E, Hide M, Yoneya Y et al. An assessment of the role of Candida albicans antigen in atopic dermatitis. J Dermatol 1999; 26: 282–7.

46. Adachi A, Horikawa T, Itchihashi M, Takashima T, Komura A. Role of Candida allergen in atopic dermatitis and efficacy of oral therapy with various antifungal agents. Arerugi 1999; 48: 719–25.

47. Ikezawa Z, Kondo M, Okajima M, Nishimura Y, Kono M. Clinical usefulness of oral itraconazole, an antimycotic drug, for refractory atopic dermatitis. Eur J Dermatol 2004; 14: 400–6.

48. Svejgaard E, Larsen PO, Deleuran M et al. Treatment of head and neck dermatitis comparing itraconazole 200 mg and 400 mg daily for 1 week with placebo. J Eur Acad Dermatol Venereol 2004; 18: 445–9.

49. Back O, Scheynius A, Johansson SGO. Ketoconazole in atopic dermatitis: therapeutic response is correlated with decrease in serum IgE. Arch Dermatol Res 1995; 287: 448–51.

50. Lintu P, Savolainen J, Kortekangas-Savolainen O, Kalimo K. Systemic ketoconazole is an effective treatment of atopic dermatitis with IgE-mediated hypersensitivity to yeasts. Allergy 2001; 56: 512–17.

51. White I, Blatchford I. The treatment of secondary bacterial infections in atopic eczema with miconazole plus hydrocortisone. Br J Clin Pract 1983: 215–16.

52. Broberg A, Faergemann J. Topical antimycotic treatment of atopic dermatitis in the head/neck area. Acta Derm Venereol 1995; 75: 46–9.

53. Schmid-Grendelmeier P, Scheynius A, Crameri R. The role of sensitization to Malassezia sympodialis in atopic eczema. Chem Immunol Allergy 2006; 91: 98–109.

54. Khosravi AR, Hedayati MT, Mansouri P et al. Immediate hypersensitivity to Malassezia furfur in patients with atopic dermatitis. Mycoses 2007; 50: 297–301.

55. Mayser P, Kupfer J, Nemetz D et al. Treatment of head and neck dermatitis with ciclopiroxolamine cream – results of a double-blind, placebo-controlled study. Skin Pharmacol Physiol 2006; 19: 153–8.

56. Casagrande BF, Flückiger S, Linder MT et al. Sensitization to the yeast Malassezia intrinsic atopic eczema. J Invest Dermatol 2006; 126: 2414–21.

8

Role of food allergens in atopic dermatitis

Ralf G Heine, David J Hill, and Clifford S Hosking

INTRODUCTION

Atopic dermatitis (AD) is a chronic relapsing inflammatory skin disorder associated with increased serum IgE levels and sensitization to food or environmental allergens.[1,2] AD affects between 10–21% of young infants[3–5] and is associated with a significant financial burden.[6] There is often a family history of allergic diseases, highlighting the importance of genetic factors in the pathogenesis of AD.[7–10]

Over the years, many studies have examined the association of AD and food hypersensitivity in children and adults.[11–45] The role of hypersensitivity to food antigens in the induction and maintenance of AD has remained an area of controversy. Several reviews by dermatologists have concluded that IgE food allergy affects only a minority of patients with AD,[46–48] whereas Sampson reported that 74% of selected children with AD deteriorated clinically on formal food challenge.[49] The Melbourne Atopy Cohort Study (MACS) has demonstrated a close association between both conditions, particularly in infants with severe AD.[27] In older children and adults, this association is less well defined, as IgE-mediated food allergies are less common than in infancy.[50]

Our understanding of the mechanisms and clinical manifestations of food allergies has improved in recent years.[51,52] In this review, the terms 'food allergy' and 'food hypersensitivity' will be used to indicate an adverse clinical reaction due to the interaction of food proteins with one or more immune mechanisms.[51,53] 'Food intolerance' is the result of non-immunological reactions to foods or food additives. Apart from the immediate-type IgE-mediated manifestations, other non-IgE mediated forms of food allergy with a delayed onset have been characterized.[53,54] This chapter will review the role of IgE- and non-IgE mediated food hypersensitivity in the pathogenesis of AD.

PREVALENCE OF FOOD ALLERGY

In recent years, the prevalence of atopic diseases and food allergies appears to have increased in many Western countries. Food allergy has its greatest incidence in infancy and early childhood.[55] It is estimated that about 8% of children will develop adverse reactions to food, most of them in the first year of life.[51] The prevalence of food allergy varies between regions and appears to be influenced by cultural and genetic factors.[3] For example, hypersensitivity to cow's milk and egg is uncommon in Southeast Asia, whereas peanut hypersensitivity is uncommon in Malaysia, Japan and the Philippines.[54] Conversely, shellfish hypersensitivity is common in children from the Philippines and Singapore where it is part of the diet from early infancy, but it is uncommon in Western children.

Despite the overall increase in the incidence of food allergies in Western countries, the spectrum of food allergens has remained relatively unchanged over the past decade, and sensitization to minor food allergens has remained uncommon.[14] In children, seven food items account for about 90% of allergic reactions to foods. These include cow's milk, egg, peanuts, soybeans, wheat, fish, and tree nuts.[56] The majority of children will develop tolerance to these food items by 3 years of age, with the exception of peanuts and tree nuts. In adults, IgE mediated food hypersensitivity is much less common. The main food allergens in adults are peanuts, tree nuts, fish, and shellfish (Table 8.1).

The prevalence of cow's milk allergy (CMA) in Australian infants under 2 years of age is 2.0% - second only to egg allergy (3.2%) (Table 8.2).[57] Prevalence figures for food allergy in that study were similar to those reported from other cohorts.[58,59] In adults, IgE-mediated food allergy is relatively uncommon. A recent Australian study investigated 1141 randomly selected young adults between 25–40 years of

Table 8.1 Major food allergens in children and adults. (Reproduced from Burks W, Helm R, Stanley S et al. Food Allergens. Curr Opin Allergy Clin Immunol 2001; 1: 243–8.)

Infants and children	Adults
Cow's milk	Peanut
Egg	Tree nuts
Peanut	Fish
Tree nuts	Shellfish
Soy	
Wheat	
Fish	

Table 8.2 Prevalence of allergy to common food proteins in Australian infants. (Reproduced from Hill DJ, Hosking CS, Zhie CY et al. The frequency of food allergy in Australia and Asia. Environ Toxicol Pharmacol 1997; 4: 101–10.)

Egg	3.2%
Cow's milk	2.0%
Peanut	1.9%
Sesame seed	0.42%
Cashew nut	0.33%
Hazelnut	0.18%
Walnut	0.16%
Brazil nut	0.07%
Almond	0.02%
Wheat	0.15%
Soy	0.10%
Fish	0.07%

age.[50] The overall prevalence of probable food allergies to cow's milk, egg white, peanut, shrimp, or wheat was 1.3%. Peanut allergy was associated with a history of asthma or eczema, but firm conclusions could not be drawn possibly due to the relatively small number of affected subjects in that study. Similarly, a Spanish study of 3034 patients over 14 years found a prevalence for food hypersensitivity of 0.98%.[60] In that study, fruit and seafood were the predominant allergens, whereas allergy to cow's milk and egg was uncommon.

GENETIC FACTORS AND ATOPIC DERMATITIS IN FOOD ALLERGY

Susceptibility for AD is most probably determined by a complex interaction of genetic and environmental factors.[7] It has been shown that children of parents with AD have a higher risk of inheriting this condition, compared with offspring of parents with asthma or rhinitis, suggesting the presence of disease-specific genetic factors for AD.[61] Further evidence for the importance of inherited factors has been gained from twin studies showing a concordance rate for monozygotic twins of 72%, compared with 23% for dizygotic twins.[62]

The search for candidate genes is hampered by the genetic complexity of AD, asthma, and atopy in general. Several strategies have been developed to unravel the genetic basis of AD, including gene linkage and association analysis. The recent completion of the first draft of the human genome has provided a large database of microsatellite genetic markers that can be utilized for linkage dysequilibrium studies between marker and disease. In order to maximize the chances of identifying specific genes involved in the pathogenesis of AD, Forrest et al studied a homogeneous group of infants with early-onset severe AD.[10] However, to date no single gene has been identified as the gene responsible for the development of AD.

Several molecules are closely involved in the allergic response. These can be mapped to several chromosomal regions of interest which, in turn, can be further examined for gene polymorphisms. Examples for these candidate regions include the chromosomal regions 5q31 (interleukin (IL) gene cluster), 6p21 (major histocompatibility complex), 7q35 (T cell receptor β subunit), 11q13 (high affinity FCE receptor), 12q14 (interferon γ), 14q11 (T cell receptor α subunit and mast cell chymase) and 16p12 (IL-4 receptor).[8] One of the regions that has attracted significant interest is the IL gene cluster on chromosome 5. This area has previously been linked to IgE production in adults with respiratory diseases.[63] Three polymorphisms in the IL-4 gene have to date been identified. Elliott et al[9] recently studied the association of polymorphisms within the promoter region of IL-4 with AD in a cohort of nuclear families with early-onset AD. A new polymorphism, −34C/T, was identified and studied with a known polymorphism, −590C/T. Neither polymorphism appeared to predispose to early-onset AD by itself, although suggestive linkage was found for the experimental −590C/−34C haplotype.[9] Further studies in humans and animal models may provide further insight into the genetic basis of AD and may ultimately lead to new therapies, such as topical administration of therapeutic antisense RNA molecules. A detailed review of the genetics of AD is provided in Chapter 2.

Table 8.3 Common food allergens. (Modified from Burks W, Helm R, Stanley S et al. Food Allergens. Curr Opin Allergy Clin Immunol 2001; 1: 243–8.)		
Food item	**Protein**	**Molecular mass [M$_r$]**
Cow's milk	*Caseins*	
	α_1-casein	27 000
	α_2-casein	23 000
	β-casein	24 000
	κ-casein	19 000
	γ-casein	21 000
	Whey proteins	
	β-lactoglobulin	36 000
	α-lactalbumin	14 400
	Bovine serum albumin (BSA)	69 000
Egg white	Ovomucoid (Gal d 1)	28 000
	Ovalbumin (Gal d 2)	45 000
	Ovotransferrin/ conalbumin (Gal d 3)	77 000
	Lysozyme (Gal d 4)	14 300
Peanut	Vicilin (Ara h 1)	63 500
	Conglutin (Ara h 2)	17 500
	Glycinin (Ara h 3)	56 000
Soy bean	Gly m 1	34 000
	Trypsin inhibitor	20 500

COMMON FOOD ALLERGENS IN CHILDREN AND ADULTS

More than 50 food allergens have been characterized.[56] In general, high-protein foods are considered to be more allergenic. Certain molecular characteristics of a food protein are believed to determine its allergenic properties. Most food allergens are water-soluble glycoproteins that appear to be particularly resistant to food processing, cooking and digestion.[64] The main protein antigens for each food allergen are summarized in Table 8.3.

Cow's milk

Cow's milk proteins can be divided by acid precipitation into caseins (milk solids) and soluble whey proteins.

Casein constitutes 80% of cow's milk protein and is considered the major allergen. Its most abundant form, α_{s1}-casein, is the basis for most cow's milk-based infant formulae. Several major and minor binding epitopes for IgE and IgG have been mapped on α_{s1}-, β- and κ-casein.[65,66] Another major allergen is the whey protein β-lactoglobulin. This protein is relatively resistant to gastric acid which may explain its properties as a food allergen. Järvinen et al demonstrated IgE and IgG binding epitopes on both major whey proteins, β-lactoglobulin and α-lactalbumin.[67]

About 80% of cow's milk allergic infants will develop tolerance to cow's milk by 3 years of age, and CMA is relatively uncommon in older children and adults.[68,69] Several specific allergenic epitopes on casein and whey proteins appear to be predictive of long-term persistence of CMA beyond childhood and may become useful prognostic markers in the future. High levels of specific IgE antibodies to linear epitopes from α_{s1}- and β-casein also have been found to be predictive for persistence of CMA.[70]

Egg

Sensitization to chicken eggs is common in children with AD. About 50% of egg allergic infants will develop tolerance in early childhood.[71] In general, egg white represents the albumin fraction of the egg and appears to be more allergenic than the yolk. Proteins in egg white include the allergens ovalbumin (Gal d 2), ovomucoid (Gal d 1), ovotransferrin (Gal d 3), ovomucin, and lysozyme (Gal d 4). The glycoprotein ovomucoid (Gal d 1) has been identified as the major allergen in egg white.[72] Previously, ovalbumin (Gal d 2) was considered the main egg allergen.[72]

Peanut

Peanuts are one of the most allergenic foods and are often implicated in food-induced anaphylaxis[73] that may, rarely, be fatal.[74] Unlike other food allergies, peanut hypersensitivity usually persists into adult life.[75-77] The main peanut allergens were first discovered in sera from patients with AD.[78,79] Ara h 1, one of the seed storage proteins in peanut, is considered the major allergen.[78] Ara h 1 has been sequenced, and at least 23 specific IgE binding epitopes identified. Two other major peanut allergens, Ara h 2 and Ara h 3, have also been characterized.[79,80]

Soy

Soy bean is a member of the legume family, and there is significant cross-reactivity with other legumes, including peanut and peas. About 15% of infants with IgE-mediated cow's milk allergy are also sensitized to soy protein.[81] Several soy bean allergens have been characterized. Gly m 1 is a protein in the 7S fraction of the peanut globulins with several soy bean-specific IgE binding epitopes. The Kunitz soybean trypsin inhibitor is considered a minor soy allergen.[82]

Fish

Codfish allergy is common in North America and Scandinavia. Most patients with fish allergy are sensitized to the main codfish allergen, Gad c 1. This allergen is a small calcium-binding protein (parvalbumin) found in fish and other vertebrates.[83,84] Five IgE epitopes have been identified on Gad c 1. Several of the IgE epitopes on parvalbumin are also present in other fish species, explaining why patients are often sensitized to several species of fish.[85]

Shellfish

In general, crustaceans (e.g. shrimp, crab, crawfish) appear to be more allergenic than molluscs (e.g. oysters, scallops). Tropomyosin (Pen a 1) is the only major allergen in shrimp, representing 20% of total protein. Immunological similarities have been demonstrated between crustaceans, cockroaches, and house dustmite, implying tropomyosin as a possible pan-allergen.[56] Several IgE epitopes on tropomyosin have been identified, showing some variability between individuals. Although there is frequent in-vitro cross-reactivity between crustaceans and molluscs, this does not appear to be associated with significant clinical cross-reactivity.[64]

PATHOPHYSIOLOGY OF FOOD ALLERGY

After birth, the gastrointestinal system of the newborn is exposed to food proteins in breast milk as well as environmental bacteria. This represents a dramatic change compared with conditions in utero where the gut was perfused with swallowed amniotic fluid that is sterile and free of antigens.[86] There is even some evidence suggesting that IgE sensitization may occur as early as during the foetal period.[86,87] The gastrointestinal system has several barrier mechanisms to protect the newborn infant from microbial invasion, including gastric acid, proteolytic digestive enzymes, epithelial tight junctions, a protective mucus layer and, most importantly, the mucosal local immune system.[88] In order to avoid immune reactions against food antigens, the gastrointestinal immune system has the ability to down-regulate its responsiveness towards ingested soluble food antigens. This phenomenon is called 'oral tolerance'.

Food allergies in infancy can be conceptualized as a failure or impairment in developing oral tolerance. The pathological mechanisms involved in the development of oral tolerance and factors leading to food antigen sensitization are not completely understood.[89] The dose and frequency of exposure as well as biological characteristics of antigens are likely to affect the development of oral tolerance. Oral tolerance involves predominantly the down-regulation of T helper-1 (Th1) responses and of cell-mediated immunity. CD4+ lymphocytes have been shown to play an integral part in the induction and maintenance of oral tolerance.[90] The deviation from a Th1- to Th2-predominant immune response is believed to be mediated by cytokines such as TGF-β, which is derived from Th3 lymphocytes in the gut. IL-4 and IL-10 are also of likely importance in the mediation of oral tolerance.[91] Factors that may predispose to impaired oral tolerance include increased antigen uptake, decreased production of secretory IgA, and an imbalance in the Th2 response.[88] Early intestinal inflammation may also predispose to food antigen sensitization due to increased gut permeability and mucosal antigen uptake.

There is increasing evidence that maternally ingested antigens, such as cow's milk, egg, and peanut, are secreted into human milk and may sensitize the breast-fed infant.[92–95] Multiple food sensitization has been described in breast-fed infants.[96] Immunological host factors are likely to mediate the infant's risk of sensitization to food allergens through breast milk. Transforming growth factor-beta (TGF-β) is considered a key molecule in promoting development of oral tolerance. During early infancy, breast milk is the main source of TGF-β. Kalliomäki et al found that TGF-β promotes specific IgA production in human colostrum.[97] IgA antibodies in human milk have a protective effect on sensitization to food allergens as they may prevent antigen entry at the intestinal surface of infants. In a study of 87 breast-fed infants, IgA concentrations in colostrum and human milk were significantly lower in mothers whose infants developed CMA in the first 12 months of life.[98] Other factors that may mediate the immune response to ingested food antigens include regulatory lymphokines such as TNF-α and IFN-γ.[99]

Timing of allergic reactions in relation to food intake

Clinical manifestations after challenge with food allergens may develop immediately after intake, but may occur as late as 24–48 hours after ingestion.[26] Three clinical patterns of food allergic reactions can be identified: immediate, intermediate, and late-onset reactions. Different pathophysiological mechanisms and clinical

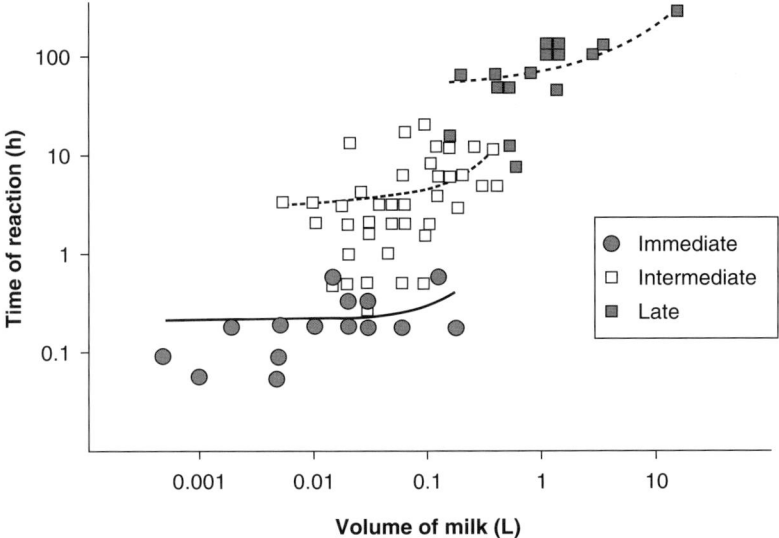

Figure 8.1   Onset of allergic reactions in relation to ingested volume of cow milk Reproduced from Hill DJ, Hosking CS, Heine RQ. Clinical spectrum of food allergy in children in Australia and South-East Asia: identification and targets for treatment. Ann Med 1999; 31: 272–81.

manifestations are associated with each type of reaction. Figure 8.1 illustrates the different timing of allergic reactions in infants with CMA.

Immediate reactions are usually IgE-mediated and present within minutes of exposure to food antigens. Manifestations range from the oral allergy syndrome, angiooedema, urticaria to bronchospasm and anaphylactic shock.[52] The *intermediate* group reacts within 1–24 hours after ingestion and presents predominantly with gastrointestinal symptoms, including vomiting and diarrhoea. They do not exhibit features of IgE sensitization.[26] The *late* group, with symptoms occurring from 24 hours up to 5 days after cow's milk challenge, presents with flares of AD or development of cough and wheeze. This group shows variable degrees of IgE sensitization and has evidence of allergen-specific T-cell proliferation.[26,29,100,101]

In infants with AD, the presence of non-IgE-mediated mechanisms appears to be of pathophysiological importance.[102] Schade et al provided evidence of T-cell activation in infants with CMA and AD.[103] In a cohort of infants with AD, all had evidence of specific T-helper cell reactivity to major cow's milk proteins. However, infants with clinical CMA showed a Th$_2$ predominant cytokine profile (high levels of IL-4, IL-5, and IL-13) whereas infants without CMA had a Th$_1$-skewed response (high level of IFNγ, low IL-4, IL-5, and IL-13). This study inferred that antigen-specific Th$_2$ cells may mediate the skin manifestations of children with AD and CMA.

ROLE OF FOOD ALLERGENS IN ATOPIC DERMATITIS

Food allergy is usually the earliest manifestation of atopy and may affect both breast- and formula-fed infants.[54,92] Early sensitization to food allergens is typically transient and followed by inhalant sensitization, as demonstrated by the appearance of specific serum IgE antibodies to inhalant allergens or positive skin prick tests (SPT).[104,105] This chapter will focus predominantly on the role of food allergens in AD, as the role of inhalant allergens will be discussed in Chapter 9.

Several studies have examined the relationship between AD and food hypersensitivity. In an early study by Sampson and McCaskill,[38] children with AD were evaluated for the presence of food allergies by double-blind placebo-controlled food challenges (DBPCFC): 85 (84%) children developed skin symptoms; of 113 children (median age 6 years, range 4 months to 24 years), 63 (56%) developed either skin, gastrointestinal, or respiratory symptoms in response to food challenge. Egg, peanut, and cow's milk accounted for 72% of all hypersensitivity reactions. The study showed that children with positive food challenges were younger than those without (median age 4.7 years vs 7.7. years), highlighting the possibility that the older children may have developed tolerance to food antigens.

Burks et al[11] performed a similar study in 46 children (mean age 5.7 years, range 9 months to 19 years) with

AD, using DBPCFC and SPT as the basis of their assessment for food allergies. They found that 28 (61%) children had positive skin tests to at least 1 food item. Again, egg, peanut, and milk accounted for the majority (78%) of food reactions. The authors concluded that the assessment for food allergies should be included in the management of persistent AD. A subsequent study by the same group has confirmed these results and has identified 7 important food items which accounted for 89% of positive challenges, including cow's milk, egg, peanut, soy, wheat, fish, and cashew nut.[12]

Eigenmann et al[19] studied the prevalence of food allergies in 63 children (median age 2.8 years) with moderately severe AD. Patients were screened for food-specific serum IgE antibodies to the six most common food allergens in childhood: milk, egg, wheat, soy, peanut, and fish. Patients were investigated for allergies by food-specific IgE levels and food challenge. Of 41 patients with positive specific IgE values, 31 were evaluated further, of whom 19 underwent a total of 50 food challenges (36 double-blind, placebo-controlled, and 14 open). Overall, the prevalence of clinically significant IgE-mediated food hypersensitivity was 37%.

In our study of 620 Australian infants (MACS) with a positive family history of food allergy, the association between sensitization to common food allergens and the presence of AD was prospectively evaluated.[27] In this cohort, the frequency of IgE-mediated hypersensitivity to cow's milk, egg, and peanut was assessed by skin prick testing in 559 infants under 16 months of age. Significantly more infants with AD had positive skin prick tests (≥ 6 mm weal) to cow's milk, egg, or peanut, compared to those without AD. Sensitization to multiple food antigens was common (Table 8.4). The calculated attributable risk for IgE-mediated food allergy as a cause of AD was 65% at 6 months, and 62% at 12 months. In the infants with severe AD, 83% had evidence of food sensitization at 6 months, and 65% at 12 months. Based on these results, infantile eczema is commonly associated with IgE-mediated hypersensitivity to foods, particularly in infants with clinically significant AD (Table 8.5).

The studies by Sampson et al,[38] Burks et al[11,12] and Eigenmann et al[19] demonstrated a lower prevalence of food allergies in AD, compared with the MACS cohort of young infants. Based on these observations it has become clearer that transient food allergies affect patients with AD mainly in the first 2 to 3 years, but particularly in the first 12 months of life, associated with sensitization to environmental and inhalant allergens. These may, in turn, contribute to ongoing skin symptoms later in older children and adults. A study of 45 adults with AD revealed sensitization to inhalant allergens in most patients, including grass pollen, house dust mite, and cat epithelium, and sensitization to food allergens was uncommon.[35] Given the relative infrequency of IgE food allergy in adults it is not surprising that food hypersensitivity is only considered to be of minor importance in adults with AD.

ANIMAL MODELS OF ATOPIC DERMATITIS

Several mouse models of food allergy and AD have been developed recently.[106–108] These mouse models may be useful in exploring the pathophysiology of food allergy and developing new experimental treatments or vaccines. The first mouse model of IgE-mediated CMA successfully mimicked some of the clinical features observed in humans.[106] In the following year, a model of peanut allergy and anaphylaxis was developed by the same group.[108] This model successfully sensitized mice to the major peanut allergens, and specific IgE antibodies to Ara h 1 and Ara h 2 were induced.

These sensitized mice also developed systemic symptoms similar to anaphylaxis on subsequent oral peanut exposure. Based on these models of IgE cow's milk and peanut allergy, a murine model of AD has recently been described.[107] Mice sensitized to cow's milk or peanut were subjected to low-grade allergen intake. About one- third of mice developed an eczematous eruption that histologically resembled AD. The lesion was positive for CD4+ lymphocytes, in keeping with AD. These findings provide further evidence for the importance of food allergens in the pathogenesis of AD and may provide new insights into the immunopathogenesis of AD.

DIAGNOSTIC INVESTIGATION

Double-blind placebo-controlled food challenge

Double-blind placebo-controlled food challenge (DBPCFC) is the definitive test for CMA.[43,109,110] DBPCFC, however, is resource-consuming and not without risks. Several studies have therefore examined to what extent specific serum IgE antibody, skin prick, or atopy patch testing (ATP) can replace formal food challenges in the diagnosis of food allergies.[32,34,41,111–120]

Food-specific IgE antibodies

Food antigen-specific IgE antibodies have been shown to be a useful tool in the assessment of immediate-type food allergy.[41,71,111–113] Sampson et al[41] measured food-specific IgE antibodies in serum samples from 196

Table 8.4 Frequency of IgE-mediated food allergy in infants with atopic dermatitis (AD). (Reproduced from Hill DJ, Hosking CS, Heine RG. Clinical spectrum of food allergy in children in Australia and South-East Asia: identification and targets for treatment. Ann Med 1999; 31: 272–81.)

No. of foods the subjects were allergic to	6 months of age MACS*						12 months of age MACS*					
	No AD		AD		Severe AD[†]		No AD		AD		Severe AD[†]	
	n	(%)	n	(%)	n	(%)	n	(%)	n	(%)	n	(%)
0	382	(95)	97	(78)	7	(17)	350	(89)	77	(64)	10	(35)
1	16	(4)	24	(19)	13	(32)	31	(8)	31	(26)	10	(34)
2	4	(1)	3	(2)	13	(32)	13	(3)	11	(9)	5	(17)
3	0	(0)	1	(1)	8	(20)	0	(0)	2	(2)	4	(2)
Total‡	20	(5)	28	(22)	34	(83)	44	(11)	44	(36)	19	(65)
Cases in total	402	(100)	125	(100)	41	(100)	394	(100)	121	(100)	29	(100)

*MACS – Melbourne Atopy Cohort Study subjects.
†This represents a separate group of infants with severe atopic dermatitis treated in a tertiary referral hospital outpatient clinic.
‡Sensitized (≥ 3+) to 1, 2 or 3 foods

Table 8.5 Incidence of IgE food sensitization in infants without and with atopic dermatitis of varying severity. (Modified from Hill DJ, Sporik R, Thorburn J et al. The association of atopic dermatitis in infancy with immunoglobulin E food sensitization. J Pediatr 2000; 137: 475–9.

	6 months of age		
	No AD	Mild to moderate AD	Severe AD
Number of patients	402	125	41
Cow's milk	4 (1)	4 (3)	21 (51)
Egg	16 (4)	23 (18)	29 (70)
Peanut	4 (1)	6 (5)	15 (37)
Any food	20 (5)	28 (22)	34 (83)
	12 months of age		
	No AD	Mild to moderate AD	Severe AD
Number of patients	394	121	29
Cow's milk	8 (2)	5 (4)	9 (31)
Egg	34 (9)	40 (33)	15 (52)
Peanut	15 (4)	14 (12)	11 (38)
Any food	44 (11)	44 (36)	19 (65)

patients with AD, allergic rhinitis or asthma, and challenge-proven food allergies. In that study, food-specific IgE cut-off levels for cow's milk, egg, peanut, and fish were determined that predicted the outcome of food challenges with more than 95% accuracy. These findings have recently been validated by the same author in a prospective study of 100 consecutive children and adolescents with suspected food allergies.[111] The previously found diagnostic cut-off levels for food-specific IgE antibodies were effective in predicting symptomatic

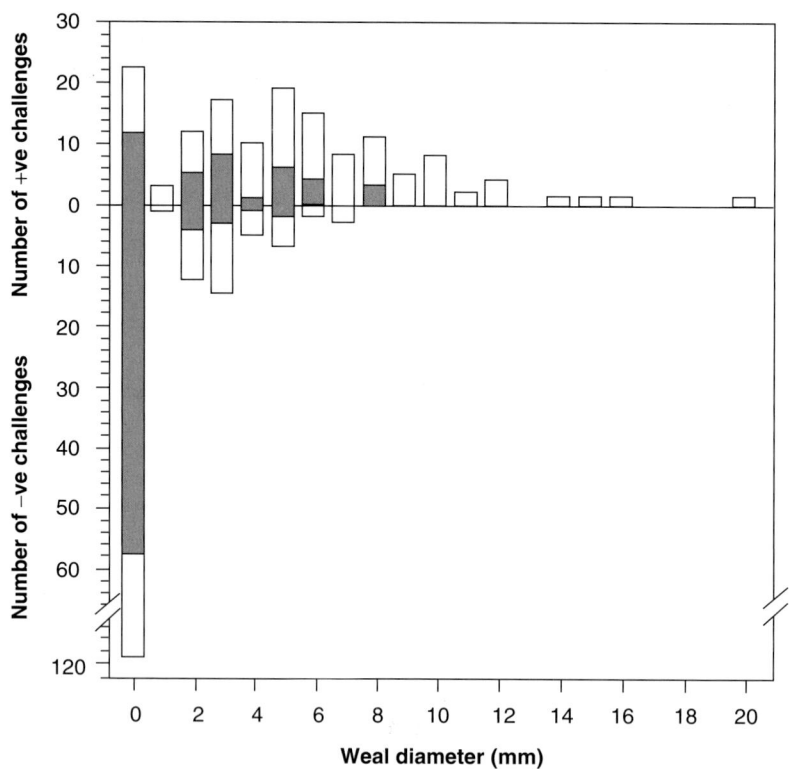

Figure 8.2a   Diagnostic skin prick test weal diameters for cow's milk. Reproduced from Sporik R, Hill DJ, Hosking CS. Specificity of allergen skin testing in predicting positive open food challenges to milk, egg and peanut in children. Clin Exp Allergy 2000; 30: 1540–6.

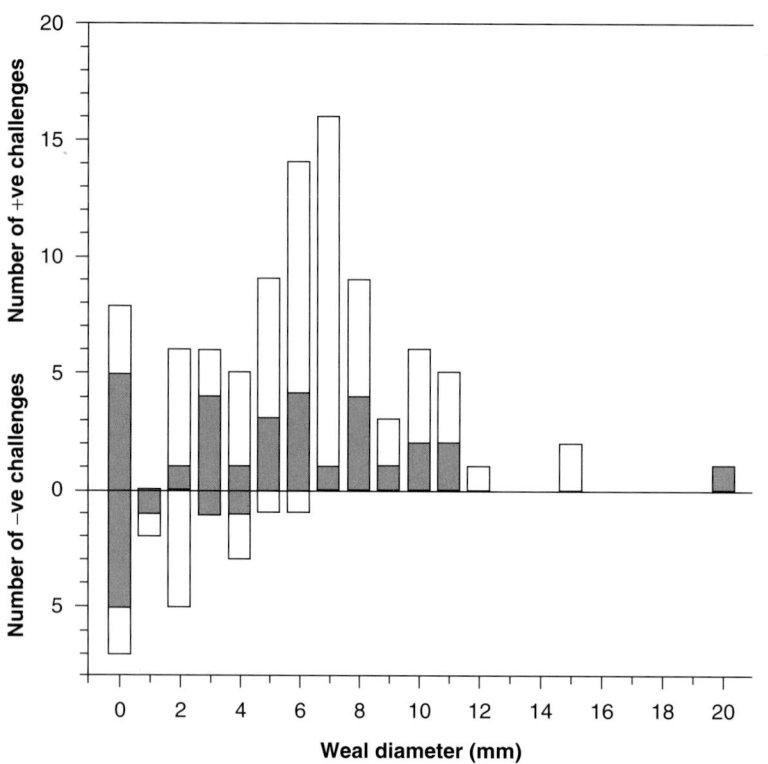

Figure 8.2b   Diagnostic skin prick test weal diameters for egg. Reproduced from Sporik R, Hill DJ, Hosking CS. Specificity of allergen skin testing in predicting positive open food challenges to milk, egg and peanut in children. Clin Exp Allergy 2000; 30: 1540–6.

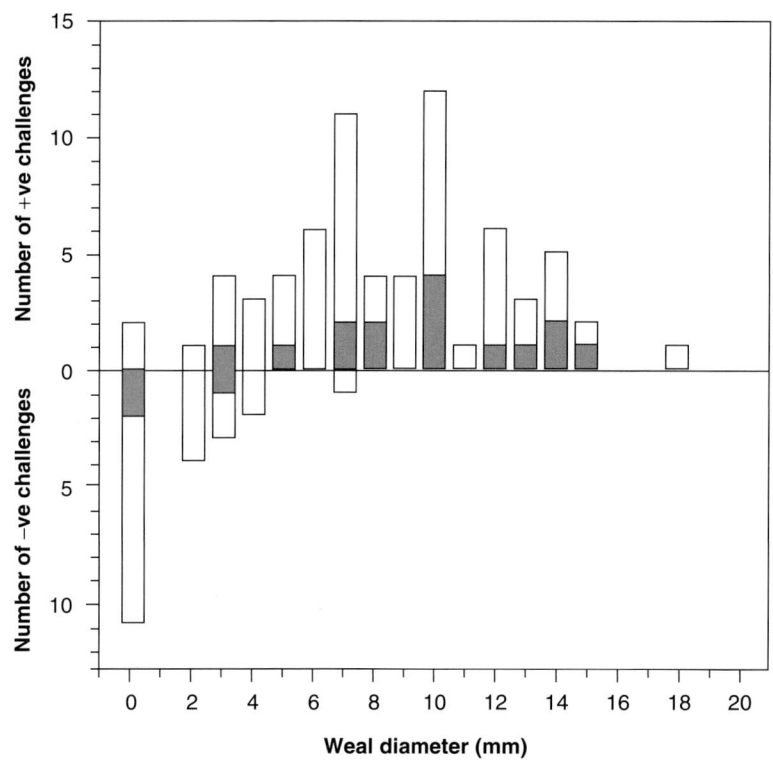

Figure 8.2c   Diagnostic skin prick test weal diameters for peanut. Reproduced from Sporik R, Hill DJ, Hosking CS. Specificity of allergen skin testing in predicting positive open food challenges to milk, egg and peanut in children. Clin Exp Allergy 2000; 30: 1540–6.

allergy to cow's milk, egg, peanut, and fish. The use of food-specific IgE testing may therefore significantly reduce the need for formal DBPCFC.

Other investigators have made similar observations. In a study of 170 infants under 12 months of age with suspected CMA, 44% had the diagnosis confirmed on subsequent challenge. A specific IgE > 2.5 KU(A)/L had a positive predictive value of 90% for immediate CMA.[112] Saarinen et al found a much lower predictive value for specific IgE antibodies, even if used in conjunction with SPT or APT.[113] These differences may, in part, be due to patient selection and different extract potencies.

Skin prick test

SPT in the diagnosis of food allergy is said to be unreliable in infancy. Hill et al studied the 'diagnostic' weal diameter to cow's milk, egg, and peanut that was 100% predictive of a positive open food challenge.[115] The cut-off weal diameter was defined as the diameter above which all children presenting with suspected food allergy reacted on food challenge (Figures 8.2 a–c). All children over 2 years with an SPT weal diameter to cow's milk > 8 mm, and those under 2 years with an SPT > 6 mm, were challenge-positive. These 'diagnostic'

cut-off weal diameters were compared with food-specific IgE antibody levels in Australian children under 2 years of age.[116] Compared with in-vitro antibody testing, use of 'diagnostic' SPT tests reduced the need for food challenges by 23%. Further studies are needed to confirm these observations.

Atopy patch test

Non-IgE mediated hypersensitivity reactions to food are difficult to diagnose as they are not reliably detected by antibody or skin prick testing.[32] The APT is an epicutaneous test that was originally developed to diagnose sensitization to aeroallergens.[117] Patch test skin reactions appear to be mediated by T-cell responses.[118] Several studies have assessed the diagnostic accuracy of the APT in relation to skin prick and serum IgE testing.[29,119,120] Isolauri et al found that the combined use of skin prick and patch testing increased the accuracy in the diagnosis of food allergies in children with AD, suggesting that IgE- and T-cell mediated phenomena can be detected independently by both tests.[29] Majamaa et al found the APT more sensitive than skin prick and IgE testing in detecting CMA in infancy.[119] A study of 75 German children (age range 4 months to 12 years) examined the diagnostic accuracy of the APT for cow's milk, egg, wheat, and soybean.[120] Findings were compared with formal DBPCFC and food-specific serum IgE antibodies. The APT was particularly useful in predicting late-phase clinical reactions (sensitivity 76%, specificity 95%). Roehr et al reported that APT, in conjunction with positive food-specific IgE levels or positive SPT, reliably predicted positive food challenges and argued that these tests may replace DBPCFC in the diagnosis of CMA.[34] There are still some difficulties in standardizing the technique and interpretation of the APT.[121,122]

PREVENTION AND TREATMENT

Dietary prevention of food allergies and atopic dermatitis

Elimination diets have long been an integral part in the treatment and secondary prevention of food allergies and AD.[30,123] There may also be a role for the delayed introduction of high-risk weaning foods, such as egg and peanut, as part of the primary prevention of food sensitization. However, while these dietary interventions may reduce the frequency of manifestations of food allergy during the period of diet exclusion, there is no conclusive evidence they prevent the development of food allergy or hasten the induction of tolerance.[124]

Data on the association of early milk feeding and AD are not conclusive, and the protective effect of breast-feeding on AD is not universally accepted. About a decade ago, a large 10-year longitudinal study from New Zealand failed to demonstrate a significant association between early cow's milk feeding and AD.[125,126] Similarly, a more recent study of 1314 infants found that breast-feeding did not prevent the onset of AD in infants with an affected parent, and the duration of breast-feeding appeared to increase the risk for AD.[127] Another study of 6209 infants also suggested that prolonged breast-feeding may increase the risk of IgE sensitization.[128]

These findings are in contrast with a recent study of 1121 infants that assessed the effect of exclusive breast-feeding and delayed introduction of solid foods on the risk of developing AD at 12 months of age.[42] In that study, the risk of AD was reduced by about 50% in infants who were exclusively breast-fed to 4 months, compared with infants who received cow's milk formula. AD was significantly associated with sensitization to cow's milk (adjusted OR 4.0, 95% CI 1.5; 10.5) and egg (adjusted OR 4.0, 95% CI 1.5; 10.5). The authors concluded that breast-feeding and delayed introduction of solid foods reduce the incidence of AD. The study was not randomized, and the formula-fed group and breast-fed group differed

significantly with regard to socioeconomic and atopic status.[42] It therefore remains unclear from this study whether early cow's milk feeding truly represents a risk factor for the development of AD or whether the early introduction of solid foods may to some extent account for the difference in AD prevalence between groups. Studies on the effect of early diet on the development of asthma have found no relationship between formula-feeding and asthma or atopy.[129] In summary, there is at this stage no conclusive evidence that exclusive breast-feeding does prevent the onset of atopy.[130]

Allergen avoidance

The treatment of food allergies follows the general principles of allergen avoidance. In breast-fed infants, maternal elimination diets have successfully been employed to reduce the food antigen exposure to the infant. Besides dietary interventions, treatment of the dermatological manifestations usually relies on topical corticosteroids and moisturizers.[131] However, in young children AD will usually relapse as soon as the topical corticosteroids are discontinued, unless the offending allergens are eliminated from the children's diet.

In order to avoid unnecessary dietary restrictions,[132] the diagnosis of food allergies should be based on established diagnostic guidelines.[53] A broad elimination diet should only be maintained for a short period of time in order to reduce the risk of growth impairment and nutritional deficiencies. In infants on therapeutic elimination diets, growth parameters need to be closely monitored, as energy and micronutrient intakes may be reduced compared with normal infants.[133] This is particularly important in infants with a past history of failure-to-thrive as a result of feeding difficulties, gastro-osophageal reflux or food protein enteropathy.[134]

Breast-feeding and maternal elimination diets in infants with atopic dermatitis

Breast-feeding is generally considered the most appropriate form of infant feeding, although it probably does not prevent food sensitization or the subsequent development of atopic disease.[17,129,130,135] In breast-fed infants, AD may develop within the first weeks of life, often while being exclusive breast-fed. Onset of AD during the early lactation period may indicate sensitization of the infant to maternally ingested food allergens.[136] Food antigens are secreted into breast milk and may cause similar immunological reactions as seen in formula-fed infants.[92]

In breast-fed infants with clinical manifestations of food allergies, including AD, a maternal exclusion diet is often effective.[18,93,137] An experienced dietitian should closely supervise the maternal diet, and a dietary calcium supplementation may be required for the mother.[138] In infants with severe AD, the maternal diet may consist of mainly vegetables, fruits, cereals, and meats. Dairy products, soy, egg, peanut, tree nuts, fish, and/or wheat are initially withheld and cautiously reintroduced into the mother's diet, while observing the infant's symptoms.

Hypoallergenic formulae

Soy formula
Soy formula is often used as a cow's milk substitute. However, a significant proportion of infants with CMA may also be sensitized to soy protein.[81,139] Soy protein may be associated with gastrointestinal or skin manifestations of food allergy. Soy allergy may manifest in infants with vomiting or worsening of eczema. In infants with soy hypersensitivity an extensively hydrolysed or amino acid-based formula should be considered, particularly if the infants are also allergic to cow's milk.[140]

Extensively hydrolysed whey- and casein-based formulae
Extensively hydrolysed formulae are commonly used in the treatment of infants with cow's milk or soy allergy. The value of partially and extensively hydrolysed formulae in preventing infants food allergy is still an area of debate.[141–143] It has been estimated that about 10–20% of infants with CMA may be intolerant of extensively hydrolysed formulae.[139,144–147] In these infants, amino acid-based formula (AAF) has proved effective and safe.[33,134,140,148]

Amino acid-based formula
Treatment of infants' multiple food protein intolerance with AAF has been shown to be effective and safe.[134,140,145,148–150] After establishing the infant on AAF the allergic manifestations usually remit within days. Infants presenting with AD and failure-to-thrive will usually achieve catch-up growth within months.[134] A recent study has demonstrated that infants with AD and multiple food allergies can successfully be treated with AAF.[33]

Hypoallergenic solid foods
In general, the introduction of non-milk foods should be delayed until after 4 months of age as early introduction of these food items may contribute to food sensitization.[42]

In our experience, the first solids to be introduced include rice cereal and apple or pear. New food items should be introduced on a weekly basis, in order that foods causing delayed reactions can be reliably identified.

Vegetables and fruit, including apple, pear, potato, pumpkin, and zucchini, are generally considered to be associated with a low risk for food allergic reactions. Meats, including chicken and lamb, can be introduced once some other solids have been successfully tolerated. Even in infants with multiple food protein allergies, several of these foods are usually tolerated.[134] The introduction of high-risk foods such as dairy products, egg, peanut, and tree nuts should be deferred until the second year of life.

Probiotics
Probiotic bacteria (*Lactobacillus* GG), if administered to mothers during pregnancy and postnatally to their infants for 6 months, have been shown to significantly reduce the risk of subsequent AD.[151,152] This protective effect may be mediated by an increase of TGF-β concentrations in breast milk.[113] Further large-scale randomized studies are needed to assess the public health benefit of this intervention.

PROGNOSIS

In most infants and young children, dietary management of food allergies and topical treatment with corticosteroids will successfully control the manifestations of AD. The severity of food allergy-related AD usually decreases towards the end of the second year. Elimination diets can be progressively relaxed as the infant develops tolerance to the offending food item. About 85% of infants with CMA and about 50% of egg allergies will develop tolerance by 3 years of age.[55,58] In contrast, only about 20% of children with allergy to peanut or tree nuts will become tolerant.[153] Although allergen avoidance appears to hasten the subsequent development of antigen tolerance it remains unclear to what extent dietary manipulations alter the course of food allergies.[143,154] Persistence of AD may be associated with sensitization to inhalant and environmental allergens, particularly to house dust mite. Infants with AD may therefore be at increased risk of other atopic manifestations in relation to inhalant sensitization, including development of asthma and allergic rhinitis.

CONCLUSION

AD affects between 10–21% of young infants and often represents the first clinical manifestation of food allergies and atopy.[3–5] Infants with clinically significant AD should therefore be investigated for the presence of food allergies. IgE-mediated food allergies may coexist with T-cell-mediated manifestations. Although the definitive test for food allergies remains the DBPCFC, the need for these resource-consuming challenges can be reduced by measurement of food-specific IgE antibodies, in combination with skin prick and atopy patch testing. In the majority of cases, food allergies remit spontaneously by 3 years of age, with the exception of peanut allergy. Persistence of AD beyond early childhood is commonly associated with sensitization to inhalant and environmental allergies, particularly to house dust mite, cat, and rye grass.

Treatment of AD in infancy relies on topical corticosteroids, immunomodulatory agents, and dietary antigen elimination. In breast-fed infants, maternal exclusion diets have been shown to be effective. In formula-fed infants, hypoallergenic formulae (soy, extensively hydrolysed or amino acid-based formulae) represent an alternative to cow's milk formula. The introduction of solids should be delayed and limited to a range of hypoallergenic vegetables, fruits, and meats. Exclusion diets may compromise the energy and micronutrient intake, and growth parameters of infants with food allergies need to be closely monitored.

REFERENCES

1. Leung DY. Atopic dermatitis: new insights and opportunities for therapeutic intervention. J Allergy Clin Immunol 2000; 105: 860–76.
2. Sicherer SH, Sampson HA. Food hypersensitivity and atopic dermatitis: pathophysiology, epidemiology, diagnosis, and management. J Allergy Clin Immunol 1999; 104: S114–22.
3. Arshad SH, Stevens M, Hide DW. The effect of genetic and environmental factors on the prevalence of allergic disorders at the age of two years. Clin Exp Allergy 1993; 23: 504–11.
4. Mar A, Tam M, Jolley D, Marks R. The cumulative incidence of atopic dermatitis in the first 12 months among Chinese, Vietnamese, and Caucasian infants born in Melbourne, Australia. J Am Acad Dermatol 1999; 40: 597–602.
5. Herd RM, Tidman MJ, Prescott RJ, Hunter JA. Prevalence of atopic eczema in the community: the Lothian Atopic Dermatitis study. Br J Dermatol 1996; 135: 18–19.
6. Su JC, Kemp AS, Varigos GA, Nolan TM. Atopic eczema: its impact on the family and financial cost. Arch Dis Child 1997; 76: 159–62.
7. Cookson WOCM, Moffatt MF. The genetics of atopic dermatitis. Curr Opin Allergy Clin Immunol 2002; 383–7.
8. Elliott K, Forrest S. Genetics of atopic dermatitis. In: Bieber T, Leung DYM, eds. Atopic Dermatitis. 1st edn. New York: Marcel Dekker, Inc., 2002: 81–110.
9. Elliott K, Fitzpatrick E, Hill D, Brown J, Adams S et al. The–590C/T and –34C/T interleukin-4 promoter polymorphisms are not associated with atopic eczema in childhood. J Allergy Clin Immunol 2001; 108: 285–7.
10. Forrest S, Dunn K, Elliott K, Fitzpatrick E, Fullerton J et al. Identifying genes predisposing to atopic eczema. J Allergy Clin Immunol 1999; 104: 1066–70.
11. Burks AW, Mallory SB, Williams LW, Shirrell MA. Atopic dermatitis: clinical relevance of food hypersensitivity reactions. J Pediatr 1988; 113: 447–51.
12. Burks AW, James JM, Hiegel A, Wilson G, Wheeler JG et al. Atopic dermatitis and food hypersensitivity reactions. J Pediatr 1998; 132: 132–6.
13. Eigenmann PA, Calza AM. Diagnosis of IgE-mediated food allergy among Swiss children with atopic dermatitis. Pediatr Allergy Immunol 2000; 11: 95–100.
14. Ellman LK, Chatchatee P, Sicherer SH, Sampson HA. Food hypersensitivity in two groups of children and young adults with atopic dermatitis evaluated a decade apart. Pediatr Allergy Immunol 2002; 13: 295–8.
15. Bohme M, Svensson A, Kull I, Nordvall SL, Wahlgren CF. Clinical features of atopic dermatitis at two years of age: a prospective, population-based case-control study. Acta Derm Venereol 2001; 81: 193–7.
16. Businco L, Meglio P, Amato G, Balsamo V, Cainelli T et al. Evaluation of the efficacy of oral cromolyn sodium or an oligoantigenic diet in children with atopic dermatitis: a multicenter study of 1085 patients. J Investig Allergol Clin Immunol 1996; 6: 103–9.
17. Chandra RK. Five-year follow-up of high-risk infants with family history of allergy who were exclusively breast-fed or fed partial whey hydrolysate, soy, and conventional cow's milk formulas. J Pediatr Gastroenterol Nutr 1997; 24: 380–8.
18. Chandra RK, Puri S, Suraiya C, Cheema PS. Influence of maternal food antigen avoidance during pregnancy and lactation on incidence of atopic eczema in infants. Clin Allergy 1986; 16: 563–9.
19. Eigenmann PA, Sicherer SH, Borkowski TA, Cohen BA, Sampson HA. Prevalence of IgE-mediated food allergy among children with atopic dermatitis. Pediatrics 1998; 101: E8.
20. Firer MA, Hosking CS, Hill DJ. Cow's milk allergy and eczema: patterns of the antibody response to cow's milk in allergic skin disease. Clin Allergy 1982; 12: 385–90.
21. Guillet G, Guillet MH. Natural history of sensitizations in atopic dermatitis. A 3-year follow- up in 250 children: food allergy and high risk of respiratory symptoms. Arch Dermatol 1992; 128: 187–92.
22. Gustafsson D, Sjöberg O, Foucard T. Development of allergies and asthma in infants and young children with atopic dermatitis – a prospective follow-up to 7 years of age. Allergy 2000; 55: 240–5.
23. Hill DJ. Effects of milk ingestion on young children with cow's milk allergy. A clinical study. Med J Aust 1984; 141: S26–9.
24. Hill DJ, Lynch BC. Elemental diet in the management of severe eczema in childhood. Clin Allergy 1982; 12: 313–15.
25. Hill DJ, Balloch A, Hosking CS. IgE responses to environmental antigens in atopic children. Clin Allergy 1981; 11: 541–7.
26. Hill DJ, Firer MA, Shelton MJ, Hosking CS. Manifestations of milk allergy in infancy: clinical and immunologic findings. J Pediatr 1986; 109: 270–6.
27. Hill DJ, Sporik R, Thorburn J, Hosking CS. The association of atopic dermatitis in infancy with immunoglobulin E food sensitization. J Pediatr 2000; 137: 475–9.
28. Iida S, Kondo N, Agata H, Shinoda S, Shinbara M et al. Differences in lymphocyte proliferative responses to food antigens and specific IgE antibodies to foods with age among food-sensitive patients with atopic dermatitis. Ann Allergy Asthma Immunol 1995; 74: 334–40.
29. Isolauri E, Turjanmaa K. Combined skin prick and patch testing enhances identification of food allergy in infants with atopic dermatitis. J Allergy Clin Immunol 1996; 97: 9–15.
30. Lever R, MacDonald C, Waugh P, Aitchison T. Randomised controlled trial of advice on an egg exclusion diet in young children with atopic eczema and sensitivity to eggs. Pediatr Allergy Immunol 1998; 9: 13–19.
31. Niggemann B, Sielaff B, Beyer K, Binder C, Wahn U. Outcome of double-blind, placebo-controlled food challenge tests in 107

children with atopic dermatitis. Clin Exp Allergy 1999; 29: 91–6.

32. Niggemann B, Reibel S, Roehr CC, Felger D, Ziegert M et al. Predictors of positive food challenge outcome in non-IgE-mediated reactions to food in children with atopic dermatitis. J Allergy Clin Immunol 2001; 108: 1053–8.

33. Niggemann B, Binder C, Dupont C, Hadji S, Arvola T et al. Prospective, controlled multi-centre study on the effect of an amino-acid-based formula in infants with cow's milk allergy/intolerance and atopic dermatitis. Pediatr Allergy Immunol 2001; 12: 78–82.

34. Roehr CC, Reibel S, Ziegert M, Sommerfeld C, Wahn U et al. Atopy patch tests, together with determination of specific IgE levels, reduce the need for oral food challenges in children with atopic dermatitis. J Allergy Clin Immunol 2001; 107: 548–53.

35. Barnetson RS, Wright AL, Benton EC. IgE-mediated allergy in adults with severe atopic eczema. Clin Exp Allergy 1989; 19: 321–5.

36. Burks AW, Williams LW, Mallory SB, Shirrell MA, Williams C. Peanut protein as a major cause of adverse food reactions in patients with atopic dermatitis. Allergy Proc 1989; 10: 265–9.

37. Sampson HA. Food antigen-induced lymphocyte proliferation in children with atopic dermatitis and food hypersensitivity. J Allergy Clin Immunol 1993; 91: 549–51.

38. Sampson HA, McCaskill CC. Food hypersensitivity and atopic dermatitis: evaluation of 113 patients. J Pediatr 1985; 107: 669–75.

39. Sampson HA. Food hypersensitivity as a pathogenic factor in atopic dermatitis. N Engl Reg Allergy Proc 1986; 7: 511–19.

40. Sampson HA. Immediate hypersensitivity reactions to foods: blinded food challenges in children with atopic dermatitis. Ann Allergy 1986; 57: 209–12.

41. Sampson HA, Ho DG. Relationship between food-specific IgE concentrations and the risk of positive food challenges in children and adolescents. J Allergy Clin Immunol 1997; 100: 444–51.

42. Schoetzau A, Filipiak-Pittroff B, Koletzko S, Franke K, von Berg A et al. Effect of exclusive breast-feeding and early solid food avoidance on the incidence of atopic dermatitis in high-risk infants at 1 year of age. Pediatr Allergy Immunol 2002; 13: 234–42.

43. Sicherer SH, Morrow EH, Sampson HA. Dose-response in double-blind, placebo-controlled oral food challenges in children with atopic dermatitis. J Allergy Clin Immunol 2000; 105: 582–6.

44. Tariq SM, Matthews SM, Hakim EA, Stevens M, Arshad SH et al. The prevalence of and risk factors for atopy in early childhood: a whole population birth cohort study. J Allergy Clin Immunol 1998; 101: 587–93.

45. Zeiger RS, Heller S. The development and prediction of atopy in high-risk children: follow- up at age seven years in a prospective randomized study of combined maternal and infant food allergen avoidance. J Allergy Clin Immunol 1995; 95: 1179–90.

46. Halbert AR, Weston WL, Morelli JG. Atopic dermatitis: is it an allergic disease? J Am Acad Dermatol 1995; 33: 1008–18.

47. Barnetson RS, Rogers M. Childhood atopic eczema. BMJ 2002; 324: 1376–9.

48. Hanifin JM. Atopic dermatitis in infants and children. Pediatr Clin North Am 1991; 38: 763–89.

49. Sampson HA. Food sensitivity and the pathogenesis of atopic dermatitis. J R Soc Med 1997; 90(Suppl 30): 2–8.

50. Woods RK, Thien F, Raven J, Walters EH, Abramson M. Prevalence of food allergies in young adults and their relationship to asthma, nasal allergies, and eczema. Ann Allergy Asthma Immunol 2002; 88: 183–9.

51. Sampson HA. Food allergy. Part 1: immunopathogenesis and clinical disorders. J Allergy Clin Immunol 1999; 103: 717–28.

52. Sicherer SH. Food allergy. Lancet 2002; 360: 701–10.

53. Sampson HA, Sicherer SH, Birnbaum AH. AGA technical review on the evaluation of food allergy in gastrointestinal disorders. American Gastroenterological Association. Gastroenterology 2001; 120: 1026–40.

54. Hill DJ, Hosking CS, Heine RG. Clinical spectrum of food allergy in children in Australia and South-East Asia: identification and targets for treatment. Ann Med 1999; 31: 272–81.

55. Bock SA. Prospective appraisal of complaints of adverse reactions to foods in children during the first 3 years of life. Pediatrics 1987; 79: 683–8.

56. Lehrer SB, Ayuso R, Reese G. Current understanding of food allergens. Ann N Y Acad Sci 2002; 964: 69–85.

57. Hill DJ, Hosking CS, Zhie CY, Leung R, Baratwidjaja K et al. The frequency of food allergy in Australia and Asia. Environ Toxicol Pharmacol 1997; 4: 101–10.

58. Høst A, Halken S. A prospective study of cow milk allergy in Danish infants during the first 3 years of life. Clinical course in relation to clinical and immunological type of hypersensitivity reaction. Allergy 1990; 45: 587–96.

59. Tariq SM, Stevens M, Matthews S, Ridout S, Twiselton R et al. Cohort study of peanut and tree nut sensitisation by age of 4 years. BMJ 1996; 313: 514–17.

60. Joral A, Villas F, Garmendia J, Villareal O. Adverse reactions to food in adults. J Investig Allergol Clin Immunol 1995; 5: 47–9.

61. Dold S, Wijst M, von Mutius E, Reitmeir R, Stiepel E. Genetic risk of asthma, allergic rhinitis and atopic dermatitis by the age of five years. Arch Dis Child 1992; 67: 1018–22.

62. Schultz-Larsen F. Atopic dermatitis: a genetic-epidemiologic study in a population-based twin sample. J Am Acad Dermatol 1993; 28: 719–23.

63. Marsh DG, Neely JD, Breazeale DR, Ghosh B, Freidhoff LR et al. Linkage analysis of IL4 and other chromosome 5q31.1 markers and total serum immunoglobulin E concentrations. Science 1994; 264: 1152–6.

64. Burks W, Helm R, Stanley S, Bannon GA. Food allergens. Curr Opin Allergy Clin Immunol 2001; 1: 243–8.

65. Chatchatee P, Järvinen K-M, Bardina L, Beyer K, Sampson HA. Identification of IgE- and IgG-binding epitopes on αs1-casein: differences in patients with persistent and transient cow's milk allergy. J Allergy Clin Immunol 2001; 107: 379–83.

66. Chatchatee P, Järvinen K-M, Bardina L, Vila L, Beyer K et al. Identification of IgE and IgG binding epitopes on β- and κ-casein in cow's milk allergic patients. Clin Exp Allergy 2001; 31: 1256–62.

67. Järvinen K-M, Chatchatee P, Bardina L, Beyer K, Sampson HA. IgE and IgG binding epitopes on alpha-lactalbumin and beta-lactoglobulin in cow's milk allergy. Int Arch Allergy Immunol 2001; 126: 111–18.

68. Høst A. Clinical course of cow's milk protein allergy and intolerance. Pediatr Allergy Immunol 1998; 9: 48–52.

69. Høst A, Jacobsen HP, Halken S, Holmenlund D. The natural history of cow's milk protein allergy/intolerance. Eur J Clin Nutr 1995; 49(Suppl 1): 13–18.

70. Vila L, Beyer K, Järvinen K-M, Chatchatee P, Bardina L et al. Role of conformational and linear epitopes in the achievement of tolerance in cow's milk allergy. Clin Exp Allergy 2001; 31: 1599–606.

71. Boyano-Martinez T, Garcia-Ara C, Diaz-Pena JM, Martin-Esteban M. Prediction of tolerance on the basis of quantification of egg white-specific IgE antibodies in children with egg allergy. J Allergy Clin Immunol 2002; 110: 304–9.

72. Bernhisel-Broadbent J, Dintzis HM, Dintzis RZ, Sampson HA. Allergenicity and antigenicity of chicken egg ovomucoid (Gal d III) compared to avalbumin (Gal d I) in children with egg allergy and in mice. J Allergy Clin Immunol 1994; 93: 1047–59.

73. Yuninger JW, Squillace DL, Jones RT, Helm RM. Fatal anaphylactic reactions induced by peanuts. Allergy Proc 1989; 10: 249–53.

74. Bock SA, Munoz-Furlong A, Sampson HA. Fatalities due to anaphylactic reactions to foods. J Allergy Clin Immunol 2001; 107: 191–3.

75. Sicherer SH. Clinical update on peanut allergy. Ann Allergy Asthma Immunol 2002; 88: 350–61.

76. Spergel JM, Beausoleil JL, Pawlowski NA. Resolution of childhood peanut allergy. Ann Allergy Asthma Immunol 2000; 85: 473–6.

77. Skolnick HS, Conover-Walker MK, Koerner CB, Sampson HA, Burks W et al. The natural history of peanut allergy. J Allergy Clin Immunol 2001; 107: 367–74.

78. Burks AW, Cockrell G, Connaughton C, Helm RM. Epitope specificity and immunoaffinity purification of the major peanut allergen, Ara h I. J Allergy Clin Immunol 1994; 93: 743–50.

79. Burks AW, Williams LW, Connaughton C, Cockrell G, O'Brien TJ et al. Identification and characterization of a second major peanut allergen, Ara h II, with use of the sera of patients with atopic dermatitis and positive peanut challenge. J Allergy Clin Immunol 1992; 90: 962–9.

80. Rabjohn P, Helm EM, Stanley JS, West CM, Sampson HA et al. Molecular cloning and epitope analysis of the peanut allergen Ara h 3. J Clin Invest 1999; 103: 535–42.

81. Zeiger RS, Sampson HA, Bock SA, Burks AW, Jr., Harden K et al. Soy allergy in infants and children with IgE-associated cow's milk allergy. J Pediatr 1999; 134: 614–22.

82. Burks AW, Cockrell G, Connaughton C, Guin J, Allen W et al. Identification of peanut agglutinin and soybean trypsin inhibitor as minor legume allergens. Int Arch Allergy Immunol 1994; 105: 143–9.

83. Elsayed S, Apol J. Immunochemical analysis of cod fish allergen M: locations of the immunoglobuin binding sites as demonstrated by the native and synthetic peptides. Allergy 1983; 38: 449–59.

84. Swoboda I, Bugajska-Schretter A, Verdino P, Keller W, Sperr WR et al. Recombinant carp parvalbumin, the major cross-reactive fish allergen: a tool for diagnosis and therapy of fish allergy. J Immunol 2002; 168: 4576–84.

85. Swoboda I, Bugajska-Schretter A, Valenta R, Spitzauer S. Recombinant fish parvalbumins: candidates for diagnosis and treatment of fish allergy. Allergy 2002; 57(Suppl 72): 94–6.

86. Jones CA, Holloway JA, Warner JO. Does atopic disease start in foetal life? Allergy 2000; 55: 2–10.

87. Kalayci Ö, Akpinarli A, Yigit S, Çetinkaya S. Intrauterine cow's milk sensitization. Allergy 2000; 55: 408–9.

88. Shah U, Walker WA. Pathophysiology of intestinal food allergy. Adv Pediatr 2002; 49: 299–316.

89. Brandtzaeg PE. Current understanding of gastrointestinal immunoregulation and its relation to food allergy. Ann N Y Acad Sci 2002; 964: 13–45.

90. Ke Y, Pearce K, Lake JP, Ziegler HK, Kapp JA. Gamma delta T lymphocytes regulate the induction and maintenance of oral tolerance. J Immunol 1997; 158: 3610–18.

91. Neurath MF, Fuss I, Kelsall BL, Presky DH, Waegell W et al. Experimental granulomatous colitis in mice is abrogated by induction of TGF-beta-mediated oral tolerance. J Exp Med 1996; 183: 2605–16.

92. Järvinen K-M, Suomalainen H. Development of cow's milk allergy in breast-fed infants. Clin Exp Allergy 2001; 31: 978–87.

93. Järvinen K-M, Mäkinen-Kiljunen S, Suomalainen H. Cow's milk challenge through human milk evokes immune responses in infants with cow's milk allergy. J Pediatr 1999; 135: 506–12.

94. Sorva R, Mäkinen-Kiljunen S, Juntunen-Backman K. Beta-lactoglobulin secretion in human milk varies widely after cow's milk ingestion in mothers of infants with cow's milk allergy. J Allergy Clin Immunol 1994; 93: 787–92.

95. Kilshaw PJ, Cant AJ. The passage of maternal dietary proteins into human breast milk. Int Arch Allergy Appl Immunol 1984; 75: 8–15.

96. de Boissieu D, Matarazzo P, Rocchiccioli F, Dupont C. Multiple food allergy: a possible diagnosis in breastfed infants. Acta Paediatr 1997; 86: 1042–6.

97. Kalliomäki M, Ouwehand A, Arvilommi H, Kero P, Isolauri E. Transforming growth factor-beta in breast milk: a potential regulator of atopic disease at an early age. J Allergy Clin Immunol 1999; 104: 1251–7.

98. Järvinen K-M, Laine ST, Järvenpää AL, Suomalainen HK. Does low IgA in human milk predispose the infant to development of cow's milk allergy? Pediatr Res 2000; 48: 457–62.

99. Järvinen K-M, Laine S, Suomalainen H. Defective tumour necrosis factor-alpha production in mother's milk is related to cow's milk allergy in suckling infants. Clin Exp Allergy 2000; 30: 637–43.

100. Firer MA, Hoskings CS, Hill DJ. Humoral immune response to cow's milk in children with cow's milk allergy. Relationship to the time of clinical response to cow's milk challenge. Int Arch Allergy Appl Immunol 1987; 84: 173–7.

101. Hill DJ, Ball G, Hosking CS, Wood PR. Gamma-interferon production in cow milk allergy. Allergy 1993; 48: 75–80.

102. Sampson HA. Food allergy. Part 1: immunopathogenesis and clinical disorders. J Allergy Clin Immunol 1999; 103: 717–28.

103. Schade RP, Ieperen-Van Dijk AG, Van Reijsen FC, Versluis C, Kimpen JL et al. Differences in antigen-specific T-cell responses between infants with atopic dermatitis with and without cow's milk allergy: relevance of TH2 cytokines. J Allergy Clin Immunol 2000; 106: 1155–62.

104. Sigurs N, Hattevig G, Kjellman NI, Nilsson L, Björksten B. Appearance of atopic disease in relation to serum IgE antibodies in children followed up from birth for 4 to 15 years. J Allergy Clin Immunol 1994; 94: 757–63.

105. Patrizi A, Guerrini V, Ricci G, Neri I, Specchia F et al. The natural history of sensitizations to food and aeroallergens in atopic dermatitis: a 4-year follow-up. Pediatr Dermatol 2000; 17: 261–5.

106. Li XM, Schofield BH, Huang CK, Kleiner GI, Sampson HA. A murine model of IgE-mediated cow's milk hypersensitivity. J Allergy Clin Immunol 1999; 103: 206–14.

107. Li XM, Kleiner G, Huang CK, Lee SY, Schofield B et al. Murine model of atopic dermatitis associated with food hypersensitivity. J Allergy Clin Immunol 2001; 107: 693–702.

108. Li XM, Serebrisky D, Lee SY, Huang CK, Bardina L et al. A murine model of peanut anaphylaxis: T- and B-cell responses to a major peanut allergen mimic human responses. J Allergy Clin Immunol 2000; 106: 150–8.

109. May CD. Objective clinical and laboratory studies of immediate hypersensitivity reactions to foods in asthmatic children. J Allergy Clin Immunol 1976; 58: 500–15.

110. Sampson HA. Food allergy. Part 2: diagnosis and management. J Allergy Clin Immunol 1999; 103: 981–9.

111. Sampson HA. Utility of food-specific IgE concentrations in predicting symptomatic food allergy. J Allergy Clin Immunol 2001; 107: 891–6.

112. García-Ara MC, Boyano Martínez TB, Díaz-Pena JM, Martín-Muñoz F, Reche-Frutos M et al. Specific IgE levels in the diagnosis of immediate hypersensitivity to cow's milk protein in the infant. J Allergy Clin Immunol 2001; 107: 185–90.

113. Saarinen KM, Suomalainen H, Savilahti E. Diagnostic value of skin-prick and patch tests and serum eosinophil cationic protein and cow's milk-specific IgE in infants with cow's milk allergy. Clin Exp Allergy 2001; 31: 423–9.

114. Hidvegi E, Cserhati E, Kereki E, Arato A. Higher serum eosinophil cationic protein levels in children with cow's milk allergy. J Pediatr Gastroenterol Nutr 2001; 32: 475–9.

115. Sporik R, Hill DJ, Hosking CS. Specificity of allergen skin testing in predicting positive open food challenges to milk, egg and peanut in children. Clin Exp Allergy 2000; 30: 1540–6.

116. Hill DJ, Hosking CS, Reyes-Benito LV. Reducing the need for food allergen challenges in young children: a comparison of in vitro with in vivo tests. Clin Exp Allergy 2001; 31: 1031–5.

117. Darsow U, Vieluf D, Ring J. The atopy patch test: an increased rate of reactivity in patients who have an air-exposed pattern of atopic eczema. Br J Dermatol 1996; 135: 182–6.

118. Wistokat-Wülfing A, Schmidt P, Darsow U, Ring J, Kapp A et al. Atopy patch test reactions are associated with T lymphocyte-mediated allergen-specific immune responses in atopic dermatitis. Clin Exp Allergy 1999; 29: 513–21.

119. Majamaa H, Moisio P, Holm K, Kautiainen H, Turjanmaa K. Cow's milk allergy: diagnostic accuracy of skin prick and patch tests and specific IgE. Allergy 1999; 54: 346–51.

120. Niggemann B, Reibel S, Wahn U. The atopy patch test (APT) – a useful tool for the diagnosis of food allergy in children with atopic dermatitis. Allergy 2000; 55: 281–5.

121. Niggemann B, Ziegert M, Reibel S. Importance of chamber size for the outcome of atopy patch testing in children with atopic dermatitis and food allergy. J Allergy Clin Immunol 2002; 110: 515–16.

122. Niggemann B. Evolving role of the atopy patch test in the diagnosis of food allergy. Curr Opin Allergy Clin Immunol 2002; 2: 253–6.

123. Juto P, Engberg S, Winberg J. Treatment of infantile atopic dermatitis with a strict elimination diet. Clin Allergy 1978; 8: 493–500.

124. Halken S, Høst A. Prevention. Curr Opin Allergy Clin Immunol 2001; 1: 229–36.

125. Fergusson DM, Horwood LJ, Shannon FT. Early solid feeding and recurrent childhood eczema: a 10–year longitudinal study. Pediatrics 1990; 86: 541–6.

126. Fergusson DM, Horwood LJ. Early solid food diet and eczema in childhood: a 10-year longitudinal study. Pediatr Allergy Immunol 1994; 5: 44–7.

127. Kulig M, Bergmann R, Niggemann B, Burow G, Wahn U. Prediction of sensitization to inhalant allergens in childhood: evaluating family history, atopic dermatitis and sensitization to food allergens. The MAS Study Group. Multicentre Allergy Study. Clin Exp Allergy 1998; 28: 1397–403.

128. Saarinen KM, Savilahti E. Infant feeding patterns affect the subsequent immunological features in cow's milk allergy. Clin Exp Allergy 2000; 30: 400–6.

129. Sears MR, Greene JM, Willan AR, Taylor DR, Flannery EM et al. Long-term relation between breastfeeding and development of atopy and asthma in children and young adults: a longitudinal study. Lancet 2002; 360: 901–7.

130. Sly PD, Holt PG. Breast is best for preventing asthma and allergies – or is it? Lancet 2002; 360: 887–8.

131. Thomas KS, Armstrong S, Avery A, Li Wan Po A, O'Neill C et al. Randomised controlled trial of short bursts of a potent topical corticosteroid versus prolonged use of a mild preparation for children with mild or moderate atopic eczema. BMJ 2002; 324: 1–7.

132. Eggesbø M, Botten G, Stigum H. Restricted diets in children with reactions to milk and egg perceived by their parents. J Pediatr 2001; 139: 583–7.

133. Isolauri E, Sütas Y, Salo MK, Isosomppi R, Kaila M. Elimination diet in cow's milk allergy: risk for impaired growth in young children. J Pediatr 1998; 132: 1004–9.

134. Hill DJ, Heine RG, Cameron DJ, Francis DE, Bines JE. The natural history of intolerance to soy and extensively hydrolyzed formula in infants with multiple food protein intolerance. J Pediatr 1999; 135: 118–21.

135. Saarinen UM, Kajosaari M. Breastfeeding as prophylaxis against atopic disease: prospective follow-up study until 17 years old. Lancet 1995; 346: 1065–9.

136. Isolauri E, Tahvanainen A, Peltola T, Arvola T. Breast-feeding of allergic infants. J Pediatr 1999; 134: 27–32.

137. Hill DJ, Hudson IL, Sheffield LJ, Shelton MJ, Menahem S et al. A low allergen diet is a significant intervention in infantile colic: results of a community-based study. J Allergy Clin Immunol 1995; 96: 886–92.

138. Arvola T, Holmberg-Marttila D. Benefits and risks of elimination diets. Ann Med 1999; 31: 293–8.

139. American Academy of Pediatrics: Committee on Nutrition. Hypoallergenic infant formulas. Pediatrics 2000; 106: 346–9.

140. Sicherer SH, Noone SA, Barnes Koerner C, Christie L, Burks AW et al. Hypoallergenicity and efficacy of an amino acid-based formula in children with cow's milk and multiple food hypersensitivities. J Pediatr 2001; 138: 688–93.

141. Nentwich I, Michková E, Nevoral J, Urbanek R, Szépfalusi Z. Cow's milk-specific cellular and humoral immune responses and atopy skin symptoms in infants from atopic families fed a partially (pHF) or extensively (eHF) hydrolyzed infant formula. Allergy 2001; 56: 1144–56.

142. Høst A, Koletzko B, Dreborg S, Muraro A, Wahn U et al. Dietary products used in infants for treatment and prevention of food allergy. Joint Statement of the European Society for Paediatric Allergology and Clinical Immunology (ESPACI) Committee on Hypoallergenic Formulas and the European Society for Paediatric Gastroenterology, Hepatology and Nutrition (ESPGHAN) Committee on Nutrition. Arch Dis Child 1999; 81: 80–4.

143. Exl BM, Fritsche R. Cow's milk protein allergy and possible means for its prevention. Nutrition 2001; 17: 642–51.

144. Vanderhoof JA, Murray ND, Kaufman SS, Mack DR, Antonson DL et al. Intolerance to protein hydrolysate infant formulas: an underrecognized cause of gastrointestinal symptoms in infants. J Pediatr 1997; 131: 741–4.

145. de Boissieu D, Matarazzo P, Dupont C. Allergy to extensively hydrolyzed cow milk proteins in infants: identification and treatment with an amino acid-based formula. J Pediatr 1997; 131: 744–7.

146. Carroccio A, Cavataio F, Montalto G, D'amico D, Alabrese L et al. Intolerance to hydrolysed cow's milk proteins in infants: clinical characteristics and dietary treatment. Clin Exp Allergy 2000; 30: 1597–603.

147. Giampietro PG, Kjellman NI, Oldaeus G, Wouters-Wessling W, Businco E. Hypoallergenicity of an extensively hydrolyzed whey formula. Pediatr Allergy Immunol 2001; 12: 83–6.

148. Isolauri E, Sütas Y, Mäkinen-Kiljunen S, Oja SS, Isosomppi R et al. Efficacy and safety of hydrolyzed cow milk and amino acid-derived formulas in infants with cow milk allergy. J Pediatr 1995; 127: 550–7.

149. Sampson HA, James JM, Bernhisel-Broadbent J. Safety of an amino acid-derived infant formula in children allergic to cow milk. Pediatrics 1992; 90: 463–5.

150. Hill DJ, Cameron DJ, Francis DE, Gonzalez-Andaya AM, Hosking CS. Challenge confirmation of late-onset reactions to extensively hydrolyzed formulas in infants with multiple food protein intolerance. J Allergy Clin Immunol 1995; 96: 386–94.

151. Kalliomäki M, Salminen S, Arvilommi H, Kero P, Koskinen P et al. Probiotics in primary prevention of atopic disease: a randomised placebo-controlled trial. Lancet 2001; 357: 1076–9.

152. Rautava S, Kalliomäki M, Isolauri E. Probiotics during pregnancy and breast-feeding might confer immunomodulatory protection against atopic disease in the infant. J Allergy Clin Immunol 2002; 109: 119–21.

153. Sicherer SH, Sampson HA. Peanut and tree nut allergy. Curr Opin Pediatr 2000; 12: 567–73.

154. Zeiger RS. Dietary aspects of food allergy prevention in infants and children. J Pediatr Gastroenterol Nutr 2000; 30(Suppl): S77–86.

9

Role of inhalant allergens in atopic dermatitis

Salima Mrabet-Dahbi and Harald Renz

INTRODUCTION

Atopic dermatitis (AD) represents a major public health problem worldwide with an estimated current incidence of 10–20% in children and 1–3% in adults.[1] Since World War II, AD prevalence has been steadily increasing in industrialized countries, but remains much lower in agricultural regions.[2] The reason for this dramatic increase has not yet been elucidated. However, the Westernized lifestyle along with insufficient microbial exposure is presently being made responsible for this phenomenon, an explanation that has been designated as the 'hygiene hypothesis'.[3]

AD patients, as diagnosed by the criteria of Hanifin et al,[4] share the same clinical features.

The unaffected skin of AD patients frequently manifests severe dryness and a greater irritant cutaneous response than healthy controls. Immunohistologically, it represents a mild hyperkeratosis and reveals a marginal perivascular T cell infiltrate[5] while in acute skin lesions spongiosis of the epidermis and a diffuse epidermal infiltrate of T cells and Langerhans cells (LCs) may be noted. In contrast, the dermis is often characterized by an evident oedema and a prominent infiltration of particularly CD4+ activated memory T cells.[6] Yet, lichenified skin lesions define the chronic stage of disease and have undergone tissue remodelling due to itching and scratching.[7] They display hyperkeratosis with minimal spongiosis and dry, fibrotic papules. The dermal infiltrate in advanced AD is mainly composed of macrophages, non-activated mast cells, and eosinophils.

AD can be classified into several subgroups, each one with diverse immunopathological features, thus underlining the heterogeneity of the disease. In this context, a subgroup of patients is characterized by IgE-mediated sensitization (immediate, type I hypersensitivity) affecting 70–80% of the individuals whereas about 20–30% of the patients are defined by a more T-cell driven feature (delayed, type IV hypersensitivity) accompanied by low serum IgE levels and the lack of IgE sensitizations.[8] Besides this strict classification some individuals combine more than one of these phenotypes whereas others do not show any of the above-mentioned features; instead non-specific cutaneous hyperreactivity is thought to be here the main precipitating factor.[9,10]

While diagnosis of AD follows relatively well-defined criteria, the underlying pathophysiology of disease is still not entirely understood. Nowadays, challenged by this puzzle, diverse studies have pointed out its multifactorial causes with activation of many immunologic and inflammatory pathways.[11] So, it is well recognized that at primary level the clinical phenotype of AD is the product of several interactions among genetic susceptibility, immune dysregulation, and defects in skin barrier function, predisposing individuals to disease, and that at a secondary level various environmental factors exacerbate the course of pre-existing lesions and therefore are considered as inflammatory triggers of AD (Figure 9.1). A broad variety of potential non-allergic and allergic triggers (inhalant, food, and bacterial antigens) have been described thus far. Among them are irritants like soap, harsh chemicals, and hard water that dehydrate the skin and thereby promote xerosis. Other non-allergic triggers include rapid temperature changes, low humidity, emotional stress, and anxiety.

Yet, many clinical studies could also support the close linkage of allergic triggers to the onset and maintenance of disease. It has been repeatedly shown that *Staphylococcus aureus* skin colonization leads to dramatic flare-ups of eczema.[12,13] One important underlying mechanism for this phenomenon might be the impaired synthesis of antimicrobial peptides providing a favourable environment for these bacteria.[14,15] Their clinical importance becomes evident as AD patients benefit by antistaphylococcal antibiotics with reduction in disease severity.[16]

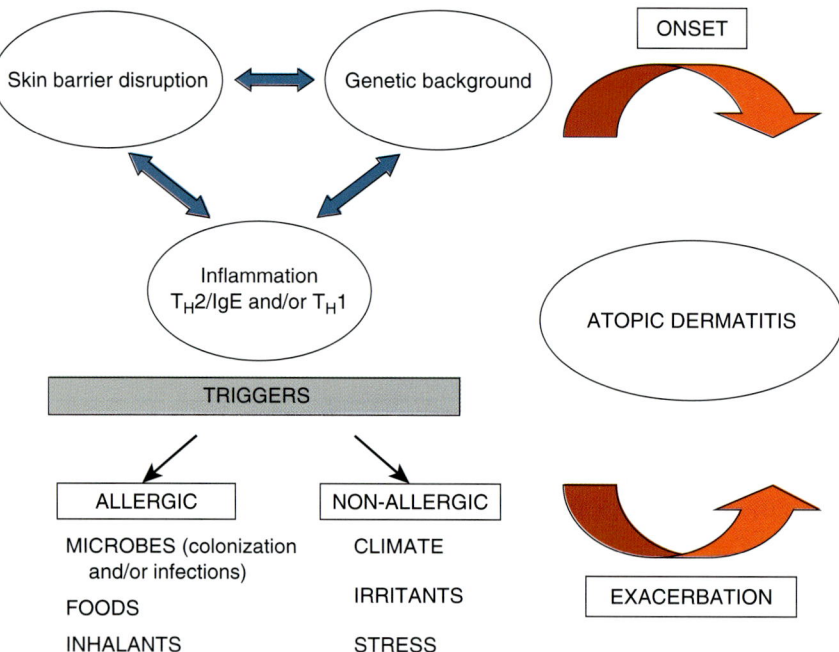

Figure 9.1 The multifactorial cause of atopic dermatitis. AD is the result of complex interactions among genetic susceptibility, immune dysregulation and skin barrier dysfunction predisposing individuals to disease and to trigger factors (either allergic or non-allergic); the latter ones are involved in disease at secondary level through exacerbation of pre-existing lesions.

In contrast, other studies have underlined the relevance of food allergens (i.e. milk, egg, and peanut) in a subgroup of AD patients as well.[17,18] Cow's milk is among the most common offending foods, and cow's milk allergy (CMA) plays a pathogenic role in approximately 35–40% of infants with AD reacting with worsening of eczema upon ingestion of cow's milk.[19] In turn, these clinical symptoms improved when the causal food allergens were removed from the diet.[20] Additionally, as shown in vitro and in vivo, PBMCs from AD patients with food allergy proliferated in response to the corresponding antigens[21] while continual oral food sensitization yielded elicitation of skin lesions in a murine model of AD.[22]

Apart from food allergens, exposure to inhalant allergens (pollen, moulds, mites, and animal dander) is also acknowledged to be relevant in particularly influencing the course of disease in infancy in some AD patients, a finding which was first reported by Walker in 1918.[23] Inhalant allergens appear to be more important in older children and adults[24] leading to aggravation of pruritus and atopic lesions after bronchial inhalation in sensitized individuals.[25] In contrast, substantial clinical improvement may occur when these patients are exposed to environments lacking the allergens to which they react.[26]

Laboratory data strengthen the role of inhalants in AD include the finding of the corresponding IgE antibodies in most patients whose degree of sensitization to mites, pollen, or animal dander is directly associated with disease severity.[27,28]

In conclusion, there are diverse groups of AD patients each of them characterized by a unique profile of disease-promoting factors (Figure 9.2). Yet, this chapter focuses solely on one of these triggers, namely the inhalant allergens, and aims to critically reflect on their pathophysiological relevance in AD.

THE IMMUNOPHENOTYPE OF ATOPIC DERMATITIS

In order to elucidate the influence of inhalant allergens in AD it is necessary to characterize some of the immunological processes of the disease. Skin lesions in AD generally evolve as the result of complex cellular interactions. One potential scenario is that IgE-bearing LCs and inflammatory dendritic epidermal cells (IDECs) present antigens which have penetrated the disrupted epidermal skin barrier[29] to receptive sensitized T cells, and mast cells, leading to their activation and release of cytokines,

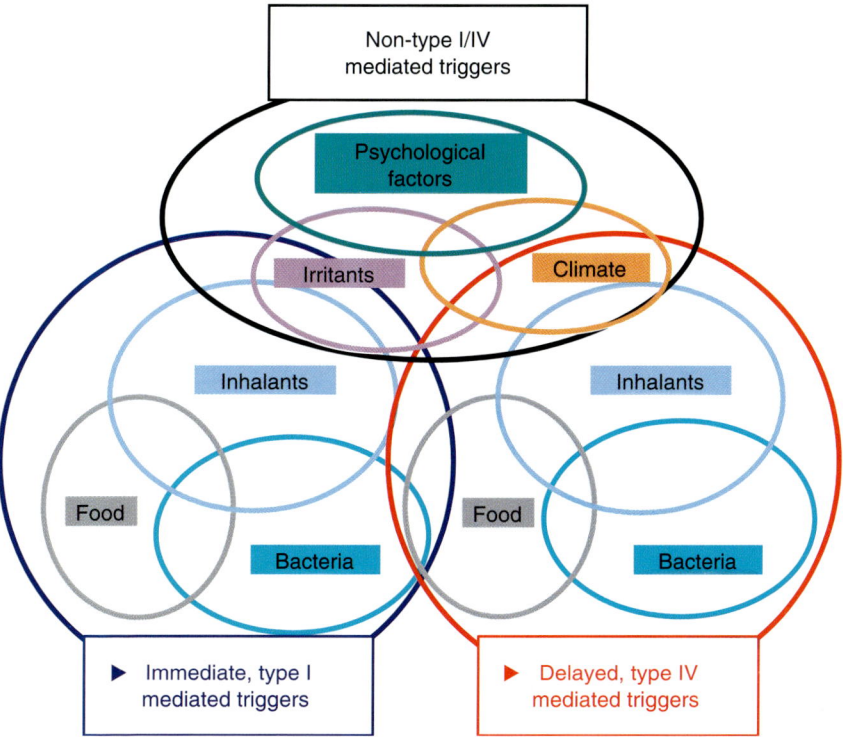

Figure 9.2   The heterogeneity of atopic dermatitis. Each patient exhibits a unique set and combination of trigger factors leading to disease exacerbation.

i.e. IL-1, IL-6, and TNF-α.[30] Simultaneously, scratching makes epithelium crucially involved in AD through aggravated chemokine and cytokine production by keratinocytes.[31] One of their most prominent secreted mediators is thymic stromal lymphopoitein (TSLP) which drives LCs to migrate into the lymph nodes and thereby contributes to the allergic phenotype.[32] In addition, TSLP-activated dendritic cells (DCs) prime naive T cells to produce IL-4, IL-5, and IL-13 and initiates chemokine production by DCs, such as macrophage-derived chemokine (MDC) or thymus and activation-regulated chemokine (TARC), both highly present in AD patients.[33] These chemokines attract T_H2 skewed cells and strongly correlate with disease severity.[34]

Other inflammatory cells such as activated mast cells, upon cross-linking of IgE, release histamine and other mediators up-regulating adhesion molecules, which in turn help to recruit eosinophils. The latter massively infiltrate the dermis and cause tissue damage through degranulation of inflammatory mediators and cytolic degeneration.[35] In this respect, high levels of these mediators have been detected in sera and urine of

AD patients correlating with disease activity and decreasing in response to therapy.[36] In addition, activated and histologically hypodense eosinophils display an enhanced survival, which is achieved by means of delayed programmed cell death.[37]

Apart from eosinophils there is overwhelming evidence for the fundamental impact of T cells in AD.[38] They express high levels of the cutaneous lymphocyte antigen (CLA), which functions as a skin homing receptor.[39] Its interaction with E-selectin localized on inflamed dermal postcapillary venules enables their immediate recruitment into the skin on invasion of foreign antigens and allergens.[40] Moreover, it has been recently shown, in vitro as well as in vivo, that the interaction of the skin-associated chemokine CCL27 and its receptor CCR10 also mediates the chemotactic response of skin-homing T cells.[41] In contrast, no respiratory tract T-cell homing receptor has been identified so far.[42] The relevance of T cells in AD pathogenesis is particularly highlighted in animal model experiments, showing that development of eczematous skin lesions depends on the presence of these cells.

THE T$_H$1/T$_H$2 PARADIGM IN AD

Although T$_H$2 cells certainly contribute to the pathogenesis of AD it is now well accepted that T$_H$1 cells also play an important role in maintaining skin inflammation. Therefore, this biphasic character represents one hallmark of AD which is defined by an initial phase with predominately T$_H$2 cytokines switching into a second T$_H$1-like chronic phase.[43] T$_H$1 cells are known to secrete IL-2 and IFN-γ, induce macrophage activation, and are very effective in controlling infection with intracellular pathogens. In contrast, T$_H$2 cells produce IL-4, IL-5, IL-9, and IL-13 as key signature cytokines and promote excellent humoral immunity, allergic reactions, and resistance to helminthic infections.[44,45]

In addition to these two main distinct T$_H$ cell populations, a further subset of regulatory T cells does exist suppressing both T$_H$1 and T$_H$2 responses. To date, several major groups of these so-called T regulatory (T$_{reg}$) cells have been described: namely, the naturally occurring CD4$^+$CD25$^+$ cells, the type 1 T regulatory cells (Tr1) and the T$_H$3 cells. The first subset accounts for 5–15% of the peripheral CD4$^+$ T cells and expresses the cytotoxic T-lymphocyte antigen 4 (CTLA-4)[46] and the glucocorticoid-induced tumour necrosis factor receptor as markers.[47] These cells are generated in the thymus and then exported to peripheral tissues, where they normally hinder potential autoimmune responses. Their mechanism of suppression relies on the inhibition of IL-2Rα chain in target T cells induced by the combined activation of CTLA-4 and membrane-bound TGF-β. Additionally, CD4$^+$CD25$^+$ cells specifically express the forkhead-winged helix transcription factor gene FoxP3 which so far is the most unambiguous marker available to identify this class of T$_{reg}$ cells. Loss of function through mutations in the FoxP3 gene results in a lack of this T-cell subset, and consequently favours the onset of various autoimmune and allergic diseases.[48] Similar to the natural T$_{reg}$ cells, Tr1 cells (adaptive T$_{reg}$ cells) also originate from the thymus but then further differentiate in the periphery under certain conditions of antigenic stimulation. They exert suppressive activity through enhanced IL-10 production whereas T$_H$3 cells mainly produce TGF-β, thereby mediating their regulatory function.

Clear evidence suggests that T$_H$1 and T$_H$2 cells can each arise from the same precursor cell (the naive T$_H$0 cell) under the influence of:

1. T-cell receptor ligation (TCR)
2. the activation of costimulatory molecules
3. the predominance of a given cytokine in the microenvironment
4. the number of postactivation cell divisions,[49] whereas the cytokine composition has emerged as key determinant in the outcome of T$_H$ responses.

For example, if the T$_H$0 cell is activated in the presence of IL-12 (from a macrophage or dendritic cell) then this cytokine initiates a process of T$_H$1 maturation. Additionally, it synergizes together with IL-2 and IL-18, another cytokine secreted by activated macrophages, to induce IFN-γ synthesis.[50] Of note, the novel IL-12 family members, such as IL-23 and IL-27, may contribute to the T$_H$1 polarization as well.[51,52] Although IL-27 is not sufficient to instruct IFN-γ production on its own, it has a profound effect in the early steps of T$_H$1 commitment by controlling IL-12 responsiveness[53] while IL-23 functions primarily on effector T cells prolonging and sustaining their IFN-γ synthesis.

Conversely, naive T cells activated in the presence of IL-4 down-regulate the IL-12 receptor and differentiate along the T$_H$2 pathway, even if the initial source of this cytokine is still a subject of debate.[54,55] However, it is suggested that APC-derived IL-6 mediates T$_H$2 development by inducing early IL-4 production.[56] Yet, generation of this phenotype also requires the interaction of two more recently discovered cytokines: namely, IL-19 and IL-25. In vitro data could show that IL-19, expressed by human peripheral blood mononuclear cells and purified monocytes after LPS stimulation,[57] up-regulated IL-4 and down-regulated IFN-γ in a dose-dependent fashion.[58] Similarly, the mast cell and T$_H$2 cell derived cytokine IL-25 induced elevated production levels of IL-4, IL-5, and IL-13.[59]

T-cell differentiation is a complex process regulated by a network of transcription factors such as GATA-3 and T-bet.[60,61] GATA-3 is expressed during T$_H$2 differentiation via pathways that probably involve the IL-4 dependent activation of the signal transducer and activator of transcription (STAT)-6. It suppresses IFN-γ, increases the transactivation of the IL-4 promoter, and also directly regulates IL-5 and IL-13 expression in T$_H$2 cells. By contrast, T-bet is exclusively expressed in T$_H$1 cells in a principally STAT-4 dependent manner, mediates IFN-γ production and maintains synthesis of the IL-12 receptor γ2 chain upon T-cell activation. Thus, a balance between T-bet and GATA-3 is believed to control T$_H$1 and T$_H$2 polarization.

With respect to AD T$_H$2 and T$_H$1 cytokines are both involved in the pathogenesis and their contribution depends on the chronicity of skin lesion. In humans, such a strong T-cell effector dichotomy does not frequently appear but can be observed in patients with autoimmune or allergic diseases as well.[62,45] Initially, AD was viewed as a prototypical T$_H$2 disease due to its mainly humoral features. One of the first studies performed in this context was carried out on PBMCs of AD patients indeed providing evidence for increased T_H2 activity (IL-4) along with diminished IFN-γ release upon mitogen stimulation.[63] Many subsequent studies could reproduce this finding even on the level of allergen-specific T cells showing an overproduction of IL-4 in response to the relevant allergen.[64,65] Presently, it is well established that T_H2 derived cytokines characterize AD patients with acute lesions[66] while T_H1 derived cytokines are predominant in patients of the chronic stage.[67]

This T_H1/T_H2 dysbalance also exists in the local environment of lesional skin and therefore critically modulates the nature, degree, and persistence of inflammation in AD. In this context analysis of skin biopsies using in-situ hybridization revealed significantly greater amounts of T_H2 cells positive for IL-4 and IL-13 mRNA whereas in chronic skin lesions IFN-γ, IL-5 and IL-12 mRNA expression predominate.[68] Furthermore, investigations on allergen patch testing followed by punch biopsies at different time points also showed these biphasic kinetics in cytokine production.[69] Figure 9.3 illustrates the acute and chronic features of AD and the involved cellular mechanisms as described above.

THE ANTIGEN SPECIFICITY OF SKIN INFILTRATING EFFECTOR T CELLS

The finding of a massive T-cell infiltrate in the lesional skin of AD patients prompted many investigators to analyse its antigen specificity, an aspect which might underline the direct involvement of environmental allergens in the onset and maintenance of eczema. Indeed, encouraged by this concept, various allergen specific T-cell clones could be generated either from blood or from naturally occurring skin lesions as well as from lesions following patch testing. In the study of Schade et al,[70] cow's milk protein (CMP) specific T-cell clones had been isolated from PBMCs of infants with AD sensitized to the corresponding allergen and thereafter compared to those T-cell clones of milk-tolerant AD infants. The data obtained from this study confirmed a key role for circulating T_H2-skewed CMP specific CD4+ T cells in food allergic AD subjects, whereas tolerance to this kind of antigen was achieved by means of low T_H2 cytokine levels. Food allergen specific T-cell clones (casein or ovalbumin) derived from PBMCs of AD patients could be generated by other investigators as well. Yet, in contrast to the aforesaid study, the authors ruled out that circulating food-specific lymphocytes were not solely restricted to the CD4+ T-cell subset and the T_H2 phenotype.[71]

The ongoing immune reaction to inhalant allergens in the skin of AD patients could be also elucidated by the existence of specifically primed T cells in this compartment. Ramb-Lindhauer et al[72] succeeded in cloning grass pollen (*Lolium perennis*) reactive T cells derived from lesional skin with a relative predominance of IL-4 secretion. Later, Reekers et al[73] examined birch pollen specific lymphocyte responses in blood and skin biopsies of AD patients with hypersensitivity to the relevant allergen. As a result, the proliferative response of birch pollen extract or Bet v1 stimulated skin derived T-cell lines was significantly higher than that of non-reactive patients. Additionally, a higher frequency of birch pollen reactive T cells was calculated from limiting-dilution assays, and a higher rate of birch pollen specific T-cell clones was generated from skin derived T-cell cultures.

In another study by van der Heijden et al[74] the authors focused on the analysis of T cells directed to the house dust mite (*Dermatophagoides pteronyssinus*), representing a perennial allergen. In this respect, a considerable number of mite specific T cells of the T_H2 phenotype could be isolated from lesional skin while many of the non-mite specific skin as well as blood derived T-cell clones produced IFN-γ. Data obtained from T-cell cloning studies of allergen patch test sites again underlined the T_H2 feature of these cells generated shortly after epicutaneous house dust mite exposure.[75] It was notable that the majority of these allergen specific T-cell clones obtained from unmanipulated, chronic skin lesions of sensitized AD patients exhibited a typical T_H1 profile.[76] However, characterization of limited numbers of mite specific T cell clones from blood or skin – as carried out previously – does not necessarily allow definite conclusions regarding their biological significance in vivo. For this reason Neumann et al[77] enrolled a large cohort of AD patients in order to perform mite specific T-cell clones from the peripheral blood, naturally occurring skin lesions, and allergen exposed skin. Their results indicated that the mass of allergen specific T cells in both skin and blood of atopic individuals failed to exhibit a restricted cytokine secretion profile and thus were classified as T_H0 cells. House dust mite specific T cells displaying a restricted secretion pattern were either of the T_H1 or the T_H2 type, whereas specific T_H2 cells were found almost exclusively in allergen patch test reactions, indicating that the T_H2 differentiation pathway is seen preferentially in allergen exposed skin.

Another important aspect in the field of allergen specific T cells is their frequency upon several studies have drawn their attention to either. While Sager et al[78] could show that mite specific T-cells appeared more

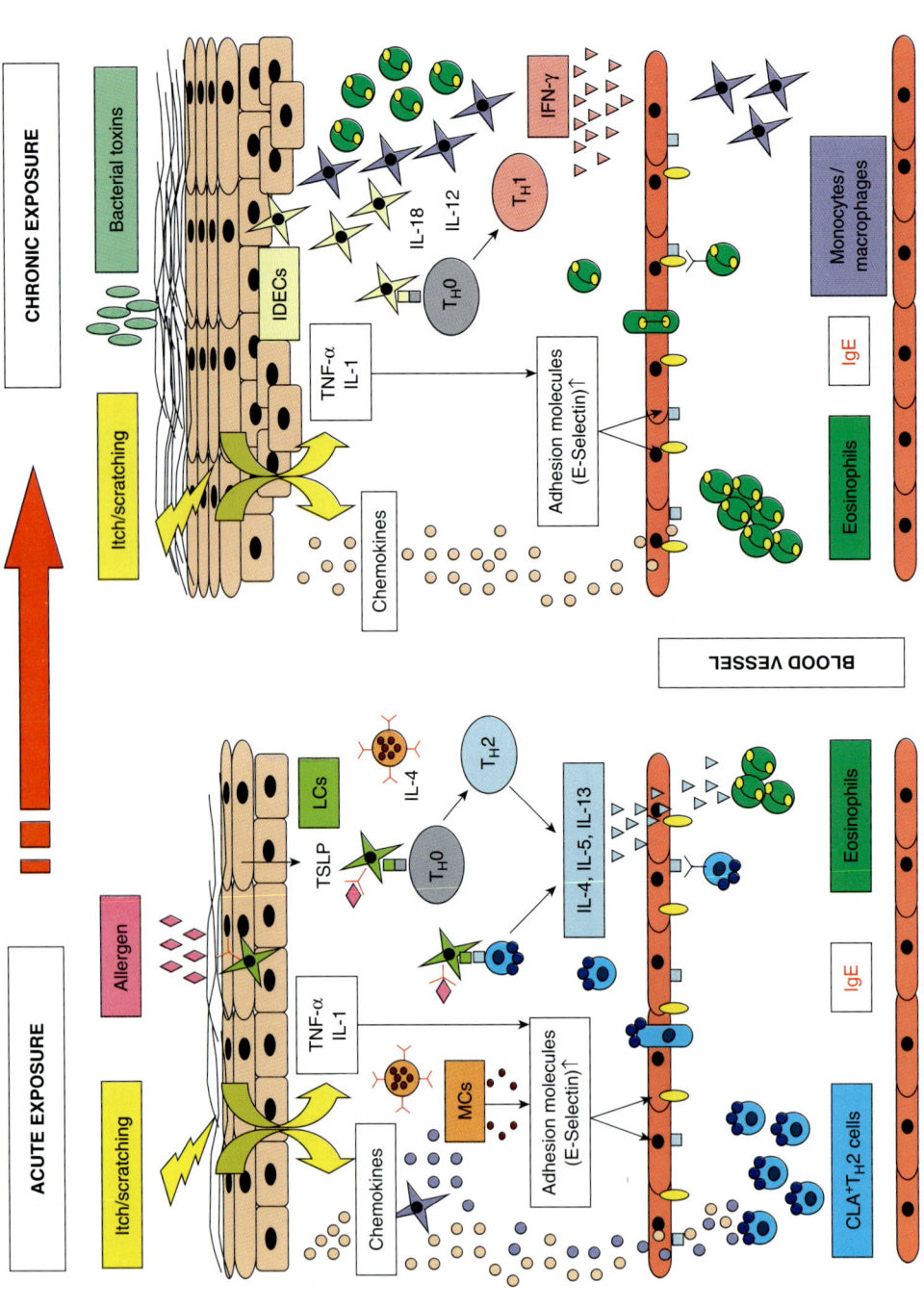

Figure 9.3   Immunological pathways in atopic dermatitis. Skin injury by scratching activates keratinocytes to release proinflammatory cytokines and chemokines followed by the expression of adhesion molecules on vascular endothelium and the facilitated extravasation of inflammatory cells into the skin. T_H2 cells circulating in the peripheral blood of AD patients express the skin homing receptor CLA, that upon interaction with these molecules, recruit into the skin on invasion of environmental allergens. Subsequently they engage allergen triggered IgE⁺ Langerhans cells (LCs) and mast cells (MCs) thus promoting T_H2 cell differentiation, a process which is additionally enhanced by keratinocyte-derived thymic stromal lymphopoietin (TSLP). In acute skin lesions T_H2 cells predominate whereas the infiltration of inflammatory dendritic epidermal cells (IDECs), macrophages and eosinophils define the chronic stage of AD. IL-12 and IL-18, produced by these various cell types, cause the switch to a T_H1- type cytokine milieu associated with increased IFN-γ expression. Furthermore, microbial toxins appear to stimulate the eosinophilic inflammation and polyclonal IgE response.

frequently in skin than in blood, Takahama et al[79] demonstrated that only a minor portion of T-cell clonotypes detected in PBMCs resembled those accumulated in AD skin lesions when comparing their TCR Vb segments with each other. Their frequency ranged from 0.5% to 1.2%, similar to the percentage of Der p specific T-cells (0.72% to 0.02%) seen in chronic AD lesions performed in the study by Werfel et al.[76] According to these data only a small number of these cells (1 or 2) show specificity to the respective allergen and are selected to expand clonally in the skin lesion by thus far unknown reasons.

Taken together, identifying allergen specific T cells particularly in lesional skin of AD patients supports the concept of a T-cell-mediated specific immune response to environmental allergens – including inhalant allergens – with clinical implications in AD.

HOW DOES SENSITIZATION TO INHALANT ALLERGENS OCCUR?

How inhalant allergens enter the body and aggravate eczema is still a matter of debate. Nevertheless, perturbation of the skin barrier may favour the invasion of these allergens into the deeper epidermal compartment. To strengthen this hypothesis of local allergen transmission, biopsy studies of AD lesions and APT reactions reveal mite allergens bound to the corresponding IgE antibodies localized on epidermal and dermal LCs of the affected patients but not of healthy volunteers.[80,81] In experimental models, eczematous skin lesions can be either provoked by the APT or by repeated epicutaneous allergen application resembling the naturally occurring eczema.[82–84] Recently, Riley et al[85] demonstrated the presence of house dust mite on the skin by vacuum cleaning. Yet, penetration of this allergen through an intact stratum corneum in AD is hard to imagine, which makes the relevance of the epidermal route in the induction of new lesions doubtful. Under these conditions the respiratory route may be relevant in a subset of patients (Table 9.1).

Indeed, early studies have shown that inhalation of house dust or pollen extract can provoke exacerbations of dermatitis.[86] More recently, Tupker et al[87] demonstrated pruritic, erythematous skin lesions in 9 of 20 AD patients after placebo-controlled bronchial provocation with house dust mite. All the responders had a history of asthma, an early bronchial reaction after allergen challenge, and an elevated total IgE level, suggesting that the respiratory route is especially relevant to this subset of AD patients. Brinkman et al[88] could extend this finding showing that skin rashes could be also triggered by inhalation of cat allergen or tree

pollen and that these flare-ups were more pronounced in patients with concomitant allergic asthma than in patients who suffered from AD alone. A possible explanation of this phenomenon is that allergen-induced inflammation in the airways might cause the release of mediators from activated inflammatory cells for possible distribution to the skin, which is already primed in AD. But it is also likely that as result of allergen exposure in the airways, allergens enter the circulation and are transported to the skin.

THE ATOPY PATCH TEST

The presence of specific T cells directed to inhalant allergens along with the effects seen in AD patients upon epicutaneous or bronchial allergen administration highlight their possible impact on AD. Therefore, a major approach to the management of this part of the disease is to avoid these potential triggers. Identification of the offending allergens on the basis of history and diagnostic testing is needed to specify avoidance recommendations for the individual patient (Table 9.2).

Many patients are highly sensitized to inhalant allergens. In this regard, a number of well-established allergologic test procedures help to verify or exclude the presence of IgE mediated hypersensitivity. However, the absence of allergen specific IgE in the serum does not necessarily indicate a lack of sensitization. Therefore, an

---

Table 9.1   Sensitization to inhalant allergens in AD

TRANSCUTANEOUS ROUTE:

- Mite allergen bound on Langerhans cells via IgE[80,81]
- Induction of eczematous skin lesion upon epicutaneous allergen application[82–84]
- Presence of house dust mite on the skin[85]

RESPIRATORY ROUTE:

- Exacerbation of AD upon inhalation[86]
- Induction of new skin lesions upon inhalation[87,88]

Table 9.2   Technical variation of the APT

- Non-standardized allergen concentration[89,103,104]
- Usage of different vehicles[106]
- Pre-treatment of the skin or not[89,100]
- Duration of patch testing[100]

extension of allergy testing is represented by the SPT that evaluates IgE bound on mast cells. Nevertheless, neither test procedure considers those AD patients characterized by cell-mediated sensitizations. Since the finding of Mitchell et al[89] that epicutaneous application of inhalant allergens on unaffected skin of AD patients elicits delayed type IV eczematous reactions, this so-called ATP, as termed by Ring in 1989,[90] has additionally gained enormous interest during the past few years in completing the test procedure spectrum. Thus the parallel use of prick and patch tests increases the rate of positive reactions. It is notable that there is even a strong correlation between both test systems pointing towards the coexistence of immediate and delayed immune responses in AD.

This has led to the concept that the APT could serve as a 'provocation' test for a subgroup of AD patients similar to the bronchial or nasal provocation tests in asthma and rhinitis.[84] It has emerged as a suitable in vivo model to study the induction of eczema by inhalant allergens after 24–72 hours. Darsow et al[91] performed the first controlled, double-blind designed multicentre study to describe significant associations of APT results and the data obtained from SPT and in vitro IgE measurement. They calculated sensitivity and specificity in 253 AD patients and found that APT had higher specificity towards inhalants (69–92%) than SPT (44–53%) and serum IgE (42–64%). Thus the classical tests may have some value as screening tests yet, specificity may be added through the APT. Additionally, APT are usually negative in patients with respiratory allergy and in healthy volunteers,[92] suggesting that this technique involves AD specific triggering mechanisms and that it may represent a specific diagnostic tool since positive reactivity is obviously not related to irritant factors present in the material.

As previously mentioned, the APT reflects the second pathophysiological aspect of AD: namely, the T-cell based and dendritic cell-mediated skin inflammation following exposure to and contact with an inhalant allergen. In this respect, it is conceivable that IDECs with the capacity of high affinity IgE receptor expression are recruited into the APT lesions of allergic AD patients although up-regulation of this receptor seems to be restricted to those with IgE sensitization.[30] In contrast, the results of Langeveld-Wildschut et al[93] demonstrated the requirement of epidermal IgE+CD1a+ cells for APT positivity. However, Wistokat-Wülfing et al[94] described the association of this test with proliferation and activation of allergen specific circulating T cells, which, along with the findings of Kerschenlohr et al,[95] definitely confirm the involvement of T-cell intervention via IDECs in the APT with a more or less prominent IgE contribution. A further criterion that strengthens the role of T cells in the APT reaction is the notion of positive results in allergic AD patients without IgE sensitization as documented by the studies of Seidenari et al,[96] Manzini et al[97] and Ingordo et al[98] The aspect of a non-IgE T-cell regulated mechanism is clearly supported by the recent finding of Manzini et al[97] showing that among 313 AD patients the agreement between APT and SPT was 58%, thus implying that allergen specific IgE is not obligatory for a positive APT reaction. Instead, the presence of allergen specific IgG4 antibodies as described by Kerschenlohr et al might reveal an important precipitating factor in this subgroup of AD patients.[95]

Former studies on APTs utilized a variety of allergenic materials (different allergen fractions) and methodologies. Potentially irritating procedures like skin abrasion, tape stripping, and detergent application were used to enhance allergen penetration, and grading of positive responses varied from centre to centre. Thus lack of uniformity yielded broadly differing positive results[99] and made the reported data difficult to interpret and to reproduce. Since even minor test modifications greatly influence the outcome of the test, much effort has been undertaken to standardize the APT procedures in terms of allergen concentration, vehicle, skin pre-treatment, and time intervals to develop a reliable diagnostic tool for routine clinical use in AD patients. Currently, the protocol of the European Task Force on Atopic Dermatitis (ETFAD) provides a standardized APT technique and therefore is the most widely used.[100]

Several studies have pointed out the importance of technical aspects in generating reliable APT results. De Groot et al[101] reviewed APT studies carried out from 1982–88 and noticed a relation between the type of allergen used and the number of positive tests. Yet, only few studies described allergen doses in units permitting comparison with environmental allergen levels.[102] One such study was from Mitchell et al[89] showing responses to house dust mites at concentrations as low as 1000 protein nitrogen units (PNU)/g whereas other researchers observed a clear dose–response relationship between allergen concentration (1000 and 10 000 PNU) and positive reactions.[103] In contrast, according to the work of Seidenari et al,[104] increase in mite allergen concentration did not improve the results in AD patients but instead was considered too irritating to the skin, thus enhancing reactivity in healthy volunteers. In addition, these proteins did not necessarily correspond to the allergenic ones and so made the concentration of the material undefinable. Therefore, to achieve a better reproducibility in multicentre studies, the ETFAD has developed a standardized approach to APT proposing a concentration between 5000 and 7000 PNU/g or 200 index of reactivity (IR)/g to obtain a useful ratio between sensitivity and specificity. In children, approximately 50% of the adult dose is sufficient.[105]

In terms of the vehicle, petrolatum is not only suitable for all inhalant allergen lyophilisates, but is even more preferred to aqueous vehicles by providing stable conditions for the preparations and inducing consistently higher positive reactions.[106] Moreover, large Finn chambers (12 mm diameter) are used instead of the smaller ones (6 mm diameter) throughout Europe which enable a better penetration and subsequent presentation of intact protein allergens. Application of these test substances occurs on clinically uninvolved skin to reflect most closely the 'real life' situation of the skin.[89] Some researchers even disrupt the epidermal barrier of the test site prior to application of the APT to improve the test condition. Yet, at the same time this procedure favours irritant reactions, explaining why the ETFAD protocol does not include any pre-treatment.

Once applied on the patient's skin, the test chambers are removed after 48 hours and the first reading is performed. Of note, reactions to patch testing on normal skin may not be maximal until 72 hours as AD patients with significantly lower specific IgE levels may react to the relevant allergen much later. Subsequently, test evaluation follows the criteria as defined by the ETFAD based on the appearance of erythema and the number as well as distribution pattern of the papules while only the latter feature along with infiltration grades a positive reaction. However, before introducing APTs in the routine diagnostic work-up of AD patients the issue of reproducibility should be also considered. Indeed, APT fulfils this criterion very well because as demonstrated in the study of Langeveld-Wildschut et al[99] repetition of the test under exactly the same conditions yielded identical clinical scores and reaction patterns in all of the investigated patients after 6 months. With reference again to the ETFAD protocol, AD patients showed a very high reproducibility of 94% of all positive APT reactions within a mean 16 months observation period.[107]

Although many studies on APT have preferentially evaluated the relevance of house dust mite, as being the most important inhalant allergen in AD, some authors have also drawn their attention to other allergens. In this respect, a German multicentre study has been patch testing AD patients with cat dander (n = 243), grass pollen (n = 243), birch pollen (n = 88) and mugwort pollen (n = 88).[91] As a conclusion, these inhalants did act as triggers for AD exacerbation upon epidermal application in certain patients. Most importantly, these findings could be underlined by the results of a very recently performed European multicentre study involving 314 AD patients distributed over 12 study centres

and following the ETFAD criteria.[108] Again cat dander, grass, and birch pollen extracts have been investigated, thereby revealing a higher specificity for the APT technique (64–91% depending on the allergen) than for SPT (50–85%) or serum IgE (52–85%).

Despite these impressive data the final scientific proof for the relevance of inhalant allergens – identified by positive APT reactions – for the clinical manifestation of AD is still missing. Thus up to now, the diagnostic value of this test appears to be controversial, as no simple correlation exists between the outcome and the clinical relevance of positive APT reactions.[93,94] The question still remains whether the APT can be really used for selection of patients who may benefit from allergen avoidance. Related to this aspect Clark et al[109] and Adinoff et al[110] found that among AD patients with moderate to severe eczema and positive prick tests to numerous inhalant allergens only those allergens known to precipitate dermatitis historically or that were identified in the surroundings of the patients elicited positive patch reactions. In a similar context, Pajno et al[111] showed that children with AD had a higher SCORAD index, and a higher rate of positive SPT and APT for mites as well as higher environmental exposure to this relevant allergen than 3 years ago at the time of first recruitment. Furthermore, reactivities have been noted to occur significantly more often in patients with a typical air-exposed predilection for the skin lesions[112] suggesting that the APT may provide an important diagnostic tool in patients with eczematous lesions of predominantly uncovered areas.[103] Nevertheless, it is important to demonstrate the clinical relevance of a positive APT; but intervention studies are still lacking in patients having been positively tested with APT.

Although the clinical relevance of the APT still remains a matter of debate, mite allergens provide the most notable results in APTs. As shown by the very recent study of Giusti et al[113] 55% of AD patients reacted positively and with a high reproducibility rate to the corresponding allergen indicating that dust mites are frequently involved in the development of such APT skin lesions. Because of these data and the fact that numerous APTs have been performed with this special kind of perennial allergen as well as the fact that mites belong to the most potent allergen sources, this subgroup of inhalants deserves to be discussed in more detail.

THE BIOLOGY OF DUST MITES AND THEIR IMPACT ON ATOPIC DERMATITIS

One historical event in allergic disease was to identify mites of the suborder Astigmata and family Pyroglyphidae as a major source of allergen in house

Table 9.3 Distinct allergen groups of *Dermatophagoides pteronyssinus*

Group	Biochemical function	MW[1] cDNA (SDS-PAGE)	IgE binding[2]
1	Cysteine protease	25 000	80–100
2	Unknown (HE1 homologue)	14 000	80–100
3	Trypsin	25 000	16–100
4	α-Amylase	57 000	40–46
5	Unknown	15 000	50–70
6	Chymotrypsin	25 000	40
7	Unknown	25 000	50
8	Glutathione-S-transferase	26 000	40
9	Collagenolytic serine protease	No cDNA (30 000)	90
10	Tropomyosin	37 000	50–95
14	Vitellogenin/apolipophorin-like	177 000 (variable)	90

[1] MW (molecular weight) calculated from cDNA.
[2] Binding frequency (% patients, variation due to patient selection).
Adapted from Thomas WR, Smith WA, Hales BJ et al. Characterization and immunobiology of house dust mite allergens. Int Arch Allergy Immunol 2002; 129: 1–18.

dust[114] encountered nowadays and the most frequent inhalant allergens in humid areas. Thirteen mite species have been detected in house dust so far, whereas *Dermatophagoides pteronyssinus* (*Der p*) and *Dermatophagoides farinae* (*Der f*) are the most common ones in homes worldwide. Beds and overstuffed furniture are the main foci for the breeding of mites, providing them ample food in form of human skin scales and other organic debris. Further principal habitats are formits (pillows, mattress, sofas, carpets, etc.) with optimal conditions for their survival (temperature of 25°C and relative humidity >70%).[115] Importantly, the airborne level of mite allergen during sleep in the bedroom is tenfold higher than that found during normal daily activities in the living rooms of the same houses, reinforcing the potential importance of the bed as a mite exposure source.[116] Of importance are Platts-Mills studies on seasonal variation revealing that mite allergens persist for months after the death of the mite.[117] Detailed characterization of *Der p* extracts reveal proteinase activity in some of the distinct allergen groups (Table 9.3) including *Der p*1 as the best documented molecule up to now.[118] It is present in mite faeces at high concentration,[119] consists of two globular domains connected by an outside loop and exhibits a mixed cysteine and serine proteinase activity.[120]

Strong circumstantial evidence suggests that *Der p* antigens are crucial precipitating factors of AD.[121] The National Institute of Environmental Health Sciences recently reported that over 45% of American homes have bedding with dust mite allergen concentrations that exceed the level necessary for allergic sensitization. In this respect, early exposure to these allergens increased the risk in developing AD;[122] conversely, several studies documented the beneficial effect of careful house dust mite avoidance on the course of disease. Roberts[123] and August[124] reported improvement of clinical symptoms in AD patients after the combination of plastic encasings, removal of carpets, and vacuum cleaning. Furthermore, Tan et al[26] performed a double-blind controlled trial on a study population of 60 AD patients for 6 months. The treatment consisted of Goretex®-covered mattresses versus light cotton bags, benzyltannate spray to kill mites versus water spray, and a high filtration vacuum cleaner versus a cheap vacuum cleaner used in bedrooms and living rooms during this period. Due to this special bedding system the dust load declined by 98% within the first month and the procedure in general yielded significantly higher changes in the severity score of the active treated group than of the placebo group. Subsequently, Friedman and Tan analysed the clinical effect of mite elimination in another collective of AD patients following the same treatment protocol. As a result bed and carpet *Der p*1 levels were reduced to minimal levels and the biggest improvements were seen in the most severely affected subjects.[125] In the study of Holm et al[126] the authors described a relationship between disease severity and CD30 in serum (expressed by allergen specific human CD4+ T cells) which was significantly decreased after a 12-month period of allergen avoidance. Yet, patients not sensitized or not exposed to mites benefited just as much from the bed covers as those who were sensitized and/or exposed to this kind of allergen. Thus, the use of active bed covers along with regular vacuum cleaning of the mattress and carpets as well as the airing of the bedroom, reduces the allergen load in bed and thereby creates a sleeping environment that can ameliorate eczema.

There is further compelling evidence supporting the involvement of house dust mites in AD pathogenesis: high titres of Der p1 specific IgE antibodies have been detected in 95% of AD patients correlating with disease severity[127] while these antibodies have been found in only 42% of asthmatic subjects.[27] When localized on LCs Der p1 specific IgE antibodies are implicated in the binding of mite allergen, thus facilitating allergen presentation with resultant T-cell activation by up to 1000-fold.[128]

Rawle et al[129] were the first to describe proliferative responses to Der p1 by peripheral blood mononuclear cells of almost all AD patients whereas later Kimura et al[65] showed the correlation between disease severity and high levels of mite-induced lymphocyte proliferation in infants with AD. The ability of Der p1 to induce T_H2 cytokine production in allergic subjects is now well established and consistent with responses seen in T-cell lines stimulated with Der p1.[130] Apart from its direct effect on T cells Der p1 pulsed dendritic cells of atopic subjects bias T_H2 development via up-regulation of TARC and MDC, thus ensuring that recently CCR4 activated T_H2 cells are attracted and do not migrate back to the draining lymph nodes.[131] Of note, dendritic cells from healthy donors exposed to this allergen preferentially attract T_H1 cells via IP-10 production.[132] Additionally, Der p1 mediates cleavage of the CD23 IgE receptor localized on human B cells and of the CD25 subunit of the T-cell IL-2 receptor, which further may enhance its allergenicity.[133] It also increases paracellular permeability through disruption of intercellular tight junctions in the respiratory epithelium,[134] hence potentiating the availability of environmental aeroallergens to dendritic cells.[135] Moreover Der p1 triggers inflammatory cytokine release from epithelial cell cultures,[136] although this aspect has not yet been confirmed in vivo.

CONCLUSION

In summary, AD is a common, inflammatory skin disorder that affects about 10% of the population, with increasing tendency and public interest in the disease during the last few years. The complex interaction between genetic and environmental mechanisms, along with an intensive network of cytokines and chemokines orchestrating the development of disease-related mechanisms, represents an active line of investigation particularly as an unifying pathogenic concept of AD has not yet been established. Besides, it is generally accepted that the course of the disease may be

Table 9.4   Evidence for the participation of inhalant allergens in AD
• Allergen specific T cells invading the skin[72–79]
• Allergen specific IgE[127]
• AD exacerbation following allergen inhalation[87,88]
• AD exacerbation following epicutaneous allergen application[99,103]
• APT skin lesions induced by the relevant allergen[89,91]
• Allergen avoidance of clinical benefit[26,123–126]

seriously pronounced following skin exposure to inhalant allergens such as mites, animal dander, mould, and pollens. Once entering the body either through the epidermal or the respiratory route they initiate a specific immune response leading to the generation and the subsequent recruitment of allergen specific T cells into the skin thereby primarily interfering in AD pathogenesis. For this reason standard testing modalities including SPT and serological assays help to identify these potential inhalants that particularly trigger the type I immune response. Additionally, the APT has emerged as an in vivo model to study the T cell-based and DC-mediated skin inflammation of AD patients reflecting a classical delayed type IV hypersensitivity. Thus, together with other diagnostic tools, the APT could be employed in the management of disease achieved by allergen avoidance. Unfortunately, minor modifications critically influence the outcome of this test procedure and therefore prevent clear interpretation and comparison of the results obtained. To address this a standardized patch test protocol has been performed by ETFAD, leading to satisfactory results in terms of specificity, sensitivity and reproducibility.

Most recently, a European multicentre study group patch testing AD patients of 12 different study centres according to the ETFAD criteria showed that mites, animal dander, and pollens acted as triggers for AD exacerbation; yet the clinical relevance of this test system has still not been fully elucidated. Nevertheless, all data on APTs consistently state the higher positivity towards house dust mites suggesting that these kinds of allergens are frequently involved in the development of such APT skin lesions and seem to be crucial precipitating factors of AD. Indeed, exposure to high doses of mite allergen in early infancy is associated with a higher incidence of developing eczema; on the other hand, efforts to create a dust mite-free environment yield significant improvement in the clinical symptoms without complete remission. The available evidence indicates that at least in a subgroup of AD patients inhalants contribute to the pathogenesis. It is possible that sensitization and subsequent disease exacerbation occurs via the respiratory route as well as through the disrupted skin barrier. However, proper diagnostic tools are urgently needed to identify this subset of AD patients with acceptable diagnostic reliability.

REFERENCES

1. Schultz Larsen F, Diepgen T, Svensson A. The occurrence of atopic dermatitis in north Europe: an international questionnaire study. J Am Acad Dermatol 1996; 34(5): 760–4.
2. Williams H, Robertson C, Stewart A et al. Worldwide variations in the prevalence of symptoms of atopic eczema in the International Study of Asthma and Allergies in Childhood. J Allergy Clin Immunol 1999; 103: 125–38.
3. Martinez FD. The coming-of-age of the hygiene hypothesis. Respir Res 2001; 2(3): 129–32.
4. Hanifin J, Rajka G. Diagnostic features of atopic dermatitis. Acta Derm Venereol 1980; 92(92): 44–7.
5. Leung DYM, Bhan AK, Schneeberger EE, Geha RS. Characterization of the mononuclear cell infiltrate in atopic dermatitis using monoclonal antibodies. J Allergy Clin Immunol 1983; 71: 47–56.
6. Wollenberg A, Bieber T. Atopic dermatitis: from the genes to skin lesions. Allergy 2000; 55: 205–13.
7. Leung DY, Boguniewicz M, Howell MD et al. New insights into atopic dermatitis. J Clin Invest 2004; 113(5): 651–7.
8. Johansson SG, Hourihane JO, Bousquet J et al. A revised nomenclature for allergy. An EACCI position statement from the EAACI nomenclature task force. Allergy 2001; 56: 813–24.
9. Imayama S, Hashizume T, Miyahara H, Tanahashi T et al. Combination of patch test and IgE for dust mite antigens differentiates 130 patients with atopic dermatitis into four groups. J Am Acad Dermatol 1992; 27: 531–8.
10. Fabrizi G, Romano A, Vultaggio P, Bellegrandi S et al. Heterogeneity of atopic dermatitis defined by the immune response to inhalant and food allergens. Eur J Dermatol 1999; 9(5): 380–4.
11. Novak N, Bieber T, Leung DYM. Immune mechanisms leading to atopic dermatitis. J Allergy Clin Immunol 2003; 112: S128–39.
12. Bunikowski R, Mielke ME, Skarabis H et al. Evidence for a disease-promoting effect of Staphylococcus aureus-derived exotoxins in atopic dermatitis. J Allergy Clin Immunol 2000; 105(4): 814–19.
13. Bunikowski R, Mielke M, Skarabis H et al. Prevalence and role of serum IgE antibodies to the Staphylococcus aureus-derived superantigens SEA and SEB in children with atopic dermatitis. J Allergy Clin Immunol 1999; 103(1): 119–24.
14. Ong PY, Ohtake T, Brandt C et al. Endogenous antimicrobial peptides and skin infections in atopic dermatitis. N Engl J Med 2002; 347(15): 1151–60.
15. Nomura I, Goleva E, Howell MD, Hamid QA et al. Cytokine mileu of atopic dermatitis, as compared to psoriasis, skin prevents induction of innate immune response genes. J Immunol 2003; 171(6): 3262–9.
16. Breuer K, Kapp A, Werfel T. Bacterial infections and atopic dermatitis. Allergy 2001; 56: 1034–41.
17. Laan MP, Tibbe GJ, Oranje AP, Bosmans EP et al. CD4+ cells proliferate after peanut extract specific and CD8+ cells proliferate after polyclonal stimulation of PBMC of children with atopic dermatitis. Clin Exp Allergy 1998; 28: 35–44.
18. Werfel T, Ahlers G, Schmidt P, Boeker M et al. Milk responsive atopic dermatitis is associated with a casein specific lymphocyte response in adolescent and adult patients. J Allergy Clin Immunol 1997; 99: 124–33.
19. Burks AW, James JM, Hiegel A, Wilson G et al. Atopic dermatitis and food hypersensitivity reactions. J Pediatr 1998; 132: 132–6.
20. Sicherer SH, Sampson HA. Food hypersensitivity and atopic dermatitis: pathophysiology, epidemiology, diagnosis, and management. J Allergy Clin Immunol 1999; 104(3Pt2): S114–22.
21. Kondo N, Agata H, Fukutomi O, Motoyoshi F et al. Lymphocyte responses to food antigens in patients with atopic dermatitis who are sensitized to foods. J Allergy Clin Immunol 1990; 86: 253–60.
22. Li XM, Kleiner G, Huang CK, Lee SY et al. Murine model of atopic dermatitis associated with food hypersensitivity. J Allergy Clin Immunol 2001; 107: 693–702.
23. Walker IC. Causation of eczema, urticaria, and angioneurotic edema by proteins other than those derived from foods. JAMA 1918; 70: 897–900.
24. Werfel T, Breuer K. Role of food allergy in atopic dermatitis. Curr Opin Allergy Clin Immunol 2004; 4(5): 379–85.
25. Friedmann PS. The role of dust mite antigen sensitization and atopic dermatitis. Clin Exp Allergy 1999; 29: 869–72.
26. Tan BB, Weald D, Strickland I, Friedmann PS. Double-blind controlled trial of effect of house dust mite allergen avoidance on atopic dermatitis. Lancet 1996; 347: 15–18.
27. Scalabrin DM, Bavbek S, Perzanowski MS, Wilson BB et al. Use of specific IgE assessing the relevance of fungal and dust mite allergens to atopic dermatitis: a comparison with asthmatic and nonasthmatic control subjects. J Allergy Clin Immunol 1999; 104: 1273–9.
28. Werfel T, Kapp A. The role of environmental allergens in the provocation of atopic dermatitis. In: Oehling AK, Huerta Lopez JG, eds. Progress in Allergy and Clinical Immunology. Seattle: Hogrefe & Huber, 1997; 4: 153–6.
29. Hara J, Higuchi K, Okamoto R, Kawashima M et al. High expression of sphingomyelin deacylase is an important determinant of ceramide deficiency leading to barrier disruption in atopic dermatitis. J Invest Dermatol 2000; 115: 406–13.
30. Kerschenlohr K, Decard S, Przybilla B, Wollenberg A. Atopy patch test reactions show a rapid influx of inflammatory dendritic epidermal cells in patients with extrinsic atopic dermatitis and patients with intrinsic atopic dermatitis. J Allergy Clin Immunol 2003; 111: 869–74.
31. Giustizieri ML, Mascia F, Frezzolini A et al. Keratinocytes from patients with atopic dermatitis and psoriasis show a distinct chemokine production profile in response to T-cell derived cytokines. J Allergy Clin Immunol 2001; 107: 871–7.
32. Toda M, Leung DYM, Molet S et al. Polarized in vivo expression of IL-11 and IL-17 between acute and chronic skin lesions. J Allergy Clin Immunol 2003; 111: 875–81.
33. Soumelis V, Reche PA, Kanzler H et al. Human epithelial cells trigger dendrtitic cell mediated allergic inflammation by producing TSLP. Nat Immunol 2002; 3: 673–80.
34. Kakinuma T, Nakamura K, Wakugawa M, Mitsui H et al. Thymus and activation regulated chemokine in atopic dermatitis: serum thymus and activation regulated chemokine level is closely related with disease activity. J Allergy Clin Immunol 2001; 107: 535–41.
35. Rothenberg ME. Eosinophilia. N Engl J Med 1998; 338: 1592–600.
36. Breuer K, Kapp A, Werfel T. Urine eosinophil protein X (EPX) is an in vitro parameter of inflammation in atopic dermatitis of the adult age. Allergy 2001; 56: 780–4.
37. Wedi B, Raap U, Lewrick H, Kapp A. Delayed eosinophil programmed cell death in vitro: a common feature of inhalant allergy and extrinsic and intrinsic atopic dermatitis. J Allergy Clin Immunol 1997; 100: 536–43.
38. Herz U, Bunikowski R, Renz H. Role of T cells in atopic dermatitis. Int Arch Allergy Immunol 1998; 115: 179.
39. Santamaria Babi LF, Picker LJ, Perez Soler MT et al. Circulating allergen-reactive T cells from patients with atopic dermatits and allergic contact dermatitis express the skin-selective homing receptor, the cutaneous lymphocyte-associated antigen. J Exp Med 1995; 181: 1935–40.

40. Akdis M, Trautmann A, Blaser K, Akdis CA et al. T cells and effector mechanisms in the pathogenesis of atopic dermatitis. Curr Allergy Asthma Rep 2002; 2: 1–3.

41. Homey B, Alenius H, Muller A et al. CCL27-CCR10 interactions regulate T cell mediated skin inflammation. Nat Med 2002; 8: 157–65.

42. Campbell JJ, Brightling CE, Symon FA, Qin S et al. Expression of chemokine receptors by lung T cells from normal and asthmatic subjects. J Immunol 2001; 166(4): 2842–8.

43. Thepen T, Langeveld-Wildschut E, Bihari I, van Wichen D et al. Biphasic response against aeroallergen in atopic dermatitis showing a switch from an initial Th2 response to a Th1 response in situ: an immunocytochemical study. J Allergy Clin Immunol 1996; 97: 828–38.

44. Abbas AK, Murphy KM, Sher A. Functional diversity of helper T lymphocytes. Nature 1996; 383(6603): 787–93.

45. O'Garra A. Cytokines induce the development of functionally heterogenous T helper cell subsets. Immunity 1998; 8: 275–83.

46. Read S, Malmstrom V, Powrie F. Cytotoxic T lymphocyte associated antigen 4 plays an essential role in the function of CD25(+)CD4(+) regulatory cells that control intestinal inflammation. J Exp Med 2000; 192: 295–302.

47. McHugh RS, Whitters MJ, Piccirillo CA, Young DA et al. CD4(+)CD25(+) immunoregulatory T cells: gene expression analysis reveals a functional role for the glucocorticoid-induced TNF receptor. Immunity 2002; 16(2): 311–23.

48. Bluestone JA, Abbas AK. Natural versus adaptive regulatory T cells. Nat Rev Immunol 2003; 3: 253–7.

49. Romagnani S. T cell subsets (Th1 versus Th2). Ann Allergy Asthma Immunol 2000; 85: 9–18.

50. El- Mezayen RE, Matsumoto T. In vitro responsiveness to IL-18 in combination with IL-12 or IL-2 by PBMC from patients with bronchial asthma and atopic dermatitis. Clin Immunol 2004; 111(1): 61–8.

51. Oppmann B, Lesley R, Blom B et al. Novel p19 protein engages IL-12p40 to form a cytokine, IL-23, with biological activities similar as well as distinct from IL-12. Immunity 2000; 13: 715–25.

52. Pflanz S, Timans JC, Cheung J et al. IL-27, a heterodimeric cytokine composed of EBI3 and p28 protein, induces proliferation of naive CD4(+) T cells. Immunity 2002; 16: 779–90.

53. Lucas S, Ghilardi N, Li J, de Sauvage FJ. IL-27 regulates IL-12 responsiveness of naive CD4+ T cells through STAT-1 dependent and independent mechanisms. Proc Natl Acad Sci USA 2003; 100(25): 15047–52.

54. Breit S, Steinhoff M, Blaser K, Heusser CH et al. A strict requirement of interleukin-4 for interleukin-4 induction in antigen stimulated human memory T cells. Eur J Immunol 1996; 26: 1860–5.

55. Sornasse T, Larenas PV, Davis KA, de Vries JE et al. Differentiation and stability of T helper 1 and 2 cells derived from naive human neonatal CD4+ T cell, analyzed at the single-cell level. J Exp Med 1996; 184: 473–83.

56. Rincon M, Anguita J, Nakamura T, Fikrig E et al. Interleukin (IL)-6 directs the differentiation of IL-4 producing CD4+ T cells. J Exp Med 1997; 185: 461–9.

57. Gallagher G, Dickensheets H, Eskdale J, Izotova LS et al. Cloning, expression and initial characterization of interleukin-19 (IL-19), a novel homologue of human interleukin-10 (IL-10). Genes Immun 2000; 1(7): 442–50.

58. Gallagher G, Eskdale J, Jordan W, Peat J et al. Human interleukin-19 and its receptor: a potential role in the induction of Th2 responses. Int Immunopharmacol 2004; 4: 615–26.

59. Ikeda K, Nakajima H, Suzuki K, Kagami S et al. Mast cells produce interleukin-25 upon Fc epsilon RI-mediated activation. Blood 2003; 101(9): 3594–6.

60. Murphy KM, Reiner SL. The lineage decisions of helper T cells. Nat Rev Immunol 2002; 2: 933–44.

61. Rengarajan J, Szabo SJ, Glimcher LH. Transcriptional regulation of Th1/Th2 polarization. Immunol Today 2000; 21: 479–83.

62. Kapsenberg ML, Wierenga EA, Bos JD, Jansen HM. Functional subsets of allergen reactive human CD4+ T cells. Immunol Today 1991; 12: 392–5.

63. Jujo K, Renz H, Abe J, Gelfand EW et al. Decreased interferon gamma and increased interleukin-4 production in atopic dermatitis promotes IgE synthesis. J Allergy Clin Immunol 1992; 90(3): 323–31.

64. Parronchi P, Macchia D, Piccinni MP, Biswas P et al. Allergen and bacterial antigen specific T cell clones established from atopic donors show a different profile of cytokine production. Proc Natl Acad Sci USA 1991; 88: 4538–42.

65. Kimura M, Tsuruta S, Yoshida T. Correlation of house dust mite specific lymphocyte proliferation with IL-5 production, eosinophilia, and the severity of symptoms in infants with atopic dermatitis. J Allergy Clin Immunol 1998; 101: 84–9.

66. Hamid Q, Boguniewicz M, Leung DYM. Differential in situ cytokine gene expression in acute versus chronic atopic dermatitis. J Clin Invest 1994; 94: 870–6.

67. Grewe M, Gyufko K, Schöpf E, Krutmann J. Lesional expression of interferon-γ in atopic eczema. Lancet 1994; 343: 25–6.

68. Hamid Q, Naseer T, Minshall EM, Song YL et al. In vivo expression of IL-12 and IL-13 in atopic dermatitis. J Allergy Clin Immunol 1996; 98: 225–31.

69. Grewe M, Bruijnzeel-Koomen CA, Schopf E, Thepen T et al. A role for Th1 and Th2 cells in the immunopathogenesis of atopic dermatitis. Immunol Today 1998; 19: 359–61.

70. Schade RP, van Ieperen-van Dijk AG, van Reijsen FC, Versluis C et al. Differences in antigen specific T cell responses between infants with atopic dermatitis with and without cow's milk allergy: relevance of Th2 cytokines. J Allergy Clin Immunol 2000; 106: 1155–62.

71. Reekers R, Beyer K, Nigemann B, Wahn U et al. The role of circulating food antigen specific lymphocytes in food allergic children with atopic dermatitis. Br J Dermatol 1996; 135(6): 935–41.

72. Ramb-Lindhauer C, Feldmann A, Rotte M, Neumann C. Characterization of grass pollen reactive T cell lines derived from lesional atopic skin. Arch Dermatol Res 1991; 283(2): 71–6.

73. Reekers R, Busche M, Wittmann M, Kapp A et al. Birch pollen related foods trigger atopic dermatitis in patients with specific cutaneous T cell responses to birch pollen antigens. J Allergy Clin Immunol 1999; 104: 466–72.

74. van der Heijden FL, Wierenga EA, Bos JD, Kapsenberg ML. High frequency of IL-4 producing CD4+ allergen specific T lymphocytes in atopic dermatitis lesional skin. J Invest Dermatol 1991; 97(3): 389–94.

75. van Reijsen FC, Bruijnzeel-Koomen CA, Kalthoff FS, Maggi E et al. Skin derived aeroallergen specific T cell clones of Th2 phenotype in patients with atopic dermatitis. J Allergy Clin Immunol 1992; 90: 184–93.

76. Werfel T, Morita A, Grewe M, Renz H et al. Allergen specificity of skin infiltrating T cells is not restricted to a type 2 cytokine pattern in chronic skin lesions of atopic dermatitis. J Invest Dermatol 1996; 107(6): 871–6.

77. Neumann C, Gutgesell C, Fliegert F, Bonifer R et al. Comparative analysis of the frequency of house dust mite specific and nonspecific Th1 and Th2 cells in skin lesions and peripheral blood of patients with atopic dermatitis. J Mol Med 1996; 74: 401–6.

78. Sager N, Feldmann A, Schilling G, Kreitsch P et al. House dust mite specific T cells in the skin of subjects with atopic dermatitis: frequency and lymphokine profile in allergen patch test. J Allergy Clin Immunol 1992; 89(4): 801–40.

79. Takahama H, Masuko-hongo K, Atsushi T, Kawa Y et al. T-cell clonotypes specific for Dermatophagoides pteronyssinus in the skin lesions of patients with atopic dermatitis. Hum Immunol 2002; 63: 558–66.

80. Maeda K, Yamamoto K, Tanaka Y, Anan S et al. House dust mite (HDM) antigen in naturally occurring lesions of atopic dermatitis (AD): the relationship between HDM antigen in the skin and HDM antigen specific IgE antibody. J Dermatol Sci 1992; 3: 73–7.

81. Tanaka Y, Anan S, Yoshida H. Immunohistochemical studies in mite antigen induced patch test sites in atopic dermatitis. J Dermatol Sci 1990; 1: 361–8.

82. Gondo A, Saeki N, Tokuda Y. Challenge reactions in atopic dermatitis after percutaneous entry of mite antigen. Br J Dermatol 1986; 115: 485–93.

83. Norris PG, Schofield O, Camp RD. A study of the role of house dust mite in atopic dermatitis. Br J Dermatol 1988; 118: 435–40.

84. Ring J, Darsow U, Gfesser M, Vieluf D. The 'atopy patch test' in evaluating the role of aeroallergens in atopic eczema. Int Arch Allergy Immunol 1997; 113: 379–83.

85. Riley G, Siebers R, Rains N, Crane J et al. House dust mite antigen on skin and sheets. Lancet 1998; 351: 649–50.

86. Tuft LA. Importance of inhalant allergen in atopic dermatitis. J Invest Dermatol 1949; 12: 211–19.

87. Tupker RA, de Monchy JG, Coenraads PJ, Homan A et al. Induction of atopic dermatitis by inhalation of house dust mite. J Allergy Clin Immunol 1996; 97: 1064–70.

88. Brinkman L, Aslander MM, Raaijmarkers JA, Lammers JW et al. Bronchial and cutaneous responses in atopic dermatitis patients after allergen inhalation challenge. Clin Exp Allergy 1997; 27: 1043–51.

89. Mitchell E, Crow J, Chapman S, Jouhal F et al. Basophils in allergen induced patch test sites in atopic dermatitis. Lancet 1982; 1: 127–30.

90. Ring J, Darsow U, Gfesser M, Vieluf D. The 'atopy patch test' with aeroallergens in atopic eczema. J Allergy Clin Immunol 1989; 82: 195.

91. Darsow U, Vieluf D, Ring J. Evaluating the relevance of aeroallergen sensitization in atopic eczema with the atopy patch test: a randomized, double-blind multicenter study. Atopy Patch Test Study Group. J Am Acad Dermatol 1999; 40: 187–93.

92. Bruijnzeel PLB, Kuijper PHM, Kapp A et al. The involvement of eosinophils in the patch test reaction to aeroallergens in atopic dermatitis: its relevance for the pathogenesis of atopic dermatitis. Clin Exp Allergy 1993; 23: 97–109.

93. Langeveld-Wildschut EG, Riedl H, Thepen T, Bihari IC et al. Modulation of the atopy patch test reaction by topical corticosteroids and tar. J Allergy Clin Immunol 2000; 106: 737–43.

94. Wistokat-Wülfing A, Schmidt P, Darsow U, Ring J et al. Atopy patch test reactions are associated with T-lymphocyte mediated allergen specific immune responses in atopic dermatitis. Clin Exp Allergy 1999; 29: 513–21.

95. Kerschenlohr K, Decard S, Darsow U, Ollert M et al. Clinical and immunologic reactivity to aeroallergens in 'intrinsic' atopic dermatitis patients. J Allergy Clin Immunol 2003; 111: 195–7.

96. Seidenari S, Manzini BM, Danese P, Giannetti A. Positive patch tests to whole mite culture and purified mite extracts in patients with atopic dermatitis, asthma, and rhinitis. Ann Allergy 1992; 69(3): 201–6.

97. Manzini BM, Motolese A, Donini M, Seidenari S. Contact allergy to Dermatophagoides in atopic dermatitis patients and healthy subjects. Contact Dermatitis 1995; 33(4): 243–6.

98. Ingordo V, Andria GD, Andria CD, Tortora A. Results of atopy patch tests with house dust mites in adults with 'intrinsic' and 'extrinsic' atopic dermatitis. J Eur Acad Dermatol Venereol 2002; 16: 450–4.

99. Langeveld-Wildschut EG, van Marion AM, Thepen T, Mudde GC et al. Evaluation of variables influencing the outcome of the atopy patch test. J Allergy Clin Immunol 1995; 96(1): 66–73.

100. Darsow U, Ring J. Airborne and dietary allergens in atopic eczema: a comprehensive review of diagnostic tests. Clin Exp Dermatol 2000; 25(7): 544–51.

101. De Groot AC, Young E. The role of contact allergy to aeroallergens in atopic dermatitis. Contact Dermatitis 1989; 21: 209–14.

102. Fitzharris P, Riley G. House dust mites in atopic dermatitis. Int J Dermatol 1999; 38: 173–5.

103. Darsow U, Vieluf D, Ring J. The atopy patch test: an increased rate of reactivity in patients who have an air-exposed pattern of eczema. Br J Dermatol 1996; 135: 182–6.

104. Seidenari S, Giusti F, Pellacani G, Bertoni L. Frequency and intensity of responses to mite patch tests are lower in nonatopic subjects with respect to patients with atopic dermatitis. Allergy 2003; 58: 426–9.

105. Darsow U. Atopie-Patch-Test: Atopisches Ekzem und Allergie. Hautarzt 2003; 54: 930–6.

106. Oldhoff JM, Bihari IC, Knol EF, Bruijnzeel-Koomen CA et al. Atopy patch test in patients with atopic eczema/dermatitis syndrome: comparison of petrolatum and aqueous solution as a vehicle. Allergy 2004; 59(4): 451–6.

107. Kerschenlohr K, Darsow U, Burdorf WHC, Ring J et al. Lessons from atopy patch testing in atopic dermatitis. Curr Sci 2004; 4: 285–9.

108. Darsow U, Laifaoui J, Kerschenlohr K, Wollenberg A et al. The prevalence of positive reactions in the atopy patch test with aeroallergens and food allergens in subjects with atopic eczema: a European multicenter study. Allergy 2004; 59(12): 1318–25.

109. Clark RA, Adinoff AD. Aeroallergen contact can exacerbate atopic dermatitis: patch tests as a diagnostic tool. J Am Acad Dermatol 1989; 21(4): 863–9.

110. Adinoff A, Tellez P, Clark R. Atopic dermatitis and aeroallergen contact sensitivity. J Allergy Clin Immunol 1988; 81: 736–42.

111. Pajno GB, Peroni DG, Barberio G, Pietrobelli A et al. Predictive features for persistence of atopic dermatitis in children. Pediatr Allergy Immunol 2003; 14: 292–5.

112. Ring J, Darsow U, Behrendt H. Role of aeroallergens in atopic eczema proof of concept with the atopy patch test. J Am Acad Dermatol 2001; 45: S49–52.

113. Giusti F, Seidenari S. Reproducibility of atopy patch tests with Dermatophagoides: a study on 85 patients with atopic dermatitis. Contact Dermatitis 2004; 50: 18–21.

114. Voorhorst R, Spieksma FTM, Varekamp N et al. House dust mite atopy and the allergens it produces: identity with the house dust allergen. J Allergy Clin Immunol 1967; 39: 325–9.

115. Wharton GW. House dust mites. J Med Entomol 1976; 12: 577–621.

116. Sakaguchi M, Inouye S, Yasueda H, Shida T. Concentration of airborne mite allergens (Der I and Der II) during sleep. Allergy 1992; 47: 55–7.

117. Platts-Mills TAE, Hayden ML, Chapman MD et al. Seasonal variation in dust mite and grass pollen allergens in dust from the houses of patients with asthma. J Allergy Clin Immunol 1986; 79: 781–91.

118. Chapman MD, Platts-Mills TA. Purification and characterization of the major allergen from Dermatophagoides pteronyssinus-antigen P1. J Immunol 1980; 125(2): 587–92.

119. Tovey ER, Chapman MD, Platt-Mills TAE. Mite faeces are a major source of house dust allergens. Nature 1981; 289: 592–3.

120. Hewitt CRA, Horton H, Jones RM, Pritchard DI. Heterogenous proteolytic specificity and activity of the house dust mite proteinase allergen Der p1. Clin Exp Allergy 1997; 27: 201–7.

121. Tupker RA, de Monchy JGR, Coentraads PJ. House dust mite hypersensitivity, eczema, and other nonpulmonary manifestations of allergy. Allergy 1998; 53(48 Suppl): 92–6.

122. Huang JL, Chen CC, Kuo ML, Hsieh KH. Exposure to a high concentration of mite allergen in early infancy is a risk factor for developing atopic dermatitis: a 3 year follow-up study. Pediatr Allergy Immunol 2001; 12(1): 11–16.

123. Roberts DL. House dust mite avoidance and atopic dermatitis. Br J Dermatol 1984; 110: 735–6.

124. August PJ. The environmental causes and management of eczema. Practitioner 1987; 231: 495–500.
125. Friedman PS, Tan BB. Mite elimination – clinical effect on eczema. Allergy 1998; 53(48 Suppl): 97–100.
126. Holm L, Öhman S, Bengtsson A, van Hage-Hamsten M et al. Effectiveness of occlusive bedding in the treatment of atopic dermatitis – a placebo-controlled trial of 12 months' duration. Allergy 2001; 56: 152–8.
127. Chapman MD, Rowntree S, Mitchell EB, Di Prisco de Fuenmajor MC et al. Quantitative assessments of IgG and IgE antibodies to inhalant allergens in patients with atopic dermatitis. J Allergy Clin Immunol 1983; 72(1): 27–33.
128. van der Heijden, van Nerven RJJ, van Katwijk M, Bos JD et al. Serum IgE facilitated allergen presentation in atopic disease. J Immunol 1993; 150: 3643–50.
129. Rawle FC, Mitchell EB, Platts-Mills TAE. T cell responses to the major allergen from the house dust mite Dermatophagoides pteronyssinus, antigen P1: comparison of patients with asthma, atopic dermatitis, and perennial rhinitis. J Immunol 1984; 133: 195–201.
130. Tsitoura DC, Verhoef A, Gelder CM, O'Hehir et al. Altered T cell ligands derived from a major house dust mite allergen enhance IFN-γ but not IL-4 production by human CD4+ T cells. J Immunol 1996; 157: 2160–5.
131. Hashimoto S, Suzuki T, Dong HY, Nagai S et al. Serial analysis of gene expression in human monocyte-derived dendritic cells. Blood 1999; 94: 845.
132. Hammad H, Smits HH, Ratajczak C, Nithiananthan A et al. Monocyte-derived dendritic cells exposed to Der p1 allergen enhance the recruitment of Th2 cells: major involvement of the chemokines TARC/CCL17 and MDC/CCL22. Eur Cytokine Netw 2003; 14(4): 219–28.
133. Shakib F, Schulz O, Swell H. A mite subversive: cleavage of CD23 and CD25 by Der p1 enhances allergenicity. Immunol Today 1998; 19: 313–16.
134. Wan H, Winton HL, Soeller C et al. Quantitative structural and biochemical analyses of tight junction dynamics following exposure of epithelial cells to house dust mite allergen Der p1. Clin Exp Allergy 2000; 30: 685–98.
135. Wan H, Winston HL, Soeller C, Tovey ER et al. Der p1 facilitates transepithelial allergen delivery by disruption of tight junctions. J Clin Invest 1999; 104: 123–33.
136. King C, Brennan S, Thompson PJ, Stewart GA. Dust mite proteolytic allergens induce cytokine release from cultured airway epithelium. J Immunol 1998; 161: 3645–51.
137. Thomas WR, Smith WA, Hales BJ, Mills KL et al. Characterization and immunobiology of house dust mite allergens. Int Arch Allergy Immunol 2002; 129: 1–18.

10

Itch – pathophysiology and treatment

Sonja Ständer, Thomas A Luger, and Martin Steinhoff

INTRODUCTION

Pruritus, regularly defined as an unpleasant sensation provoking the desire to scratch,[1] is a diagnostic hallmark of atopic dermatitis (AD).[2,3] As a cutaneous sensory perception, itch is excited on neuropeptide-containing free nerve endings of unmyelinated nociceptor fibres. It is known that several mediators such as neuropeptides, proteases, or cytokines provoke itch by direct binding to itch receptors or indirectly via histamine release. Although great efforts have been made during the last years, the pathophysiology of pruritus in AD is not fully understood but several facts explain its intensity and therapy refractoricity demanding a specific management.

NERVOUS SYSTEM AND ITCH TRANSMISSION

Sensory cutaneous nerves

The skin is equipped with an effective communication and control system designed to protect the organism in a constantly changing environment. For this purpose a dense network of highly specialized afferent sensory and efferent autonomic nerve branches occurs in all cutaneous layers. Recent studies have clearly shown that the sensation of itch is transmitted by a subpopulation of unmyelinated, histamine-sensitive C-polymodal nociceptive neurons to different areas of the brain including the cerebellum, motor areas, and postcentral sensory gyrus.[4–7] Cutaneous terminals are free nerve endings located in the papillary dermis and around skin appendages. The nerve endings are covered by a variety of specialized receptors which contribute to the induction of itch and burning pain. After activation of the receptor by binding of the corresponding ligand, the nerve fibre either transmits an electrical signal to the central nervous system (CNS) or may directly elicit an inflammatory reaction by antidromic propagation of these impulses. The effector function of a nerve may be determined by secreted neuropeptides and the corresponding receptors of target structures.[8] In addition, there is accumulating evidence that neuropeptides exert multiple effects on immunocompetent cells suggesting a strong interaction between the nervous and the immune system.[4,5,9–11]

Autonomic cutaneous nerves

In contrast to sensory nerve fibres, the distribution of autonomic nerves is restricted to the dermis, innervating blood vessels, arteriovenous anastomoses, lymphatic vessels, glands, hair follicles, and stimulating immune cells to release neurotransmitters. Although autonomic nerves represent only a minority of cutaneous fibres which predominantly generate neurotransmitters such as acetylcholine (ACh) and catecholamines, recent observations revealed a potential role for neuropeptides released from sympathetic and parasympathetic neurons during cutaneous inflammation. Moreover, autonomic nerve fibres participate in the regulation of vascular effects in the skin by releasing ACh and vasoactive intestinal peptide (VIP).[12–16] In addition, muscarinic and nicotinergic acetylcholine receptor expression has been described on keratinocytes, melanocytes, fibroblasts, and lymphocytes indicating a regulatory role of the autonomic nervous system in the induction of inflammation.[17–20]

Nervous system in atopic dermatitis

Several investigators demonstrated that cutaneous nerve fibres in atopic skin lesions are altered in number and morphology. An increase of sensory but decrease of adrenergic autonomic nerve fibres was observed[21] indicating a differential role of primary afferent and autonomic nerve fibres in pruritus pathophysiology. Mihm et al[22] described cutaneous myelinated nerves appearing demyelinated and sclerotic. However, other groups were not able to confirm these pathological changes upon light microscopical level.[23,24] Furthermore lesional atopic skin showed an increased number of neurofilament-, PGP 9.5-, calcitonin gene related peptide (CGRP)-, and substance P (SP)-positive nerve fibres in the papillary dermis,[25] at the dermoepidermal junction,[23,26] in the epidermis,[21] and around sweat glands.[27] At the ultrastructure level, the axons contained many mitochondria and neurofilaments with abundant neurovesicles[25] confirming immunohistological findings. In a semiquantitative analysis, Sugiura et al[25] found different densities of PGP-positive peripheral nerves. Highest density was in prurigo lesions, followed by lichenified lesions, and subacute lesions. Early acute lesions of AD showed almost the same density as non-involved skin of patients with AD. These results were confirmed by electron microscopical investigation. Lesional AD skin revealed an increased content of hyperplastic nerve fibres with enlarged axons.[23,25] Terminal Schwann cells seem to migrate closer to the epidermis as in normal controls.[23] In addition, axons lost their surrounding cytoplasm of Schwann cells in some areas and may thus communicate directly with dermal cells.[25]

The hyperplasy of nerve fibres and increased content of neuropeptides in AD may be explained by increase in nerve growth factor (NGF) as found in the blood[28] and skin.[29–31] NGF is essential for the development and function of peripheral and central neurons. An increase of NGF stimulates nerve fibre proliferation in lesional AD skin and contributes to the altered nociception. Together, a higher immunoreactivity for most neuropeptides like CGRP and SP and altered nerve structures suggests that peripheral nerve fibres may play a role in the pathophysiology of itching in AD.[26]

Central transmission and central sensitization

Pruritic information is transmitted via the dorsal root ganglion to the spinal cord. At the spinal level, spinothalamic projection neurons were found to be selectively excited by histamine and thus probably participate in the transmission of pruriceptive information in a dedicated neuronal pathway.[6,32] In addition, PET (positron emission tomography) studies in humans could show activation of the primary sensory cortex after cutaneous histamine application.[7,33] Motor-associated areas were activated which correlates to the desire to scratch. In contrast to pain, itch does not provoke a spinal reflex. The scratching movement is governed by a centre in the distal medulla close to the bottom of the IV ventricle being under control of midbrain structures.[34] The observation that rubbing, scratching, and pressing temporarily relieve the sensation of itch may be explained by the 'gate-control-theory': painful sensations transmitted via fast conducting A-fibres suppress slow conducted pruritic sensations on the spinal level.

Interestingly, recent observations suggest a central sensitization for itch in AD patients.[35,36] After application of noxious stimuli in lesional skin of patients with AD, itch was evoked instead of burning pain. The authors concluded that the chronic barrage of pruriceptive input may elicit central sensitization for itch, so that painful sensations no longer inhibit itch but on the contrary is perceived as itch. In contrast to the well-known A-fibre-mediated allokinesis and hyperkinesis, this type of central sensitization appears to be elicited by C-nociceptors. This also explains the fact that, in AD, itch is also evoked by weak mechanical stimulation, like the contact of wool on the skin, which is at variance with the insensitivity of pruriceptors to mechanical stimulation.

CUTANEOUS NEURORECEPTORS AND MEDIATORS: INDUCTION OF PRURITUS

Itching is induced by a large variety of chemical mediators binding to specialized receptors on free nerve endings. Several studies could demonstrate that itch in individuals with AD follow different pathways as compared to non-atopic individuals. For example, while normal volunteers experience intense pruritus after injection of histamine or substance P, patients with AD only remark weak itch sensations (Table 10.1). The following section gives an overview about the mediators and receptors playing a role in the cutaneous elicitation of pruritus in AD.

Histamine

Many mediators triggering itch have been investigated in AD. Among them, histamine has been a persistent candidate and has been the most thoroughly studied pruritogen for decades. About 80 years ago, Lewis reported that intradermal injections of histamine provoke redness, weal, and flare (so called triple response of neurogenic inflammation) accompanied with pruritus.[37,38] Williams[39] suggested that histamine may play a role in the pathogenesis of AD since intramuscular histamine injections resulted in pruritus. Elevated histamine levels in both lesional and uninvolved skin in AD patients were also reported.[40,41] However, recent investigations were not able to detect increased histamine levels in the skin.[42] Uehara et al[43–46] noticed reduced itch sensations in response to either intracutaneously injected or iontophoretically applied histamine when compared to non-atopic healthy subjects. Furthermore, intradermally injected substance P (SP) releases histamine and provokes diminished itch perception in patients with AD in comparison to healthy subjects which underlines the minor capacity of histamine to induce pruritus in AD.[47] These conflicting results of elevated levels of histamine and diminished itching after histamine application may

Table 10.1   Cutaneous basis of itch in atopic dermatitis

Substrate	Provocation of itch	Mechanism
	Cutaneous inductors of itch	
Histamine	(+)	Binding to histamine receptors on sensory nerve fibres
Neuropeptides (e.g. substance P)	+	Mast cell degranulation, increased concentration in lesional skin
Acetylcholine	+	Central sensitization?
Tryptase	+	Binding to PAR-2 on sensory nerve fibres
Cytokines: Interleukin 2	+	Possible release of various mediators
Interleukin 8	−	
Neurotrophin-4	+	m.n.n.
Eosinophils	+	Release mediators like PAF, leucotrines; histamine, proteinase liberation
Platelet-activating factor (PAF)	+	Histamine liberators
Leukotrienes	+	m.n.n.
	Cutaneous suppressors of itch	
Cannabinoids	Interruption of itch transmission	Binding to CB1 and CB2 on cutaneous sensory nerve fibres
Opioid peptides	Induction of itch-inhibiting neurons on spinal level; suppression in the skin?	Binding to opioid receptors
Vanilloids, calcineurin inhibitors	Interruption of itch transmission	Binding to TRPV1 on cutaneous sensory nerve fibres
Interferon gamma	Suppression of pruritus	m.n.n.

−, no induction of itch; (+), induction of weak itch; +, clear induction of itch; m.n.n., mechanism not known.

indicate either an intrinsic down-regulation of neuronal H_1-receptor density or affinity, or increased histamine degradation in atopic skin.[48] Consequently, antihistamines are often not efficient in AD, as demonstrated in experimental studies as well as double-blind, cross-over trials.[49,50] These results support the idea that mediators other than histamine play the dominant role in the pathophysiology of itch response in AD.

Neuropeptides

Several observations support the idea that an imbalance of cutaneous neuropeptides such as SP, vasoactive intestinal peptide (VIP), somatostatin, and neurotensin is one basis for the pathophysiology of itching in AD.[10,11,20,51] For example, in patients with AD, alterations in the nerve fibre containing neuropeptide profile could be demonstrated. Somatostatin-immunoreactive nerve fibres were decreased in AD patients.[52] Neuropeptide Y (NPY)-positive nerve fibres and LCs are increased as compared

to healthy controls.[21,26,52] Moreover, tissue concentrations of VIP were decreased while SP concentrations were increased in lesional skin.[53–55] SP induced effects are mediated via activation of the neurokinin receptor (NKR) 1.[56,57] Experimental studies showed that intradermally injected SP releases histamine via binding to NKR on mast cells and thereby acts as a pruritogen.[58] Accordingly, in animal models, the effect of a NK1 antagonist, BIIF 1149 CL, on scratching behaviour in an AD mouse model was determined. Immediately after application a significantly inhibited scratching behaviour was observed suggesting an important role of tachykinins such as SP in AD.[59] However, despite these preliminary results, the complex role of neuropeptides in AD has to be clarified in further experimental studies.

Acetylcholine

Acetylcholine (ACh) was speculated during past years to play an important role in the elicitation of itch sensations in patients suffering from AD. ACh is not only a neurotransmitter in glandular epithelium like eccrine sweat glands, it has also been shown to activate muscarinic receptors on cultured human keratinocytes and can be synthesized, released, and degraded in an autocrine, paracrine, and endocrine fashion by human keratinocytes in vitro.[60–62] Interestingly, Scott[63] found increased ACh levels in biopsies of patients with AD suggesting that increased production or release of ACh is involved in the pathophysiology of pruritus in AD.

Recent investigations showed that intradermal application of ACh elicits pruritus instead of pain in lesional AD skin[16,46] while all healthy control subjects reported on burning pain. These results suggested that ACh may induce pruritus in AD in a cholinergic, histamine-independent mechanism. Moreover, this finding may explain the generalized itching after sweating of AD patients since ACh is a major neurotransmitter activating sweat glands. However, since recently a central sensitization in AD patients was identified,[35,36] it may also be speculated that this explains the results of these experimental studies. It seems likely that it is not the ACh administration that is responsible for the induction of itch, but the injection along with a painful stimulus and the 'translation' of the pain sensation into a pruritic sensation on the spinal level that produces itch. Further studies have to clarify this issue.

Tryptase

A role of proteinases such as trypsin as pruritogenic agents has been proposed for over 40 years[64] based on the observation that intradermal injection of mast cell tryptase into human and rabbit skin results in pruritus, vasodilatation, and erythema.[65,66] Recently, it has been demonstrated that tryptase mediates its cellular effects by activating a proteinase-activated receptor-2 (PAR-2). A recent study showed that in AD skin tryptase was increased up to fourfold and PAR-2 was markedly enhanced on primary afferent nerve fibres.[66–71] This suggests enhanced PAR-2 signalling as a new link between inflammatory and sensory phenomena in AD patients. PAR-2 therefore represents a promising therapeutic target for the treatment of cutaneous neurogenic inflammation and pruritus.

CUTANEOUS NEURORECEPTORS AND MEDIATORS: SUPPRESSION OF PRURITUS

Cannabinoids

Endogenous as well as synthetic cannabinoids are known for their analgetic potency. Recently, the cannabinoid receptor agonist HU210 was shown to suppress experimental histamine-induced pruritus and also to reduce axon reflex erythema after topical application.[72] These findings suggest functional active cannabinoid receptors are present on cutaneous nerve fibres. In fact, both cannabinoid receptors CB1 and CB2 were found to be expressed on sensory nerve fibres and mast cells in human skin.[73] In sum, these studies suggest cannabinoid receptors mediate antipruritic effects after activation on sensory nerve fibres. This offers a new therapy modality of pruritus in AD. In preliminary studies, a cream containing the cannabinoid palmitoylethanolamin has already showed anti-inflammatory and antipruritic effects in AD.[74]

Opioids

Opioid peptides such as β-endorphin, enkephalins, and endomorphins play a major role in the nociceptive pathway in the central nervous system by interacting with opioid receptors (μ-, δ-, κ-, orphan-receptor). Systemically administered morphins reduce pain but induce pruritus on the spinal level.[75–80] Accordingly, opioid receptor antagonists may significantly diminish itch in several pruritic diseases including AD.[81–87]

Several findings suggest a role of opioids in the pathogenesis of AD pruritus. β-endorphin serum levels were demonstrated to be significantly elevated in children with pruritic AD.[88] Skin biopsies from AD patients revealed a significant downregulation of epidermal mu-opiate receptor expression.[89] Previous studies revealed the presence of mu-opiate receptors on cutaneous sensory nerve fibres[90] and that opioids act upon nerve fibres to inhibit the release of inflammatory neuropeptides such as SP, neurokinin A and CGRP[65,91] suggesting that peripheral opioids diminish sensitivity of peripheral nerve endings. It may therefore be speculated that the reduced expression of mu-opioid receptors increases the peripheral sensitivity in AD and contributes to histamine-unrelated chronic pruritus.

Vanilloids and calcineurin inhibitors

Capsaicin, heat, and protons bind to a receptor of the TRP family, the TRPV1. This receptor was recently described on peripheral cutaneous nerve fibres with constant expression also in AD skin biopsies.[92] Along with repeated topical application of capsaicin, the release and the reaccumulation of neuropeptides such as SP are inhibited in unmyelinated, polymodal C-type cutaneous nerves. Moreover, the nerve fibre is desensitized and itch sensations are not transmitted to the CNS.[93–98] Consequently, topical application of capsaicin proved to be an effective treatment in otherwise intractable pruritus of AD.[97,98] Interestingly, the calcineurin inhibitors tacrolimus[99] and pimecrolimus[100] were recently demonstrated also to bind to the TRPV1 which explains their significant antipruritic effect.

CYTOKINES AND INFLAMMATORY CELLS

Cytokines are released from various cutaneous and immune cells during inflammation. Certain cytokines have been demonstrated to induce pruritus and activate neuropeptide release from sensory nerves in the skin of patients with AD.

Interleukins

While interleukin (IL)-1 does not seem to correlate with itching, IL-2 is claimed to be a potent inducer of pruritus. As observed upon therapeutical application, high doses of recombinant IL-2, as given to cancer patients, frequently provoke redness and cutaneous itching.[101] Furthermore, AD patients treated with oral cyclosporin A, a drug that inhibits the production of various cytokines including IL-2, experience attenuation of itch.[102,103] Additionally, a single intracutaneus injection of IL-2 induced a low-intensity intermittent local itch with maximal intensity between 6 h and 48 h as well as erythema in both atopic and healthy individuals.[104,105] Interestingly, in patients with AD, this reaction tends to appear earlier than in healthy controls. Moreover, bradykinin appears to enhance the effect of IL-2-induced pruritus on sensory nerves.[106] Upon prick testing, supernatants of mitogen-stimulated leucocytes were pruritic in AD patients but not in controls, probably due to increased concentration of IL-2 and Il-6.[107] The mechanism for the induction of itch by IL-2 remains to be established, but the latency preceding the itch response after injection in AD patients suggests an indirect pruritogenic effect of IL-2 via other mediators.

Recently, various studies revealed increased levels of the proinflammatory chemokine IL-8 in lesional skin,[108] plasma,[109] and blood mononuclear cells[110, 111] especially eosinophils,[112] of AD patients. However, the capacity of IL-8 to induce pruritus is questionable since prick testing with Il-8 does not induce wealing or pruritus.[110] Further studies will have to clarify the influence of IL-8 in the pathophysiology of pruritus.

Interferon gamma

Interferon gamma (INF-γ) appears to have a beneficial effect on pruritus in AD.[113] In a double-blind study, pruritus was reduced by 50% even 1–2 years after long-term treatment with recombinant human interferon gamma.[114] It is well known that INF-γ production is profoundly diminished in peripheral blood mononuclear cells of AD patients[115] which may contribute to the development of pruritus. Although an important role of INF-γ in the pathophysiology of pruritus in AD is likely, the underlying mechanism by which low INF-γ levels induce pruritus, however, has to be identified.

Neurotrophin-4 (NT-4)

Recent observations indicate that neurotrophin-4 may be involved in inflammatory and itch responses of patients with AD. NT-4 is a keratinocyte-derived agent which is highly expressed under inflammatory conditions and which exerts growth-promoting effects on nerve cells. Accordingly, NT-4 expression was found to be significantly increased in lesional skin of patients with AD and in prurigo lesions of AD skin.[116] Interestingly, NT-4 production can be induced by INF-γ, which itself is known to have a beneficial effect on pruritus. These findings suggest a close relationship between immune and neurotrophic factors in the pathophysiology of pruritus in AD.

Eosinophils and basophils

Although a role of eosinophils in the pathogenesis of AD is well established, their role in the pathophysiology of pruritus during AD is still an enigma. Eosinophils release factors which may have a direct pruritogenic effect such as platelet-activating factor, leucotrienes, prostanoids, kinins, cytokines, and proteases.[117–122] They may also exert an indirect itch response by activating mast cells to release histamine or proteinases from eosinophils. In summary, although some reports are in favour of a role for eosinophils during pruritus in various diseases,[117–119] direct evidence for a role of eosinophils for itch responses during AD is still lacking. In patients with AD, peripheral blood basophils are normal in number, but in vitro studies revealed abnormal function with increased or faster histamine releasability.[123,24] However, Bull et al could demonstrate that basophils and basophil release of histamine do not contribute to induction of itch and erythema in patients with AD.[125]

Platelet-activating factor

Platelet-activating factor (PAF) is a lipid mediator with a potent proinflammatory activity. PAF is released by several inflammatory cells such as mast cells, eosinophils, basophils, and neutrophils.[67] PAF could be demonstrated to increase vascular permeability. Consequently, a weal and flare reaction as well as pruritus resulted after intradermal injection suggesting release of histamine by

PAF.[126] Several PAF antagonists have been developed so far, and preliminary results of a double-blind study applying a synthetic PAF antagonist topically could demonstrate a statistically significant reduction of pruritus in patients with AD during the first 2 weeks of therapy.[127] However, further studies will have to clarify the practicability of PAF antagonists upon daily use.

Leukotrienes

So far, the role of leukotrienes in the pathogenesis of pruritus is speculative, although there is increasing evidence about their relevance in elicitation of itch. Andoh et al[128] demonstrated that intradermal injected leukotriene E4 is able to provoke scratching in mice. Additionally, a correlation of nocturnal itch and high urinary leukotriene E4 levels was demonstrated suggesting that increased production of leukotrienes may contribute to nocturnal itch induction in AD.[129] Preliminary studies showed reduction of pruritus in patients with AD during treatment with the leukotriene receptor antagonists zafirlukast and zileuton.[130–132]

TRIGGER FACTORS AGGRAVATING PRURITUS PERCEPTION IN ATOPIC DERMATITIS

The skin of AD patients reveals a higher tendency to itch upon minimal provocation, due to reduced itch threshold and prolonged itch duration to pruritic stimuli as compared to healthy skin.[133–135] A series of pruritus triggering factors are known[135] which release mast cell mediators or vasomotor and sweat reactions to cause itch, and all may be subjected to emotional influences.[134]

Scratching

It is frequently debated if scratching itself leads to the induction of AD or if itch along with scratching is a consequence of the presence of eczemas. However, the influence of the itch-scratch response on the pathophysiology of AD has not been precisely elucidated. A recent animal study addressing this issue suggests that scratching behaviour contributes to the development of dermatitis by enhancing various immunological responses.[136] In a murine AD model, capsaicin-sensitive sensory nerves of mice were ablated by neonatal capsaicin treatment, and the development of spontaneous dermatitis in the ablated mice was compared with that in non-treated AD mice. Interestingly, scratching behaviour was almost completely prevented in the capsaicin-treated mice, and – more importantly – the development of dermatitis, elevation of the serum IgE level, and the numbers of

infiltrating eosinophils and mast cells were significantly suppressed. Immunological studies showed that the capability of spleen T cells to produce both T-helper (Th) 1 (interferon-gamma) and Th2 (IL-5 and IL-13) cytokines was diminished. These findings suggested that the prevention of the itch sensation and/or itch-associated scratching behaviour may be an additional important step in the basic treatment of AD.

Epidermal barrier

Xerosis of the skin in patients with AD reflects a disturbed epidermal barrier and is a well-known activator of pruritus in AD patients of all ages. An increased transepidermal water loss and a decreased ability of the stratum corneum to bind water were measured[137] which may result from incomplete arrangement of intercellular lipid lamellae in the stratum corneum.[138,139] A decrease of water content below 10% seems to be crucial for induction of itch and scratching.[140] This generalized dryness of the skin triggers pruritus by unknown mechanisms.[137,138] One possibility may be that an impaired barrier function in the skin supports the entrance of irritants and itchy agents.[141,142] Additionally, pH changes within the skin may activate itch receptors.[95]

Interestingly, a recent study showed that psychological stress induces alterations in the epidermal barrier homeostasis and stratum corneum integrity.[143] In animal studies, psychological stress results in decreased lamellar body formation and secretion, as well as in decreased corneodesmosome production. These findings suggested a correlation between stress factors and decreased barrier function.

Stress

In general, itch can be induced or modified by cognitive stress perception like fatigue, anxiety, and repressed emotions as well as psychiatric diseases like depression.[144–151] Consequently, in AD, a correlation between the intensity of pruritus, scratching, and mental stress factors could be demonstrated upon experimental studies.[146,147,152–154] Consistently, upon clinical examination, up to 81% of AD patients acknowledge their pruritus to be aggravated by emotional stress.[155] Relaxation therapies like autogenic training or hypnosis indirectly prove these findings by revealing a significant improvement of itching and eczema in AD patients.[156,157]

An activation of the psycho-neuroendocrine system seems likely to contribute to stress-induced itch in AD.[146,147] In a rat model, it was demonstrated that immobilization stress triggers mast cell degranulation.[158] Thus, increased release of pruritogenic mediators by mast cells may result in scratching and skin lesions following stress tension.[146] This is underlined in a study demonstrating increased blood eosinophils, IgE, interferon-gamma and IL-4 levels 24 h after the stress test in AD patients.[159] The present findings suggest that stress may be associated with atopy-relevant immunological changes in AD sufferers. Pruritus intensity may also be increased by vasodilator responses and increased skin temperature to emotional stress as demonstrated by psychophysiological studies.[134,160]

Sweating

Generalized itching initiated by any stimulus to sweating (thermal, emotional stimuli) is a typical hallmark and represents the most common trigger factor of itch in patients with AD.[134,161,162] Interestingly, increased sweating in lichenified skin was observed in AD patients suggesting a decreased threshold for sweat stimulation in chronic pruritic and altered skin.[163] The underlying mechanism of sweat-induced pruritus remains to be explored, but there is increasing evidence that ACh is involved. ACh induces eccrine sweating,[8] is found to be increased in the skin of AD patients,[63] and finally acts pruritogenic in AD patients.[16]

Microcirculation

There is considerable evidence that the cutaneous microvasculature contributes to pruritus. Clinically, itching is mostly associated with erythema and hyperthermia. Most mediators for itching such as histamine, tryptase, ACh, SP, and prostaglandins are potent vasodilatators, rarely vasoconstrictors such as NPY (neuropeptide Y) or catecholamines. Interestingly, while neuropeptide-induced itching does not vary between atopic and non-atopic patients, vascular responses obviously show a significant difference between these two groups. Moreover, patients with AD were more susceptible to stress and showed increased vasodilatation as compared to controls.[164]

Exogenous factors

Pruritus produced by direct contact with wool in patients with AD is a characteristic and reproducible phenomenon.[165,166] It is likely that the irritation is caused by the spiky nature of wool fibres themselves while wearing wool garments close to the skin. Mechanical vibration seems not to be responsible for induction of itch since it inhibits experimental, histamine-induced itch.[167] Thicker wool fibres were found to provoke more intense itching than thinner fibres and an additional redness after application of wool samples.[168] Other irritants like lipid solvents and disinfectants[169] may additionally contribute to aggravate xerosis. Contact- and aero-allergens as dust mites or pollens[161] may also provoke pruritus. Microbiological agents like bacteria (*Staphylococcus aureus*) or yeast may exacerbate both dermatitis and pruritus.[135,161]

Pruritus and erythema may be also triggered by substances increasing blood flow, induce vasodilatation, or release histamine. Among those, heat, hot and spicy foods, hot drinks, and alcohol are most likely to generate itch in AD patients.[135,161,170] In early childhood, food allergies exacerbate eczematous skin lesions, although food allergies mostly resolve during ageing in older children and adults.[170]

MANAGEMENT OF ITCH IN ATOPIC DERMATITIS (TABLE 10.2)

The handling and treatment of severe itch is one of the major challenges in the management of patients with AD. To effect a successful suppression of pruritus, several levels have to be considered. First of all, *identification and elimination of individual trigger factors* must be appreciated as the primary goal of the management.[148,171] Since patients frequently develop some harmful self-treatments, e.g. alcohol-containing solutions, these misleading therapies must be eliminated. *Lotions and creams lubricating the skin* have to be recommended. To combat skin dryness, application of hydrophilic emollients and bathing with oily bath additives is additionally helpful.[171] Adding substances such as *urea, menthol, camphor, and polidocanol* to these creams leads to an immediate short-term interruption of the itch. These creams can be applied by the patients each time the itch starts to worsen.[172] Unspecific physical modalities are described to be beneficial like acupuncture,[173] and cutaneous field stimulation.[174]

Another level of therapy is the handling of the *scratch artefacts*. Chronic pruritus induces chronic scratching or rubbing. Accordingly, erosions, ulcerations, bleeding, crusts, and lichenifications up to prurigo nodularis may develop. Stage-dependent, disinfections, antimicrobials, and topical corticosteroids have to be applied. In patients with prurigo nodularis or lichen simplex associated with AD, frequently an automatic scratching behaviour develops. These patients additionally need education to control scratch behaviour.[175] For example, the behaviour method 'habit reversal' can be employed.[176] First, patients become aware of their scratching behaviour by counting scratch movements. In a second step, they learn a new behaviour by reacting to scratch impulses. Scratch-induced skin damage caused by nocturnal scratch movements may be improved by using cotton gloves. Also controlled physical exercise like gymnastics or ball

Table 10.2 Therapeutic strategies combating pruritus in atopic dermatitis	
Therapeutic modalities	**Examples**
Elimination of trigger factors	Perspiration, xerosis, emotional stress, scratching, wearing wool fibres, using soaps, detergents, hot, spicy food, hot drinks, alcohol
Lubrication, short-term interruption of itch	Emollients Bathing with oily additives Lotions, creams or sprays containing menthol, camphor, polidocanol, urea Skin care to reduce sweating-induced itch
Therapy of scratch artefacts	Disinfections, antimicrobials, topical steroids Interruption of itch-scratch-cycle: behaviour method in automatic scratching Physical exercise Acupuncture Cutaneous field stimulation
Symptomatic therapy: **Anti-inflammatory therapy**	Corticosteroids, topical, and systemical Cyclosporin A Tacrolimus, pimecrolimus Interferon gamma Immunoglobulin therapy Ultraviolet light
Symptomatic therapy: **Interfering with pathophysiology of** **pruritus in AD**	Leukotriene antagonists Opiate antagonists Capsaicin Cannabinoid agonists
Contradictory results	Antihistamines, Doxepin (but: contact allergy upon long-term application) Mycophenolate mofetil

games were demonstrated in a controlled study to teach patients to cope better with itch attacks.[177]

Since chronic scratching represents also a trigger factor and maintains the itch-scratch-cycle, the most important step in the management of the AD patients is the interruption of itch by an effective symptomatical topical and/or systemical therapy.

Symptomatical topical and systemical therapy

Studies concerning the pathophysiology of pruritus clearly demonstrated that different nociceptive mechanisms are involved in AD. Thus, conventional therapeutic modalities like *antihistamines* often fail to ameliorate pruritus in AD.[178] This is comprehensive with the idea that histamine is not the major mediator of pruritus in AD.[49] Placebo-controlled studies concerning the antipruritic effect of oral antihistamines have shown conflicting results in AD. In some studies, no superior effect was observed as compared to placebo[50,179,180] while others showed a significant antipruritic effect.[46,181,182] In recent experimental studies, the H_1-antihistamine cetirizine could be demonstrated to focally reduce itch.[46] However, an evidence-based review concerning the efficacy of antihistamines in relieving pruritus in AD concluded that little objective evidence exists for H_1-antihistamines to demonstrate improvement of pruritus.[178] Topical application of the tricyclic antidepressant doxepin is suggested to have antipruritic effects because of its high affinity to H_1 histamine receptors. In fact, 5% doxepin cream revealed improvement of histamine-induced and SP-mediated cutaneous responses but also evoked sedative effects in some patients.[183,184] Unfortunately, doxepin was accompanied by contact allergies after long-term application.[185]

In general, anti-inflammatory, *immunomodulating therapies* as regularly applied in AD often result also in cessation of pruritus, since they suppress the inflammatory mechanisms underlying the induction of itch. So far, most effective and consistent antipruritics remain systemic immunomodulators such as glucocorticoids, cyclosporin A (CyA), tacrolimus, pimecrolimus, and ultraviolet light therapy.[102,186–189] Moreover, there are no evident and efficient alternatives to topical application of corticosteroids for the control of acute episodes in AD.[189–191] With reduction of skin lesions, a decreased itch intensity results probably due to reduction of inflammatory cells and protection of depolarization of nerve fibres mediated directly by the steroid.[192] CyA, a cyclic polypeptide with potent immunosuppressive effects, has been reported to have a considerable itch-relieving effect in various diseases including AD. In a randomized study, CyA was demonstrated to significantly reduce itch intensity.[102] After discontinuation of this therapy, pruritus recurred immediately. Since oral cyclosporin A has demonstrated to be effective in AD, a topical CyA formulation has been developed to avoid adverse systemic effects. However, no significant improvement of AD was found upon clinical application.[193]

Recently, much interest has been drawn to tacrolimus and pimecrolimus, both effective immunomodulators and calcineurin inhibitors. Although the mode of action is similar to that of CyA, the molecular weight is lower and their potency of inhibiting T-cell activation is higher. Multiple, large randomized studies in recent years confirmed the ability of topical administration of tacrolimus and pimecrolimus to interrupt acute attacks of AD, quickly reduce pruritus, and prevent exacerbation after cessation of eczemas in adults and even children with AD.[194–196] Treatment with interferon gamma has been shown to be effective not only for the improvement of erythema, excoriations, and lichenifications, but also of pruritus.[114,197,198] In addition, this effect was maintained up to 2 years after therapy.[114] Amelioration of pruritus has also been described under intravenous immunoglobulin therapy in few cases of AD.[199,200] As of yet, however, no controlled studies have been performed.

Other therapeutical modalities such as capsaicin,[97,98] opiate receptor antagonists,[82,86,87] and leukotriene antagonists[130–132] also appear to be promising new approaches in the therapy of AD, but will have to prove their safety and practicability in further controlled studies. In conclusion, the pathophysiology of pruritus in AD has not been evaluated completely. Accordingly, no specific antipruritic agent has been developed, and management of itch in AD is confined mainly to immunomodulating therapies. However, the consideration of several levels may improve this distressing situation for the patients. Further investigations are necessary to establish antipruritic substances influencing the centrally and peripherally altered itch perception in order to interfere with the complex pathophysiology of pruritus in AD.

REFERENCES

1. Rothman S. Physiology of itching. Physiol Rev 1941; 21: 357–81.
2. Hanifin JM, Rajka G. Diagnostic features of atopic dermatitis. Acta Derm Venereol Suppl (Stockh) 1980; 92: 44–7.
3. Koblenzer CS. Itching and the atopic skin. J Allergy Clin Immunol 1999; 104: 109–13.
4. Handwerker HO. Sixty years of C-fiber recordings from animal and human skin nerves: historical notes. Prog Brain Res 1996; 113: 39–51.
5. Schmelz M, Schmidt R, Bickel A et al. Specific C-receptors for itch in human skin. J Neurosci 1997; 17: 8003–8.
6. Andrew D, Craig AD. Spinothalamic lamina I neurons selectively sensitive to histamine: a central neural pathway for itch. Nat Neurosci 2001; 4: 72–7.
7. Darsow U, Drzezga A, Frisch M et al. Processing of histamine-induced itch in the human cerebral cortex: a correlation analysis with dermal reactions. J Invest Dermatol 2000; 115: 1029–33.
8. Metze D, Luger T. Nervous system in the skin. In: Freinkel RK, Woodley DT, eds. The Biology of the Skin. New York: Parthenon, 2001: 153–76.
9. Schmelz M, Michael K, Weidner C et al. Which nerve fibres mediate the axon reflex flare in human skin? Neuroreport 2000; 11: 645–8.
10. Scholzen T, Armstrong CA, Bunnett NW et al. Neuropeptides in the skin: interactions between the neuroendocrine and the skin immune systems. Exp Dermatol 1998; 7: 81–96.
11. Steinhoff M, Armstrong C, Scholzen T et al. Neurocutaneous control of inflammation. In: Norris DA, ed. Immune Mechanisms in Cutaneous Disease, 2nd edn. New York: Marcel Dekker, 2001.
12. Kaji A, Shigematsu H, Fujita K et al. Parasympathetic innervation of cutaneous blood vessels by vasoactive intestinal polypeptide-immunoreactive and acetylcholinesterase-positive nerves: histochemical and experimental study on rat lower lip. Neuroscience 1988; 25: 353–62.
13. Advenier C, Devillier P. Neurokinins and the skin. Allerg Immunol Paris 1993; 25: 280–2.
14. Brain SD, TJ Williams TJ. Inflammatory oedema induced by synergism between calcitonin gene-related peptide (CGRP) and mediators of increased vascular permeability. Br J Pharmacol 1985; 86: 855–60.
15. Wallengren J, Badendick K, Sundler F et al. Innervation of the skin of the forearm in diabetic patients: relation to nerve function. Acta Derm Venereol 1995; 75: 37–42.
16. Heyer G, Vogelsang M, Hornstein OP. Acetylcholine is an inducer of itching in patients with atopic eczema. J Dermatol 1997; 24: 621–5.
17. Schallreuter KU. Epidermal adrenergic signal transduction as part of the neuronal network in the human epidermis. J Investig Dermatol Symp Proc 1997; 2: 37–40.
18. Röcken M, Schallreuter K, Renz H et al. What exactly is "atopy"? Exp Dermatol 1998; 7: 97–104.
19. Grando SA. Biological functions of keratinocyte cholinergic receptors. J Investig Dermatol Symp Proc 1997; 2: 41–8.
20. Slominski A, Wortsman J. Neuroendocrinology of the skin. Endocr Rev 2000; 21: 457–87.
21. Tobin D, Nabarro G, Baart de la Faille H et al. Increased number of immunoreactive nerve fibers in atopic dermatitis. J Allergy Clin Immunol 1992; 90: 613–22.
22. Mihm MC, Soter NA, Dvorak HF et al. The structure of normal skin and the morphology of atopic eczema. J Invest Dermatol 1976; 67: 305–12.

23. Urashima R, Mihara M. Cutaneous nerves in atopic dermatitis. A histological, immunohistochemical and electron microscopic study. Virchows Arch 1998; 432: 363–70.

24. Prose PH, Sedlis E. Morphologic and histochemical studies of atopic eczema in infants and children. J Invest Dermatol 1960; 34: 149–65.

25. Sugiura H, Omoto M, Hirota Y et al. Density and fine structure of peripheral nerves in various skin lesions of atopic dermatitis. Arch Dermatol Res 1997; 289: 125–31.

26. Pincelli C, Fantini F, Massimi P et al. Neuropeptides in skin from patients with atopic dermatitis: an immunohistochemical study. Br J Dermatol 1990; 122: 745–50.

27. Ostlere LS, Cowen T, Rustin MH. Neuropeptides in the skin of patients with atopic dermatitis. Clin Exp Dermatol 1995; 20: 462–7.

28. Toyoda M, Nakamura M, Makino T et al. Nerve growth factor and substance P stimulate plasma disease activity in atopic dermatitis. Br J Dermatol 2002; 147: 71–9.

29. Horiuchi Y, Bae S, Katayama I. Nerve growth factor (NGF) and epidermal nerve fibers in atopic dermatitis model NC/Nga mice. J Dermatol Sci 2005; 39: 56–8.

30. Albers KM, Wright DE, Davis BM. Overexpression of nerve growth factor in epidermis of transgenic mice causes hypertrophy of the peripheral nervous system. J Neurosci 1994; 14: 1422–32.

31. Pincelli C, Sevignani C, Manfredini R et al. Expression and function of nerve growth factor and nerve growth factor receptor on cultured keratinocytes. J Invest Dermatol 1994; 103: 13–18.

32. Carstens E. Responses of rat spinal dorsal horn neurons to intracutaneous microinjection of histamine, capsaicin, and other irritants. J Neurophysiol 1997; 77: 2499–514.

33. Drzezga A, Darsow U, Treede RD et al. Central activation by histamine-induced itch: analogies to pain processing: a correlational analysis of O-15 H_2O positron emission tomography studies. Pain 2001; 92: 295–305.

34. Ghez C. Voluntary movement. In: Kandel ER, Schwartz JH, eds. Principles of Neural Science, 2nd edn. New York: Elsevier, 1985; Chap 38: 756–81.

35. Ikoma A, Fartasch M, Heyer G et al. Painful stimuli evoke itch in patients with chronic pruritus: central sensitization for itch. Neurology 2004; 62: 212–17.

36. Ikoma A, Rukwied R, Ständer S et al. Neuronal sensitization for histamine-induced itch in lesional skin of patients with atopic dermatitis. Arch Dermatol 2003; 139: 1455–8.

37. Lewis T. The Blood Vessels of the Human Skin and Their Responses. London: Shaw and Sons, 1927.

38. Lewis T, Grant RT, Marvin HM. Vascular reactions of the skin to injury. Heart 1929; 14: 139–60.

39. Williams DH. Skin temperature reaction to histamine in atopic dermatitis (disseminated neurodermatitis). J Invest Dermatol 1938; 1: 119–29.

40. Johnson HH, DeOreo GA, Lascheid WP et al. Skin histamine levels in chronic atopic dermatitis. J Invest Dermatol 1960; 34: 237–8.

41. Juhlin L. Localization and content of histamine in normal and diseased skin. Acta Derm Venereol 1967; 47: 383–91.

42. Ruzicka T, Glück S. Cutaneous histamine levels in histamine releasability from the skin in atopic dermatitis and hyper-IgE-syndrome. Arch Dermatol Res 1983; 275: 41–4.

43. Heyer G, Hornstein OP, Handwerker HO. Skin reactions and itch sensation induced by epicutaneous histamine application in atopic dermatitis and controls. J Invest Dermatol 1989; 93: 492–6.

44. Uehara M. Reduced histamine reaction in atopic dermatitis. Arch Dermatol 1982; 118: 244–5.

45. Heyer G, Koppert W, Martus P et al. Histamine and cutaneous nociception: histamine-induced responses in patients with atopic eczema, psoriasis and urticaria. Acta Derm Venereol 1998; 78: 123–6.

46. Heyer GR, Hornstein OP. Recent studies of cutaneous nociception in atopic and non-atopic subjects. J Dermatol 1999; 26: 77–86.

47. Heyer G, Hornstein OP, Handwerker HO. Reactions to intradermally injected substance P and topically applied mustard oil in atopic dermatitis patients. Acta Derm Venereol 1991; 71: 291–5.

48. Heyer G. Abnormal cutaneous neurosensitivity in atopic skin. Acta Derm Venereol Suppl (Stockh) 1992; 176: 93–4.

49. Rukwied R, Lischetzki G, McGlone F et al. Mast cell mediators other than histamine induce pruritus in atopic dermatitis patients: a dermal microdialysis study. Br J Dermatol 2000; 142: 1114–20.

50. Wahlgren CF, Hägermark Ö, Bergström R. The antipruritic effect of a sedative and a non-sedative antihistamine in atopic dermatitis. Br J Dermatol 1990; 122: 545–51.

51. Ansel JC, Kaynard AH, Armstrong CA et al. Skin–nervous system interactions. J Invest Dermatol 1996; 106: 198–204.

52. Pincelli C, Fantini F, Massimi P et al. Neuropeptide Y-like immunoreactivity in Langerhans cells from patients with atopic dermatitis. Int J Neurosci 1990; 51: 219–20.

53. Anand P, Springall DR, Blank MA et al. Neuropeptides in skin disease: increased VIP in eczema and psoriasis but not axillary hyperhidrosis. Br J Dermatol 1991; 124: 547–9.

54. Pincelli C, Fantini F, Romualdi P et al. Skin levels of vasoactive intestinal polypeptide in atopic dermatitis. Arch Dermatol Res 1991; 283: 230–2.

55. Fantini F, Pincelli C, Romualdi P et al. Substance P levels are decreased in lesional skin of atopic dermatitis. Exp Dermatol 1992; 1: 127–8.

56. Andoh T, Nagasawa T, Satoh M et al. Substance P induction of itch-associated response mediated by cutaneous NK1 tachykinin receptors in mice. J Pharmacol Exp Ther 1998; 286: 1140–5.

57. Scholzen TE, Steinhoff M, Bonaccorsi P et al. Neutral endopeptidase terminates substance P-induced inflammation in allergic contact dermatitis. J Immunol 2001; 166: 1285–91.

58. Thomsen JS, Sonne M, Benfeldt E et al. Experimental itch in sodium lauryl sulphate-inflamed and normal skin in humans: a randomized, double-blind, placebo-controlled study of histamine and other inducers of itch. Br J Dermatol 2002; 146: 792–800.

59. Ohmura T, Hayashi T, Satoh Y et al. Involvement of substance P in scratching behaviour in an atopic dermatitis model. Eur J Pharmacol 2004; 491: 191–4.

60. Grando SA, Kist DA, Qi M et al. Human keratinocytes synthesize, secrete and degrade acetylcholine. J Invest Dermatol 1993; 101: 32–6.

61. Grando SA, Zelickson BD, Kist DA et al. Keratinocyte muscarinic acetylcholine receptors: immunolocalization and partial characterization. J Invest Dermatol 1995; 104: 95–100.

62. Kurzen H, Schallreuter KU. Novel aspects in cutaneous biology of acetylcholine synthesis and acetylcholine receptors. Exp Dermatol 2004; 13(suppl 4): 27–30.

63. Scott A. Acetylcholine in normal and diseased skin. Br J Dermatol 1962; 74: 317–22.

64. Shelley WB, Arthur RP. The neurohistology and neurophysiology of the itch sensation in man. AMA Arch Derm 1957; 76: 296–323.

65. Bernstein JE. Capsaicin in dermatologic disease. Semin Dermatol 1988; 7: 304–9.

66. Steinhoff M, Vergnolle N, Young SH et al. Agonists of proteinase-activated receptor 2 induce inflammation by a neurogenic mechanism. Nat Med 2000; 6: 151–8.

67. Jarvikallio A, Naukkarinen A, Harvima IT et al. Quantitative analysis of tryptase- and chymase-containing mast cells in atopic dermatitis and nummular eczema. Br J Dermatol 1997; 136: 871–7.

68. Harvima IT, Naukkarinen A, Harvima RJ et al. Enzyme- and immunohistochemical localization of mast cell tryptase in psoriatic skin. Arch Dermatol Res 1989; 281: 387–91.

69. Naukkarinen A, Harvima IT, Aalto ML et al. Mast cell tryptase and chymase are potential regulators of neurogenic inflammation in psoriatic skin. Int J Dermatol 1994; 33: 361–6.

70. Damsgaard TE, Olesen AB, Sorensen FB et al. Mast cells and atopic dermatitis. Stereological quantification of mast cells in atopic dermatitis and normal human skin. Arch Dermatol Res 1997; 289: 256–60.

71. Steinhoff M, Neisius U, Ikoma A et al. Proteinase-activated receptor-2 mediates itch: a novel pathway for pruritus in human skin. J Neurosci 2003; 23: 6176–80.

72. Dvorak M, Watkinson A, McGlone F et al. Histamine induced responses are attenuated by a cannabinoid receptor agonist in human skin. Inflamm Res 2003; 52: 238–45.

73. Ständer S, Schmelz M, Metze D et al. Distribution of cannabinoid receptor 1 (CB1) and 2 (CB2) on sensory nerve fibers and adnexal structures in human skin. J Dermatol Sci 2005; 38: 177–88.

74. Kemény L. Comparative study of S236 cream and hydrocortisone 1% in patients with atopic dermatitis. J Am Acad Dermatol 2005; 52(suppl): (abstr) p68.

75. Fjellner B, Hägermark Ö. The influence of the opiate antagonist naloxone on experimental pruritus. Acta Derm Venereol 1984; 64: 73–5.

76. Stein C. The control of pain in peripheral tissue by opioids. N Engl J Med 1995; 332: 1685–90.

77. Bernstein JE, Swift RM. Relief of intractable pruritus with naloxone. Arch Dermatol 1979; 115: 1366–7.

78. Fjellner B, Hägermark Ö. Potentiation of histamine-induced itch and flare responses in human skin by the enkephalin analogue FK 33-824, β-endorphin and morphine. Arch Dermatol Res 1982; 274: 29–37.

79. Summerfield JA. Pain, itch and endorphins. Br J Dermatol 1981; 105: 725–6.

80. Hägermark Ö. Peripheral and central mediators of itch. Skin Pharmacol 1992; 5: 1–8.

81. JA Summerfield JA. Naloxone modulates the perception of itch in man. Br J Clin Pharmacol 1980; 10: 180–3.

82. Metze D, Reimann S, Beissert S et al. Efficacy and safety of naltrexone, an oral opiate receptor antagonist, in the treatment of pruritus in internal and dermatological diseases. J Am Acad Dermatol 1999; 41: 533–9.

83. Bernstein JE, Grinzi RA. Butorphanol-induced pruritus antagonized by naloxone. J Am Acad Dermatol 1981; 5: 227–8.

84. Penning JP, Samson B, Baxter AD. Reversal of epidural morphine-induced respiratory depression and pruritus with nalbuphine. Can J Anaesth 1988; 35: 599–604.

85. Bergasa NV, Alling DW, Talbot TL et al. Effects of naloxone infusions in patients with the pruritus of cholestasis. A double-blind, randomized, controlled trial. Ann Intern Med 1995; 123: 161–7.

86. Metze D, Reimann S, Luger TA. Effective treatment of pruritus with naltrexone, an orally active opiate antagonist. Ann N Y Acad Sci 1999; 885: 430–2.

87. Brune A, Metze D, Luger T et al. Antipruritic therapy with the oral opioid receptor antagonist naltrexone. Open, non-placebo controlled administration in 133 patients. Hautarzt 2004; 55: 1130–6.

88. Georgala S, Schulpis KH, Papaconstantinou ED et al. Raised β-endorphin serum levels in children with atopic dermatitis and pruritus. J Dermatol Sci 1994; 8: 125–8.

89. Bigliardi-Qi M, Lipp B, Sumanovski LT et al. Changes of epidermal mu-opiate receptor expression and nerve endings in chronic atopic dermatitis. Dermatology 2005; 210: 91–9.

90. Ständer S, Gunzer M, Metze D et al. Localization of mu-opioid receptor 1A on sensory nerve fibers in human skin. Regul Pept 2002; 110: 75–83.

91. Hägermark Ö, Rajka G, Bergvist U. Experimental itch in human skin elicited by rat mast cell chymase. Acta Derm Venereol 1972; 52: 125–8.

92. Ständer S, Moormann C, Schumacher M et al. Expression of vanilloid receptor subtype 1 in cutaneous sensory nerve fibers, mast cells, and epithelial cells of appendage structures. Exp Dermatol 2004; 13: 129–39.

93. Bernstein JE, Parish LC, Rapaport M et al. Effects of topically applied capsaicin on moderate and severe psoriasis vulgaris. J Am Acad Dermatol 1986; 15: 504–7.

94. Ellis CN, Berberian B, Sulica VI et al. A double-blind evaluation of topical capsaicin in pruritic psoriasis. J Am Acad Dermatol 1993; 29: 438–42.

95. Caterina MJ, Schumacher MA, Tominaga M et al. The capsaicin receptor: a heat-activated ion channel in the pain pathway. Nature 1997; 389: 816–24.

96. Dray A. Neuropharmacological mechanisms of capsaicin and related substances. Biochem Pharmacol 1992; 44: 611–15.

97. Reimann S, Luger T, Metze D. Topical administration of capsaicin in dermatology for treatment of itching and pain. Hautarzt 2000; 51: 164–72.

98. Ständer S, Luger T, Metze D. Treatment of prurigo nodularis with topical capsaicin. J Am Acad Dermatol 2001; 44: 471–8.

99. Senba E, Katanosaka K, Yajima H et al. The immunosuppressant FK506 activates capsaicin- and bradykinin-sensitive DRG neurons and cutaneous C-fibers. Neurosci Res 2004; 50: 257–62.

100. Ständer S, Luger TA. Antipruritic effects of pimecrolimus and tacrolimus. Hautarzt 2003; 54: 413–17.

101. Gaspari AA, Lotze MT, Rosenberg SA et al. Dermatologic changes associated with interleukin 2 administration. JAMA 1987; 258: 1624–9.

102. Wahlgren CF, Scheynius A, Hägermark Ö. Antipruritic effect of oral cyclosporin A in atopic dermatitis. Acta Derm Venereol 1990; 70: 323–9.

103. van Joost T, Stolz E, Heule F. Efficacy of low-dose cyclosporine in severe atopic skin disease. Arch Dermatol 1987; 123: 166–7.

104. Wahlgren CF, Tengvall Linder M, Hägermark Ö et al. Itch and inflammation induced by intradermally injected interleukin-2 in atopic dermatitis patients and healthy subjects. Arch Dermatol Res 1995; 287: 572–80.

105. Darsow U, Scharein E, Bromm B et al. Skin testing of the pruritogenic activity of histamine and cytokines (interleukin-2 and tumour necrosis factor-alpha) at the dermal-epidermal junction. Br J Dermatol 1997; 137: 415–17.

106. Martin HA. Bradykinin potentiates the chemoresponsiveness of rat cutaneous C-fibre polymodal nociceptors to interleukin-2. Arch Physiol Biochem 1996; 104: 229–38.

107. Cremer B, Heimann A, Dippel E et al. Pruritogenic effects of mitogen-stimulated peripheral blood mononuclear cells in atopic eczema. Acta Derm Venerol 1995; 75: 426–8.

108. Sticherling M, Bornscheuer E, Schröder JM et al. Immuno-histochemical studies on NAP-1/IL-8 in contact eczema and atopic dermatitis. Arch Dermatol Res 1992; 284: 82–5.

109. Kimata H, Lindley I. Detection of plasma interleukin-8 in atopic dermatitis. Arch Dis Child 1994; 70: 119–22.

110. Lippert U, Hoer A, Möller A et al. Role of antigen-induced cytokine release in atopic pruritus. Int Arch Allergy Immunol 1998; 116: 36–9.

111. Hatano Y, Katagiri K, Takayasu S. Increased levels in vivo of mRNAs for IL-8 and macrophage inflammatory protein-1 alpha (MIP-1 alpha), but not RANTES mRNA in peripheral blood mononuclear cells of patients with atopic dermatitis (AD). Clin Exp Immunol 1999; 117: 237–43.

112. Yousefi S, Hemmann S, Weber M et al. IL-8 is expressed by human peripheral blood eosinophils. Evidence for increased secretion in asthma. J Immunol 1995; 154: 5481–90.

113. Reinhold U, Kukel S, Brzoska J et al. Systemic interferon gamma treatment in severe atopic dermatitis. J Am Acad Dermatol 1993; 29: 58–63.

114. Stevens SR, Hanifin JM, Hamilton T et al. Long-term effectiveness and safety of recombinant human interferon gamma therapy for atopic dermatitis despite unchanged serum IgE levels. Arch Dermatol 1998; 134: 799–804.
115. Reinhold U, Wehrmann W, Kukel S et al. Evidence that defective interferon-gamma production in atopic dermatitis patients is due to intrinsic abnormalities. Clin Exp Immunol 1990; 79: 374–9.
116. Grewe M, Vogelsang K, Ruzicka T et al. Neurotrophin-4 production by human epidermal keratinocytes: increased expression in atopic dermatitis. J Invest Dermatol 2000; 114: 1108–12.
117. Velazquez JR, Lacy P, Moqbel R. Replenishment of RANTES mRNA expression in activated eosinophils from atopic asthmatics. Immunology 2000; 99: 591–9.
118. Akdis CA, Akdis M, Trautmann A et al. Immune regulation in atopic dermatitis. Curr Opin Immunol 2000; 12: 641–6.
119. Yamamoto J, Adachi Y, Onoue Y et al. CD 30 expression on circulating memory CD4+ T cells as a Th2-dominated situation in patients with atopic dermatitis. Allergy 2000; 55: 1011–18.
120. Czarnetzki BM, Csato M. Comparative studies on human eosinophil migration towards platelet-activating factor and leukotriene B4. Int Arch Allergy Appl Immunol 1989; 88: 191–3.
121. Sigal CE, Valone FH, Holtzmann MJ et al. Preferential human eosinophil chemotactic activity of the platelet-activating factor (PAF) 1-0-hexadecyl-2-acetyl-sn-glyceryl-3-phosphocholine (AGEPC). J Clin Immunol 1987; 7: 179–84.
122. Weller PF, Lee CW, Foster DW et al. Generation and metabolism of 5-lipoxygenase pathway leukotrienes by human eosinophils: predominant production of leukotriene C4. Proc Natl Acad Sci U S A 1983; 80: 7626–30.
123. Lebel B, Venencie PY, Saurat JH et al. Anti-IgE induced histamine release from basophils in children with atopic dermatitis. Acta Derm Venereol Suppl (Stockh) 1980; 92: 57–9.
124. von der Helm D, Ring J, Dorsch W. Comparison of histamine release and prostaglandin E2 production of human basophils in atopic and normal individuals. Arch Dermatol Res 1987; 279: 536–42.
125. Bull HA, Courtney PF, Bunker CB et al. Basophil mediator release in atopic dermatitis. J Invest Dermatol 1993; 100: 305–9.
126. Fjellner B, Hägermark Ö. Experimental pruritus evoked by platelet activating factor (PAF-acether) in human skin. Acta Derm Venereol 1985; 65: 409–12.
127. Abeck D, Andersson T, Grosshans E et al. Topical application of a platelet-activating factor (PAF) antagonist in atopic dermatitis. Acta Derm Venereol 1997; 77: 449–51.
128. Andoh T, Kuraishi Y. Intradermal leukotriene B4, but not prostaglandin E2, induces itch-associated responses in mice. Eur J Pharmacol 1998; 353: 93–6.
129. Miyoshi M, Sakurai T, Kodama S. Clinical evaluation of urinary leukotriene E4 levels in children with atopic dermatitis. Arerugi 1999; 48: 1148–52.
130. Carucci JA, Washenik K, Weinstein A et al. The leukotriene antagonist zafirlukast as a therapeutic agent for atopic dermatitis. Arch Dermatol 1998; 134: 785–6.
131. Zabawski EJ, Kahn MA, Gregg LJ. Treatment of atopic dermatitis with zafirlukast. Dermatol Online J 1999; 5: 10.
132. Woodmansee DP, Simon RA. A pilot study examining the role of zileuton in atopic dermatitis. Ann Allergy Asthma Immunol 1999; 83: 548–52.
133. Rajka G. Essential Aspects of Atopic Dermatitis. Berlin: Springer, 1989: 57–69.
134. Hanifin JM. Pharmacophysiology of atopic dermatitis. Clin Rev Allergy 1986; 4: 43–65.
135. Morren MA, Przybilla B, Bamelis M et al. Atopic dermatitis: triggering factors. J Am Acad Dermatol 1994; 31: 467–73.
136. Mihara K, Kuratani K, Matsui T et al. Vital role of the itch-scratch response in development of spontaneous dermatitis in NC/Nga mice. Br J Dermatol 2004; 151: 335–45.
137. Werner Y. The water content of the stratum corneum in patients with atopic dermatits. Measurement with the Corneometer CM 420. Acta Derm Venereol 1986; 66: 281–4.
138. Werner Y, Lindberg M, Forslind B. Membrane-coating granules in "dry" non-eczematous skin of patients with atopic dermatitis. A quantitative electron microscopic study. Acta Derm Venereol 1987; 67: 385–90.
139. Fartasch M, Diepgen TL. The barrier function in atopic dry skin. Disturbance of membrane-coating granule exocytosis and formation of epidermal lipids? Acta Derm Venereol Suppl (Stockh) 1992; 176: 26–31.
140. Hägermark Ö. The pathophysiology of itch. In: Ruzicka T, Przybilla B, Ring J, eds. Handbook of Atopic Eczema. Berlin: Springer, 1991: 278–86.
141. Wahlgren CF. Itch and atopic dermatitis: an overview. J Dermatol 1999; 26: 770–9.
142. Yoshiike T, Aikawa Y, Sindhvananda J et al. Skin barrier defect in atopic dermatitis: increased permeability of the stratum corneum using dimethyl sulfoxide and theophylline. J Dermatol Sci 1993; 5: 92–6.
143. Choi EH, Brown BE, Crumrine D et al. Mechanisms by which psychologic stress alters cutaneous permeability barrier homeostasis and stratum corneum integrity. J Invest Dermatol 2005; 124: 587–95.
144. Griesemer RD. Emotionally triggered disease in a dermatological practice. Psychiatr Ann 1978; 8: 49–56.
145. Niemeier V, Kupfer J, Gieler U. Observations during an itch-inducing lecture. Dermatol Psychosom 2000; 1: 15–18.
146. Fjellner B, Arnetz BB, Eneroth P et al. Pruritus during standardized mental stress. Relationship to psychoneuroendocrine and metabolic parameters. Acta Derm Venereol 1985; 65: 199–205.
147. Fjellner B, Arnetz BB. Psychological predictors of pruritus during mental stress. Acta Derm Venereol 1985; 65: 504–8.
148. Metze D, Reimann S, Luger T, Juckreiz-Symptom oder Krankheit. In: Plewig G, Przybilla B, eds. Fortschritte der praktischen Dermatologie und Venerologie. Berlin: Springer, 1997: 77–86.
149. Koblenzer CS. Psychocutaneous Disease. Orlando: Grune & Stratton, 1987: 281–310.
150. Gupta MA, Gupta AK, Schork NJ et al. Depression modulates pruritus perception. A study of pruritus in psoriasis, atopic dermatitis, and chronic idiopathic urticaria. Psychosom Med 1994; 56: 36–40.
151. Cormia FE. Experimental histamine pruritus. I. Influence of physical and psychological factors on threshold reactivity. J Invest Dermatol 1952; 19: 21–34.
152. Arnetz BB, Fjellner B, Eneroth P et al. Endocrine and dermatological concomitants of mental stress. Acta Derm Venereol Suppl (Stockh) 1991; 156: 9–12.
153. Buhk H, Muthny FA. Psychophysiologische und psychoneuroimmunologische Ergebnisse zur Neurodermitis. Übersicht und kritische Bilanz, Hautarzt 1997; 48: 5–11.
154. Hermanns N, Scholz OB. Kognitive Einflüsse auf einen histamininduzierten Juckreiz und Quaddelbildung bei der atopischen Dermatitis. Verhaltensmod Verhaltensmed 1992; 13: 171–94.
155. Wahlgren CF. Pathophysiology of itching in urticaria and atopic dermatitis. Allergy 1992; 47: 65–75.
156. Ehlers A, Stangier U, Gieler U. Treatment of atopic dermatitis: a comparison of psychological and dermatological approaches to relapse prevention. J Consult Clin Psychol 1995; 63: 624–35.
157. Shenefelt PD. Hypnosis in dermatology. Arch Dermatol 2000; 136: 393–9.
158. Singh LK, Pang X, Alexacos N et al. Acute immobilization stress triggers skin mast cell degranulation via corticotropin releasing hormone, neurotensin, and substance P: a link to neurogenic skin disorders. Brain Behav Immun 1999; 13: 225–39.

159. Buske-Kirschbaum A, Gierens A, Hollig H et al. Stress-induced immunomodulation is altered in patients with atopic dermatitis. J Neuroimmunol 2002; 129: 161–7.

160. Münzel K, Schandry R. Atopic eczema: psychophysiological reactivity with standardized stressors. Hautarzt 1990; 41: 606–11.

161. Beltrani VS. The clinical spectrum of atopic dermatitis. J Allergy Clin Immunol 1999; 104: S87–98.

162. Hanifin JM. Basic and clinical aspects of atopic dermatitis. Ann Allergy 1984; 52: 386–95.

163. Rovensky J, Saxl O. Differences in the dynamics of sweat secretion in atopic children. J Invest Dermatol 1964; 43: 171–6.

164. Graham DT, Wolf S. The relation of eczema to attitude and to vascular reactions of the human skin. J Lab Clin Med 1953; 42: 238–54.

165. Wahlgren CF, Hägermark Ö, Bergstrom R. Patients' perception of itch induced by histamine, compound 48/80 and wool fibres in atopic dermatitis. Acta Derm Venereol 1991; 71: 488–94.

166. Bendsoe N, Bjornberg A, Asnes H. Itching from wool fibres in atopic dermatitis. Contact Dermatitis 1987; 17: 21–2.

167. Ekblom A, Fjellner B, Hansson P. The influence of mechanical vibratory stimulation and transcutaneous electrical nerve stimulation on experimental pruritus induced by histamine. Acta Physiol Scand 1984; 122: 361–7.

168. Fisher AA. Nonallergic "itch" and "prickly" sensation to wool fibers in atopic and nonatopic persons. Cutis 1996; 58: 323–4.

169. Hogan DJ, Dannaker CJ, Maibach HI. Contact dermatitis: prognosis, risk factors, and rehabilitation. Semin Dermatol 1990; 9: 233–46.

170. Sicherer SH, Sampson HA. Food hypersensitivity and atopic dermatitis: pathophysiology, epidemiology, diagnosis, and management. J Allergy Clin Immunol 1999; 104: S114–22.

171. Bueller HA, Bernhard JD. Review of pruritus therapy. Dermatol Nurs 1998; 10: 101–7.

172. Vieluf D, Matthias C, Ring J. Trockene juckende Haut – ihre Behandlung mit einer neuen Polidocanol-Harnstoff-Zubereitung. Z Hautkr 1992; 67: 816–21.

173. Lundeberg T, Bondesson L, Thomas M. Effect of acupuncture on experimentally induced itch. Br J Dermatol 1987; 117: 771–7.

174. Nilsson HJ, Levinsson A, Schouenborg J. Cutaneous field stimulation (CFS): a new powerful method to combat itch. Pain 1997; 71: 49–55.

175. van der Schaar WW, Lamberts H. Scratching for the itch in eczema; a psychodermatologic approach. Ned Tijdschr Geneeskd 1997; 141: 2049–51.

176. Melin L, Frederiksen T, Norén P et al. Behavioural treatment of scratching in patients with atopic dermatitis. Br J Dermatol 1986; 115: 467–74.

177. Hornstein OP, Gall K, Salzer B et al. Controlled physical exercise in patients with chronic neurodermitis. Dtsch Z Sportmed 1998; 49: 39–45.

178. Klein PA, Clark RA. An evidence-based review of the efficacy of antihistamines in relieving pruritus in atopic dermatitis. Arch Dermatol 1999; 135: 1522–5.

179. Henz BM, Metzenauer P, O'Keefe E et al. Differential effects of new-generation H1-receptor antagonists in pruritic dermatoses. Allergy 1998; 53: 180–3.

180. Berth-Jones J, Graham-Brown RA. Failure of terfenadine in relieving the pruritus of atopic dermatitis. Br J Dermatol 1989; 121: 635–7.

181. Doherty V, Sylvester DG, Kennedy CT et al. Treatment of itching in atopic eczema with antihistamines with a low sedative profile. BMJ 1989; 298: 96.

182. Hannuksela M, Kalimo K, Lammintausta K et al. Dose ranging study: cetirizine in the treatment of atopic dermatitis in adults. Ann Allergy 1993; 70: 127–33.

183. Sabroe RA, Kennedy CT, Archer CB. The effects of topical doxepin on responses to histamine, substance P and prostaglandin E2 in human skin. Br J Dermatol 1997; 137: 386–90.

184. Drake LA, Millikan LE. The antipruritic effect of 5% doxepin cream in patients with eczematous dermatitis. Doxepin Study Group. Arch Dermatol 1995; 131: 1403–8.

185. Shelley WB, Shelley ED, Talanin NY. Self-potentiating allergic contact dermatitis caused by doxepin hydrochloride cream. J Am Acad Dermatol 1996; 34: 143–4.

186. Hanifin JM, Ling MR, Langley R et al. Tacrolimus ointment for the treatment of atopic dermatitis in adult patients. Part I, efficacy. J Am Acad Dermatol 2001; 44: S28–38.

187. Jekler J, Larkö O. Combined UVA-UVB versus UVB phototherapy for atopic dermatitis: a paired-comparison study. J Am Acad Dermatol 1990; 22: 49–53.

188. Luger T, van Leent EJ, Graeber M et al. SDZ ASM 981: an emerging safe and effective treatment for atopic dermatitis. Br J Dermatol 2001; 144: 788–94.

189. Hoare C, Li Wan Po A, Williams H. Systematic review of treatments for atopic eczema. Health Technol Assess 2000; 4: 1–191.

190. Aliaga A, Rodriguez M, Armijo M et al. Double-blind study of prednicarbate versus flucortin butyl ester in atopic dermatitis. Int J Dermatol 1996; 35: 131–2.

191. Maloney JM, Morman MR, Stewart DM et al. Clobetasol propionate emollient 0.05% in the treatment of atopic dermatitis. Int J Dermatol 1998; 37: 142–4.

192. Yosipovitch G, Szolar C, Hui XY et al. High-potency topical corticosteroid rapidly decreases histamine-induced itch but not thermal sensation and pain in human beings. J Am Acad Dermatol 1996; 35: 118–20.

193. De Rie MA, Meinardi MM, Bos JD. Lack of efficacy of topical cyclosporin A in atopic dermatitis and allergic contact dermatitis. Acta Derm Venereol 1991; 71: 452–4.

194. Alomar A, Berth-Jones J, Bos JD et al. The role of topical calcineurin inhibitors in atopic dermatitis. Br J Dermatol 2004; 151(suppl 70): 3–27.

195. Novak N, Kwiek B, Bieber T. The mode of topical immunomodulators in the immunological network of atopic dermatitis. Clin Exp Dermatol 2005; 30: 160–4.

196. Ashcroft DM, Dimmock P, Garside R et al. Efficacy and tolerability of topical pimecrolimus and tacrolimus in the treatment of atopic dermatitis: meta-analysis of randomised controlled trials. BMJ 2005; 330: 516. Epub 2005 Feb 24.

197. Hanifin JM, Schneider LC, Leung DY et al. Recombinant interferon gamma therapy for atopic dermatitis. J Am Acad Dermatol 1993; 28: 189–97.

198. Jang IG, Yang JK, Lee HJ et al. Clinical improvement and immunohistochemical findings in severe atopic dermatitis treated with interferon gamma. J Am Acad Dermatol 2000; 42: 1033–40.

199. Kimata H. High dose gammaglobulin treatment for atopic dermatitis. Arch Dis Child 1994; 70: 335–6.

200. Gelfand EW, Landwehr LP, Esterl B et al. Intravenous immune globulin: an alternative therapy in steroid-dependent allergic diseases. Clin Exp Immunol 1996; 104(suppl 1): 61–6.

11

Psychosomatic aspects of atopic dermatitis

Gereon Heuft and Gudrun Schneider

THE HISTORICAL DEVELOPMENT OF PSYCHOSOMATIC DERMATOLOGY

Embryologically, skin and the central nervous system (CNS) have the same origin in the ectoderm and are functionally closely related. One speaks of the skin as 'reflecting the soul'. Skin is a communication organ and plays an important role in the development and socialization over a whole life span. Skin is sensitive to tactile stimuli and responds to emotional stimuli. Skin diseases have a direct influence on communication, physical experience, as well as sexuality. Since skin is subject to one's own perception as well as those of others, skin diseases provoke reactions from the social environment and have an influence on self-confidence as well as relationships to other people culminating in either real or alleged stigmatization. Because of the immediate availability of their skin manifestation, patients have access to their lesions at all times, so that behavioural aspects (such as scratching, touching, exaggeration or neglect of the required skin care) may lead to new lesions and complications in the course of the disease. Personality aspects, certain coping strategies as well as mechanisms, lifestyle, support, and acceptance through the social environment also play an important role.

Psychosomatic aspects of different skin diseases have a long tradition in the scientific literature. Since 1933, when Sack[1] founded psychosomatic dermatology in Germany with his article 'Skin and Psyche', papers have been published describing individual clinical case reports, approaching the subject, e.g. through psychodynamic/psychoanalytic interpretations ('anecdotal phase') (e.g. MacKenna 1944; Kalz 1945; Engels 1982).[2–4] First psychophysiological measurements may be found in Deutsch (1952).[5] A phase of systematic investigations in larger samples in some cases applying psychometric instruments and with control group design followed. The question was researched as to whether certain skin diseases may be associated with certain conspicuous personality traits and intrapsychic conflicts (hypothesis of conflict or personality specificity), also whether certain life events ('life-event-research') or stress trigger skin diseases or their exacerbation; the influence of skin disease on self-perception and quality of life was also researched. In the past 20 years, research has led to important insights into the psychophysiological and psychoneuroimmunological relationship of many dermatoses because of the apparent close relationship between psyche, neuroendocrine, and the immune system.[6–8]

PSYCHOSOMATIC ASPECTS OF ATOPIC DERMATITIS

Atopic dermatitis (AD) is a frequently found skin disease characterized by chronic or chronic relapsing itching lesions; in children these are especially eczematous-exudative with a scratch effect, crusts, and lichenification. The frequency in the population has increased in recent years, and hereditary disposition has been proven.[9] In atopics, disorders of the humoral and cellular immunity (raised serum IgE, defect of the T-suppressor cells, low natural killer cell activity), vegetative regulation disorders with a reduced sebaceous gland production, and a disorder in perspiration have been verified. At present, a multifactorial pathogenesis is assumed,[10] whose course may be decisively influenced by psychic factors.

Rook et al[11] introduced their chapter 'Psychocutaneous Disorders' in the 'Textbook of Dermatology' as follows: '... the role of emotional factors on diseases of the skin is of such significance that, if they are ignored, the effective management of at least 40% of the patients attending departments of dermatology is impossible.' Obermayer[12] reported 66% and Medansky et al[13] even 80% of dermatologic patients as 'psychogenically influenced'.

The prevalence of anxiety and depression was mostly investigated. Depression scores and suicidal reflections were mostly found in the cases of disfiguring skin diseases: Gupta et al[14] found suicidal thoughts in 7.2% of the inpatient psoriatic patients, in 5.6% of the patients with (non-cystic) acne, in 2.1% of AD and outpatient psoriatic patients, while alopecia areata patients reported no suicidal thoughts at all. In an investigation in German departments of dermatology, 23.2% of the heads of the departments found psychotherapeutic therapy to be a necessary requirement in addition to dermatological treatment.[15]

The relevance of developmental psychology and personality for atopic dermatitis

Cutaneous stimulation during childhood seems to be an important factor in cell growth and CNS maturation; this has been shown both in animal models as well as for premature children.[16] Dermatosis influences tactile stimuli early on; it stands to reason that primary objects develop a special relationship to those babies who suffer from dermatosis, who are being 'tortured' by the chronic itching and who cannot be calmed down. This puts into perspective earlier 'discoveries' on the pathology of a mother–child relationship especially in the context of 'rejecting' mothers.[17] It is possible that such a possible rejection may also develop due to the illness the child has developed, so that a disturbed parent–child relationship may in turn worsen the dermatosis, the child ending up in a circulus vitiosus by scratching excessively to compensate non-fulfilled needs.[18] Qualitative evaluation of interviews in 5 families with neurodermatitis children demonstrated illness-related burdens for the family; however, family-typical and not illness-typical coping patterns could be found.[19]

Even controlled studies have presented inconsistent results for mothers with distinct psychological traits and with neurodermitis children: mothers of babies and small children with atopic eczema described themselves as more depressed, more hopeless, more anxiously over-protective, and their child as being less positive in its emotional behaviour than mothers of a control group with healthy children. Pauli-Pott et al[20] and Ring et al[21] described 14 mothers of neurodermitis children as being 'less spontaneous, more controlled and less emotional than a normal collective'. 'Strictness' as a method for raising children was described by the neurodermitis children as being more evident in mothers, while the fathers were less conspicuous. These results, however, could not be replicated in the controlled investigation carried out by Langfeldt[22] with 50 mothers in each group. Absolon et al[23] also found no striking differences.

A child may also be influenced in its further development: e.g. itching may lead to sleeping disorders, may reduce concentration, and may lead to a worsening in school achievement. The altered physical appearance may also lead to an altered self-perception and a lowering of self-awareness.[24] Whereas Ring et al[21] found no psychometric differences in school children with AD when compared to a control group, Absolon et al[23] found psychically conspicuous behaviour twice as often in children with an average or severe case of atopic eczema than was the case for children with only a slight case of neurodermitis or a healthy control group.

Conspicuous personality behaviour has been repeatedly reported for neurodermitis patients: raised values for neuroticism, raised values for anxiety and depression have been found,[25,26] raised excitability, and inadequate coping with stress;[27] however, these may also be found in other psychosomatically determined illnesses as well and are therefore not specific for neurodermitis. Considering the burden involved in pruritus and the obvious skin disease, visible to all, as well as the early beginnings of the disease, there is every reason to believe that certain personality traits develop in the course of the illness and may interact with the course of the disease. All in all no specific personality types could be consistently described for neurodermitis patients.[28] However, there are indications that subgroups may be found that are psychically conspicuous.[25,29]

Atopic eczema and life events and/or stress

The basis of life-event-research in the 1960s was the model that the sum of 'critical' life events (without taking the context and the person involved into consideration) leads to illness. The 1970s and 1980s emphasized the inclusion of subjective burdens due to situations/events, the role of personality aspects, and the experienced social support in coping; this was expanded in the 1990s to include the salutogenetic perspective. Today, the sum of everyday burdens is considered to be a chronic life-event. Chronic psychosocial burdens influence the activity of the hypothalamus–hypophyseal–adrenal cortex system and the sympatic nervous system[30,31] and lead to molecular and structural changes in the brain.[32] In the present life-event and stress research the following question is considered: 'Which life event influences which person with what characteristics at which point in time under the impact of what factors in what way, i.e. which disorders are evoked in what way and which mechanisms play a role?' (Seikowski et al, p. 57[33]).

Psychosocial stressors like burdening life-events and psychic burdens are regarded to be important factors triggering exacerbations of AD. To research the relation between stress and neurodermitis, retrospective interviews, life-event research, experimental stress reactions, and chronologic serial analyses as well as psychotherapy evaluation studies were applied. Despite the many published papers on the relation between neurodermitis and emotional factors, only a few papers actually satisfy scientific methodology standards.[34] The largest sample up to now (1457 patients with AD) was investigated by applying a questionnaire after the earthquake in Hanshin, Japan on January 17, 1995. 38% of the neurodermitis patients from the area most severely affected (A) and 34% from the area less severely affected (B) reported worsening of their skin disease as compared to 7% in the control group. Improvement was reported by 9% from A, 5% from B, and 1% in the control group. Subjectively felt stress was reported by 63% from A, 48% from B, and 19% from the undamaged area. In the multiple logistic regression analyses, subjective stress was the best predictor for the exacerbation of the skin disease.[35]

In serial analyses the explicit influence of stress factors on the severity of skin alterations and different immunological parameters could be demonstrated.[36] It was interesting that 24 hours later an increase in psychic burdens was associated with a distinct worsening of dermatologic symptoms; however, patients also reported an increase in burdens 24 h after skin exacerbation. This could refer to the fact that in the sense of a circulus vitiosus psychosocial burdens were both the cause as well as the result of dermatologic illness. Correlations between the degree of severity of the self-evaluated itching and the level of depression for the different itching dermatoses, among others the atopic eczema, could be shown.[37]

Psychophysiological and psychoneuroimmunologic aspects of atopic eczema

As serial analyses have proven, the relationship between stress and skin alterations is conveyed by different neuroendocrine, immunologic, and vegetative regulation mechanisms.[8] In a meta-analysis, clinical depression went hand in hand with a variety of relevant alterations of cellular immunity.[38] Embryologic development (both the epidermis as well as the CNS develop via the neural tube from the neural plate) already accounts for the close functional connection between CNS and the skin organ. Deformation syndromes quite often concern both skin and CNS. Emotions trigger skin reactions: to blush, to pale, to perspire, etc. Many common function systems such as hormones, neurotransmitters, and receptors correspond both in skin and CNS.[39] Numerous neuropeptides have been found in the skin, e.g. substance P (SP), calcitonin-gene-related-peptide (CGRP), vasoactive intestinal peptide (VIP), neuropeptides Y (NPY), neurokinin, neurotensin, etc. Neuropeptides are found in the myelinized A-fibres and the non-myelized C-fibres both in sensitive as well as

autonomous nerve fibres. The skin organ is extensively supplied with various nerve fibres the sensoric nerves not only conduct afferent nerves from the skin to the CNS but also fulfil efferent neurosecretory functions. Ascending conduction pathways supply information to the thalamus, where the switching to the higher cortical centres takes place, which are responsible for the transformation of cognitive information. Descending pathways lead the sensoric information back to the spinal cord to effect the peripheral autonomous answers (perspiration, vasodilatation, etc.) The effect of some neuropeptides (SP, CGRP, VIP, NPY) are known: SP, for example, is a potent vasodilator and raises the permeability of blood vessels; intradermal injection of SP leads to reddening of the skin and urticaria, whereby the effect of SP is 100 times more potent than histamine. SP-induced secretion from cutaneous mast cells raises the leukocyte count in the tissue, strengthens the phagocytosis through macrophages and neutrophils, increases the in-vitro production of IgA through lymphocytes of Peyer plaques by more than 300%, potentiates the activity of other mediators, etc. It has been discussed that through the mechanism of the axon reflexes, in emotional stress neuropeptides are released in the skin that lead to neurogenic inflammations. Effects of emotional stress on the skin physiology could thus be explained; however, up to now, raised concentrations of certain peptides could be proven for experimental stress in the CNS but not for the skin. Psychophysiological comparative investigations on experimental stress between patients with neurodermitis and healthy probands have led to contradicting results: Faulstich et al[40] have determined significant differences, with a raised reactivity of heart frequency, EMG, and fluctuation of the skin resistance in patients with neurodermitis. Arnetz et al[41] and Köhler et al[42] found no general psychophysiological hyperreactivity in patients with neurodermitis compared to healthy individuals. Possibly there are subgroups in patients with AD concerning the psychophysiological irritability.

The psychophysiological differences found at first for atopic, psoriatic patients, and healthy individuals may be due to the differences in coping, mood, or cognition. If these factors were controlled then the only difference found was a significantly lower secretion of growth hormones under stress in the skin patients. Functional changes in the hypothalamus–hypophyseal–adrenal cortex axis are discussed. Scheich et al[27] reported on relations between level of serum IgE and irritability/excitability in patients with neurodermitis. Psychophysiological relations were demonstrated for a raised self-perception and leukocyte count and for the influence of cognitive evaluation of the investigative situation on skin reaction;[43] this was valid for both healthy individuals and patients. Of 30 inpatient neurodermitis patients, 90% reacted after dramatizing instructions in a standardized histamine prick test with increased itching and/or urticaria as opposed to a more soothing instruction. The influence of sensoric nerves on allergic inflammations has been presented by Undem et al.[7]

Psychosocial burdens due to atopic eczema and chronic dermatoses

Chronic skin diseases lead to severe psychosocial burdens that are quite frequently underestimated, since as a rule these diseases are not life-threatening.[44] Specific dermatologic burdens are itching, and a visible impairment in the case of atopic eczema. The itching may be extensive, so that a reflexive scratching may be the case which then leads to a circulus vitiosus of tissue damage and subsequent itching. This itching-scratching circle is perceived as a loss of control and is often accompanied by extensive feelings of guilt. The visible skin alterations may be experienced as a stigma, which may contribute to a negative self-concept and to avoidance and social withdrawal to reduce the anxiety of being stigmatized by the social environment.[45] The feeling of being stigmatized correlates with the extent of brooding, i.e. a strong inner preoccupation with the dermatosis.[46] Women are more influenced by skin diseases than men; patients with an atopic eczema or psoriasis had a more impaired sex-life than healthy individuals, and here psoriatic patients more than neurodermitis patients. Localization and morphology of skin appearance have an influence on the reactions of healthy individuals; however, for the extent of the subjectively felt disfigurement cognitive coping processes are more important than the extent of the symptoms. Neurodermitis patients with emotion-related coping strategies (avoidance of negative emotions, high self-acceptance, low stress vulnerability, avoidance of generalizations and brooding) were less impaired by the skin disease whereas a high disposition of personal self-attentiveness contributed to a higher burdening through the disease. In a longitudinal study, coping behaviour that included expressing emotions, looking for social support, and diversions led to a reduction in anxiety and depression; less medical treatment was necessary, and better physical health could be found 1 year later. Coping strategies explained higher variance in psychic health and life quality than in physical health.

These empirical results show that skin diseases themselves may be seen as psychosocial stressors that demand coping possibilities from the individual and that these may also be overtaxing. As a result, clinically relevant adjustment and depressive disorders, anxiety, etc., may develop. In the context of comorbidity, these must be diagnosed with care and must be treated in addition to the AD.

PSYCHOSOMATIC THERAPY OF CHRONIC SKIN DISEASES

Psychosomatic therapy of AD includes promotion of coping processes as well as the treatment of the psychic comorbitidy (e.g. anxiety or depression).

Coping

The problems of coping are also defined as somatopsychosomatic disorders. On a symptom level, one speaks of an acute stress reaction (ICD-10: F43.0) if the psychic symptoms last no longer than 4 weeks. A longer duration of problems in coping is, according to ICD-10 (F43.2), defined as adjustment disorders: for example, a 25-year-old patient with neurodermitis since childhood, who has not left her home for 4 months because of an exacerbation and is therefore socially isolated. These psychosocial symptoms may be related solely to the severity of the skin disease, since no further (neurotic) conflicts could be found.

Such burdens quite often overtax the individual's regulation systems that would otherwise regulate the individual coping competence and the demands made on the individual from the environment: the patient experiences the limits of his personal and social resources. The world is no longer as it once was and the individual is no longer the same person he once was prior to the illness.

Coming to terms with such a situation may be doomed to failure because the patient, according to the model of learned helplessness[47] (Figure 11.1), experiences the skin phenomena, for example, as something he cannot control and thus allowing negative future expectations to arise. The objective of psychotherapeutic treatment in such cases should be to support the patient and his family in their endeavours to adapt; these endeavours may in turn be subdivided into inner psychic processes and psychosocial coping processes. The goal of both is to maintain the capability to act or to re-attain this capability. As Figure 11.1 demonstrates, subjective illness concepts play an important role (external attribution: 'That what is happening to me, comes uninfluenced from the outside').

Every illness also signifies a narcissistic insult; if self-esteem problems have already existed prior to the illness, then an adaptive reaction to the illness may prove difficult. For example, a 33-year-old neurodermitis patient was enraged every morning when looking into the mirror; however, at the same time she was also

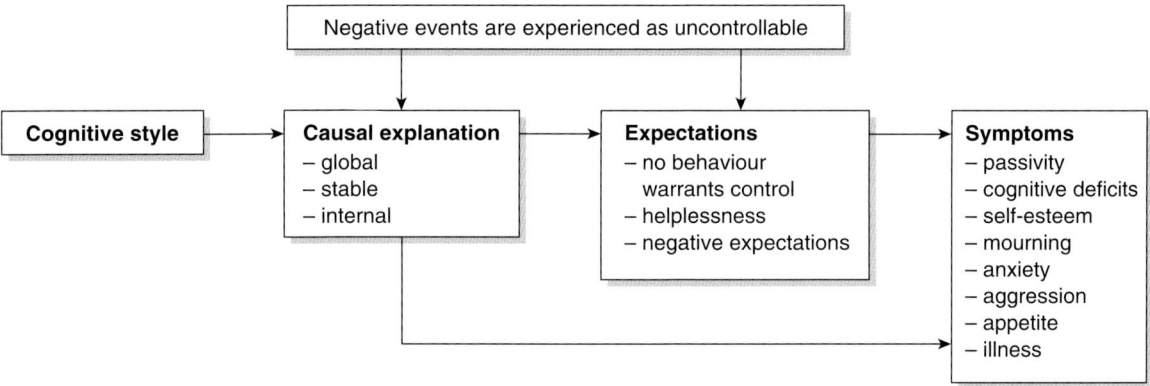

Figure 11.1   Model of learned helplessness. (Adapted according to Hautzinger M. Depression im Alter. Weinheim: Psychologie Verlags Union, 2000.[55])

someone who reacted angrily when she was challenged during the times without visible skin problems. Such repetitive dysfunctional conflict patterns make it necessary to take other treatment possibilities, e.g. psychodynamic psychotherapy, into consideration (see below).

Special programmes for patients to learn to cope with AD include behavioural therapeutic methods such as psycho-educative elements, training in handling stress, training in social competences, learning relaxation methods all with the following goal: assistance in coping with the illness, assistance in coping with the fear of losing control and penetration of the itch-scratch circle.[48,49] These programmes are usually carried out as group programmes on an inpatient or outpatient basis. In practical experience, these programmes have proven to be quite useful[50] and in controlled studies in patients with atopic eczema their efficacy with regard to dermatologic findings and psychosocial parameters when compared to a solely dermatological treatment has also been well documented.[51]

Cognitive behavioural psychotherapy (CBT)

The indication for behavioral therapeutic measures is based on symptoms, disorders, and available resources. Changes are either achieved by learning or relearning processes or by active environmental changes. Figure 11.2 demonstrates the basic model of cognitive therapy according to *Beck*.[52] In dealing with dysfunctional assumptions (e.g. 'I am ugly'), those thoughts that automatically come to mind ('no one wants to have anything to do with me') are changed with regard to the external trigger, e.g. the skin disease, so that depressive symptoms for example may be reduced. The afflicted learn to recover their feeling of internal control.

The sessions take place once a week; between the sessions 'homework' is assigned that is previously agreed on in the sessions. This may include practical exercises and may include e.g. phobic avoidance behaviour or changes in cognitive processes.

Psychodynamic psychotherapy

If in addition to AD, repetitive dysfunctional conflicts exist since early childhood development then the indication for psychodynamic psychotherapy (PDP) is given. As a rule, these sessions also take place once a week. Psychoanalytic treatment with a higher frequency (2–3/week) are more seldom and usually indicated in patients with an additional personality or ego-structural disorder.

Psychodynamic treatment procedures in dermatologic patients have been described for smaller samples in an outpatient setting[6] or, depending on the severity of the disorder, in an integrative inpatient setting.[53] The pre-post evaluation of integrative inpatient treatment in 40 neurodermitis patients demonstrated satisfactory results.[54] The advantages of inpatient treatment are:

- A continuous change between doctors/therapists and treatment concepts can be stopped.
- Patients are given a feedback in the intensive inpatient treatment programme through both the patient and the therapist group, thus experiencing an emotionally corrective experience ('I am not that repulsive at all') and are allowed new insights ('I can change something').
- Inpatient treatment allows a more 'external' perspective in cases of difficult personal or familial conflict relations and may thus be solved more easily.

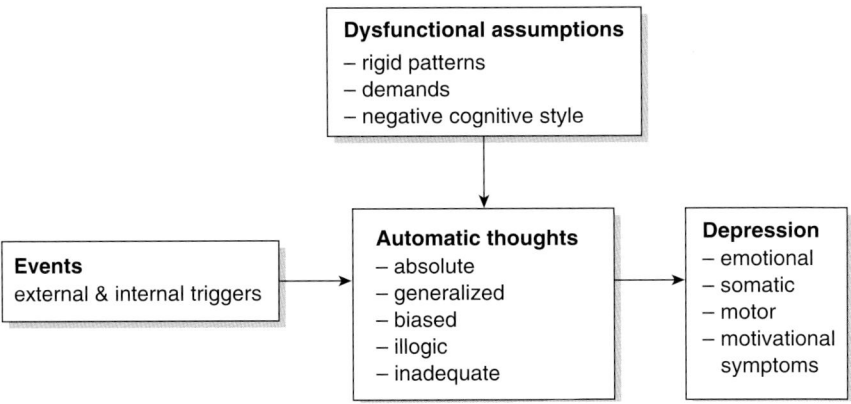

Figure 11.2   Beck's cognitive model (Adapted according to Hautzinger M. Depression im Alter. Weinheim: Psychologie Verlags Union. 2000.[55])

Traumatic experiences in the biography of a patient present a special therapeutic problem. Even if the patients insist on speaking about these severe psychic burdens, it must be ensured that they are able to control their emotions. In these cases, an internal 'secure spot' is first practised with the patient. Only when the patient has gained enough confidence during treatment, should an extensive trauma-specific treatment follow.

Psychotropic medication

In those problems that arise in coping with illness discussed here, *antidepressive medication* is only indicated if in addition severe depressive symptoms or anxiety persist. This medication must then be applied in an adequate dosage for at least 2–4 weeks before one can declare them to be effective or non-effective. If the psychic disorders are due to neurotic conflicts, then antidepressive medication is only helpful in those cases where severe psychovegetative symptoms such as sleep disorders or a severe inner unrest prevail.

In acute anxiety or agitated depression *tranquillizers* may be considered as a highly effective emergency medication; as a rule they have a swift effect and may be applied orally. They should, however, be applied no longer than 4 weeks because of the pronounced risk of dependency. This is also valid for a low-dose tranquillizer dependency often found in older people and leading to chronic dysphoria and lack of interest. *Low-potent neuroleptic* drugs are indicated in psychotic crises or severe states of unrest; they should however only be applied within the context of a psychiatric liaison service.

In summary it may be stated that we have a broad repertoire for both of the psychotherapeutic models addressed here (CBT and PDP) at our disposal depending on the differential indication for therapy and the goals aimed for (coping vs cognitive restructuring vs handling conflicts). These psychotherapeutic approaches may be supported by medication, in most cases antidepressant drugs, where indicated.

REFERENCES

1. Sack W. Haut und Psyche. In: Jadassohn J, ed. Handbuch der Haut- und Geschlechtskrankheiten. Berlin Heidelberg: Springer, 1933.
2. MacKenna RMB. Psychosomatic factors in cutaneous disease. Lancet 1944; 247: 679–81.
3. Kalz F. Psychological factors in skin disease. Journal of the Canadian Medical Association 1945; 53: 247–53.
4. Engels WD. Dermatologic disorders. Psychosomatic illness reviews. Psychosomatics 1982; 23: 1209–19.
5. Deutsch F. Some psychodynamic considerations of psychosomatic skin disorders. Plethysmographic and psychoanalytic observations. Psychosom Med 1952; 14: 287–94.
6. Koblenzer PJ. A brief history of psychosomatic dermatology. Dermatol Clin 1996; 14: 395–7.
7. Undem BJ, Kajekar R, Hunter DD, Myers AC. Neural integration and allergic disease. J Allergy Clin Immunol 2000; 106: 213–20.
8. Buske-Kirschbaum A, Geiben A, Hellhammer D. Psychobiological aspects of atopic dermatitis: an overview. Psychother Psychosom 2001; 70: 6–16.
9. Schultz-Larsen F, Hanifin JM. Secular change in the occurence of atopic dermatitis. Acta Derm Venereol 1992; 176: 7–12.
10. Niemeier V, Kupfer J, Al-Abesie S, Schill WB, Gieler U. Hauterkrankungen zwischen psychoneuroimmunologischer Forschung und psychosomatischer Therapie. Z Dermatol 1999; 185: 62–6.
11. Rook A, Wilkinson DS. Psychocutaneous disorders. In: Rook A, Wilkinson DS, Ebling FJG, eds. Textbook of Dermatology. Oxford: Blackwell Scientific Publications, 1979: 2023–35.

12. Obermayer ME. Psychocutaneous Medicine. Springfield, IL: Charles C. Thomas, 1955.

13. Medansky RS, Handler RM. Psychosomatic dermatology. Int J Dermatol 1981; 20: 42–3.

14. Gupta MA, Gupta AK. Depression and suicidal ideation in dermatology patients with acne, alopecia areata, atopic dermatitis and psoriasis. Br J Dermatol 1998; 139: 846–50.

15. Gieler U, Niemeier V, Kupfer J, Brosig B, Schill W. Psychosomatische Dermatologie in Deutschland. Eine Umfrage an 69 Hautkliniken. Hautarzt 2001; 52: 104–10.

16. Field TM, Schanberg SM, Scafid F. Tactile kinesthetic stimulation effects on preterm neonates. Pediatrics 1986; 77: 654–8.

17. Miller H, Baruch DW. A study of hostility in allergic children. Am J Orthopsychiat 1950; 10: 506–19.

18. Howlett S. Emotional dysfunction. child-family-relationships and childhood atopic dermatitis. Br J Dermatol 1999; 140: 381–4.

19. Fegert JM, Probst M, Vierlböck S. Das an Neurodermitis erkrankte Kind in der Familie. Eine qualitative Untersuchung zu Auswirkungen und zur Bewältigung der Erkrankung. Prax Kinderpsychol Kinderpsychiat 1999; 48: 677–93.

20. Pauli-Pott U, Darui A, Beckmann D. Infants with atopic dermatitis: maternal hopelessness, child-rearing attitudes and perceived infant temperament. Psychother Psychosom 1999; 68: 39–45.

21. Ring J, Palos E, Zimmermann F. Psychosomatische Aspekte der Eltern-Kind-Beziehung bei atopischem Ekzem im Kindesalter. I. Psychodiagnostische Testverfahren bei Eltern und Kinder und Vergleich mit somatischen Befunden. Hautarzt 1986; 37: 560–7.

22. Langfeldt H. Sind Mütter von Kindern mit Neurodermitis psychisch auffällig? Hautarzt 1995; 46: 615–19.

23. Absolon CM, Cottrell D, Eldrige SM, Glover MT. Psychological disturbance in atopic eczema: the extent of the problem in school-aged children. Br J Dermatol 1997; 137: 241–5.

24. Rauch PK, Jellinek MS. Pediatric dermatology: some developmental and psychological issues. Adv Dermatol 1998; 4: 143–58.

25. Gieler U, Ehlers A, Höhler T, Burkhard G. Die psychosoziale Situation der Patienten mit endogenem Ekzem. Eine clusteranalytische Studie zur Korrelation psychischer Faktoren mit somatischen Befunden. Hautarzt 1990; 41: 416–23.

26. Hashiro M, Okumura M. The relationship between the psychological and immunological state in patients with atopic dermatitis. J Derm Sci 1998; 16: 231–5.

27. Scheich G, Florin I, Rudolph R, Wilhelm S. Personality characteristics and serum IgE-levels in patients with atopic dermatitis. J Psychosom Res 1993; 37: 637–42.

28. Musgrove K, Morgan JK. Infantile eczema: a long-term follow-up study. Br J Dermatol 1976; 95: 365–72.

29. Mohr W, Bock H. Persönlichkeitstypen und emotionale Belastung bei Patienten mit atopischer Dermatitis. Z Klin Psychol 1993; 12: 302–14.

30. Schubert C, Lampe A, Rumpold G, Geser W, Noisterning B et al. Der Einfluß von Alltagsbelastungen und assoziierten Emotionen auf den dynamischen Verlauf von Cortisol und Neopterin bei Patientinnen mit systemischem Lupus Erythematodes: Ergebnisse aus zwei "integrativen Einzelfallstudien". Z Psychosom Med Psychother 2001; 47: 58–79.

31. Doering S, Wedekind D, Pilz J, Bandelow B, Adler L et al. Cortisolbestimmung im Nachturin – Vorstellung einer Methode für die psychoneuroendokrinologische Forschung. Z Psychosom Med Psychother 2001; 47: 42–57.

32. Fuchs E, Flügge G. Psychosoziale Belastung als Ursache molekularer und struktureller Veränderungen im Gehirn. Z Psychosom Med Psychother 2001; 47: 80–97.

33. Seikowsky K, Gollek S. Belastende Lebensereignisse bei hautkranken Personen. Z Dermatol 1999; 185: 56–61.

34. Ginsburg IH, Prystowsky JH, Kornfeld DS, Wolland H. Role of emotional factors in adults with atopic dermatitis. Int J Dermatol 1993; 32: 656–60.

35. Kodama A, Horikawa T, Suzuki T, Ajiki W, Takashima T et al. Effect of stress on atopic dermatitis: investigation in patients after the great Hanshin earthquake. J Allergy Clin Immunol 1999; 104: 173–6.

36. Buske-Kirschbaum A, Jobst S, Wustmans A, Kirschbaum C, Rauh W et al. Attenuated free cortisol to psychosocial stress in children with atopic dermatitis. Psychosom Med 1997; 59: 419–26.

37. Gupta MA, Gupta AK, Schork NJ, Ellis CN. Depression modulates pruritus perception. A study of pruritus in psoriasis, atopic dermatitis and chronic idiopatic urticaria. Psychosom Med 1994; 56: 36–40.

38. Herbert TB, Cohen S. Depression and immunity: a meta-analytic review. Psychol Bull 1993; 113: 472–86.

39. Panconesi E, Hautmann G. Psychophysiology of stress in dermatology. Dermatol Clin 1996; 14: 399–421.

40. Faulstich ME, Williamson DE, Duchman EG, Conerly SL, Branley PL. Psychophysiological analysis of atopic dermatitis. J Psychosom Res 1985; 29: 415–17.

41. Arnetz BB, Fjellner B, Eneroth P, Kallner A. Stress and psoriasis. Psychoendocrine and metabolic reactions in psoriatic patients during standardized stress exposure. Psychosom Med 1985; 47: 528–41.

42. Köhler T, Weber D. Psychophysiological reactions of patients with atopic dermatitis. J Psychosom Res 1992; 36: 391–4.

43. Hermanns N, Scholz OB. Kognitive Einflüsse auf einen histamininduzierten Juckreiz und Quaddelbildung bei atopischer Dermatitis. Verhaltensmod Verhaltensmed 1992; 13: 171–94.

44. Ginsburg IH, Link B. Feelings of stigmatization in patients with psoriasis. J Am Acad Dermatol 1989; 20: 53–63.

45. Harlow D, Poyner T, Finlay AY, Dykes PJ. Impaired quality of life of adults with skin disease in primary care. Br J Dermatol 2000; 143: 979–82.

46. Schmid-Ott G, Kuensebeck H, Jaeger B, Werfel T, Frahm K et al. Validity study for the stigmatization experience in atopic dermatitis and psoriatic patients. Acta Derm Venereol 1999; 79: 443–7.

47. Seligman MEP. Learned helplessnes. Munich: Psychologie Verlags Union, 1986.

48. Niebel G. Verhaltensmedizin der chronischen Hautkrankheit. Bern: Huber, 1995.

49. Stangier U, Gieler U, Ehlers A. Neurodermitis bewältigen. Berlin: Springer, 1996.

50. Stangier U. Zur Praxis der Verhaltenstherapie bei dermatologischen Störungen. Z Dermatol 1999; 185: 82–6.

51. Ehlers A, Stangier U, Gieler U. Treatment of atopic dermatitis. A comparison of psychological and dermatological approaches to relapse prevention. J Consult Clin Psychol 1995; 3: 624–35.

52. Beck AT. The development of depression. A cognitive model. In: Friedmann RJ, Katz MM, eds. The psychology of depression. New York: Wiley, 1974: 3–28.

53. Simmich T, Traenckner I, Gieler U. Integrative Kurzzeitpsychotherapie bei Hauterkrankungen. Hautarzt 1998; 49: 203–8.

54. Löwenberg H, Peters M. Evaluation einer stationären psychotherapeutisch-dermatologischen Behandlung bei Neurodermitispatienten. Psychother Psychosom med Psychol 1994; 44: 267–72.

55. Hautzinger M. Depression im Alter. Weinheim: Psychologie Verlags Union, 2000.

12

Quality of life in atopic dermatitis patients

Matthias Augustin and Marc A Radtke

HISTORICAL DEVELOPMENT IN QUALITY OF LIFE ASSESSMENT

Taking the patient's quality of life (QoL) into account in dermatological therapy has only become a matter of course over the past two decades. The ethical basis for this is found in the conception that it is necessary in taking any therapeutic decision to determine whether the benefit of treatment justifies the risks and the cost of therapy and whether the patient will benefit from the measures applied.[1] This is based on the patient's perspective and recording of how he experiences the treatment which he undergoes. Therapy decisions were often not made *with* the patient but *about* the patient. A patient movement has only arisen in the recent past in several countries whose activity is expressed in both self-help groups and in public lobbying and which has vehemently made clear to research that the relevance for the patient must be proven both in clinical studies and in basic research.

One great hurdle in the path was to make a person's QoL depictable and to develop methods of objectifying it.[2] Unlike objectifiable parameters like blood pressure, pulse, skin findings, eczema score, EASI, the patient's statements about his well-being, and his QoL rest on his subjective judgement. The fact that this cannot be measured by an objective doctor or scientist was long a source of uneasiness among methods developers and medical researchers. The same sort of subjectivity problems occurred, however, in recording pain and itching, so that acceptance now exists for course parameters which must be recorded from the patient's point of view.

The quality of life as a parameter in evaluating health goals in medicine has only become important during the past two decades, so that reliable methods of data recording are still undergoing development, as is the case in other areas of medicine. The first areas in which 'Quality of Life' was taken into account in clinical studies and in research were oncology and internal

medicine. Especially in oncology, the basic question quickly arose after development of the numerous chemo- and chemo-immunotherapies, as to the extent to which the not inconsiderable side effects of the therapy could be justified by an increase in the quality versus quantity of life. The frequent demand from patients for more *quality* rather than more *quantity* of life was addressed in the 1980s, and the clinical parameters 'increased survival time' and 'recurrence-free time' set against the parameter 'quality of life'. It became necessary to develop reproducible methods for valid and reliable measurement of the parameter 'Quality of Life'. Many of the now renowned research groups for quality of life and a variety of instruments for recording QoL were the result.

An additional impetus for research into QoL was given in medical economics.[3] This likewise new research area addresses the question of how the limited financial resources in the health system can be fairly distributed where they are needed. In this area, it is also mandatory to redefine the criteria for evaluating therapeutic procedures. The patient's increased QoL was recognized as one of the criteria for fair distribution of means.[3] Hence, the health goals in pharmacoeconomics address not only the length of life or the pathological deviation of real values of physiological variables from certain norm values but also the quality of life over time.

Meanwhile there has been great QoL research activity in nearly all areas of clinical medicine. In many countries, recording of quality of life is demanded for licensing or cost-reimbursement of drugs (for example, USA, Australia, Finland, Great Britain,[4]) or recommended by the responsible authorities (EU Regulatory, Italy, France). In some countries, guidelines have now been published by medical societies which require equal attention to QoL, costs, and clinical efficacy in clinical studies (for example Germany, The Netherlands, Switzerland).

In summary, the historical development shows that QoL and corresponding research have been gaining in importance through social as well as health-political legislative and last but not least medical demands.

DEFINITION OF QUALITY OF LIFE

QoL can be divided into two subsections. On the one hand, general quality of life which addresses basic needs and supports a person in the social structure. Among the components are, for example, food, housing, work, education, culture, social security, an intact environment, or also the right to free self-determination, as defined in the UN Charter.

Health-related quality of life (HR-QoL) is differentiated from this and comprises physical and emotional well-being, social relationships, and functionality in everyday living with respect to a person's health.[5] This, in turn, is divided into a 'general health-related QoL (generic quality of life)' and a 'disease-specific quality of life'. Many authors emphasize that the QoL consists less of the objective availability of material and immaterial things than of the degree to which an individual actually achieves his desired status of physical, emotional, and social well-being.[6] In psychological terminology, QoL is a multidimensional construct,[7] which cannot directly be measured but assessed by reflecting its individual dimensions. General well-being, defined as the general level of satisfaction and overall health status, is among the dimensions of QoL. Another component is physical functional capacity, for example mobility, the ability to cope with daily activities, pain, and physical symptoms. Emotional functional capacity, as well as social and cognitive functionality (memory, learning ability, judgement) are also part of QoL. Feelings like depression, rage, helplessness or also participation in social activities, family relationships, and leisure activities are subheadings of emotional capacity (Table 12.1).

Looking at patient-related individual benefit of QoL recordings, it can be assumed that the measured results based on valid, change-sensitive instruments will be reflected in individualized therapy planning and decision-making, as well as in appropriate outcome evaluation.[8] There is a need for valid instruments to record QoL which include not only the clinical and biochemical aspects of the disease, but even more the physical, emotional, and psychosocial factors which are affected by the disease.[7] Due to this necessity, various instruments to record QoL have already been developed which record disease-related aspects of a certain diagnosis or general factors of dermatological disease.

Table 12.1   Areas of recording in quality of life
a) Physical well-being
b) Emotional well-being
c) Social life
d) Functional ability in professional, everyday living, and leisure activities
e) Spirituality

Moreover, QoL in health economics and health politics is decisive as a decisional parameter for the fairest possible according-to-need allocation of the limited resources in the health system.[8] It is a declared health-political goal in all Western countries to provide the necessary financial resources to maintain or reinstate QoL for chronically ill patients. In order to do this, reliable data will be needed in future on which this cost allocation can be based.

RECORDING QUALITY OF LIFE

It is generally agreed that recording QoL is an essential part of disease evaluation for individualized therapy planning and assessment of therapeutic outcomes.[9,10] We differentiate between clinical recording on the one hand and scientific recording on the other.

An essential component of clinical recording is the detailed history and consultation with the patient and, where necessary or desirable, his family. This is the basis for the initial estimation of the patient's suffering and should go beyond the physical examination. The patient can often give very precise and exact answers to targeted questions on the effect on everyday living exerted by the severity of the disease and the situation which led him to consult a therapist. The questioning should also address the secondary effects of the treatment by itself on QoL. It has proven beneficial to create a doctor–patient relationship which enables including psychosocial examination in addition to recording only the skin disease.

Secondly, despite methodical limitations, QoL can be meaningfully recorded and reproduced during the course of the disease for scientific purposes. Methods for recording QoL are available in the form of questionnaires for rating by self and others of various components.[11–13] The questionnaires on QoL generally consist of individual statements (items), to which the patient ticks a preferred response, e.g. 'applies to me – doesn't apply to me.' Several questions are usually

| Table 12.2   Questionnaires for recording quality of life in allergic skin diseases |||||
Questionnaire	Author	Year	Disease	Items
Dermatology Life Quality Index (DLQI)	Finlay et al	1994	Skin diseases in general	10
Children's Dermatology Life Quality Index (CDLQI)	Lewis-Jones et al	1995	Skin diseases in general	10
Dermatology Quality of Life Scales (DQOLS)	Morgan et al	1996	Skin diseases in general	29
Skindex	Chren et al	1996	Skin diseases in general	61
Marburger Hautfragebogen	Stangier et al	1996	Skin diseases in general, atopic eczema	51
Dermatology Specific Quality of Life Instrument (DSQL)	Anderson et al	1997	Acne, contact dermatitis	52
Freiburg Life Quality Assessment for dermatoses (FLQA-d/short form	Augustin et al	2000	Skin diseases in general, atopic eczema	51/28
Infant's Dermatitis Quality of Life Index	Lewis-Jones et al	2001	Skin diseases in general	10
Deutsches Instrument zur Erfassung der LQ bei Hauterkrankungen (DIELH)	Schäfer et al	2001	Skin diseases in general, atopic eczema	36

asked in each area of QoL, and their mean is then the 'score' for the corresponding scale.

Both questionnaires related to general health (so-called generic instruments) and disease-specific questionnaires are used in recording QoL (Table 12.2). Among the generic instruments are, for example, the SF-36, the Nottingham Health Profile or the EQ5-D (Euroqol) Questionnaire.[14–16] Examples of disease-specific QoL questionnaires in dermatology are the Dermatology Life Quality Index developed in the UK[17] (Table 12.3), the Skindex from the USA,[18,19] and the Dermatology-Specific Quality of Life Instrument, also developed in the USA.[20] The Freiburger Life Quality Assessment (FLQA) is a combined German questionnaire with both disease-specific and general health-related parts.[21,22]

The advantages of a disease-specific questionnaire are greater differentiation capacity within subgroups of patients and greater sensitivity for changes over the course of disease. Special stress of the disease can thus be better identified. They are also better suited for discrimination of therapeutic effects in clinical studies.

In contrast, generic questionnaires enable comparisons with other diseases and with healthy persons, thus permitting better decision making on a general basis.[9] Most recommendations today by health-economics and clinical-pharmacological societies thus

include reference to the combined use of both disease-specific and general QoL questionnaires.[10,23] The inventories are filled out by the patient himself or – if impossible – by his family members or other competent persons (proxy questioning).[24] The development of such questionnaires is time-consuming and makes high demands with respect to meeting criteria of high test quality. A specific guideline on the use of QoL instruments in dermatology has been published by the German Society for Dermatology.[23,25]

QUALITY OF LIFE IN ATOPIC DERMATITIS

Quality of life for patients with atopic dermatitis

Atopic and allergic diseases of the skin and mucosae have been increasing in prevalence in industrialized countries over the past several decades. According to recent studies, about 10–20% of schoolchildren in EU countries are affected by symptoms of atopic eczema (European Allergy White Paper: The UCB Institute of Allergy. Brussels, 1998). Clinical experience has shown that AD is associated with a considerable detriment to QoL, affecting all areas of everyday living, physical, and emotional well-being (Figure 12.1).[17,18,21,22,26–31] The proportion of patients showing clinically significant levels of impairment

Table 12.3   Excerpt from the DLQI

Dermatologischer Lebensqualitäts-Index (DLQI)

(Dermatology Life Quality Index; Copyright: AY Finlay, GK Kahn, 1992* dt Übersetzung: M Augustin, 1997)

Patienten-Nr.: _____   Datum:_____   DLQI-Score: _____

In diesem Fragebogen soll ermittelt werden, wie sehr Ihre Hautprobleme in der vergangenen Woche Ihr Leben beeinfluβt haben. Bitte kreuzen Sie pro Frage ein Kästchen an. Wenn eine Aussage für Sie gar nicht zutrifft, dann kreuzen Sie bitte "Entfällt" an.

1. Wie **juckend, schmerzhaft, wund** oder **brennend** war Ihre Haut in der letzten Woche?	Sehr stark Stark Etwas Gar nicht	O O O O	
2. Wie sehr haben Sie sich in der letzten Woche wegen Ihrer Haut **geschämt** oder **verunsichert** gefühlt?	Sehr stark Stark Etwas Gar nicht	O O O O	
3. Wie stark hat Sie Ihre Haut in der letzten Woche beim **Einkaufen**, oder bei der **Haus**- und **Gartenarbeit** gestört?	Sehr stark Stark Etwas Gar nicht	O O O O	Entfällt O
4. Wie stark hat Ihre Haut in der letzten Woche die **Auswahl Ihrer Kleidung** beeinflubt?	Sehr stark Stark Etwas	O O O	Entfällt O

is even higher in AD than in psoriasis.[18,21,22] QoL impairment also include the patient's family[32] and interferes with the perception of treatment.[33]

The extent of QoL impairment for patients with chronic skin diseases is even sometimes greater than the stress of chronic internal-medical diseases and tumours (Figure 12.2).[34,35] Despite that fact that there is usually no vital threat, skin diseases rank high among diseases, which justifies appropriate monetary expense for their treatment.

The QoL for patients with AD was significantly improved in controlled clinic studies by various dermatological treatment procedures. Among these are cyclosporin A, tacrolimus, standard dermatological therapy with topical steroids, standard dermatological therapy with behaviour therapy, balneotherapy, and UV-therapy/photopheresis.[36–44]

Feldman[45] coined the term 'patient-centered care' in which the patient's QoL plays an integral role, and permanent communication and exchange with the patient are important components for the clinician and the approach to the disease. Clinical and therapeutic decisions depend on a number of different factors. The patient's QoL does not always directly correlate with the severity of the disease as reflected in the skin findings and degree of area affected. It is therefore very important to include these factors in the evaluation of a disease and in the evaluation of the severity. Decisions concerning therapies can then be taken individually and patient-appropriately with the patient's direct involvement. Investigation into QoL may help to document the result of medical measures scientifically in a way which the patient can understand.

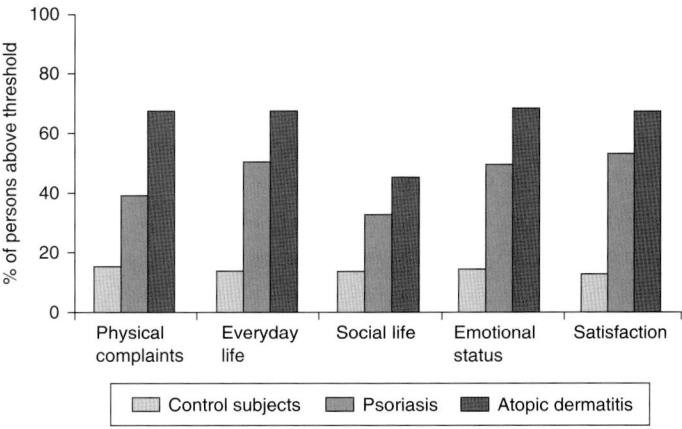

Figure 12.1   Proportion of patients with marked detriment to QoL (from: Augustin M et al. Eur J Dermatol 2004; 14: 1–8).

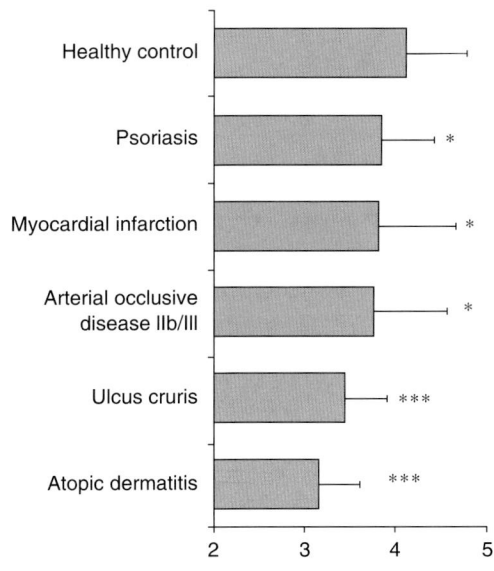

*p < 0.05, **p < 0.01, ***p < 0.001   QoL scale (mean+SD)

Figure 12.2   Quality of life in patients with atopic dermatitis compared to other chronic diseases, measured by the questionnaire on everyday life (n = 726, Bullinger M, Kirchberg I, von Steinbüchel N. The questionnaire on everyday life – a methodology on the evaluation of health related to quality of life. Z Med Psychol 1993; 3: 121–31; data by Augustin M, Zschocke I, Lange S, Schöpf E et al. The Freiburg questionnaire on quality of life in skin diseases: Validation and clinical results on 1865 patients. Plettenberg Meigel, Moll: Dermatologie an der Schwelle Zuin neuch Jahrtausend S. Berlin: Springer, Verlag, Berlin, 2000: 722–4). High values indicate good quality of life.

Quality of life in patients with atopic dermatitis compared to other skin diseases

In a cohort study published in 2001 by Augustin et al,[35] significant reductions to QoL were found in all scales for patients with AD (Figure 12.3). In this study, for comparative recording of AD, a random sample of 2021 consecutive patients at the University Dermatology Clinic Freiburg was examined, including 165 patients with AD undergoing treatment in the outpatient clinic. Patients with AD showed the greatest reductions of QoL among all patients, followed by other chronic skin diseases such as chronic leg ulcer, psoriasis, and chronic urticaria.

Patients with medication intolerances showed no significant detriment to QoL compared to age-matched controls. In patients with insect toxin allergy, there was only impaired QoL in the area of therapy (hyposensitization treatment), but not in the other areas of life. These findings can be understood clinically, since patients who are allergic to medications or to insect toxins have a high degree of control over the occurrence of interolance reactions and have no symptoms when they avoid the corresponding substances or situations. By contrast, patient with AD are continuously disturbed by their symptoms or by potential impairment. Also, the uncertainty is greater for patients with food allergies and with chronic urticaria, due to anxiety and fear of unexpected reactions.

Quality of life in patients with atopic dermatitis compared to other chronic diseases

Very few state-of-the-art direct comparison studies have yet been published to cover a broad spectrum of

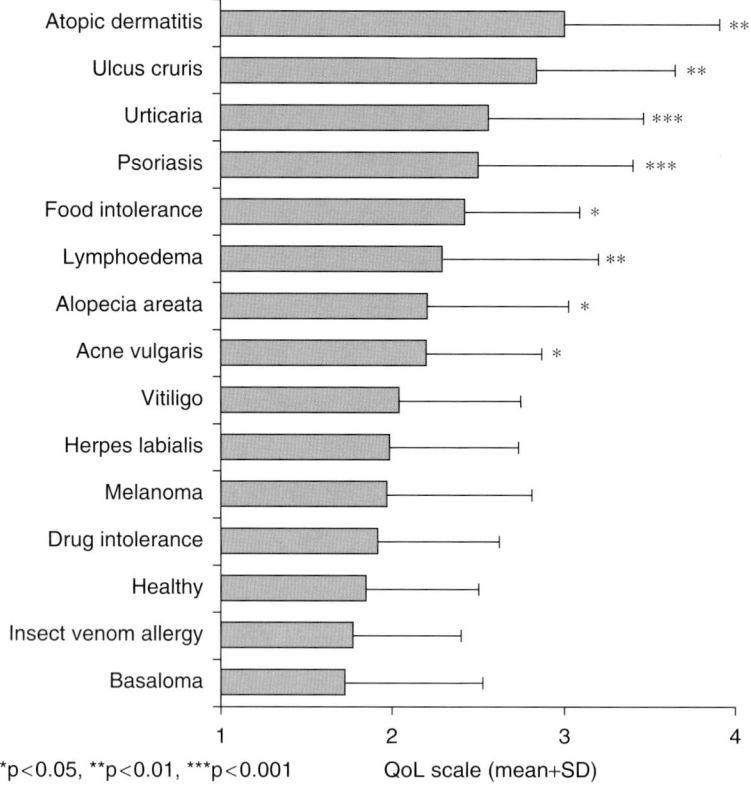

Figure 12.3 Quality of life in various skin diseases compared to patients with atopic dermatitis (AD) in Germany, measured with the FLQA (n = 2021, data from Augustin M, Zschocke I. Lebensqualität und Ökonomie bei allergischen Hauterkrankungen. Allergologie 2001; 24(9): 433–42). High values indicate great impairment of quality of life.

allergic skin diseases and internal medical diseases. Our own data comparing AD and other chronic diseases show that the extent of detriment to QoL for patients with AD is greater than that for patients following cardiac infarction (in rehabilitation) and for patients with arterial occlusive diseases in Stages II to IV (Figure 12.2). The results show that the degree of detriment to QoL depends less on the danger to life than on the symptoms associated with the disease and the social and emotional limitations.

Predictors of quality of life

According to an international consensus, QoL is a construct which cannot be directly measured but evaluated in different subdimensions. It is of particular interest to understand which patient-related factors contribute to high or low QoL. Investigations by Lange et al[46] indicate that quality of life in AD is mainly predicted by 4 factors:

1. physical complaints
2. social anxiety
3. helplessness
4. coping with disease

Consecutively, a high impairment of QoL is found in patients with high burden of symptoms (itching, burning skin, sleeplessness), problems in social life, feelings of being helpless, and in depressive forms of coping with illness.

These predictors underline the necessity of a comprehensive disease management, including consequent and early treatment of symptoms; training of social competence; and active coping strategies (e.g. in educational programmes).

NOTES FOR PRACTICE

Recording QoL as a diagnostic tool is as yet not widespread in practical dermatology. Specialist psychological measuring instruments are usually better suited to clarify concrete emotional questions (such as emotional distress), since QoL in such cases is a complex, multidimensional construct from a psychological point of view. However, recording QoL as part of quality management may be meaningful both in practical dermatology both in the doctor's office and in the hospital. As part of quality management, recordings could be made using short questionnaires, for example the Dermatology Life Quality Index (DLQI), in a pre–post comparison in order to document the outcomes of dermatological practice. This procedure is already the rule in clinical trials.

The question of how the patient's QoL can be improved is even more relevant for practical dermatology. An improvement in QoL is not only a high priority ethical goal but also a competitive factor for the dermatologist against other specialist areas in which dermatological patients are treated.

To improve the QoL of dermatological patients, it is necessary to determine which factors influence the QoL. As demonstrated in the predictor study, QoL of patients with AD is particularly influenced by social anxiety and physical symptoms.

These areas could be special targets in therapy. Appropriate dermatological treatment coupled with additional psychosocial support measures should be considered as the primary means of improving QoL.

Going beyond dermatological treatment, targeted measures to support coping with the disease can also contribute to improving the QoL in many diseases. Such measures include thoroughly informing the patient, which can be promoted by well-written information sheets. Clear, well-structured patient management can also set boundaries for demanding, time-consuming patients, without withdrawing the support they need. Patient training with dermatological information and behaviour training has already been found to be significantly effective with respect to improvement in physical symptoms, coping and QoL of patients with AD.[47] Another supportive measure may be participation in a self-help group, in which exchange of experience and information is possible.

FURTHER PERSPECTIVES

In light of the current health-economics situation and the still-increasing research activity in the area of QoL research and pharmacoeconomics, it can be assumed that these areas will increase in importance in the coming years. Meanwhile, efforts are apparent in Europe, North America and in Asian countries to harmonize the methods for recording QoL and to reach a consensus on the procedures for clinical studies. The German Dermatological Society has already published a corresponding guideline for recording QoL. Based on this consensus agreement, the recording of QoL and also of resultant costs have become fixed components of good clinical studies (Good Clinic Retrospective) and have already been included in national laws governing marketing authorization and reimbursement of drugs in several countries.[4]

Dermatology can especially benefit from these activities, since QoL studies clearly emphasize that some skin diseases rank highly and thus justify qualified, specialist dermatological treatment, even from a cost point of view. Thanks to QoL studies, the focus will be directed away from only preserving life, which is usually of subordinate importance in inflammatory skin diseases, to the quality of the remaining years of life. In cost discussions, it will be helpful to be able to present the high detriment experienced by patients with chronic skin diseases.

REFERENCES

1. Editorial. Quality of life in clinical trials. Lancet 1995; 346: 1–2.
2. Revicki DA. Relationship of pharmaeconomics and health-related quality of life. In: Spilker B (ed.). Quality of life and pharmaeconomics in clinical trials. Philadelphia: Lippincott-Raven, 1996, 1077–84.
3. Feeny DH, Torrance GW, Labelle R. Integrating economics evaluations and quality of life assessments. In: Spilker B (ed.): Quality of life and pharmacoeconomics in clinical trials. Philadelphia: Lippincott-Raven, 1996: 85–95.
4. Zentner A, Velasco-Garrido M, Busse R. Methoden zur vergleichenden Bewertung pharmazeutischer Produkte. Methods for the comparative evaluation of pharmaceuticals. DIMDI, Köln 2005 http://gripsdb.dimdi.de/de/hta/hta_berichte/hta122_bericht_de.pdf
5. Bullinger M, Hasford J. Evaluating Quality of life measures for German clinical trials. Control Clin Trials 1991; 12: 914–1055.
6. Augustin M, Amon U, Braathen L, Bullinger M, Gieler U et al. Assessment of Quality of Life in Dermatology (guideline) (Erfassung von Lebensqualität in der Dermatologie (Leitlinie)). J Dtsch Dermatol Ges 2004; 9: 802–6.
7. Hays RD, Sherbourne CD, Bozzette SA. Pharmacoeconomics and quality of life research beyond the randomized clinical trial. In: Spilker B (ed.): Quality of Life and pharmacoeconomics in clinical trials. Philadelphia: Lippincott-Raven, 1996: 155–9.
8. Rychlik R, Wertheimer A, Rusche H, Augustin M, Nelles S et al. Policy decision making and outcomes research in drug utilization. Zeitschrift für Gesundheitswissenschaften/J Public Health 2005: 1–14.
9. Brecht JG, Jenke A, Köhler ME, Harder S. Empfehlungen der Deutschen Gesellschaft für Klinische Pharmakologie und Therapie zur Durchführung und Bewertung pharmakoökonomischer Studien. In: Kori-Lindner (Hrsg.) Pharmakoökonomie in Deutschland. Editio Cantor, Aulendorf 1995: 211–24.
10. von der Schulenburg JM, Greiner W. "Hannover Guidelines" für die ökonomische Evaluation von Gesundheitsgütern und –Dienstleistungen. In: Kori-Linder (Hrsg.) Pharmakoökonomie in Deutschland. Editio Cantor, Aulendorf 1995: 225–32.

11. McDowell I, Newell C. Measuring Health: A Guide to Rating Scales and Questionnaires. New York: Oxford University Press, 1987.

12. Teeling-Smith G. Measuring Health a Practical Approach. Wiley: Chihester 1988.

13. Walker SR, Rosser RM. Quality of Life Assessment and Application. Lancaster: MTP Press, 1988.

14. Ware JE, Snow KK, Kosinski M, Gandek B. SF-36 Health Survey: Manual and Interpretation Guide. Boston, MA: The Health Institute, New England Medical Center, 1993.

15. Hunt SM, McKenna SP, McEwen J, Williams J, Papp E. The Nottingham Health Profile: Subjective health status and medical consultations. Soc Sci Med 1981; 15A: 221.

16. Rabin R, de Charro F. EQ-5D: a measure of health status from the EuroQol Group. Ann Med 2001; 33(5): 337–43.

17. Finlay AY, Kahn GK. Dermatology Life Quality Index (DLQI): a simple practical measure for routine clinical use. Clin Exp Dermatol 1994; 9: 210–16.

18. Chren MM, Lasker RJ, Quinn LM, Mostow EN, Zyzanski SJ. Skindex, a Quality-of-Life measure for patients with skin diseases: reliability, validity and responsiveness. J Invest Dermatol 1996; 107: 707–13.

19. Augustin M, Wenninger K, Gieler U, Schroth MJ, Chren M et al. German adaption of the Skindex-29-Questionnaire on quality of life in dermatology: validation and clinical results. Dermatology 2004; 209: 14–20.

20. Anderson RT, Rajagopalan R. Development and validation of a quality of life instrument for cutaneous diseases. J Am Acad Dermatol 1997; 37: 41–50.

21. Augustin M, Zschocke I, Seidenglanz K, Lange S, Schiffler A et al. Validation and clinical results of the FLQA-d, a quality of life questionnaire for patients with chronic skin diseases. Dermatol Psychosom 2000; 1: 12–17.

22. Augustin M, Lange S, Wenninger K, Seidenglanz K, Amon U et al. Validation of a comprehensive Freiburg Life Quality Assessment (FLQA) core questionnaire and development of a threshold system. Eur J Dermatol 2004; 14(2): 107–13.

23. Augustin M, Amon U, Bullinger M, Gieler U et al. Erfassung von Lebensqualität in der Dermatologie (Leitlinie). J Dtsch Dermatol Ges 2004; 9: 802–6.

24. Hays RD, Bickery BG, Hermann BP, Perrine K, Cramer J et al. Agreement between self reports and proxy reports of quality of life in epilepsy patients. Qual Life Res 1995; 4: 159–68.

25. Augustin M, Amon U, Bullinger M, Gieler U. Recommendations for the assessment of quality of life in dermatology. Dermatol Psychosom 2000; 1: 84–7.

26. Finlay AY. Measurement of disease activity and outcome in atopic dermatitis. Br J Dermatol 1996; 135: 509–15.

27. Linnet J, Jemec GB. An assessment of anxiety and dermatology life quality in patients with atopic dermatitis. Br J Dermatol 1999; 140: 268–72.

28. Lundberg L, Johannesson M, Silverdahl M, Hermansson C, Lindberg M. Health-related quality of life in patients with psoriasis and atopic dermatitis measured with SF-36, DLQI and a subjective measure of disease activity. Acta Derm Venereol 2000; 80: 430–4.

29. Lundberg L, Johannesson M, Silverdahl M, Hermansson C, Lindberg M. Quality of life, health-state utilities and willingness to pay in patients with psoriasis and atopic eczema. Br J Dermatol 1999; 141: 1067–75.

30. Zachariae R, Zachariae C, Ibsen H, Mortensen JT, Wulf HC. Dermatology life quality index: data from Danish inpatients and outpatients. Acta Derm Venereol 2000; 80: 272–6.

31. Schäfer T, Staudt A, Ring J. Entwicklung des Deutschen Instruments zur Erfassung der Lebensqualität bei Hauterkrankungen (DIELH) Hautarzt 2001; 52: 492–8.

32. Chamlin SL, Cella D, Frieden IJ, Williams ML, Mancini AJ et al. Development of the Childhood Atopic Dermatitis Impact Scale: initial validation of a quality-of-life measure for young children with atopic dermatitis and their families. J Invest Dermatol 2005; 125(6): 1106–11.

33. Augustin M, Zschocke I, Fölster-Holst G, Ravens-Sieberer U, Bullinger M et al. Attitudes on the use of steroids among parents of children with atopic dermatitis. Dermatol Psychosom 2000; 4: 155–61.

34. Petersen C, Schmidt S, Power M, Bullinger M. The DISABKIDS Group. Development and pilot-testing of a health-related quality of life chronic generic module for children and adolescents with chronic health conditions: a European perspective. Qual Life Res 2005; 14(4): 1065–77.

35. Augustin M, Zschocke I. Lebensqualität und Ökonomie bei allergischen Hauterkrankungen. Allergologie 2001; 24(9): 433–42.

36. Salek MS, Finlay AY, Luscombe DK, Allen BR, Berth-Jones J et al. Cyclosporin greatly improves the quality of life of adults with severe atopic dermatitis. A randomized, double-blind, placebo-controlled trial. Br J Dermatol 1993; 129: 422–30.

37. Berth-Jones J, Finlay AY, Zaki I, Tan B, Goodyear H et al. Cyclosporine in severe childhood atopic dermatitis: a multicenter study. J Am Acad Dermatol 1996; 34: 1016–21.

38. Kubota K, Machida I, Tamura K, Take H, Kurabayashi H et al. Treatment of refractory cases of atopic dermatitis with acidic hot-spring bathing. Acta Derm Venereol 1997; 77: 452–4.

39. Blessing C, Garbe C. Atopische Dermatitis: Klassische dermatologische Externatherapie führt zu guter Abheilung und Verbesserung der Lebensqualität. Eine Untersuchung. Deutscher Dermatologe 1998; 46: 2–8.

40. Mohla G, Horvath N, Stevens S. Quality of life improvement in a patient with severe atopic dermatitis treated with photopheresis. J Am Acad Dermatol 1999; 40: 780–2.

41. Czech W, Brautigam M, Weidinger G, Schopf E. A body-weight-independent dosing regimen of cyclosporine microemulsion is effective in severe atopic dermatitis and improves the quality of life. J Am Acad Dermatol 2000; 42: 653–9.

42. Thompson AK, Finn AF, Schoenwetter WF. Effect of 60 mg twice-daily fexofenadine HCl on quality of life, work and classroom productivity, and regular activity in patients with chronic idiopathic urticaria. J Am Acad Dermatol 2000; 43: 24–30.

43. Granlund H, Erkko P, Remitz A, Langeland T, Helsing P et al. Comparison of cyclosporin and UVAB phototherapy for intermittent one-year treatment of atopic dermatitis. Acta Derm Venereol 2001; 81: 22–7.

44. Drake L, Prendergast M, Maher R, Breneman D, Korman N et al. The impact of tacrolimus ointment on health-related quality of life of adult and pediatric patients with atopic dermatitis. J Am Acad Dermatol 2001; 44: 65–72.

45. Feldman S, Behnam SM, Behnam SE, Koo JY. Involving the patient: impact of inflammatory skin disease and patient-focused care. J Am Acad Dermatol 2005; 53(1Suppl 1): S78–85.

46. Lange S, Zschocke I, Seidenglanz K, Schiffler A, Zöllinger A et al. Predictors of the quality of life in patient with atopic dermatitis. Dermatol Psychosom 2000; 1: 66–70.

47. Staab D, Diepgen TL, Fartasch M, Kupfer J, Lob-Corzilius T et al. Age related, structured educational programmes for the management of atopic dermatitis in children and adolescents: multicentre, randomised controlled trial. BMJ 2006; 332: 933–8.

13

General management of patients with atopic dermatitis

Mark Boguniewicz and Noreen Nicol

EDUCATION OF PATIENTS AND CAREGIVERS

Education of patients and their caregivers is a crucial component in caring for patients with atopic dermatitis AD. Learning about the chronic or relapsing nature of AD, exacerbating factors, and therapeutic options is important for both patients and caregivers. Just as asthma action plans are integral to the management of asthmatic patients, so too, clinicians treating patients with AD need to provide both verbal and written information that includes general disease information along with detailed skin care recommendations (Figure 13.1). Patients or caregivers may forget or confuse skin care recommendations given them without a written step-care plan. This should be reviewed and modified at follow-up visits. There are many ways to customize care plans so that they meet the individual patient and family needs. Factors including severity of disease, age, patient history, and current environment all need to be considered. Development of a skin care programme that is agreed upon by the clinician, patient, and caregivers requires open communication. In-depth discussions can rarely be accomplished in an abbreviated clinic visit and adequate time needs to be set aside for proper education or they need to be coordinated with special classes. Presentations at international meetings have touted the benefits of attending eczema schools. At the National Jewish Medical and Research Center in Denver, Colorado, a weekly in-depth class on all aspects of AD is taught by the nursing staff to supplement teaching that occurs in the clinic, day hospital, or inpatient settings.

When patients with AD present with suboptimal response to prescribed therapy, the clinician's reaction often is to substitute another medication without

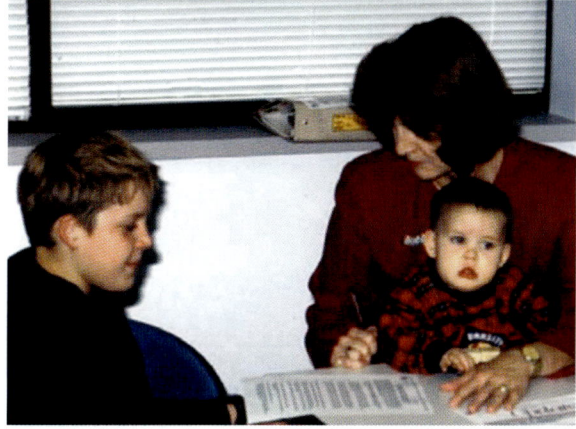

Figure 13.1 Education involves a written atopic dermatitis care plan.

any attempt to evaluate the whole picture. After several such encounters, patients may seek help elsewhere or are labelled as therapeutic failures. The experience of the authors at a national referral centre is that the vast majority of patients sent with a diagnosis of recalcitrant AD or treatment failure can be helped with conventional therapy when appropriate attention is given to the individual patient.[1] Direct demonstration of specific skin care techniques is very useful and often revealing when done on follow up to help understand when a patient may not be showing the expected therapeutic response. The patient or caregiver needs to show an appropriate level of understanding to help ensure a good outcome. Illustrative examples of treatment failures that were easily corrected with appropriate review and education include a patient referred as a failure of hydration therapy who demonstrated by applying a thick coat of petrolatum to her body prior to soaking her skin, rather than after the bath. Another patient sent as a failure of topical corticosteroid therapy demonstrated his approach to using the topical medication by applying a minute quantity from a small-sized tube and rubbing it in over a large area. When asked how long he had been using the same tube of medicine (which should have lasted no more than one week as discussed below in Practical aspects of using topical corticosteroids), the patient related that he had in fact been using it for several months. Another common mistake is the application of a high potency corticosteroid (e.g. beclomethasone dipropionate 0.05%) to an area of the body such as the face or axillae, while using a lower potency corticosteroid (e.g. hydrocortisone 2.5%) to the trunk or extremities, based on the patient's or caregiver's perception that corticosteroid potency is based solely on the assigned percent value (i.e. 0.05% vs 2.5%), rather than on the specific corticosteroid preparation (i.e. beclomethasone dipropionate vs hydrocortisone). This can be avoided through education as well as careful prescription writing by the clinician.

The patient and family with chronic AD have often seen multiple health care providers who may have given them confusing or conflicting information. This may set up a cycle of frustration and search for a straightforward solution to their problem. Practitioners of unproven therapies may take advantage of these patients, even promising a cure. Thus, it becomes imperative to convey the message that at present, treatment is directed at levels of control, not a cure. Stepwise management as proposed in the PRACTALL consensus report should be considered.[2] Adequate time is needed to discuss this chronic illness, potential triggers, along with diagnostic and treatment options irrespective of degree of disease severity. However, in the patient with severe, difficult to control disease, education is an especially critical part of illness management.

Patients who are 'failing' conventional therapy may benefit from hospitalization (as discussed later in this chapter). The significant and sustained clinical improvement often seen with this intervention may in large part be due to in-depth, hands-on education, along with changes in environmental exposures, reduction in stressors, and assurance of adherence with therapy. At the National Jewish Medical and Research Center, patients from across the US and abroad are treated in a variety of settings including the outpatient clinic, day hospital programme, and inpatient service. A high percentage of these patients experience significant improvement even when treated with medications that they previously believed were ineffective, when the treatment is integrated into a comprehensive and individualized management programme with thorough understanding as the foundation.

It is imperative to offer patients good references otherwise they will find their own, potentially less reliable ones. Patients with chronic AD may benefit from contacting national organizations, which provide education. In the US, educational brochures and videos can be obtained from the *National Eczema Association* (800-818-7546 or www.eczema-assn.org) and information, instruction sheets, and brochures from the National Jewish Medical and Research Center Lung Line (800-222-LUNG or www.njc.org). In Europe, educational brochures and videos can be obtained from the *National Eczema Society* (0870-241-3604 or www.eczema.org). The National Eczema Society has also endorsed the book *Eczema and your child: a parent's guide*. It is important to stress to patients and caregivers that they should review advice or tips gained through outside sources with their clinicians. Often, even small changes to a care regimen can either be detrimental or of little benefit, but can add to the cost of the treatment regimen. An open and ongoing dialogue between the clinician, patient, and caregivers improves the likelihood of adherence with the treatment plan and leads to improved outcomes.

Patients and caregivers should also be counselled regarding the natural history and prognosis of the disease with appropriate vocational counselling. Hand eczema is an important cause of occupational disability in patients with a history of AD, and patients and caregivers need to recognize that even those who appear to outgrow their AD may be prone to hand eczema.[3] Thus, jobs requiring wet work or frequent hand washing may not be good choices for patients with significant AD.

PSYCHOSOCIAL ISSUES IN THE CONTEXT OF GENERAL MANAGEMENT OF ATOPIC DERMATITIS

Given the significant impact of AD on quality of life (QoL) of patients and families, addressing psychosocial issues is of great importance in managing this illness (see also Chapters 11 and 12).[4] A key component of AD is the sleep disruption that affects not only patients, but caregivers as well. The fragmented sleep results in daytime fatigue, which can impact school and job performance. Patients will occasionally drop out of school or be unable to maintain employment, and caregivers may give up their jobs due to this aspect of the AD. This in fact can contribute to the high economic burden of this disease.[5] Despite the significance of this chronic problem, patients and caregivers find that sleep disruption is often not adequately addressed by clinicians. Use of sedating antihistamines, sedatives, or hypnotics may be appropriate, especially in the acute setting. Counselling, relaxation, or bio-feedback may all be helpful, especially in patients with habitual scratching.[6,7] Select patients may benefit from insight-oriented psychotherapy.[8]

Studies to explore the application of behavioural management techniques to aid patients in the management of their child's eczema have been conducted.[9] It is well recognized that patients with chronic AD have a learned behaviour component that perpetuates their itch-scratch cycle. One behavioural management strategy to consider is habit reversal. This method involves an alternative or competing behaviour adopted in place of the undesirable behaviour. The patient and caregivers need to integrate the new behaviours into their daily routines. Simple examples to replace scratching behaviours include patting the site rather than scratching, or application of a cool washcloth or a moisturizer to the involved area. Involving the patient/caregivers in this process and addressing their concerns will promote not only self-esteem, but will also assist in the development of life skills to promote long-term self-management.

AVOIDANCE OF IRRITANTS

Patients with AD have a lowered threshold of irritant responsiveness and need to avoid irritants.[10] Irritants are substances which cause direct toxic damage to the skin without preceding allergic sensitization. In addition, patients with AD have an abnormal stratum corneum, even in non-involved skin, that contributes to diffusional water loss after application of a topical irritant, confirming a functional abnormality.[11] Additionally, inflammatory changes including spongiosis, perivenular mononuclear infiltrate, and activated eosinophils can be seen after application of the irritant. Thus, non-specific triggers may contribute to chronic inflammation in AD. Common irritants include soaps, detergents, solvents, acids, alkalis, particulate dusts, and 'wet work'. Cotton gloves can be used as a barrier against irritants such as newspaper ink (Figure 13.2). These allow patients to maintain manual dexterity and are available even for young children (Figure 13.3a and 13.3b). In addition, cotton gloves can decrease trauma to the skin caused by scratching.

Since soaps and detergents are potential irritants, clinicians often advise patients to completely avoid them. This may be inappropriate advice as cleansers may be useful, especially in patients with frequent skin infections. In a double-blind, placebo-controlled study, daily bathing with an antimicrobial soap containing 1.5% triclocarban resulted in reduction in *Staphylococcus aureus* colonization and significantly greater clinical improvement than with the placebo soap.[12] Thus, the potential benefit of such cleansers needs to be weighed against possible irritant effects.

Most of the irritancy of cleansers, soaps, and detergents resides in the surfactant. In addition, the effect of pH on the irritancy of cleansers has been debated for some time.

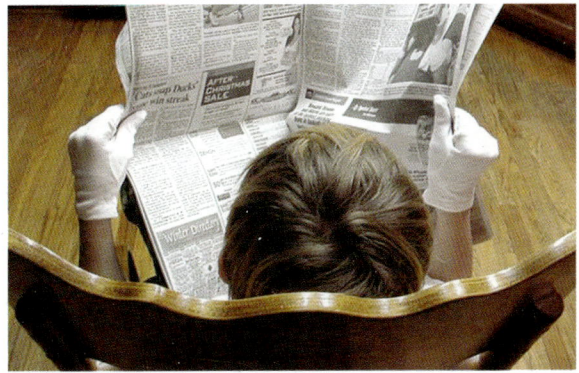

Figure 13.2 Use of cotton gloves as a barrier against irritants such as newsprint ink.

Current recommendations usually include using cleansers with minimal defatting activity and a neutral pH. Commercial soaps may contain, in addition to surfactant, a number of additives including optical whiteners, suds-controlling agents, germicidal agents, perfumes, abrasive agents, and dyes. Of these, perfumes and dyes frequently contribute to skin irritation. Perfume- and dye-free products are often identified as 'sensitive skin formulations' and may be better tolerated by patients with AD. In a comparative study of 18 soaps and cleansers using a chamber test, Dove® was found to be the mildest with respect to erythema, scaling, and fissuring.[13] Alcohol and astringents in skin care products can be drying and their use should be minimized. Laundry detergents present similar problems. However, presence of enzymes in detergents did not appear to make a difference with respect to clinical outcomes in one controlled trial.[14] Use of a liquid rather than powder detergent can result in more complete rinsing or adding a second rinse cycle may facilitate removal of residual detergent. New clothing should be laundered prior to wearing to remove formaldehyde and other chemicals.

Environmental factors that can modulate the effect of irritants include temperature, humidity, and texture of fabrics. Temperature in home and work environments should be temperate with moderate humidity to minimize sweating. Patients tend to do better in an air-conditioned environment. Occlusive clothing should be avoided and loose-fitting cotton or cotton blend garments substituted to help with overheating. The most important quality of the fabric may be non-abrasiveness and breathability and many blended fabrics are well-tolerated. Two randomized controlled studies found that texture or roughness, rather than fabric type (natural vs synthetic) determined tolerability and skin irritancy.[15,16]

Intense sun exposure can lead to overheating and evaporation, along with perspiration, which can

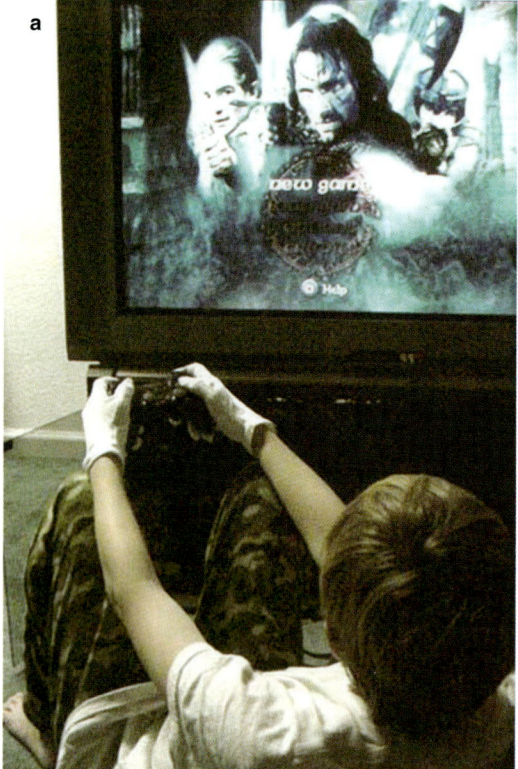

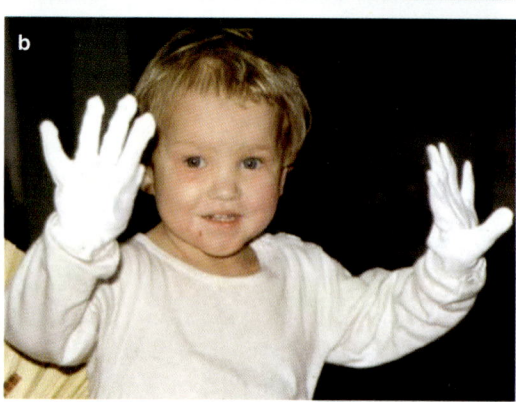

Figure 13.3a and 13.3b   Use of cotton gloves by children allows them to play or perform normal activities and is usually readily accepted. Gloves can also minimize skin trauma from scratching.

contribute to skin irritation. Although ultraviolet rays in sunlight have some beneficial properties with regards to AD, they can cause photodamage and sunburn. Patients and caregivers need to be educated as to the risks and benefits of natural sunlight and proper use of sunscreens. Sunscreens made specifically for the face due to their 'facial formulation' are often the ones best tolerated by patients with AD.

While patients are often counselled to avoid swimming in chemically treated pools, such activity can in fact improve the dermatitis of some patients. It is important to instruct patients or caregivers to use gentle cleansers afterwards to effectively remove the chlorine or bromine rather than simply rinsing off, and then to apply a moisturizer.

AVOIDANCE OF ALLERGENS

Food allergens have been shown to play a role in a subset of patients with AD (discussed in Chapter 8).[17] In children who have undergone double-blind, placebo-controlled food challenges, milk, egg, peanut, soy, wheat, and fish account for approximately 90% of the food allergens found to exacerbate AD.[18] Food challenges are usually done after first clearing up the patient's eczema or at least having a stable baseline and the specifics of this procedure have been described.[19] Food challenges were first reported at the authors' centre in the 1970s recognizing that a positive skin test to a food allergen did not necessarily define clinical relevance.[20] Removal of *proven* food allergens on the other hand from the patient's diet can lead to significant clinical improvement.[18,21] It is important for patients to completely avoid implicated foods, as even small amounts of the food allergen can contribute to food-specific IgE synthesis. Organizations such as Food Allergy and Anaphylaxis Network) can provide valuable information on hidden sources of common food allergens, recognizing specific food proteins by various names on food labels and methods of preparing certain foods with safe substitution of allergenic ingredients. Following the natural history of food-related AD is important as most patients will become tolerant to food allergens such as milk or egg protein, even in the face of positive skin tests. Typically, labour-intensive food challenges have been required to help define the natural history of food allergy. Recently, quantitation of specific IgE levels for 4 food allergens measured by the Pharmacia CAP System FEIA (egg $\geq 7\,kU_A/L$, milk $\geq 15\,kU_A/L$, peanut $\geq 14\,kU_A/L$, and fish $\geq 20\,kU_A/L$) have been shown to be associated with a $> 95\%$ chance of clinical reaction (Figure 13.4, Table 13.1).[22] Thus, a child with AD and a milk-specific IgE of $15\,kU_A/L$ or greater would not need to undergo an oral milk challenge. Serial IgE measurements using the Pharmacia CAP System FEIA to these food allergens has also proven to be of value in following the natural history of patients' food allergies to help determine when a food could be reintroduced.

The issue of prevention of AD with dietary manipulation is often raised by expectant parents. In a prospective study, Zeiger et al[23] found that restricting

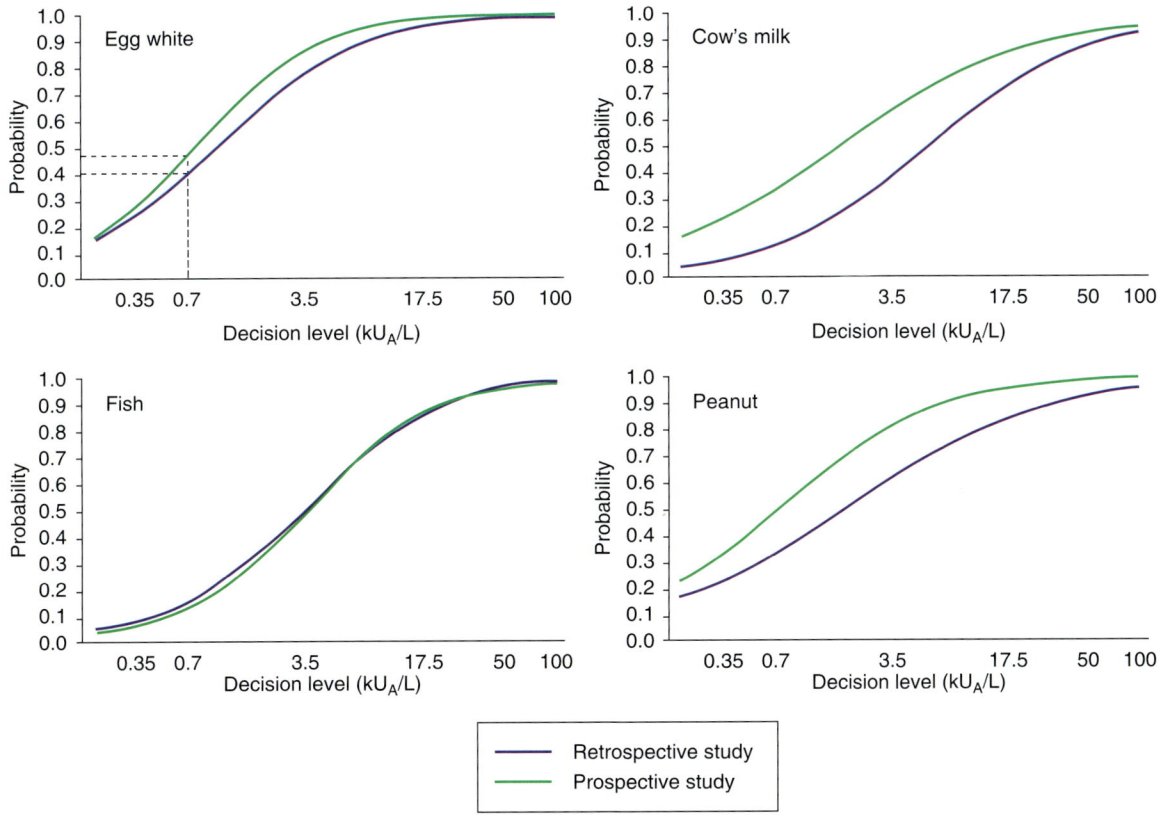

Figure 13.4   Probability of reacting to a food allergen based on allergen-specific IgE measured by Pharmacia CAP System FEIA (from ref 22).

the mother's diet during the third trimester of pregnancy and during lactation and the child's diet during the first 2 years of life resulted in decreased prevalence of AD in the prophylaxis group compared with a control group at 12 months of age but not at 24 months. Follow-up through 7 years of age showed no difference between the prophylaxis and control groups for AD or respiratory allergy.[24] Kay et al[25] also found that breast-feeding did not affect the lifetime prevalence of AD in a large ethnically and socially diverse group of children in England. In contrast, one 17-year prospective cohort study found that infants who were breast-fed exclusively for more than 6 months had a significantly lower prevalence of eczema at 1 year (all infants) and 3 years (infants with a family history of atopy) compared to infants who were breast-fed for less than 1 month or intermittently breast-fed.[26]

While the benefits of breast-feeding infants with AD have been touted, sensitization to allergens in the mother's diet transferred through breast milk is a potential problem for at-risk infants. Isolauri et al[27] investigated the extent and severity of allergic sensitization in a group of exclusively breast-fed infants with

AD. Cessation of breast feeding and institution of an amino acid formula compared to continued breast-feeding, even with maternal elimination, resulted in improvement in a number of clinical parameters including extent and intensity of eczema and Scoring atopic dermatitis (SCORAD) (p<0001). In addition, nutritional and growth parameters also improved when breast-feeding was discontinued in this population.

In some studies, the degree of sensitization to aeroallergens has also been shown to be associated with the severity of AD (see Chapter 9).[28] Isolation of Der p 1-specific T cells from skin lesions and allergen patch test sites of AD patients sensitized to dust mite allergen provides supportive evidence that the inflammatory response in AD can be elicited by inhalant allergens.[29] Importantly, environmental control measures aimed at reducing dust mite allergen load including the use of dust mite-impermeable covers for pillows and mattresses have been shown to improve AD in patients with specific IgE to dust mite allergen in some controlled studies.[30–32] While some studies have not found such benefit,[33,34] this may reflect the need to reduce allergen exposure in other environments or other factors

Table 13.1   Recommended interpretation of food allergen-specific IgE levels (kU$_A$/L) in the diagnosis of food allergy (Sampson HA. Utility of food-specific IgE concentrations in predicting symptomatic food allergy. J Allergy Clin Immunol 2001; 107: 891–6.)

	Egg	Milk	Peanut	Fish	Soy	Wheat	
Reactive if =(no challenge necessary)	7	15	14	20	65	80	Probability
Possibly reactive (physician challenge*)					30†	26†	of
Unlikely reactive if < (home challenge*)	0.35	0.35	0.35	0.34	0.35	0.35	reaction

*In patients with a strongly suggestive history of an IgE-mediated food allergic reaction, food challenges shoul be performed with physician supervision, regardless of food-specific IgE value. If the food-specific IgE level is less than 0.35 kU$_A$/L and the skin prick test response is negative, the food challenge can be performed at home unless there is a compelling history of reactivity.

†

contributing to chronic skin inflammation. Of note, in one 12-month study of adults with AD, the use of polyurethane-coated cotton encasings was compared to cotton encasings.[35] Eczema severity was more pronounced in the patients using the treated covers. House dust mite exposure and specific IgE both decreased significantly in this group. Of interest, patients not sensitized to house dust mite also benefited from use of the mite-proof covers, suggesting that impermeable covers may reduce exposure to other allergens, irritants or possibly superantigens. Dust mite-impermeable covers for pillows and mattresses appears to be a simple and relatively low cost environmental control measure.[36] While no controlled studies have looked at avoidance of furred animals in homes of patients with AD, in sensitized patients avoidance of such indoor allergens makes sense based on our current understanding of allergic inflammation (see Chapters 4 and 9).

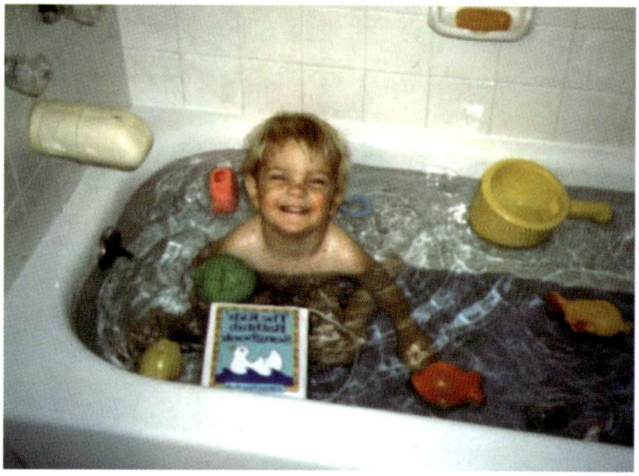

SKIN HYDRATION

Atopic skin shows enhanced transepidermal water loss associated with impaired function of the epidermal barrier.[37] Patients may also have decreased ceramide levels in their skin, resulting in reduced water binding capacity, higher transepidermal water loss, and decreased water content.[38] Re-hydrating the skin is best accomplished through soaking baths, although showers may be appropriate for patients with milder disease. Bathing may also remove allergens from the skin surface and reduce colonization by *S. aureus*. Of note, balneotherapy in acidic hot springs has been shown to help patients with refractory AD.[39,40] Unfortunately, some clinicians have confused wetting of skin, which is typically followed by evaporation and microfissuring,

Figure 13.5   Bathing is the best way to re-hydrate the skin and adding toys will help younger patients cooperate with the soak.

with soaking of skin which leads to re-hydration in conjunction with sealing in the moisture. Thus, water avoidance is often recommended even for patients with severe xerosis. At the authors' centre, 'soak and seal' are central to proper skin care.

Bathing or soaking the affected area should be done for approximately 15 minutes in warm water making sure that involved areas are covered to avoid evaporation (Figures 13.5 and 13.6). Water temperature should feel comfortable to the patient, as the oft-recommended 'tepid' is usually too cool for most patients. Adding age-appropriate toys will help young children cooperate with the bath. A wet washcloth or towel can be used for hydration of the face or neck (Figure 13.7). Cutting out eye and mouth holes allows older patients to read or

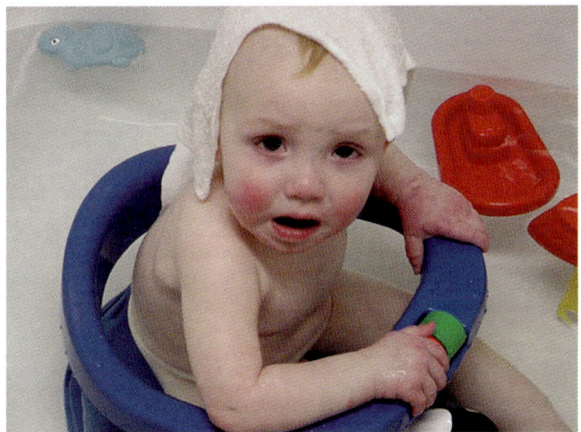

Figure 13.6   Infant in tub with proper support.

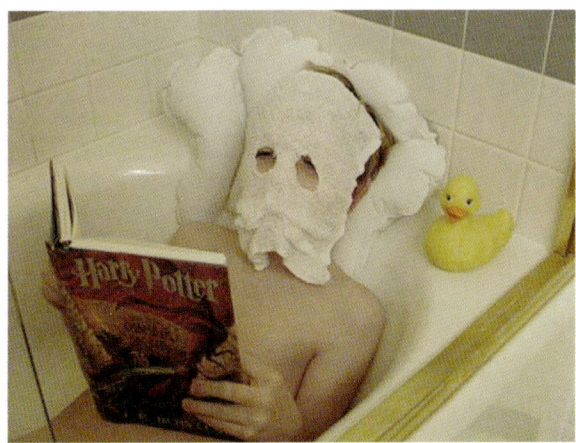

Figure 13.8   Hydration of the face with a wet mask while reading can be done in a tub, bed or chair.

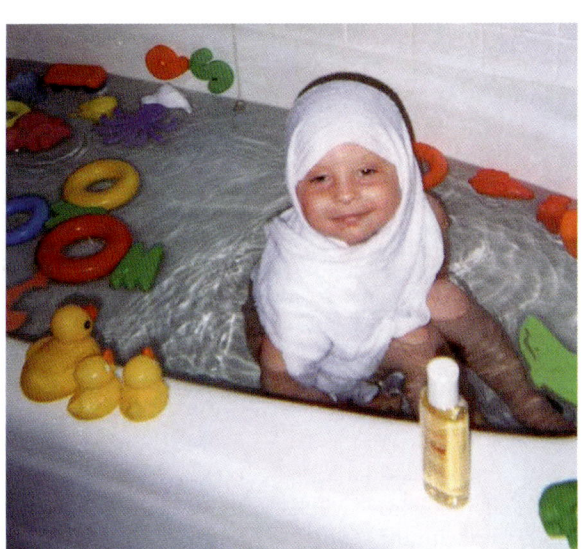

Figure 13.7   Wet towels can be used on exposed areas of eczema during baths to allow for hydration.

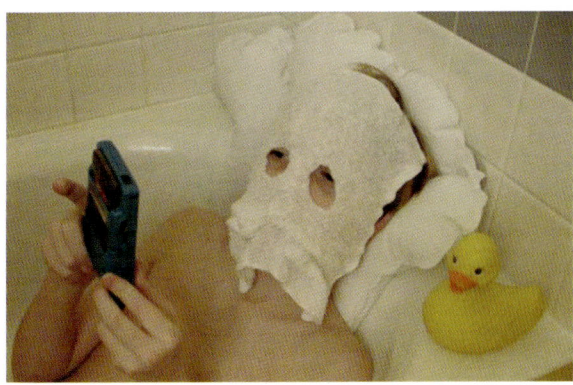

Figure 13.9   Hydration of the face with a wet mask may be more readily acceptable by allowing the patient to play a video game.

engage in other tub-safe activities (Figures 13.8 and 13.9). A basin can be used for eczema of the hands or feet (Figure 13.10). Baths can be increased to several times daily during flares of AD. Addition of oatmeal to the bath water may be soothing to patients but does not promote skin hydration, while bath oils may give the patient a false sense of lubrication and can make the tub slippery. Recently, addition of rice starch to bath water was shown to improve barrier function in patients with AD.[41] After hydrating the skin, patients should gently pat away excess water with a soft towel and *immediately* apply an occlusive preparation to prevent evaporation.

MOISTURIZERS

Use of moisturizers together with hydration may help re-establish and preserve the stratum corneum barrier.[42] Daily moisturizer therapy can also increase high-frequency conductance, a parameter for the hydration state of the skin surface.[43] This allows for ranking the efficacy of moisturizers according to the duration of effects or the magnitude of increase in the hydration level of the stratum corneum. In another study, the effect of a urea-containing moisturizer on the barrier properties of atopic skin was investigated by

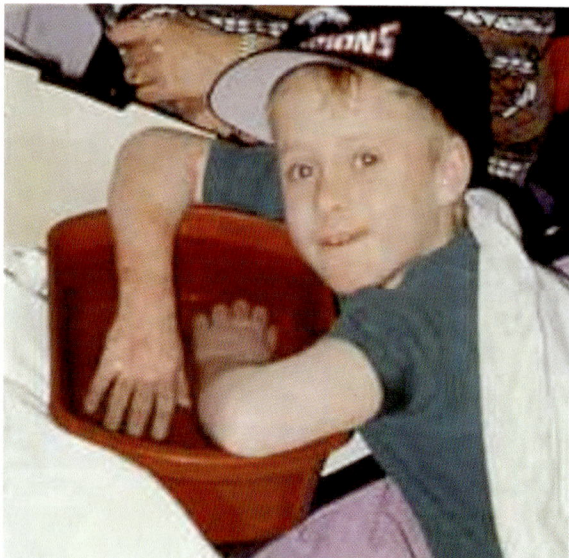

Figure 13.10   Involved body areas can be soaked selectively in a basin, even during clinic visit to demonstrate technique.

measuring skin capacitance and transepidermal water loss.[44] The skin was then exposed to an irritant (sodium lauryl sulphate) and the irritant reaction was measured non-invasively. The urea treatment significantly increased skin capacitance, indicating increased skin hydration. The water barrier function, reflected by transepidermal water loss values, improved while skin susceptibility to sodium lauryl sulphate was significantly reduced. Thus, certain moisturizers could improve skin barrier function and reduce susceptibility to irritants. Adding a moisturizer to a low potency topical corticosteroid was shown to improve clinical parameters in 2 studies of patients with AD.[45,46] Moisturizers have also been shown to decrease the need for topical corticosteroids.[47]

Alpha-hydroxy acids impact keratinization by affecting corneocyte cohesion and stratum corneum formation. In addition, they increase dermal mucopolysaccharides and collagen formation. The efficacy and safety of 12% ammonium lactate emulsion has been assessed by clinical criteria and by non-invasive methods including electrical capacitance of stratum corneum, skin surface lipids, transepidermal water loss (TWEL), skin surface topography as well as the biomechanical properties of the skin.[48] All patients tested showed a significant increase in electrical capacitance, skin surface lipids, extensibility and firmness of the skin, and an improvement in the skin barrier function and skin surface topography. Of potential clinical importance, 12% ammonium lactate has been shown to

mitigate the epidermal and dermal atrophy associated with application of a potent topical corticosteroid.[49] However, ammonium lactate should not be applied to open lesions as this results in significant burning and stinging.

As discussed above, a number of studies suggest that AD is associated with decreased levels of ceramides, contributing not only to a damaged permeability barrier, but also making the stratum corneum susceptible to colonization by *S. aureus*.[50] In a recent study, a ceramide-dominant emollient was added to standard therapy in place of their moisturizer in 24 children with 'stubborn-to-recalcitrant' AD.[51] SCORAD values improved significantly in 22 of the 24 children by 3 weeks with further progressive improvement in all of the patients between 6 and 21 weeks. TEWL decreased concomitantly with SCORAD and stratum corneum integrity (cohesion) and hydration also improved slowly. Finally, ultrastructure of the stratum corneum revealed extracellular lamellar membranes, which were largely absent in baseline samples. Several ceramide-dominant creams are marketed as barrier-repair creams. Other non-steroidal creams with unique mechanisms of action include Atopiclair® and Mimyx®.[52]

Moisturizers are available in ointments, creams, lotions, and oils. In general, ointments are formulated with the fewest additives and are the most occlusive, although in a hot, humid environment, they may trap perspiration, which may result in increased pruritus. Lotions and creams may be irritating due to added preservatives or fragrances. In addition, lotions contain more water than creams and may have a drying effect due to evaporation. While oils may go on easily, they are often less effective moisturizers. Moisturizers should be obtained in the largest size available (typically one pound/480 g jars) since they typically need to be applied several times each day on a chronic basis. Of note, even young patients can be taught to apply their moisturizer, which allows them to participate in their skin care (Figures 13.11a and 13.11b). Vegetable shortening can be used as an inexpensive moisturizer. Petroleum jelly is not a moisturizer, but can be used as a sealer after hydrating the skin.

PRACTICAL ASPECTS OF USING TOPICAL CORTICOSTEROIDS

Topical corticosteroids have been the mainstay of treatment for AD, showing efficacy in both acute and chronic disease. By acting on multiple resident and infiltrating cells, primarily through suppression of inflammatory genes, they are effective in reducing inflammation and pruritus.[53] In addition, topical corticosteroids may

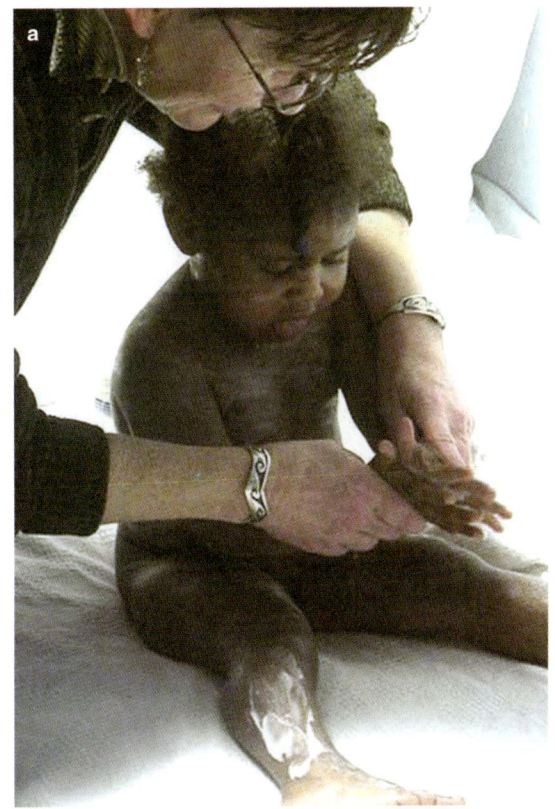

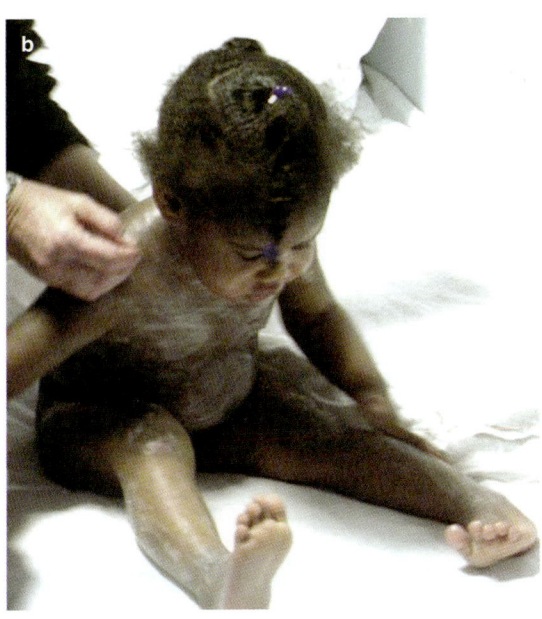

Figure 13.11a and 13.11b   Involving children in their therapy is important. Young children may participate readily at an early age, applying their moisturizer.

Table 13.2   Representative topical corticosteroid preparations

Group 1*	Clobetasol propionate (Temovate) 0.05% ointment/cream
	Betamethasone dipropionate (Diprolene) 0.05% ointment/cream
	Halobetasol propionate (Ultravate) 0.05% ointment/cream
Group 2	Mometasone furoate (Elocon) 0.1% ointment
	Halcinonide (Halog) 0.1% cream
	Fluocinonide (Lidex) 0.05% ointment/cream
	Desoximetasone (Topicort) 0.25% ointment/cream
Group 3	Fluticasone propionate (Cutivate) 0.005% ointment
	Halcinonide (Halog) 0.1% ointment
	Betamethasone valerate (Valisone) 0.1% ointment
Group 4	Mometasone furoate (Elocon) 0.1% cream
	Triamcinolone acetonide (Kenalog) 0.1% ointment/cream
	Fluocinolone acetonide (Synalar) 0.025% ointment
Group 5	Fluocinolone acetonide (Synalar) 0.025% cream
	Hydrocortisone valerate (Westcort) 0.2% ointment
Group 6	Desonide (DesOwen) 0.05% ointment/ cream/lotion
	Alclometasone dipropionate (Aclovate) 0.05% ointment/cream
Group 7	Hydrocortisone (Hytone) 2.5% & 1% ointment/cream

*Steroids listed by group from 1 (super potent) through 7 (least potent).
Adapted from Stoughton RB. Vasoconstrictor assay-specific applications. In: Maibach HI, Surber C, eds. Topical Corticosteriods, Basel: Karger, 1992.

have an effect on bacterial colonization in AD, reducing the density of *S. aureus*.[54,55]

Topical corticosteroids are available in potencies ranging from extremely high (class 1) to low (class 7) (Table 13.2).[56] Of note, the vehicle the product is formulated in can alter the potency of the corticosteroid and move it up or down in this classification. While generic formulations are required to have the same active ingredient and concentration as the original product, many do not have the same formulation of the vehicle and their bioequivalence can vary significantly.[57] In general, a steroid molecule will be most potent in an ointment base.

Topical corticosteroids are available in a variety of bases including ointments, creams, lotions, solutions, gels, sprays, foam, oil, and even steroid-impregnated tape. Thus, there is no need to compound these medications. In addition, use of an emollient immediately prior to or on top of a topical corticosteroid may decrease the effectiveness of the latter. Ointment-based preparations are most occlusive, have the fewest additives, provide better delivery of the medication, and decrease evaporative losses. During periods of excessive heat or humidity, cream formulations may be better tolerated since the increased occlusion may contribute to pruritus or folliculitis. In general, however, creams and lotions, while easier to apply, may contribute to skin irritation and xerosis. Solutions are useful on the scalp or other hirsute areas, although the alcohol in them can be quite irritating when used on inflamed or excoriated lesions. Ingredients used to formulate the different bases may be irritating to individual patients and may cause sensitization. In addition, the corticosteroid molecule itself can induce an allergic contact dermatitis.[58] This diagnosis is often difficult to establish on clinical grounds since it can present as acute or chronic eczema. Patch testing has been done primarily with tixocortol pivalate and budesonide, although this approach can miss allergic sensitization in a subset of patients. Expanded testing, on the other hand, has been associated with both false-positive and false-negative reactions.[59]

Choice of which topical corticosteroid preparation to prescribe will depend in large part on the severity and distribution of eczematous lesions. Patients need to be informed about the potency and potential side effects of their prescribed topical corticosteroid. Patients may erroneously assume that the potency of a topical corticosteroid is defined by the percent stated after the compound name (as discussed above under Education of Patients and Caregivers). In general, using the least potent corticosteroid that is effective should be the rule. This approach needs to be balanced by the possibility that initiation of therapy with a topical corticosteroid that is too weak may result in persistence or worsening of AD, which in turn can lead to decreased adherence with the treatment regimen. Thus, a step-care approach starting with a mid or high potency preparation (except to eczema of the face, axillae or groin) followed by a lower potency preparation with clinical improvement may be a more effective strategy. All too often,

Area	Single application (g)	Twice-daily application for 2 weeks (g)
Face, hands, genital area	2	60
Arm, anterior or posterior trunk	3	80
Leg	4	120
Entire body	30–60	840–1680

Table 13.3 Amount of topical corticosteroid to dispense for an average-sized adult

Modifed from Weston WL, Lane AT, Morelli JG. Color Textbook of Pediatric Dermatology, 2nd edn. St Louis, Mosby, 1996.

patients are prescribed a high potency corticosteroid with instructions to discontinue it within 7 to 14 days, without a plan to step down, resulting in rebound flaring of their AD, similar to what is frequently seen after oral corticosteroids. In some cases, therapy-resistant lesions may require a potent topical corticosteroid under occlusion, although this approach should be used cautiously and be reserved primarily for severe eczema of the hands or feet.[60,61] It is important to remember that Lotrisone contains both clotrimazole, an antifungal, and beclomethasone dipropionate, a high potency corticosteroid, and should rarely be used for treating AD and never applied to the face, groin or axillae.

Prescribing topical corticosteroids in inadequate amounts can also contribute to suboptimally controlled AD, especially in patients with widespread disease (Table 13.3). It is worth remembering that it takes approximately 30 grams of medication to cover the entire body of an average adult.[62] Thus, patients who have to refill prescriptions frequently may undertreat their eczema or become non-adherent with their prescribed regimen. In addition, obtaining medications in larger quantities can result in significant savings for patients. The fingertip unit (FTU) defined as the amount of topical medication extending from the tip to the first joint on the palmar aspect of the index finger has been studied in children with AD as a measure for applying topical corticosteroids.[63] It takes approximately 1 FTU to cover the hand or groin, 2 FTUs for the face or foot, 3 FTUs for an arm, 6 FTUs for the leg, and 14 FTUs for the trunk.

Topical corticosteroids have typically been applied twice daily and using them more frequently may increase side effects and cost without a significant clinical benefit. Of note, once daily treatment has been shown to be effective for certain corticosteroid preparations, including fluticasone propionate[64] and mometasone furoate.[65] Once daily application may improve adherence with the treatment regimen. Given the concern with side effects associated with chronic use, topical corticosteroids have not been considered appropriate for 'maintenance therapy' especially to normal-appearing skin. More recent studies with fluticasone propionate in patients as young as 3 months of age[66,67] have shown that once control is achieved with a once daily regimen, long-term control can be maintained with twice weekly therapy. Of note, during the maintenance phase of the study, the corticosteroid preparation was applied to areas that appeared to have healed, which resulted in delayed relapses compared with placebo therapy.

Patients with AD may not respond appropriately to their topical corticosteroid. Reasons for this may include S. aureus superinfection, inadequate potency of the preparation, or insufficient amount dispensed as discussed above. Other causes for apparent treatment failure include steroid allergy and possibly corticosteroid insensitivity. However, a much more practical reason for therapeutic failure with topical corticosteroids is non-adherence with the treatment regimen. As with any chronic disease, patients or caregivers often expect a quick and permanent resolution of their illness and become disillusioned with the lack of a cure. In addition, a significant number of patients or caregivers admit to non-adherence with topical corticosteroids due to fear of adverse effects.[68,69]

PRACTICAL ASPECTS OF ORAL CORTICOSTEROID THERAPY

The use of oral corticosteroids should be avoided as much as possible in a chronic, relapsing disease such as AD. Although patients may experience rapid and dramatic relief from their eczema, this is often followed by rebound flaring. Short courses of an oral corticosteroid are at times used with the initiation of other treatment measures. Gradual tapering of the oral corticosteroid with intensification of topical skin care may dampen rebound flaring.

TAR PREPARATIONS

While the anti-inflammatory properties of tars are not as pronounced as those of topical corticosteroids, they may be useful in reducing the need for topical corticosteroids in chronic maintenance therapy of AD. In a comparison with a moderate potency topical corticosteroid, tar therapy was found to be comparable in its inhibitory effect on the influx of a number of pro-inflammatory cells, as well as on the expression of adhesion molecules in response to epicutaneous allergen challenge.[70] Currently, tars are used primarily in shampoos for scalp inflammation or as bath additives. Coal tar products have been developed which are better tolerated with respect to odour and staining of clothes. A moisturizer applied over the tar product will decrease the drying effect on the skin. Some patients prefer a tar compounded in an ointment or cream base such as 5% LCD (Liquor Carbonis detergents) in Aquaphor ointment to avoid the need for multiple layers. Tar preparations may be used primarily at bedtime to allow the patient to remove the preparation in the morning and limiting staining to a few pairs of pyjamas and bed sheets. Tar preparations should not be used on acutely inflamed skin, since this may result in irritation. Side effects associated with tars include folliculitis and photosensitivity.

PRACTICAL ASPECTS OF ANTI-INFECTIVE THERAPY

Systemic antibiotic therapy is usually necessary to treat lesions secondarily infected with S. aureus that are widespread. First- or second-generation cephalosporins given for 7–10 days are usually effective (e.g. cephalexin 500 mg twice daily or 25–50 mg/kg divided twice daily for paediatric patients). A semisynthetic penicillin can also be used. Since erythromycin-resistant organisms are common, erythromycin and other macrolides are of limited usefulness. Patients become rapidly re-colonized after a course of antibiotics;[71] however, long-term maintenance antibiotic therapy should be avoided as it may predispose to colonization by methicillin-resistant organisms. The topical anti-staphylococcal antibiotic mupirocin (Bactroban) applied 3 times daily to affected areas for 7–10 days can be used to treat localized areas of involvement.[72] Treatment twice daily for 5 days with a nasal preparation of mupirocin may reduce nasal carriage of S. aureus.[73] On the other hand, use of topical neomycin can result in allergic contact dermatitis as neomycin is among the more common allergens causing contact dermatitis.[74]

Patients with eczema herpeticum, also referred to as Kaposi's varicelliform eruption, usually require treatment with systemic aciclovir in a hospital setting.[75] Recurrent cutaneous herpetic infections can be suppressed with a prophylactic oral antiviral (e.g. aciclovir 400 mg twice daily). Superficial dermatophytosis and M. sympodialis can be treated with topical or rarely systemic antifungal drugs. A subset of patients with AD may respond to treatment with antifungal agents.[76]

PRACTICAL ASPECTS OF ANTIHISTAMINE AND ANXIOLYTIC THERAPY

Pruritus is the cardinal symptom of AD and the associated scratching can contribute to open, superinfected lesions, bleeding, lichenification, or nodular changes, sleep deprivation and impact on quality of life (QoL). Eliminating triggers of pruritus whenever possible is critical. Systemic antihistamines and anxiolytics may be useful in the management of patients with AD primarily through their tranquillizing and sedative effects and can be dosed in the evening to avoid daytime drowsiness. The tricyclic antidepressant doxepin is both a histamine H_1- and H_2- receptor antagonist with a long half-life and may be dosed 10–50 mg once in the evening. If nocturnal itching and scratching remain severe, short-term use of a sedative to allow adequate rest may be appropriate. In general, second-generation antihistamines have been less useful in AD, especially in controlling pruritus. However, they may still help with allergic triggers. Of interest, treatment of children with AD with cetirizine reduced the number developing asthma in the subgroups sensitized to house dust mite or pollen.[77]

Treatment of AD with topical antihistamines and local anaesthetics should be avoided because of potential sensitization. Although in a 1 week multicentre, double-blind, vehicle-controlled study, topical 5% doxepin cream significantly reduced pruritus and sensitization was not reported, rechallenge with the drug after the 7-day course of therapy was not evaluated.[78] Since then, several case reports have documented allergic contact dermatitis to doxepin cream.[79]

MANAGEMENT OF RECALCITRANT DISEASE

Wet wrap dressings

Wet wrap dressings reduce pruritus and inflammation by cooling of the skin and improve penetration of topical corticosteroids. They also act as a protective barrier from the trauma associated with scratching. One form of this treatment modality involves using tubular bandages applied over diluted topical corticosteroids. In a study of erythrodermic children, clinical improvement was noted within 2–5 days with no relapses on follow up 2 weeks later.[80] Mean serum cortisol levels were depressed, but normalized after 2 weeks. In a more recent study, children with severe AD showed significant clinical improvement after 1 week of treatment.[81] Of note, there was no significant difference noted using several dilutions of the mid-potency topical corticosteroid. This suggests that clinical benefit can be obtained with this treatment in more severe patients even with the use of lower potency corticosteroids. Of note, in a long-term maintenance trial in 21 children with severe AD using wet tubular dressings over a weak topical corticosteroid 2 times per week or less for 3 months, all of the children improved and in addition their sleep disturbance and topical corticosteroid use were both reduced.[82]

An alternative approach used for many years with success at the National Jewish Medical and Research Center in Denver employs wet clothing, such as long underwear and cotton socks, applied over an undiluted layer of topical corticosteroids with a dry layer of clothing on top.[83] It is important to emphasize that these are wet, not wet-to-dry, dressings that are used for debridement of wounds. Specifics of the procedure are described in Table 13.4 with selective steps demonstrated in Figures 13.12a–k. Alternatively, the face, trunk, or extremities can be covered by wet, followed by dry, gauze and secured in place with a dressing such as Spandage® elastic bandage or pieces of tube socks. Wraps may be removed when they dry out (typically after 1–3 hours) or they may be re-wet. However, it is often practical to apply them at bedtime and most patients are able to sleep with them on. Patients occasionally will complain of feeling chilled, which can be prevented by appropriate bundling and use of blankets. Maceration of the skin, folliculitis, and secondary infection are uncommon in the authors' experience. In fact, S. aureus colonization was found to be decreased in a recent controlled study of wet wrap dressings with topical corticosteroid.[84] Given the cumbersome nature of this therapy, it is probably best reserved for acute exacerbations of AD, although it can also be used selectively to limited areas of resistant dermatitis with minimal inconvenience.

HOSPITALIZATION

AD patients who are erythrodermic or who appear toxic may require hospitalization either as inpatients or in a day hospital. In addition, patients who appear to be treatment failures or resistant to a number of conventional therapies should be considered for hospitalization. Removing the patient from environmental triggers or stressors, together with intense education and assurance of adherence with the treatment regimen, results in marked clinical improvement in many cases. The patient can also undergo appropriately controlled provocative challenges to help identify potential allergic triggers.

Table 13.4   Stepped approach to wet wrap therapy

SUPPLIES

1. Topical medications and moisturizers.
2. Tap water at comfortable body temperature.
3. Basin for dampening of dressings.
4. Clean dressings of approximate size to cover involved area:
   a. **Face:** 2 to 3 layers of wet Kerlix® gauze held in place with SurgiNet.
   b. **Arms, legs, hands & feet:** 2 to 3 layers of wet Kerlix® gauze held in place with Ace bandages or tube socks, or cotton gloves, or wet tube socks followed by dry tube socks.
   c. **Total body:** Combination of above, or wet pyjamas or long underwear covered by dry pyjamas, or sweatsuit.
5. Blankets to prevent chilling.
6. Non-sterile gloves if desired.

PROCEDURE

1. Be certain that the patient's room is warm and ensure privacy.
2. If wraps are to be applied to a large portion of the body, work with two people if possible. It is necessary to work rapidly to prevent chilling.
3. Explain the procedure to the patient and parent.
4. Fill the basin with warm tap water.
5. Soak the dressings. Squeeze out excess water. Dressings should be wet, not dripping.
6. Usually, the patient will have had a soaking bath prior to this procedure. Pat skin dry with a towel.
7. Apply the appropriate topical medications to affected areas and moisturizer to non-affected areas immediately after pat drying the skin.
8. Cover an area with w`raps using 2 to 4 layers of wet gauze or other material. Immediately after wrapping, cover with appropriate dry material such as an Ace bandage, socks, or pyjamas. Start at the feet and move upward. Use wet, long underwear or wet pyjamas covered by dry pyjamas or sweatsuit with total body involvement in place of wet gauze.
9. Observe for chilling. Blanket can be put in a drier to warm up and cover patient, but do not overheat the patient. Wraps can be removed after 1–3 hours or can be re-wet.
10. If patient is known or suspected to have an infection of the involved areas, place dressings in appropriate bag and dispose according to infection control procedure.
11. After all dressings are removed, moisturizers may be applied to the entire body.
12. Special considerations with latex sensitive patients:
    A. Provide hydration therapy in tub rooms.
       a. Use built-in mechanical stopper in tub, not a rubber one.
       b. No rubber/latex toys should be used in the bathtub.
    B. Apply creams with latex free gloves or ungloved hands as appropriate.
    C. Apply wet wraps using Kerlix® 1 wet layer followed by 2 dry layers only to areas of body requiring wet wraps. Avoid use of wet clothing, which may contain elastic bands or elastic fibres as dressing material. Even covered elastic may cause a reaction when wet. Wash all clothing before use.
13. Documentation should include charting of topical medications used, patient's skin assessment with special attention to worsening of skin, and tolerance for procedure.

Figure 13.12   Various stages of applying wet wrap dressings. The complete procedure is described in Table 13.4. Wraps should be applied selectively to involved areas.

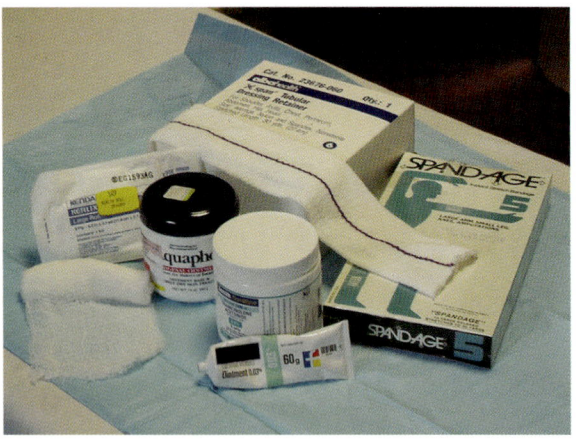

Figure 13.12a   Supplies gathered prior to beginning procedure.

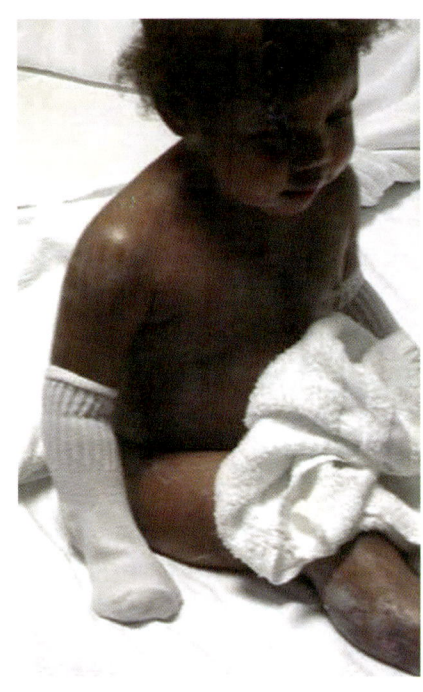

Figure 13.12b   Wet tube socks can be used to hands and feet in place of dressings.

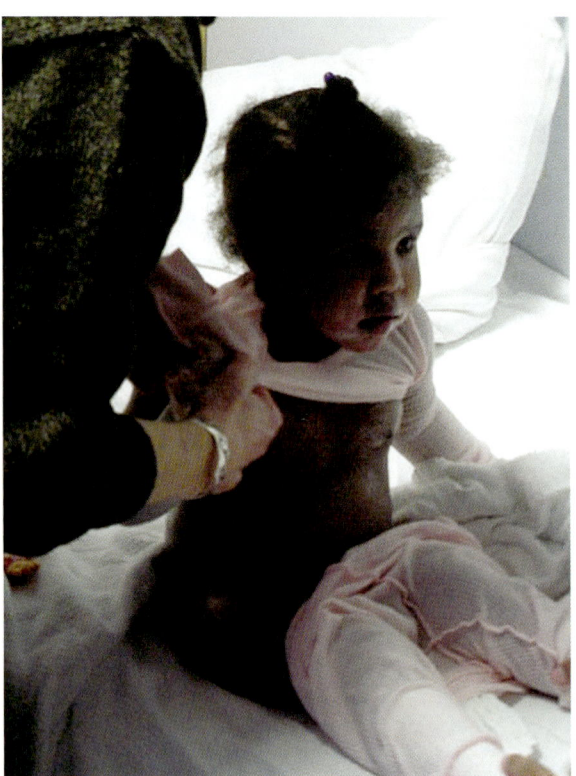

Figure 13.12c   Wet wraps to body can be accomplished with an initial layer of wet cotton-blend underwear.

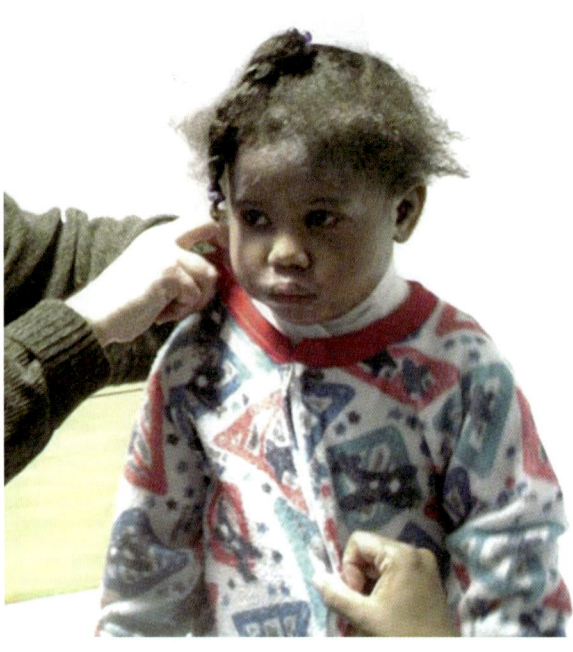

Figure 13.12d   Wet layer of clothing should be covered by a dry layer. One-piece footie pyjamas work well in small children. Additionally, when the neck is involved, a turtleneck shirt or a dressing can be added.

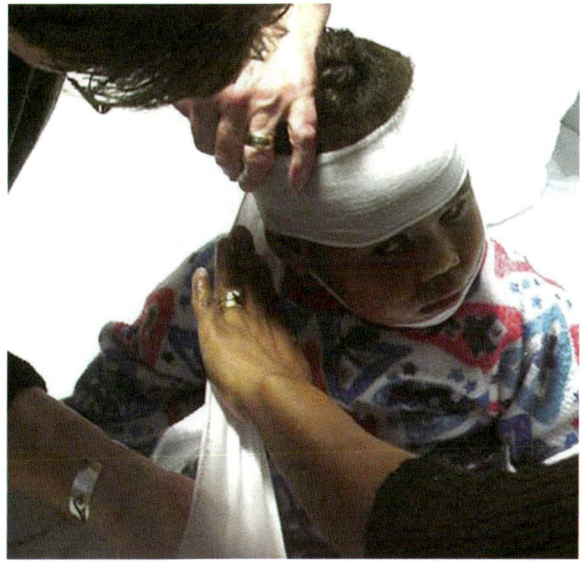

Figure 13.12e   Wet Kerlix® wrapped around forehead and chin.

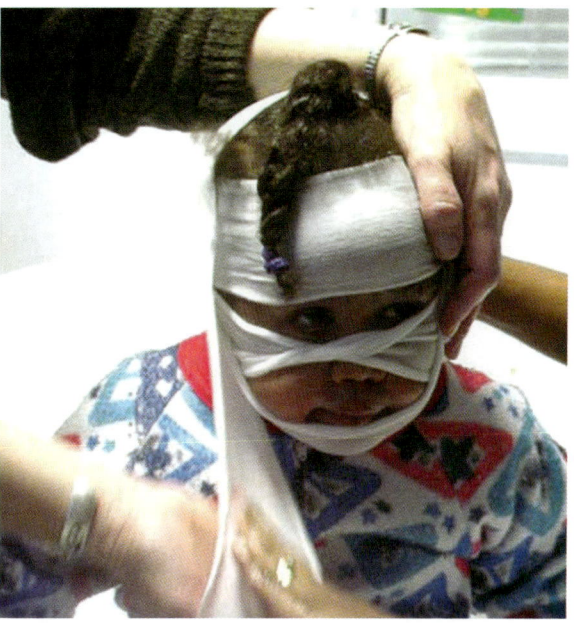

Figure 13.12f   Wet Kerlix® applied to facial area for perioral and cheek involvement, twisting Kerlix® around the nasal area.

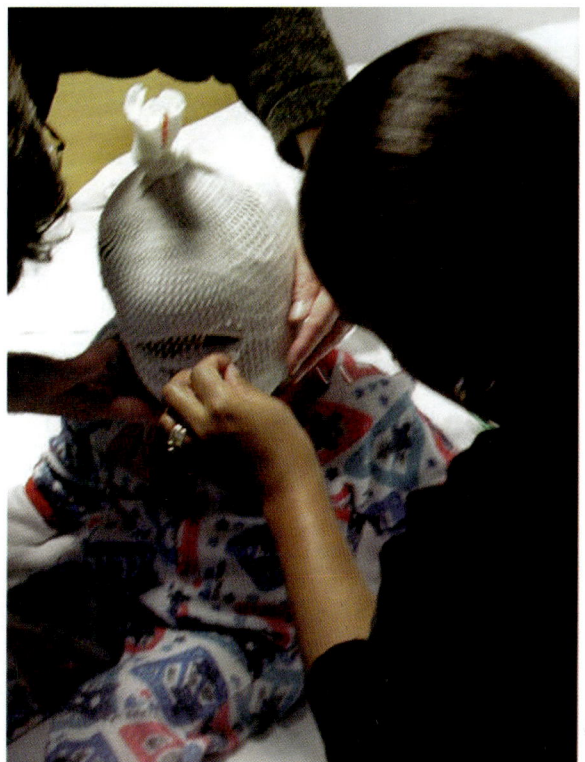

Figure 13.12g   Spandage® (burn netting) applied over wet Kerlix® with small openings for eyes, nose, and mouth cut out when cheeks and perioral area are involved.

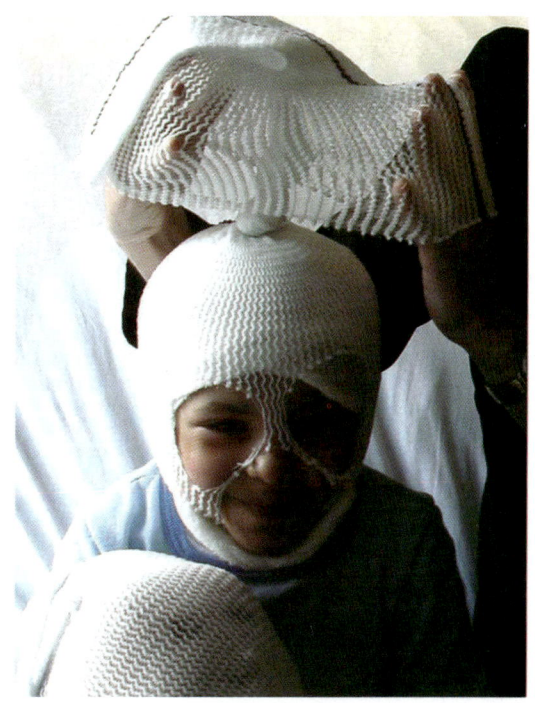

Figure 13.12h   Larger opening can be made with Spandage® or burn netting when cheeks or perioral area are not involved.

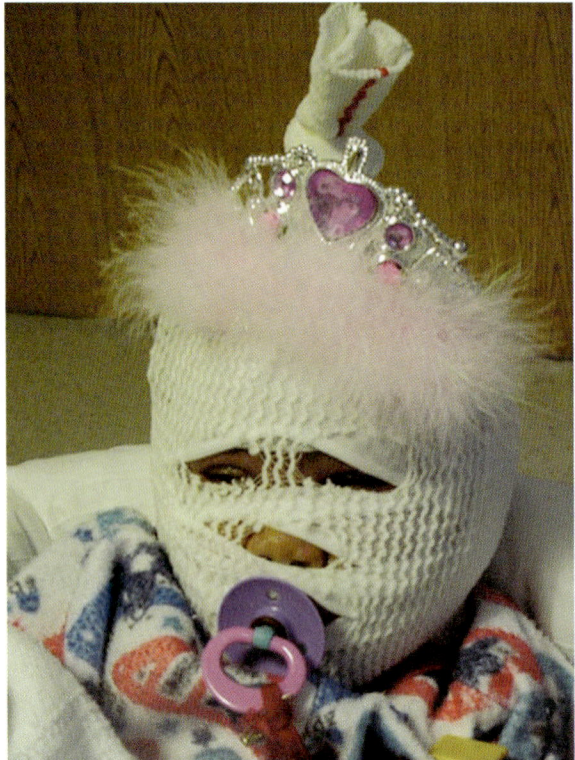

Figure 13.12i Completed head wrap, which can be appropriately adorned.

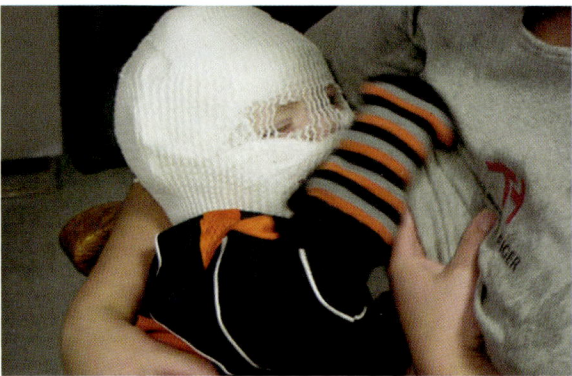

Figure 13.12j Head wrap allows for routine nursing.

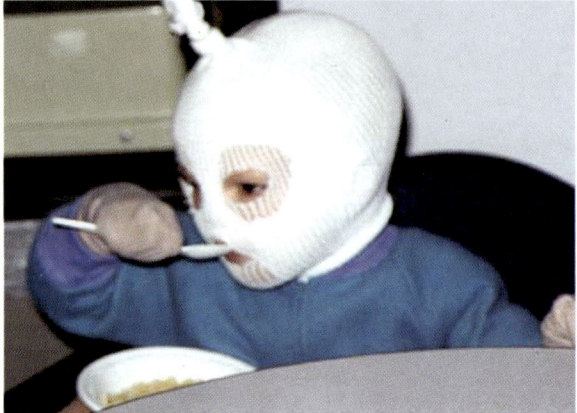

Figure 13.12k Total body wrap allows for routine activities.

REFERENCES

1. Boguniewincz M, Nicol N. Conventional therapy. In: Boguniewicz M, ed. Immunology and Allergy Clinics of North America, Atopic Dermatitis, Philadelphia: WB Saunders 2002: 107–24.
2. Akdis CA, Akdis M, Bieber T et al. Diagnosis and treatment of atopic dermatitis in children and adults: European Academy of Allergology and Clinical Immunology/American Academy of Allergy, Asthma and Immunology/PRACTALL Consensus report. Allergy 2006; 61: 969–87.
3. Lammintausta K, Kalimo K, Raitala R et al. Prognosis of atopic dermatitis: a prospective study in early adulthood. Int J Dermatol 1991; 30: 563–8.
4. Bender BG. Psychological dysfunction associated with atopic dermatitis. In: Boguniewicz M, ed. Immunology and Allergy Clinics of North America, Atopic Dermatitis. Philadelphia: WB Saunders 2002: 43–53.
5. Ellis CN, Drake LA, Prendergast MM et al. Cost of atopic dermatitis and eczema in the United States. J Am Acad Dermatol 2002; 46: 361–70.
6. Noren P, Melin L. The effect of combined topical steroids and habit-reversal treatment in patients with atopic dermatitis. Br J Dermatol 1989; 121: 359–66.
7. Horne DJ, White AE, Varigos GA. A preliminary study of psychological therapy in the management of atopic eczema. Br J Med Psychol 1989; 62: 241–8.
8. Koblenzer CS. Psychotherapy for intractable inflammatory dermatoses. J Am Acad Dermatol 1995; 32: 609–12.
9. Bridgett C. Psychodermatology and atopic skin disease in London 1989–99 – helping patients to help themselves. Dermatol Psychosom 2000; 1: 183–6.
10. Nassif A, Chan SC, Storrs FJ et al. Abnormal skin irritancy in atopic dermatitis and in atopy without dermatitis. Arch Dermatol 1994; 130: 1402–7.
11. Tabata N, Tagami H, Kligman AM. A twenty-four-hour occlusive exposure to 1% sodium lauryl sulfate induces a unique histopathologic inflammatory response in the xerotic skin of atopic dermatitis patients. Acta Derm Venereol 1998; 78: 244–7.
12. Breneman DL, Hanifin JM, Berge CA et al. The effect of antibacterial soap with 1.5% triclocarban on Staphylococcus aureus in patients with atopic dermatitis. Cutis 2000; 66: 296–300.

13. Forsch PJ, Kligman AM. The soap chamber test, a new method for assessing the irritancy of soaps. J Am Acad Dermatol 1979; 1: 35–41.

14. Andersen PH, Bindslev-Jensen C, Mosbech H et al. Skin symptoms in patients with atopic dermatitis using enzyme-containing detergents. Acta Derm Venereol 1998; 78: 60–2.

15. Diepgen TL, Salzer B, Tepe A et al. A study of skin irritations caused by textiles under standardized sweating conditions in patients with atopic eczema. Melliand Deutsch/English 1995; 12: E268–9.

16. Bendsoe N, Bjornberg A, Asnes H. Itching from wool fibres in atopic dermatitis. Contact Dermatitis 1987; 17: 21–2.

17. Sicherer SH, Sampson HA. Food hypersensitivity and atopic dermatitis: pathophysiology, epidemiology, diagnosis, and management. J Allergy Clin Immunol 1999; 104: 114–22.

18. Sampson HA, McCaskill CC. Food hypersensitivity and atopic dermatitis: evaluation of 113 patients. J Pediatr 1985; 107: 669–75.

19. Bock SA, Sampson HA, Atkins FM et al. Double-blind, placebo-controlled food challenge (DBPCFC) as an office procedure: a manual. J Allergy Clin Immunol 1988; 82: 986–97.

20. May CD. Objective clinical and laboratory studies of immediate hypersensitivity reactions to foods in asthmatic children. J Allergy Clin Immunol 1976; 58: 500–15.

21. Sampson HA, Broadbent K, Bernhisel-Broadbent J. Spontaneous basophil histamine release and histamine-releasing factor in patients with atopic dermatitis and food hypersensitivity. N Engl J Med 1989; 321: 228–32.

22. Sampson HA. Utility of food-specific IgE concentrations in predicting symptomatic food allergy. J Allergy Clin Immunol 2001; 107: 891–6.

23. Zeiger R, Heller S, Mellon M et al. Genetic and environmental factors affecting the development of atopy through age 4 in children of atopic parents: a prospective randomized study of food allergen avoidance. Pediatr Allergy Immunol 1992; 3: 110–27.

24. Zeiger RS, Heller S. The development and prediction of atopy in high-risk children: follow-up at age seven years in a prospective randomized study of combined maternal and infant food allergen avoidance. J Allergy Clin Immunol 1995; 95: 1179–90.

25. Kay J, Gawkrodger DJ, Mortimer MJ et al. The prevalence of childhood atopic eczema in a general population. J Am Acad Dermatol 1994; 30: 35–9.

26. Saarinen UM, Kajosaari M. Breast-feeding as prophylaxis against atopic disease: prospective follow-up study until 17 years old. Lancet 1995; 346: 1065–9.

27. Isolauri E, Tahvanainen A, Peltola T et al. Breast-feeding of allergic infants. J Pediatr 1999; 134: 27–32.

28. Schafer T, Heinrich J, Wjst M et al. Association between severity of atopic eczema and degree of sensitization to aeroallergens in schoolchildren. J Allergy Clin Immunol 1999; 104: 1280–4.

29. van Reijsen FC, Bruijnzeel-Koomen CA, Kalthoff FS et al. Skin-derived aeroallergen-specific T-cell clones of Th2 phenotype in patients with atopic dermatitis. J Allergy Clin Immunol 1992; 90: 184–93.

30. Tan BB, Weald D, Strickland I et al. Double-blind controlled trial of effect of house dust-mite allergen avoidance on atopic dermatitis. Lancet 1996; 347: 15–18.

31. Ricci G, Patrizi A, Specchia F et al. Effect of house dust mite avoidance measures in children with atopic dermatitis. Br J Dermatol 2000; 143: 379–84.

32. Friedmann PS, Tan BB. Mite elimination – clinical effect on eczema. Allergy 1998; 53: 97–100.

33. Oosting AJ, de Bruin-Weller MS, Terreehorst I et al. Effect of mattress encasings on atopic dermatitis outcome measures in a double-bind, placebo-controlled study: the Dutch mite avoidance study. J Allergy Clin Immunol 2002; 110: 500–6.

34. Gutgesell C, Heise S, Seubert S et al. Double-blind placebo-controlled house dust mite control measures in adult patients with atopic dermatitis. Br J Dermatol 2001; 145: 70–4.

35. Holm L, Bengtsson A, van Hage-Hamsten M et al. Effectiveness of occlusive bedding in the treatment of atopic dermatitis – a placebo-controlled trial of 12 months' duration. Allergy 2001; 56: 152–8.

36. Arlian LG, Platts-Mills TA. The biology of dust mites and the remediation of mite allergens in allergic disease. J Allergy Clin Immunol 2001; 107: 406–13.

37. Werner Y, Lindberg M. Transepidermal water loss in dry and clinically normal skin in patients with atopic dermatitis. Acta Derm Venereol 1985; 65: 102–5.

38. Imokawa G, Abe A, Jin K et al. Decreased level of ceramides in stratum corneum of atopic dermatitis: an etiologic factor in atopic dry skin. J Invest Dermatol 1991; 96: 523–6.

39. Kubota K, Machida I, Tamura K et al. Treatment of refractory cases of atopic dermatitis with acidic hot-spring bathing. Acta Derm Venereol 1997; 77: 452–4.

40. Inoue T, Inoue S, Kubota K. Bactericidal activity of manganese and iodide ions against Staphylococcus aureus: a possible treatment for acute atopic dermatitis. Acta Derm Venereol 1999; 79: 360–2.

41. De Paepe K, Hachem JP, Vanpee E et al. Effect of rice starch as a bath additive on the barrier function of healthy but SLS-damaged skin and skin of atopic patients. Acta Derm Venereol 2002; 82: 184–6.

42. The role of therapeutic moisturizers and cleansers in the treatment of various skin conditions: Report from a consensus roundtable. Cutis 2005; 76(6S): 2–33.

43. Tabata N, O'Goshi K, Zhen YX et al. Biophysical assessment of persistent effects of moisturizers after their daily applications: evaluation of corneotherapy. Dermatology 2000; 200: 308–13.

44. Loden M, Andersson AC, Lindberg M. Improvement in skin barrier function in patients with atopic dermatitis after treatment with a moisturizing cream (Canoderm). Br J Dermatol 1999; 140: 264–7.

45. Hanifin JM, Hebert AA, Mays SR et al. Effects of a low-potency corticosteroid lotion plus a moisturizing regimen in the treatment of atopic dermatitis. Curr Ther Res 1998; 59: 227–33.

46. Kantor I, Milbauer J, Posner M et al. Efficacy and safety of emollients as adjunctive agents in topical corticosteroid therapy for atopic dermatitis. Today Ther Trend 1993; 11: 157–66.

47. Lucky AW, Leach AD, Laskarzewski P et al. Use of an emollient as a steroid-sparing agent in the treatment of mild to moderate atopic dermatitis in children. Pediatr Dermatol 1997; 14: 321–4.

48. Vilaplana J, Coll J, Trullas C et al. Clinical and non-invasive evaluation of 12% ammonium lactate emulsion for the treatment of dry skin in atopic and non-atopic subjects. Acta Derm Venereol 1992; 72: 28–33.

49. Lavker RM, Kaidbey K, Leyden J. Effects of topical ammonium lactate on cutaneous atrophy from a potent topical corticosteroid. J Am Acad Dermatol 1992; 26: 535–44.

50. Arikawa J, Ishibashi M, Kawashima M et al. Decreased levels of sphingosine, a natural antimicrobial agent, may be associated with vulnerability of the stratum corneum from patients with atopic dermatitis to colonization by Staphylococcus aureus. J Invest Dermatol 2002; 119: 433–9.

51. Chamlin SL, Kao J, Frieden IJ et al. Ceramide-dominant barrier repair lipids alleviate childhood atopic dermatitis: changes in barrier function provide a sensitive indicator of disease activity. J Am Acad Dermatol 2002; 47: 198–208.

52. Abramovits W, Boguniewicz M for the Adult Atopiclair Study Group. A multicenter, randomized, vehicle-controlled clinical study to examine the efficacy and safety of MAS063DP (Atopiclair) in the Management of mild to moderate atopic dermatitis in adults. J Drugs Dermatol 2006; 5: 236–44.

53. Barnes PJ. New directions in allergic diseases: mechanism-based anti-inflammatory therapies. J Allergy Clin Immunol 2000; 106: 5–16.

54. Nilsson EJ, Henning CG, Magnusson J. Topical corticosteroids and Staphylococcus aureus in atopic dermatitis. J Am Acad Dermatol 1992; 27: 29–34.

55. Stalder JF, Fleury M, Sourisse M, Rostin M, Pheline F et al. Local steroid therapy and bacterial skin flora in atopic dermatitis. Br J Dermatol 1994; 131: 536–40.

56. Stoughton RB. Vasoconstrictor assay-specific applications. In: Maibach HI, Surber C, eds. Topical Corticosteroids. Basel: Karger, 1992: 42–53.

57. Stoughton RB. The vasoconstrictor assay in bioequivalence testing: practical concerns and recent developments. Int J Dermatol 1992; 31: 26–8.

58. Matura M, Goossens A. Contact allergy to corticosteroids. Allergy 2000; 55: 698–704.

59. Seukeran DC, Wilkinson SM, Beck MH. Patch testing to detect corticosteroid allergy: Is it adequate? Contact Dermatitis 1997; 36: 127–30.

60. Volden G. Successful treatment of therapy-resistant atopic dermatitis with clobetasol propionate and a hydrocolloid occlusive dressing. Acta Derm Venereol Suppl (Stockh) 1992; 176: 126–8.

61. McLean C, Lobo R, Brazier D. Cataracts, glaucoma, femoral avascular necrosis caused by topical corticosteroid ointment. Lancet 1995; 345: 3330.

62. Weston WL, Lane AT, Morelli JG. Color Textbook of Pediatric Dermatology, 2nd edn St Louis: Mosby, 1996.

63. Long CC, Mills CM, Finlay AY. A practical guide to topical therapy in children. Br J Dermatol 1998; 138: 293–6.

64. Wolkerstorfer A, Strobos MA, Glazenburg EJ et al. Fluticasone propionate 0.05% cream once daily versus clobetasone butyrate 0.05% cream twice daily in children with atopic dermatitis. J Am Acad Dermatol 1998; 39: 226–31.

65. Lebwohl M. A comparison of once-daily application of mometasone furoate 0.1% cream compared with twice-daily hydrocortisone valerate 0.2% cream in pediatric atopic dermatitis patients who failed to respond to hydrocortisone: mometasone furoate study group. Int J Dermatol 1999; 38: 604–6.

66. Van Der Meer JB, Glazenburg EJ, Mulder PG et al. The management of moderate to severe atopic dermatitis in adults with topical fluticasone propionate. Br J Dermatol 1999; 140: 1114–21.

67. Hanifin J, Gupta AK, Rajagopalan R. Intermittent dosing of fluticasone propionate cream for reducing the risk of relapse in atopic dermatitis patients. Br J Dermatol 2002; 147: 528–37.

68. Charman CR, Morris AD, Williams HC. Topical corticosteroid phobia in patients with atopic eczema. Br J Dermatol 2000; 142: 931–6.

69. Zuberbier T, Orlow SJ, Paller AS et al. Patient perspectives on the management of atopic dermatitis. J Allergy Clin Immunol 2006; 118: 226–32.

70. Langeveld-Wildschut EG, Riedl H, Thepen T et al. Modulation of the atopy patch test reaction by topical corticosteroids and tar. J Allergy Clin Immunol 2000; 106: 737–43.

71. Boguniewicz M, Sampson H, Leung S et al. Effects of cefuroxime axetil on Staphylococcus aureus colonization and superantigen production in atopic dermatitis. J Allergy Clin Immunol 2001; 108: 651–2.

72. Luber H, Amornsiripanitch S, Lucky AW. Mupirocin and the eradication of Staphylococcus aureus in atopic dermatitis. Arch Dermatol 1988; 124: 853–4.

73. Doebbeling BN, Reagan DR, Pfaller MA et al. Long-term efficacy of intranasal mupirocin ointment. A prospective cohort study of Staphylococcus aureus carriage. Arch Intern Med 1994; 154: 1505–8.

74. Albert MR, Gonzalez S, Gonzalez E. Patch testing reactions to a standard series in 608 patients tested from 1990 to 1997 at Massachusetts General Hospital. Am J Contact Dermat 1998; 9: 207–11.

75. Bork K, Brauninger W. Increasing incidence of eczema herpeticum: analysis of seventy-five cases. J Am Acad Dermatol 1988; 19: 1024–9.

76. Boguniewicz M, Schmid-Grendelmeien P, Leung DYM. Clinical Pearls: Atopic dermatitis. J Allergy Clin Immunol 2006; 118: 40–3.

77. Allergic factors associated with the development of asthma and the influence of cetirizine in a double-blind, randomised, placebo-controlled trial: first results of ETAC. Early Treatment of the Atopic Child. Pediatr Allergy Immunol 1998; 9: 116–24.

78. Drake LA, Fallon JD, Sober A et al. Relief of pruritus in patients with atopic dermatitis after treatment with topical doxepin cream. J Am Acad Dermatol 1994; 31: 613–16.

79. Shelley WB, Shelley ED, Talanin NY. Self-potentiating allergic contact dermatitis caused by doxepin hydrochloride cream. J Am Acad Dermatol 1996; 34: 143–4.

80. Goodyear HM, Spowart K, Harper JI. "Wet wrap" dressings for the treatment of atopic eczema in children. Br J Dermatol 1991; 125: 604.

81. Wolkerstorfer A, Visser RL, de Waard-van der Spek FB et al. Efficacy and safety of wet-wrap dressings in children with severe atopic dermatitis: influence of corticosteroid dilution. Br J Dermatol 2000; 143: 999–1004.

82. Mallon E, Powell S, Bridgman A. "Wet wrap" dressings for the treatment of atopic eczema in the community. J Dermatol Treat 1994; 5: 97–8.

83. Nicol NH. Atopic dermatitis: the (wet) wrap-up. Am J Nurs 1987; 87: 1560–3.

84. Schnopp C, Holtmann C, Sybille S et al. Topical steroids under wet-wrap dressings in atopic dermatitis – a vehicle-controlled trial. Dermatology 2002; 204: 56–9.

14

Mode of action of glucocorticoids

Ekkehard May, Thomas Zollner, Heike Schäcke, Stefanie Schoepe, Hartmut Rehwinkel,
Wolfram Sterry, and Khusru Asadullah

INTRODUCTION

Glucocorticosteroids (GCs) are the most widely used drugs in dermatology and remain the mainstay therapy for a multitude of indications. The frequency of systemic, intralesional, and in particular topical application of GCs in daily dermatological practice is thus not surprising (Table 14.1). Soon after its introduction more than 50 years ago, GC therapy became a cornerstone in the therapy of atopic dermatitis (AD) and application of topical GC is frequently the therapy of choice in AD to date, while systemic GC therapy is rarely indicated due to its higher side-effect potential.

The introduction of topical hydrocortisone in the early 1950s signified a great advance as compared to previously available therapies. Yet, it was triamcinolone acetonide, the first of the halogenated corticosteroids, that sparked a revolution in GC development which ultimately led to the very potent agents available now. The enthusiasm for these highly effective agents peaked during the 1960s and 1970s, and perhaps inevitably, the more potent GCs were often used inappropriately and indiscriminately. Adverse effects became apparent and the subsequent backlash of opinion against GCs created confusion and prejudice against all steroid-containing preparations, whose extreme may be termed 'steroid phobia'.[1] Even today, disaffirmation of corticosteroids is considerable.[2,3]

However, topical GCs are successfully and commonly used for the treatment of AD and numerous other cutaneous inflammatory diseases. Since the strongest anti-inflammatory compounds belong to the GCs, they show great advantages in certain indications, localizations, and types of disease. However, due to their high potencies, they may have deleterious effects when used improperly (Figure 14.1). Their adequate use thus belongs to the 'art of treatment' in dermatology, requiring profound personal experience as well as solid knowledge of mode of action, indications as well

Table 14.1 Examples of GC therapy in dermatology	
Application	**Indication**
Topical	Atopic dermatitis
	Contact eczema
	Psoriasis
	Prurigo
Intralesional	Prurigo
	Keloids
Systemic	Bullous diseases
	Connective tissue diseases
	Anaphylactic reactions

as contraindications, different types of GCs available, possible combinations, and finally side effects. This review gives an overview of these aspects.

CLASSIFICATION AND MOLECULAR ASPECTS

Chemical structure

Cortisol or hydrocortisone has a steroidal structure characterized by a keto group at position 3, a double bond at position 4, a β-hydroxyl group at position 11, an α-hydroxyl group, and a substituted carbon side chain at position 17. Oxidation of the hydroxyl group at position 11 gives cortisone, an inactive compound. (Figure 14.2).[4] To achieve therapeutic efficacy, the chemical structure has to be modified. Fluorination at positions 6 and/or 9 generally increases activity. The most commonly introduced chemical modifications are:

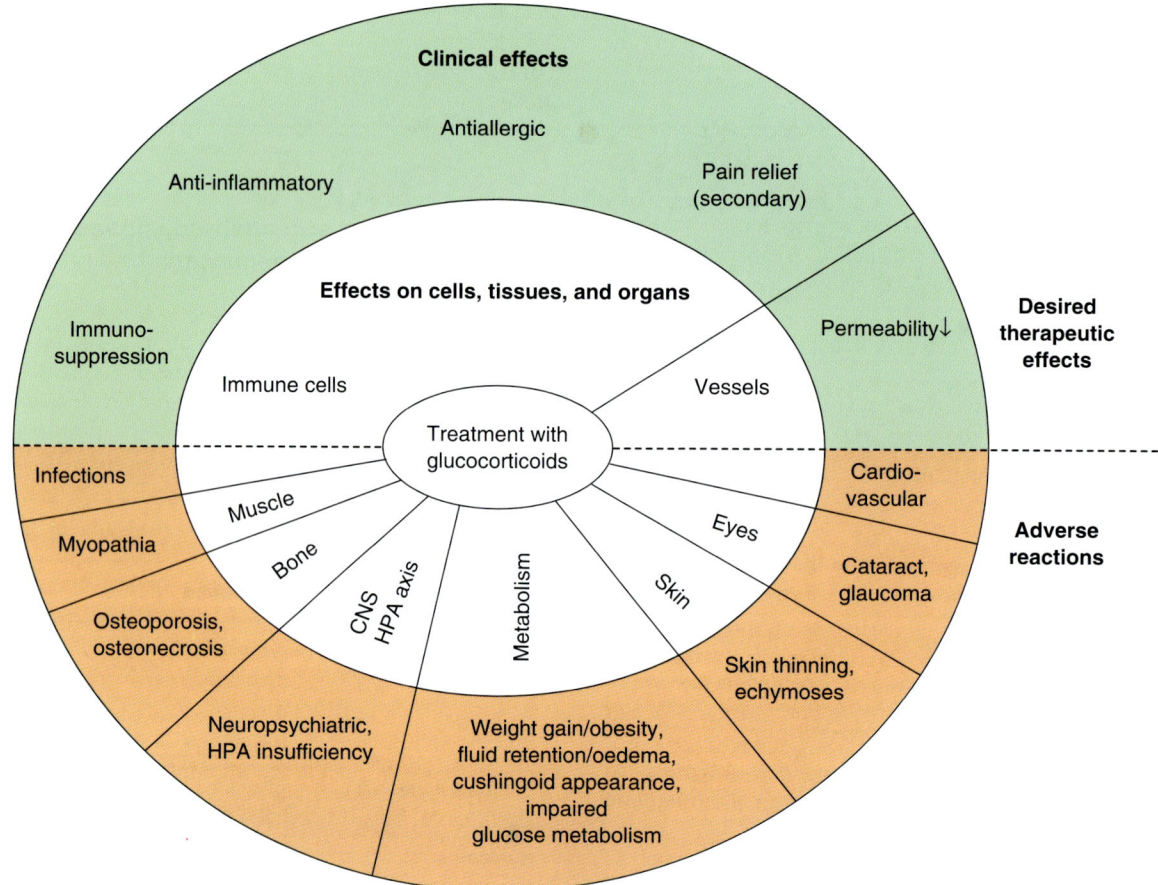

Figure 14.1　Most important clinical effects of glucocorticoids. Examples for desired therapeutic effects as well as side effects of GCs on different organs are shown. CNS = central nervous system, HPA = hypothalamic–pituitary axis. (Reprinted from Buttgereit F, Burmester GR, Lipworth BJ. Optimised glucocorticoid therapy: the sharpening of an old spear: Lancet 2005; 365(9461): 801–3,[90] by courtesy of F. Buttgereit and Elsevier.)

1. Introduction of a double bond at position 1 affords prednisolone.
2. Introduction of a double bond at position 1, an α-fluorine at position 9 and an α-methyl group at position 16 leads to dexamethasone.
3. Introduction of a double bond at position 1, an α-fluorine at position 9 and an α-hydroxyl group at position 16 gives triamcinolone.
4. Introduction of a double bond at position 1, an α-fluorine at position 9 and a β-methyl group at position 16 yields betamethasone.
5. Both triamcinolone and betamethasone require increased lipophilic properties for full activity. This can be achieved by structural variations. In the case of triamcinolone the hydroxyl groups at the positions 16 and 17 have been transformed in an acetonide giving triamcinolone acetonide. Regarding betamethasone, esterification is possible: in the case of betamethasone dipropionate the hydroxyl groups at positions 17 and 21 have been esterified. Introduction of a double bond at position 1, an α-fluorine at position 9, a β-methyl group at position 16, a substitution of the hydroxyl group at position 21 by a chlorine and the oxidation of the hydroxyl group at position 11 gives after esterification of the hydroxyl group at position 17 clobetasone butyrate. The substitution of the hydroxyl group at position 11 by a ketone group limits the potential of systemic absorption of this otherwise powerful topical steroid.[5]

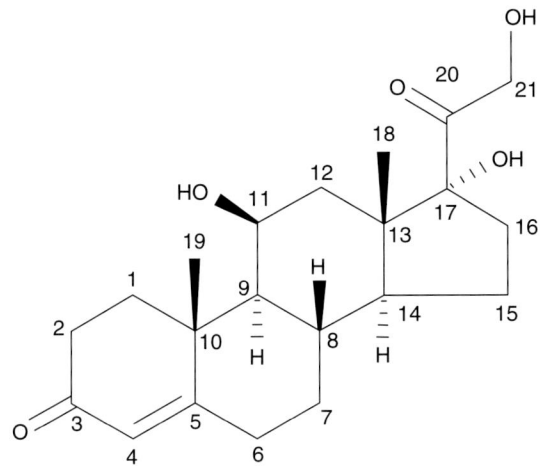

Figure 14.2   Structure of cortisol (hydrocortisone).

Table 14.2 Four categories of topical glucocorticoids according to strength: typical examples		
Class	**Potency**	**Example***
I	Low	Dexamethasone 0.1%
		Hydrocortisone acetate 1.0%
		Hydrocortisone 1–2.5%
II	Moderate	Methylprednisolone aceponate 0.1%
		Prednicarbate 0.25%
		Mometasone furoate 0.1%
III	Strong	Halcinonide 0.1%
		Betamethasone valerate 0.1%
		Fluocionide 0.05%
		Amcinonide 0.1
IV	Very strong	Clobetasol propionate 0.05%

*Potency is given for creams. Potency may differ for other formulations.

Potency: assessment and classification

The potency of GCs is usually determined by measuring surrogate markers such as vasoconstriction. After application of a topical GC onto the normal forearm, blanching occurs after 4–7 hours, and may persist 8–48 hours. The effects seen in the vasoconstriction assay correlate reliably with the clinical potency of classical GCs.[6,7]

The predominant classification of topical GCs is based on their potencies (Table 14.2). In clinical use, GCs are placed into 4 groups according to their clinical effects, both wanted and unwanted. Group I contains mild, group II moderate, group III strong, and group IV very strong topical GCs (Table 14.2). Since brand names as well as chemical entities differ in various countries, the reader is referred also to local reviews. Being familiar with several pharmaceutical products from each group is a prerequisite to be able to treat adequately in different clinical situations.

The local potency of a given GC is determined by its concentration, its penetration profile as well as its molecular structure; the latter will determine the interaction with the steroid receptor as well as the interaction of the steroid–receptor complex with the DNA of the target cell.

More recently, the therapeutic index (TIX) has been introduced for topical GCs[8] describing the benefit:risk ratio evaluation based on in vitro and in vivo data concerning both efficacy and safety.[9] The clinical part of the concept has in particular been based on a communication by Schäfer-Korting.[10,11] The TIX indicates the ratio of desired and adverse effects of several GCs. Since a TIX of 1–2 reflects an equal ratio of desired and adverse effects, a TIX of 2–3 indicates a GC with improved benefit:risk ratio. For example mometasone furoate, a class III GC with a TIX of 2 shows predominance of desired effects over side effects. The TIX considers atrophogenicity (Table 14.3) and further side effects as well as a series of beneficial effects of a given GC and thus integrates its advantages and limitations.[8] Local administration of metabolically unstable compounds and introduction of the prodrug principle represent major steps in the development of GCs with an improved benefit:risk ratio (see Perspectives on Optimizing Glucocorticoids Therapy and Novel Approaches to Target the Glucocorticoid Receptor).

Mode of action

Topical GCs are absorbed by lipophilic structures of the epidermis. They penetrate the lower epidermis as well as the upper dermis while concentrations decrease with increasing depth. GCs enter cells of the epidermis and dermis by diffusion through the cell membrane and possibly by receptor-mediated processes.[12] In the cytoplasm, they bind to the glucocorticosteroid receptor (GR). This receptor belongs to a group of DNA binding molecules that includes the receptors for sexual, mineralosteroid and, thyroid hormones as well as vitamin A, retinoids, and vitamin D. Their effects are mainly exerted by up- and/or down-regulation of gene expression. Among the numerous genes having GC response

Table 14.3   Therapeutic index (TIX) based on therapeutic strength and atrophogenicity

TIX	Skin atrophy	Class	Glucocorticoid
1	1	I	Hydrocortisone
1.06	2	II	Triamcinolone acetonide
1.2	2	III	Betamethasone valerate
1.4	1	II	Hydrocortisone butyrate
1.5	2	IV	Clobetasol propionate
2	1	II	Prednicarbate
2	1	II	Methylprednisolone acep(onate
2	1	II	Mometasone furoate

TIX of 1–2, Relation of desired and adverse effect is balanced; 2–3, GC with improved benefit:risk ratio. Skin atrophy: 1, GC induces little skin atrophy; 2, strong induction of skin atrophy. Modified from Luger T et al. Topische Dermatotherapie mit Glukokortikoiden Therapeutischer Index. J Dtsch Dermatol Ges 2004; 2(7): 629–34; Garbe C, Wolf G. Topische Therapie. In: Braun-Falco O et al, eds. Dermatologie and Venerologie. Berlin: Springer, 2005: 1431–61.

elements (GREs) in their promotor regions are genes encoding structural proteins (collagens), enzymes (phospholipase A2), adhesion molecules, cytokines (interleukins, transforming growth factor alpha[13]) and many others. These complex interactions cause 4 effects that are relevant in clinical treatment:[5]

1. Vasoconstriction
2. Immunomodulation
3. Anti-inflammation
4. Anti-proliferation.

The vasoconstrictive effect is clinically useful in acute inflammation, when the infiltration of additional inflammatory cells from the circulation needs to be blocked. Reduced drug clearance from the skin due to diminished blood supply and circulation is considered another beneficial consequence of vasoconstriction. Immunomodulation may depend on functional changes of GR-expressing immunocytes such as T cells (TC) or various antigen-presenting cells (APC), or on GC-mediated block of mitosis, e.g. halted proliferation and clonal TC expansion. Immunomodulatory and anti-proliferative effects are therefore partially overlapping, and both contribute to the beneficial anti-inflammatory efficacy of GCs. Taking these effects together, the outstandingly broad and efficacious clinical profile of many GCs becomes comprehensible.

Molecular mechanisms of the glucocorticoid receptor activity

GC bind to cytosolic GR, a member of the nuclear receptor superfamily which generally functions as a ligand-activated transcription factor. The GR consists of a C-terminal ligand binding domain (LBD), a DNA binding domain with a dimerization interface in the centre of the molecule and the two transcription activation (AF) domains AF-1 and AF-2.[14] In the absence of a ligand, the cytosolic GR is associated with molecular chaperones, co-chaperones and immunophilins. Binding of ligands to the GR releases the protein complex and induces translocation of the ligand receptor complex to the nucleus where it modulates gene expression either positively (transactivation) or negatively (transrepression).

GC-induced transactivation has been shown to be DNA-dependent, i.e. the activated receptor homodimer binds to specific sequences in the promoter or enhancer region of GC sensitive genes, termed GREs, thereby inducing gene transcription. Three different types of GREs requiring different types of binding have been described: simple, composite, and tethering GREs. While simple and composite GREs attract direct binding of the activated GR to the DNA, tethering GREs recruit GRs that are engaged in protein–protein interaction with other DNA-binding transcription factors.[15]

Dimerization of the GR is considered a prerequisite for activation of gene transcription. Thus, introduction of a point mutation into the dimerization domain of the GR suppresses the transactivation function of the receptor in vitro.[16] These results were supported by findings from a mouse carrying a mutated GR.[17] In this model, a GR A458T mutation within the dimerization domain abolishes or strongly reduces the ability of the receptor to induce the transcription of several genes in these animals. Thus, the dimerization domain of the GR is supposed to be an important domain for positive regulation of gene expression by the GR. However, a recent screen to determine different sets of primary transactivated GR targets implies that not only an intact dimerization domain is required for full transactivation activity of the GR, but also AF-1 and AF-2 in a promoter-specific fashion.[18] Importantly, there is good evidence that major side effects of GC therapy, such as diabetes, glaucoma, muscle atrophy, etc., are predominantly depending on transactivation mechanisms[19] (Table 14.4). These findings provide a promising rationale for the development of novel GR targeting drugs with superior effect:side effect ratios (see below).

GR-induced negative regulation (transrepression) is as variable as positive regulation. First, GR binding to negative GREs (nGREs) in promoter or enhancer regions of sensitive genes may suppress transcription of

Table 14.4	Side effects of classical GCs
Organ	**Side effect of GC treatment**
Skin	Atrophy, striae, acne, perioral dermatitis
Skeleton/muscle	Muscle dystrophy, osteoporosis, bone necrosis
Eye	Glaucoma, cataract
CNS	Depression, anxiety
Endocrine system	Diabetes, adrenal atrophy, growth retardation
Cardiovascular system	Hypertension, thrombosis
Gastrointestinal system	Ulcer/gastric bleeding

these genes. In contrast to GREs associated with the positive regulation modus, negative GREs are not particularly conserved. A second mechanism of transrepression is conferred by liganded GR that binds closely to the starting point of transcription, thus interfering with the general transcription initiation complex and resulting in inhibition of gene transcription. Third, the activated GR can bind via protein–protein interaction as a monomer to other transcription factors such as AP-1 or NF-κB and thus inhibit their activity.[20] Expression of numerous pro-inflammatory cytokines, chemokines, adhesion molecules, and enzymes is regulated by these two transcription factors.[21–23] Therefore, this mechanism is supposedly the major mechanism of anti-inflammatory and immunosuppressive effects of GCs.

Studies with histone deacetylase (HDAC) inhibitors, which usually relieve negative regulation of other nuclear receptors, provided conflicting results.[24–28] AP-1 though, as a downstream target of JNK, can be inhibited via suppression of C-Jun N-terminal kinases (JNK) kinase activity by the GR.[29,30] GCs are also known to interfere with the extracellular signal-regulated protein kinase (ERK-1 and ERK-2) and p38 MAP kinases pathways via increased expression of the dual-specificity MAP kinase phosphatase (MKP-1).[31,32]

In addition, negative regulation of pro-inflammatory proteins via the activated GR may be due to decreased mRNA stability and/or translation of e.g. IL-2, IL-1, VEGF, TNF-α, IL-6, IL-8, and COX-2. Such mechanisms of regulation may include protein–protein interactions of the activated GR with RNA-binding proteins similar to its interaction with subunits of transcription factors. Alternatively, they might rely on GC-mediated synthesis of new proteins with mRNA-destabilizing properties.[33]

Co-factors bind to the carboxy-terminal portion of the LBD of the GR in a ligand-dependent fashion. They either promote transcriptional activation (co-activators) or repress promoter activity (co-repressors).[34,35] While co-activator binding is hormone-dependent, co-repressors bind to ligand-free or antagonist-liganded receptor.[36–38] For both types of co-regulators, enzymatic activities have been described[35] and they are also suggested to be important for cell and tissue specificity of GC effects.

Percutaneous penetration

Penetration

Penetration is the sum of processes that allow a steroid to find its way through the horny layer into epidermis and dermis. Penetration depends on several factors inherent to normal or inflamed skin and on the physicochemical properties of the steroid, and is further influenced by the vehicle. Methods to investigate the steroid penetration include the use of radiolabelled molecules, but also advanced tape stripping techniques in combination with analytical techniques.

Resorption

Resorption is defined as the systemic uptake of steroids following topical application. While treatment of small areas will not cause any problem related to steroid resorption, the use of high potency steroids, in particular in conjunction with occlusion using plastic foils, is associated with the risk of systemic side effects of GCs such as depression of endogenous cortisol production, adrenal cortex atrophy, bone demineralization, and growth retardation in children.

It is important to realize that different sites of the skin differ dramatically regarding penetration of topical steroids. As compared to palms and soles, a GC molecule will penetrate 40 times more efficiently when applied to the forehead. Other areas with a high resorption are eyelids, scalp, axilla, and genital areas.

Modern pharmacology has synthesized steroid molecules that are cleaved into relatively low potency steroids when they enter systemic circulation, thereby reducing or even abrogating the risk of resorption and systemic side effects.

PRINCIPLES OF TREATMENT

One must keep in mind that AD as a chronic disease needs treatment over decades. Therefore, care has to be taken to avoid long-term side effects that may accumulate over the years. Therapy of AD should always pay attention to several aspects to reduce GC consumption. Such multimodal therapy should include:

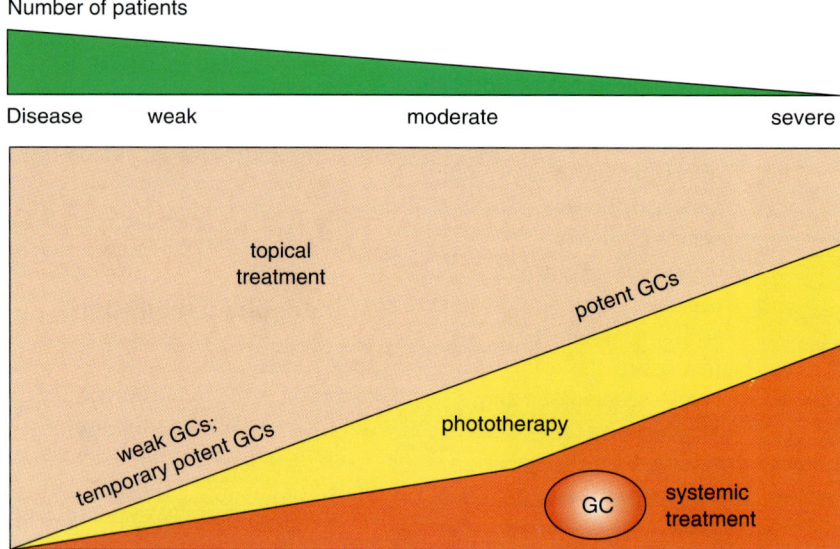

Figure 14.3 GCs in the therapy of eczema. Whereas topical GCs are frequently applied in mild to moderate AD (either by using weak GC over longer periods of time or potent GCs over limited periods), systemic GCs are usually only applied (if at all) temporarily in patients with severe disease and often in combination with other regimens.

1. Avoidance of individual provocation factors, such as irritants (e.g. dry air, detergents, wool), allergens (e.g. house dust mites, pollen, microbial factors including *Pityrosporum orbiculare*)
2. Use of adjunctive agents such as emollients and balneotherapy
3. Phototherapy
4. Antiseptics, in case of superinfection.

When treating AD with GCs several aspects need special consideration, including:

1. Topical or systemic treatment
2. Severity (extent and activity) of the disease
3. Age of the patient
4. Control of compliance
5. Combination with other treatment modalities
6. Possible side effects.

Figure 14.3 schematically indicates the place of GC therapy in AD. Some 'golden rules' to avoid topical GC-induced side effects are summarized in Box 14.1.

Topical or systemic treatment?

Systemic application of GC will control the disease in almost all cases in a very short time period. Fast onset of action and short treatment period make this treatment modality appealing at least for adults. Large affected

---

Box 14.1 Golden rules to prevent frequent problems of GC therapy

- Make the right diagnosis
- Don't treat infections with GCs
- No long-term therapies of infants with potent steroids
- Caution with potent steroids in special location (genital, face)
- Don't prescribe more than 50 g of class III and IV steroids on one prescription
- Consider re-examination of patients who need prescriptions periodically – consider alternative therapy

Side effects mediated by topical GCs occur only rarely when GCs are applied correctly!

---

body surface area (at least > 20%) or resistance to alternative therapy/ies may indicate a systemic treatment option. However, the multitude of partially severe side effects require careful benefit:risk analyses, especially since AD is a chronic disease. Patients with or prone to diabetes mellitus, arterial hypertension, osteoporosis, gastric ulcer, or glaucoma have an increased risk when treated with systemic GCs. In general, treatment with 0.75–1 mg/kg body weight/day (prednisolone, methyl prednisolone) is effective. The daily dose should be applied once in the morning to reduce suppressive effects on the HPA axis. Usually, the initial dose can be rapidly reduced (e.g. every other day) and a treatment period exceeding 10 days should be an exception.

Mostly, even in severe cases of AD, systemic GC therapy is not needed and experienced dermatologists manage to control the disease with topical treatment. The following aspects therefore focus on topical GC therapy.

Severity of atopic dermatitis

High potency GCs are prone to more severe side effects, especially skin atrophy. Furthermore, even in severe forms of AD, daily (or twice daily) application of moderate to strong potency topical GCs can control the disease and avoid side effects caused by very strong potency GCs. Daily application is in general preferred and sufficient, since the stratum corneum serves as a reservoir that releases the active agent over a prolonged period of time. This allows for additional use of complementary adjunctive therapy such as emollients to reduce the overall amount of GCs ('tandem therapy'). We recommend that patients treat early manifestations rather than waiting for full blown exacerbation, and predominantly use one moderate potency GC (e.g. methylprednisolone aceponate, prednicarbate, or mometasone furoate). Dependent on the severity of the exacerbation, it should initially be applied (twice) daily and reduced to every other day and twice a week, when the symptoms are controlled ('interval therapy'). Although such an interval therapy is not well documented in randomized, placebo-controlled, prospective studies, there are a few examples demonstrating its value. Prolonged therapy of AD with fluticasone propionate ointment (0.005%) on 2 days per week for 16 weeks was significantly effective over placebo in stabilizing the disease remission. Similar effects have been observed in chronic hand eczema. Intermittent application of mometasone furoate ointment (0.1%) on 3 days per week significantly reduced the reoccurrence rate over placebo or twice weekly application.[39]

Location

The sensitivity for GCs is different at different sites. As mentioned above, the skin sites differ dramatically regarding the penetration potential of topical steroids. As compared to palms and soles, GC molecules will penetrate much more efficiently when applied to the forehead, eyelids, scalp, axilla, or genital area. Consequently, caution is necessary when treating such regions (shorter treatment periods, use of lower potency GCs). Topical unwanted side effects have not been reported associated with steroid treatment of the scalp.

Age of patient

GC penetration is enhanced in young children. In addition, they have a higher relative body surface area. Children are therefore at special risk of developing systemic side effects such as growth retardation, Cushing's syndrome and intracranial hypertension.[40,41] Also, they may develop local side effects, in particular steroid acne or striae distensae. Since several inflammatory skin diseases such as AD characteristically show an early onset, repetitive treatment over prolonged periods of time are likely. One should therefore consider the use of steroids in children carefully[42] and utilize all treatment options including avoidance of provocation factors. In addition, modern moderate potency GC such as methylprednisolone aceponate or prednicarbate should be used due to their better effect/side effect ratio as compared to older compounds. But even with these compounds, application should be restricted to a minimum and not exceed 3 weeks of continuous application.

Control of compliance

Use of topical steroids requires strict control of compliance. Thus, 'golden rules' have been defined repeatedly.[5,43] These include:

1. Regular clinical observation
2. No unsupervised repeated prescriptions
3. Limitation of the quantity prescribed to the affected area and the time period expected to be necessary for clearing or expected therapeutic effect
4. Periods of steroid-free treatment
5. Use of high potency steroids only under control of dermatologists.

Control of compliance is not only necessary to avoid the unrestricted excessive use, which may cause severe side effects, but also with regard to the widespread steroid phobia. It is thus not uncommon that patients do not use the prescribed GCs because of personal concerns. It is the physician's task to explain the effect/potential side effect profile of a given GC to the patient in order to achieve a realistic perception of the regimen.

Steroid phobia

This phenomenon of steroid phobia initially occurred in the 1960s–70s and is still of considerable concern. A questionnaire-based study of 200 dermatology outpatients with atopic eczema (age range 4 months–67.8 years) assessed the prevalence of topical corticosteroid phobia in Great Britain. Overall, 72.5% of people worried about using topical corticosteroids on their own or their child's skin. Twenty-four per cent of people admitted to having been non-compliant with topical corticosteroid treatment because of such worries. The most frequent cause for concern was the perceived risk of skin thinning (34.5%). In addition, 9.5% of patients worried about systemic absorption leading to effects on growth and development. This indicates that a considerable number of patients indeed worry about using their prescribed GC.[1]

SIDE EFFECTS

Systemic side effects

The use of systemic GCs is limited by their potential to induce severe and sometimes irreversible undesired effects, such as osteoporosis, diabetes, Cushing's syndrome, glaucoma, muscle atrophy, and many others, especially after long-term treatment (Table 14.4). This is the reason why systemic GC therapy is only exceptionally used in AD (e.g. for very severe exacerbation). In contrast, topical GC therapy generally induces systemic side effects very rarely. With the advent of potent and highly potent topical GCs, however, reports of systemic side effects became more frequent. Two clinical situations – treatment of children and the use of occlusive techniques in larger areas – demand special care and attention since systemic side effects with suppression of plasma cortisol may occur. For instance, halcinonide cream applied for 5 days suppressed plasma cortisol levels in patients with extensive psoriasis with and without occlusion. This was attributed to the increased absorption of steroids through the defective horny layer barrier situation in psoriatics. In contrast, no adrenal suppression was observed when halcinonide cream was applied to more than 50% of the body surface in normal healthy individuals.[44]

When highly potent steroids were used in hospitalized patients with psoriasis and eczema, clobetasol had a higher potency than betamethasone dipropionate or diflorasone diacetate in suppressing plasma cortisol.[4] It is our clinical experience that systemic side effects correlate with topical potency; dermatologists treating large areas of the body for any skin disease should be thus be aware of the fact that systemic GC effects may occur, and that those may in part be relevant for both the therapeutic effect as well as for unwanted side effects.

Local side effects

Steroid acne

Prolonged treatment with steroids may result in the development of steroid acne (Figure 14.4). Most commonly, this will occur in adjunction of scalp treatment in the nuchal region as well as on the forehead. The localization and the lack of blackhead formation allow differentiation from normal acne. Treatment should include informing the patient and avoidance of contact

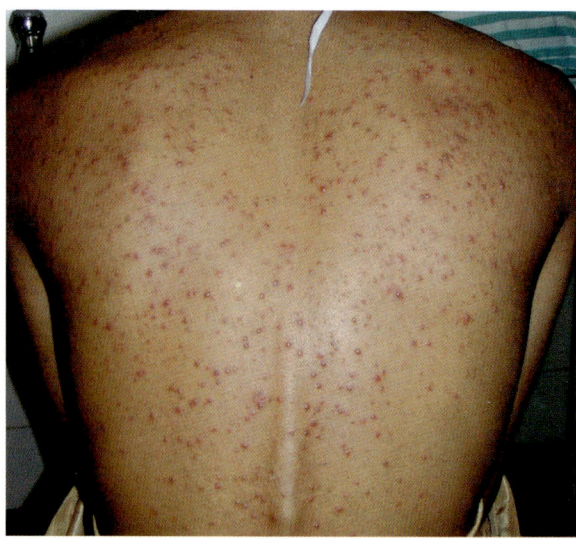

Figure 14.4 Steroid acne. Steroid-induced red papular eruption on the back, chest, and face of an 18-year-old man a month after starting oral ciclosporine and prednisone (to prevent renal graft rejection). (With permission from S. Paramoo, Dermatlas; http://www.dermatlas.org.)

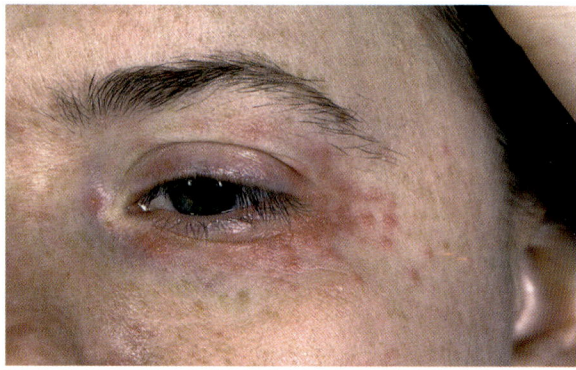

Figure 14.5 Steroid-induced dermatitis. Periocular steroid-induced dermatitis. (From Zollner TM, Boehncke WH., Kaufmann R (eds). Atopische Dermatitis). Berlin: Blackwell, Science, 2002.

with steroid ointment outside the areas intended to be treated rather than formal topical acne treatment.

Perioral dermatitis

Perioral and periocular dermatitis occur frequently after uncontrolled use of topical steroid formulations by patients suffering from a facial skin disease (Figure 14.5). Seborrhoeic dermatitis may be the most frequent skin disorder associated with steroid abuse in males, while cosmetogenic folliculitis prevails in females.

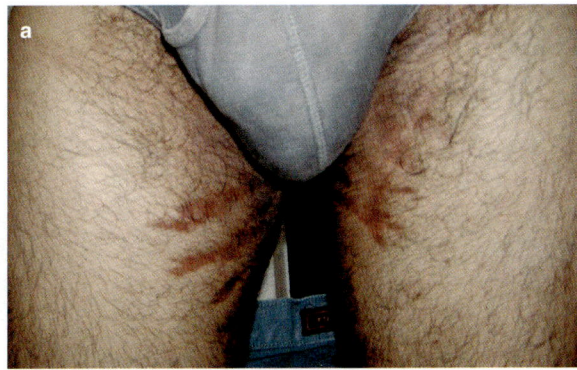

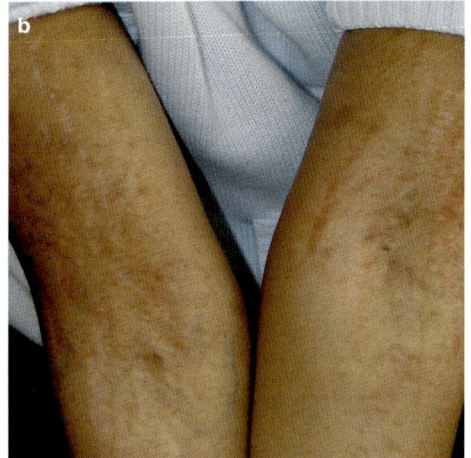

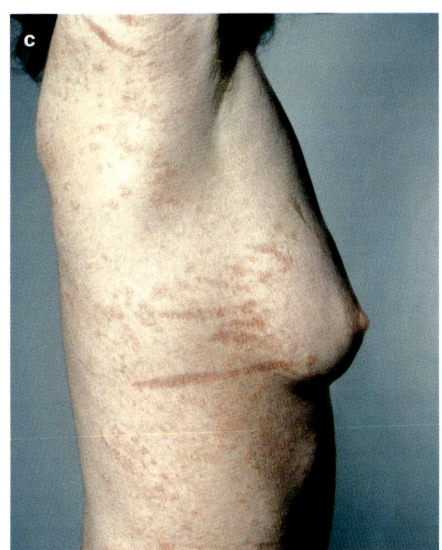

Figure 14.6   Striae rubrae distensae (stretch marks). (a) A 28–year-old man developed itchy erythematous circinate lesions of the groins which he treated with a fluorinated steroid and miconazole for several months. Striae were noted on examination of the anterior thighs and groin creases. (With permission from: S. Paramoo, Dermatlas; http://www.dermatlas.org). (b) Striae formation on the arm creases of an adolescent girl following a year of application of a high potency topical steroid for atopic dermatitis. (With permission from B. Cohen, Dermatlas; http://www.dermatlas.org). (c) Severe striae formation on the trunk of a young women after extensive use of topical steroids.

Striae distensae

In adolescent patients with prolonged use of steroids in certain areas, particularly the axillary regions and the thighs, striae distensae will develop as a result of decreased collagen production along with increased connective tissue tension during body growth (Figure 14.6). Therefore, intertriginous psoriasis in adolescents should be treated, if at all, only with great care: short-term use and selection of middle or low potency steroids. Also, in such patients the 'golden rules' should be followed strictly.

Glaucoma

Potent topical steroids may cause glaucoma when applied around the eyelids.[45] Such preparations should not be used around the eyelids or on the patient's face.

Allergic contact dermatitis

Allergic contact dermatitis may occur in reaction to many topical glucocorticosteroids.[46] The allergen is either the steroid molecule itself or resides in the vehicle. Careful observation of the patient and the therapeutic effects, particular those that are unexpected, will help an early detection of sensitization of the patient, and to identify the eliciting agent by patch testing.

Skin atrophy

Skin atrophy is the most important cutaneous side effect of GC therapy,[47,48] since a major function of the skin, the formation of a permeability barrier between the external milieu and the organism, is compromised.[49] GC-induced skin atrophy is characterized by profound increase of skin transparency, occurring as a cigarette-paper-like consistency accompanied by increased fragility, tearing, bruising ('steroid purpura'),[50] and a thin, shiny, and telangiectatic surface[51,52] (Figure 14.7). The first original description of the phenomenon was published in 1963 by Epstein et al[53] reporting 5 patients with atrophic striae in the groin, who had topically received Mycolog cream (containing triamcinolone acetonide, neomycin, gramicidin, and nystatin). Histopathologically, in GC-induced skin atrophy, flat dermal–epidermal junctions,[50] reduced thickness of the epidermis,[52] decreased size of keratinocytes,[54] and reduced number of fibroblasts[54,55] occurs. Rearrangement of the

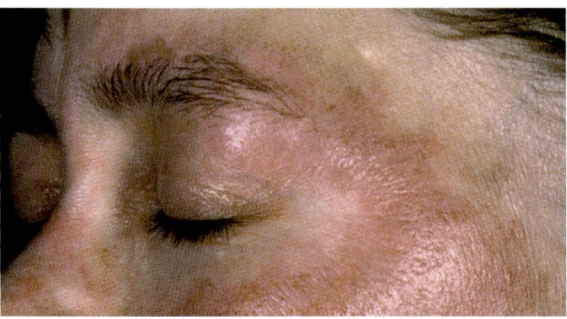

Figure 14.7 Skin atrophy after treatment with topical GC. Atrophy and erythema after topical steroid application in the face. (From Zollner TM, Boehncke WH, Kaufmann R (eds). Atopische Dermatitis. Berlin: Blackwell, 2002; Vol 14.[91])

geometry of the dermal fibrous network[56] and diminution of stratum corneum intercellular lipid lamellae are found.[57]

Both systemic as well as topical GC therapy can induce skin atrophy. Factors that determine the atrophogenic potential of a given topical GC are its potency, duration of therapy, frequency of application,[58] and further unknown factors. Different formulations may also markedly influence both the clinical efficacy of a GC as well as its atrophogenic potential simply due to the differing potential of the vehicle to release the drug into the stratum corneum.[59] The area size of GC application is an important factor contributing to the development of GC-induced skin atrophy. Atrophy is more common in areas of the body where humidity and occlusion results in greater penetration of the steroid such as groin and axillae.[60] The face or intertriginous areas are more sensitive to corticosteroid penetration,[61] whereas kapillitum, palmae, and plantae are less sensitive for GC-induced skin atrophy.[8]

PERSPECTIVES ON OPTIMIZING GLUCOCORTICOID THERAPY AND NOVEL APPROACHES TO TARGET THE GLUCOCORTICOID RECEPTOR

Several approaches have been made to identify strategies to improve the effect/side-effect profile of GCs. Progress in preclinical, sensitive, and predictive determination of the side-effect potential (e.g. atrophogenic potential) and insight into the molecular mechanisms of GC-mediated effects and side effects will have impact on the identification and development of novel drugs.

The atrophogenic potential of existing topical GC varies to some degree; however, the pro-atrophogenic potential of a given conventional GC in general closely correlates with its anti-inflammatory potency.[62] To selectively address both the anti-inflammatory and pro-atrophic factors of GC activity, one may consider strategies based on pharmacokinetics and pharmacodynamics separately. Dermato-pharmacokinetics focus on temporal, histological, and spatial aspects, including those related to drug delivery, while strategies that involve pharmacodynamics aim at exploiting mechanistic aspects and modes of action that result from intrinsic pharmacological properties of a compound. Both types of approaches should ultimately favour suppressive effects on immunocytes over pro-atrophic effects on keratinocytes and fibroblasts. Whereas with the first group of approaches novel topical therapies may be identified, the second group of approaches may eventually lead to the discovery of GR ligands which are really distinct from classical GCs and show a dissociated profile with the separation of effects and side effects making them suitable for improved topical as well as systemic therapy.

Optimizing treatment regimen

A relatively trivial approach to minimize GC-mediated atrophy is to simply limit the period of skin exposure by intermittent treatment schedules. Some reduction of skin atrophy can thereby be achieved even when strongly atrophogenic GCs are applied. This is indicated by reduced decrease of procollagen I and III under intermittent usage of topical hydrocortisone.[63] Yet, to improve the overall outcome of anti-inflammatory treatment, interruption of therapy might not be appropriate. Rotational treatment with topical GC and alternative regimen, e.g. topical calcineurin inhibitors, topical vitamin D_3, or retinoids, may therefore be a better choice. Continuous immunosuppression may be achieved by addressing complementary anti-inflammatory pathways.[64] Other strategies include intermittent use of the GC only every second day (tandem therapy),[65–67] intermittent treatment twice weekly,[68,69] or use of very potent GCs only for a very few days with subsequent switch to less potent GCs as soon as a response is observed.[70,71]

Optimizing pharmacokinetics and biotransformation

Rather than limiting periods of exposure, selective addressing of target cells and tissues may be a more straightforward approach to achieve immunomodulation while avoiding atrophy. The major players in AD, psoriasis, and allergic contact dermatitis are T cells. Those may initially be activated by antigen presenting cells of the skin such as Langerhans cells (LCs), plasmocytoid dendritic cells, inflammatory dendritic epidermal cells, or macrophages. Atrophy, on the other hand, is caused mainly by effects on dermal fibroblasts and epidermal keratinocytes. Yet, after decades of GC research, the ostensive lack of potent anti-inflammatory but non-atrophogenic GR ligands clearly illustrates the challenge to hit the respective target cells differentially. This may partly be ascribed to the fact that, under inflammatory conditions, T cells and antigen presenting cells are present and acting in both epidermis and dermis. Thus, a spatial separation of atrophy and inflammation is virtually not possible. The atrophogenic effects of dermal fibroblasts may outweigh those of epidermal keratinocytes, while epidermal immunocytes may significantly contribute to skin inflammation. This perception underlies efforts to optimize the physicochemical properties of topical GC towards high lipophilicity and high molecular size. Increased lipophilicity (logP > 3) may facilitate partitioning into the skin while increased molecular weight (> 500 Da) may slow down transdermal permeation into the bloodstream, providing skin-selective treatment, especially of the upper skin layers.[72,73] Retention of active drug in the tissue with comparably high inflammatory activity but relatively low contribution to atrophy may therefore lead to a superior drug profile. This principle might explain the favourable benefit:risk ratio, e.g. of prednicarbate (PC; prednisolone 17-ethylcarbonate, 21-propionate), a topical GC with reduced atrophogenic potential. It is assumed that the advantage of PC relies in its rapid hydrolysation to prednisolone 17-ethylcarbonate in the epidermis, a metabolite with high GR affinity and anti-inflammatory activity.[74] PC as well as this metabolite permeates the skin slowly; thus, most of the drug is decomposed before lower skin levels, the dermis with its more atrophy-sensitive fibroblasts, is ever reached. Similarly, the active metabolite of mometasone furoate was found to have higher GR binding affinities in the epidermis than in the dermis.[75] Aiming at increased drug permeation into the skin and reduced risk of systemic side effects, optimization of PC parameters as well as the prodrug–drug–antedrug concept has extensively been pursued in topical GC development, as exemplified by PC or methylprednisolone aceponate (MPA). The prodrug properties, achieved by for example esterification, generally also increase lipophilicity and therefore facilitate drug uptake into the stratum corneum.[76] The prodrug may have reduced or no pharmacological activity. Within the skin, the prodrug becomes activated by ester-cleavage through cutaneous esterases or spontaneous

hydrolysis, as in the case of MPA or the inhaled GC budesonide.[77] To prevent the body from systemic GC mediated effects, the active drug requires biotransformation into an inactive or significantly less active metabolite (antedrug) in the systemic circulation or, with some protraction, even within the skin. This principle is widely accepted and applied. Screening for metabolically unstable corticoids, e.g. those that contain carboxamide moieties on the side-chain or at the C-16 position of prednisolone[78] is therefore a standard approach. Overall, improved physicochemical properties and biotransformation is highly rewarding regarding reduction of systemic side effects and may also lessen a compound's atrophogenic potential. Yet, due to the obvious co-localization of atrophy-prone fibroblasts and keratinocytes with the various kinds of immunocytes in the dermis and the epidermis, both its use to counter atrophy and its effect on the pro-inflammatory milieu in the deeper skin layers is logically limited. More sophisticated adaptations of biotransformation approaches are required to achieve intracutaneous cell type specific activation or deactivation. PC, for instance, is metabolized and activated to only a minor degree in fibroblasts (about 1% per hour) whereas it is rapidly and almost completely activated in keratinocytes in vitro.[79] This example shows that cell type-specific properties can in principle be exploited. However, it is obviously not representing the perfect solution, since both cell types account for atrophy and should ideally deal with the drug similarly. Differential metabolization of the compound should clearly be sought to affect immunocytes vs keratinocytes and fibroblasts. So far, however, findings of this kind are fortuitous, and stringent strategies to rationally exploit such differences are not established. In addition, keratinocytes and fibroblasts may contribute also to the pro-inflammatory cascade, e.g. by releasing stimulatory cytokines such as TNF-α and IL-1.[80,81] Complete barring of those cell populations from GC action may therefore not be appropriate.

Optimizing formulation

Besides physicochemistry and biotransformation, drug interaction with physical parameters such as skin hydration and formulation properties may also significantly influence atrophy. The importance of delivery issues becomes apparent, e.g. when PC is applied under occlusion. Its superiority regarding induction of atrophy is then abrogated.[82] Use of transferosomes, highly flexible lipid vesicles, may on the other hand favourably modulate skin atrophy.[83] The clinical use of liposome encapsulation of betamethasone dipropionate has been analysed in a phase II trial in atopic eczema with an outcome supporting the concept.[84] Another

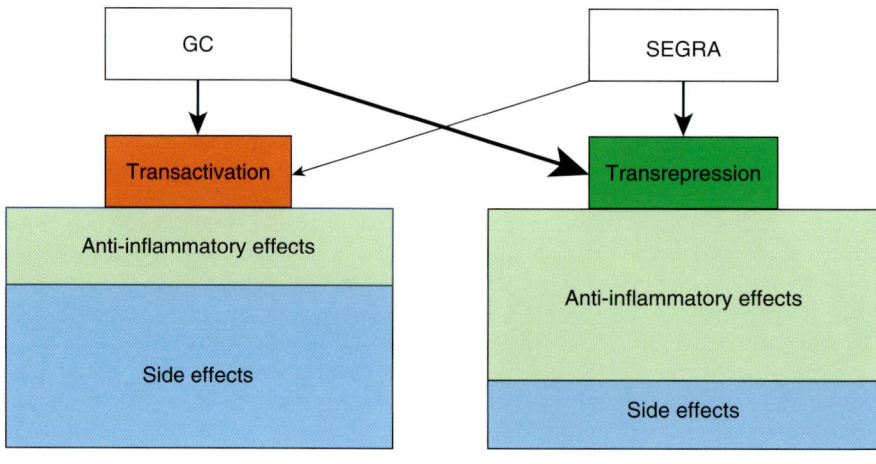

Figure 14.8   Mechanisms of GCs and SEGRAs mode of action. Simplistic model underlying the development of selective glucocorticoid receptor agonists (SEGRA) compounds. Reduction of primarily transactivation-dependent side effects and increase of anti-inflammatory transrepression effects will lead to drugs with a benefit:risk ratio superior to conventional GCs. (Adapted from Schäcke H et al. SEGRAs: a novel class of anti-inflammatory compounds. Ernst Schering Res Found Workshop 2002; 40: 357–71.[88])

approach might involve the use of nanoparticles. These solid lipid particles might also favour epidermal drug delivery and retention versus dermal delivery.[85] It is moreover very tempting to speculate whether such drug-loaded particles would be engulfed by cutaneous phagocytes. If so, this might offer an appropriate way to direct anti-inflammatory compounds straight to crucial immunocytes such as macrophages.

Novel pharmacological approaches

The most ambitious and most promising approach to separate beneficial effects and side effects of GR ligands addresses differential molecular modes of action that might underlie anti-inflammatory or undesired properties, respectively. Such mechanisms obviously do not obey clear-cut rules since GR ligands may activate and suppress gene activation in several different ways (see above). There is evidence, however, that for side-effect induction, GC-driven gene transactivation is more relevant than gene transrepression. In contrast, immunomodulation seems to primarily depend on GC-mediated transrepression, i.e. silencing of pro-inflammatory genes.[86] Thus, GR ligands primarily leading to transrepression and only to a lower extent to transactivation should have a better therapeutic index (Figure 14.8). First, GR ligands with dissociated properties, termed selective GR agonists (SEGRA) have recently been identified.[87–89] SEGRA clearly differ from GCs both structurally and

functionally. They are non-steroidal, not hormone-derived and orchestrate molecular pathways differently from GCS. SEGRA compounds thus show great potential to reduce side effects of GC while being equipotent regarding immunosuppression. Consistently rats treated with a SEGRA compound showed significantly reduced systemic side effects and skin atrophy when compared to prednisolone-treated animals. Dissociated GR ligands therefore bear great potential to achieve an improved benefit:risk ratio.

CONCLUSION

Amongst the most potent therapeutics for AD are glucocorticoids. Since hydrocortisone was launched in the 1950s, a multitude of chemical modifications have been tested and introduced leading to the widely used standard GCs of today that provide a great benefit for many AD patients. However, the flip side of the coin is obvious – potentially strong side effects, both systemic and cutaneous, especially when used inappropriately. Professional attendance and advice is therefore indispensable regarding prescription of GCs. Most importantly, the physician has to choose from a large palette of GCs with individual potencies and benefit:risk ratios and is responsible for an adequate treatment scheme according to the severity and location of the disease and depending on the age of the patient. The reason for the potent induction of both wanted and unwanted effects of GCs is certainly based on several molecular mechanisms that underlie GC activity – such as transactivation and transrepression of genes – as well as on the large variety of GC-sensitive tissues and genes.

Intensive research over past decades has led to the identification of various steroids with properties far superior to first-generation GCs. Therapeutic effects have been improved first and foremost by increasing potencies, while side effects were reduced by optimization of pharmacokinetic properties, by biotransformation (e.g. the prodrug principle), or by the advancement of formulations.

Yet, completely dissociated GR ligands, i.e. compounds that mediate exclusively anti-inflammatory effects over side effects based on their molecular mode of action are not available on the market at present. Recently however, the GR-targeting SEGRA concept proved to be successful in rodent immune disease models and may open new roads in the treatment of AD and many other inflammatory diseases.

ACKNOWLEDGEMENT

The authors published several reviews focusing on similar topics recently. Parts of this manuscript are similar to such reviews.

REFERENCES

1. Charman CR, Morris AD, Williams HC. Topical corticosteroid phobia in patients with atopic eczema. Br J Dermatol 2000; 142(5): 931–6.
2. Rao VU, Apter AJ. Steroid phobia and adherence – problems, solutions, impact on benefit/risk profile. Immunol Allergy Clin North Am 2005; 25(3): 581–95.
3. Green C et al. Topical corticosteroids for atopic eczema: clinical and cost effectiveness of once-daily vs. more frequent use. Br J Dermatol 2005; 152(1): 130–41.
4. Amin S et al. eds. Topical corticoids. In: Roenigk HH, Maibach HI, eds. Psoriosis, 3rd edn. Berlin: Springer, 1998: New York Basel Hong Kong. 453–67.
5. Higgins EM DuVivier A. Glucocorticosteroids. In: Dubertret L., ed. Psoriasis. Brescia: ISED, 1994: 102–11.
6. MacKenzie AW, Stoughton RB, Method for comparing percutaneous absorption of steroids. Arch Dermatol 1962; 86: 608–10.
7. Cornell RC, Stoughton RB. Correlation of the vasoconstriction assay and clinical activity in psoriasis. Arch Dermatol 1985; 121(1): 63–7.
8. Luger T et al. Topische Dermatotherapie mit Glukokortikoiden Therapeutischer Index. J Dtsch Dermatol Ges 2004; 2(7): 629–34.
9. Schackert C, Korting HC, Schäfer-Korting M. Qualitative and quantitative assessment of the benefit-risk ratio of medium potency topical corticosteroids in vitro and in vivo: characterisation of drugs with an increased benefit-risk ratio. BioDrugs 2000; 13(4): 267–7.
10. Schäfer-Korting M et al. Prednicarbate activity and benefit/risk ratio in relation to other topical glucocorticoids. Clin Pharmacol Ther 1993; 54(4): 448–56.
11. Korting HC, Kerscher MJ, Schafer-Korting M. Topical glucocorticoids with improved benefit/risk ratio: do they exist? J Am Acad Dermatol 1992; 27(1): 87–92.
12. Daufeldt S et al. Membrane initiated steroid signaling (MISS): computational, in vitro and in vivo evidence for a plasma membrane protein initially involved in genomic steroid hormone effects. Mol Cell Endocrinol 2006; 246(1–2): 42–52.
13. Lee SW et al. Autocrine stimulation of interleukin-1 alpha and transforming growth factor alpha production in human keratinocytes and its antagonism by glucocorticoids. J Invest Dermatol 1991; 97(1): 106–10.
14. Warnmark A et al. Activation functions 1 and 2 of nuclear receptors: molecular strategies for transcriptional activation. Mol Endocrinol 2003; 17(10): 1901–9.
15. Lefstin JA, Yamamoto KR. Allosteric effects of DNA on transcriptional regulators. Nature 1998; 392(6679): 885–8.
16. Heck S et al. A distinct modulating domain in glucocorticoid receptor monomers in the repression of activity of the transcription factor AP-1. EMBO J 1994; 13(17): 4087–95.
17. Reichardt HM et al. DNA binding of the glucocorticoid receptor is not essential for survival. Cell, 1998; 93(4): 531–41.
18. Rogatsky I et al. Target-specific utilization of transcriptional regulatory surfaces by the glucocorticoid receptor. Proc Natl Acad Sci U S A 2003; 100(24): 13845–50.
19. Schäcke H, Docke WD, Asadullah K. Mechanisms involved in the side effects of glucocorticoids. Pharmacol Ther 2002; 96(1): 23–43.
20. Cato AC, Wade E. Molecular mechanisms of anti-inflammatory action of glucocorticoids. Bioessays 1996; 18(5): 371–8.
21. Barnes PJ, Molecular mechanisms of corticosteroids in allergic diseases. Allergy 2001; 56(10): 928–36.
22. Adcock IM, Caramori G. Cross-talk between pro-inflammatory transcription factors and glucocorticoids. Immunol Cell Biol 2001; 79(4): 376–384.
23. Karin M, Yamamoto Y, Wang QM. The IKK NF-kappa B system: a treasure trove for drug development. Nat Rev Drug Discov 2004; 3(1): 17–26.
24. Ito K, Barnes PJ, Adcock IM. Glucocorticoid receptor recruitment of histone deacetylase 2 inhibits interleukin-1beta-induced histone H4 acetylation on lysines 8 and 12. Mol Cell Biol 2000; 20(18): 6891–903.
25. Ito K et al. p65-activated histone acetyltransferase activity is repressed by glucocorticoids: mifepristone fails to recruit HDAC2 to the p65–HAT complex. J Biol Chem 2001; 276(32): 30208–15.
26. Ito K et al. Histone deacetylase 2–mediated deacetylation of the glucocorticoid receptor enables NF-kappaB suppression. J Exp Med 2006; 203(1): 7–13.
27. Vanden Berghe W et al. Induction and repression of NF-kappa B-driven inflammatory genes. Ernst Schering Res Found Workshop 2002; (40): 233–78.
28. Nissen RM, Yamamoto KR. The glucocorticoid receptor inhibits NFkappaB by interfering with serine-2 phosphorylation of the RNA polymerase II carboxy-terminal domain. Genes Dev 2000; 14(18): 2314–29.
29. Caelles C, Gonzalez-Sancho JM, Munoz A, Nuclear hormone receptor antagonism with AP-1 by inhibition of the JNK pathway. Genes Dev 1997; 11(24): 3351–64.
30. Bruna A et al. Glucocorticoid receptor-JNK interaction mediates inhibition of the JNK pathway by glucocorticoids. EMBO J 2003; 22(22): 6035–44.

31. Kassel O et al. Glucocorticoids inhibit MAP kinase via increased expression and decreased degradation of MKP-1. EMBO J 2001; 20(24): 7108–16.

32. Lasa M et al. Dexamethasone causes sustained expression of mitogen-activated protein kinase (MAPK) phosphatase 1 and phosphatase-mediated inhibition of MAPK p38. Mol Cell Biol 2002; 22(22): 7802–11.

33. Stellato C, Post-transcriptional and nongenomic effects of glucocorticoids. Proc Am Thorac Soc, 2004; 1(3): 255–63.

34. McKenna NJ, O' Malley BO. Minireview: nuclear receptor coactivators – an update. Endocrinology 2002; 143(7): 2461–5.

35. Khan OY, Nawaz Z. Nuclear hormone receptor co-regulators. Curr Opin Drug Discov Devel 2003; 6(5): 692–701.

36. Robyr D,Wolffe AP, Wahli W. Nuclear hormone receptor coregulators in action: diversity for shared tasks. Mol Endocrinol 2000; 14(3): 329–47.

37. Aranda A, Pascual A. Nuclear hormone receptors and gene expression. Physiol Rev 2001; 81(3): 1269–304.

38. Xu J, O'Malley BW. Molecular mechanisms and cellular biology of the steroid receptor coactivator (SRC) family in steroid receptor function. Rev Endocr Metab Disord 2002; 3(3): 185–92.

39. Gille J. Atopische Dermatitis In: Zollner TM, Boehncke WH, Kaufmann R., (eds). Berlin: Blackwell Science, 2002. 2002; Blackwell Science: Berlin.

40. Freiwel M. Percutaneous absorption of topical steroids in children. Br J Dermatol 1969; 81(Suppl. 4): 113–16.

41. Guy RH, MH, Calculations of body exposure from percutaneous absorption data. In: Bronaugh RL, Maibach HI. (eds). Percutaneous Absorption. New York: Dekker, 1985: 461–6.

42. Rasmussen E. Psoriasis in children. Dermatol Clin 1986; 4: 99–106.

43. Sterry W. Therapy with topical corticosteroids. Arch Dermatol Res 1992; 284(Suppl 1): 27–9.

44. Gomez EC, Kaminester L, Frost P. Topical halcinonide and betamethasone valerate effects on plasma cortisol. Arch Dermatol 1977; 113: 1196–1202.

45. Cubey RB, Glaucoma following the application of corticosteroids to the skin of the eyelids. Br J Dermatol 1976; 95: 207–208.

46. Alani MD, Alani SD, Allergic contact dermatitis to corticosteroids. Ann Allergol 1972; 30: 181–5.

47. Sterry W, Asadullah K, Topical glucocorticoid therapy in dermatology. Ernst Schering Res Found Workshop 2002; (40): 39–54.

48. Schoepe S et al. Glucocorticoid-induced skin atrophy. Exp Dematol 2006; 15(16): 406–20.

49. Kao JS et al. Short-term glucocorticoid treatment compromises both permeability barrier homeostasis and stratum corneum integrity: inhibition of epidermal lipid synthesis accounts for functional abnormalities. J Invest Dermatol 2003; 120(3): 456–64.

50. Kimura T, Doi K. Dorsal skin reactions of hairless dogs to topical treatment with corticosteroids. Toxicol Pathol 1999; 27(5): 528–35.

51. Booth BA et al. Steroid-induced dermal atrophy: effects of glucocorticosteroids on collagen metabolism in human skin fibroblast cultures. Int J Dermatol 1982; 21(6): 333–7.

52. Mills CM, Marks R. Side effects of topical glucocorticoids. Curr Probl Dermatol 1993; 21: 122–31.

53. Epstein NN, Epstein WL, Epstein JH. Atrophic striae in patients with inguinal intertrigo. Arch Dermatol 1963; 87: 450–7.

54. Kolbe L et al. Corticosteroid-induced atrophy and barrier impairment measured by non-invasive methods in human skin. Skin Res Technol 2001; 7(2): 73–7.

55. Saarni H, Hopsu-Havu VK. The decrease of hyaluronate synthesis by anti-inflammatory steroids in vitro. Br J Dermatol 1978; 98(4): 445–9.

56. Lehmann P et al. Corticosteroid atrophy in human skin. A study by light, scanning, and transmission electron microscopy. J Invest Dermatol 1983; 81(2): 169–76.

57. Sheu HM et al. Depletion of stratum corneum intercellular lipid lamellae and barrier function abnormalities after long-term topical corticosteroids. Br J Dermatol 1997; 136(6): 884–90.

58. Garbe C, Wolf G. Topische Therapie. In: Braun-Falco et al, eds. Dermatologie und Venerologie. Berlin: Springer, 2005: 1431–61.

59. Smith EW, Haigh JM, Surber C. Quantification of corticosteroid-induced skin vasoconstriction: visual ranking, chromameter measurement or digital imaging analysis. Dermatology 2002; 205(1): 3–10.

60. Cornell RC, Stoughton RB. The use of topical steroids in psoriasis. Dermatol Clin 1984; 2: 397–408.

61. Stoughton RB, Cornell RC. Corticosteroids, In: Fitzpatrick TB, eds. Dermatology in General Medicine. New York: McGraw-Hill, 1993: 2846–50.

62. Brazzini B, Pimpinelli N. New and established topical corticosteroids in dermatology: clinical pharmacology and therapeutic use. Am J Clin Dermatol 2002; 3(1): 47–58.

63. Nuutinen P et al. Modulation of collagen synthesis and mRNA by continuous and intermittent use of topical hydrocortisone in human skin. Br J Dermatol 2003; 148(1): 39–45.

64. McMichael AJ et al. Concurrent application of tretinoin (retinoic acid) partially protects against corticosteroid-induced epidermal atrophy. Br J Dermatol 1996; 135(1): 60–4.

65. Frosch PJ. Local corticoid treatment – possibilities and recommendations. Z Hautkr 1987; 62(12): 919–24.

66. du Vivier A, Phillips H, Heir M. Applications of glucocorticosteroids. The effects of twice-daily vs once-every-other-day applications on mouse epidermal cell DNA synthesis. Arch Dermatol 1982; 118(5): 305–8.

67. Fukaya Y et al. A study of systemic and topical effects of topical steroid application through the comparison of two application schedules. J Dermatol 1990; 17(1): 28–33.

68. Korting HC et al. Maintenance treatment and early intervention – the new paradigm in the management of atopic eczema. J Dtsch Dermatol Ges 2005; 3(7): 519–23.
Intermittent dosing of fluticasone propionate cream for reducing the risk of relapse in atopic dermatitis patients. J Dtsch Dermatol Ges 2005; 3(7): 519–23.

69. Hanifin J, Gupta AK, Rajagopalan R. Intermittent dosing of fluticasone propionate cream for reducing the risk of relapse in atopic dermatitis patients. Br J Dermatol 2002; 147(3): 528–37.

70. Furue M et al.Clinical dose and adverse effects of topical steroids in daily management of atopic dermatitis. Br J Dermatol 2003; 148(1): 128–33.

71. Prawer SE, Katz HI. Guidelines for using superpotent topical steroids. Am Fam Physician 1990; 41(5): 1531–8.

72. Billich A et al. Percutaneous absorption of drugs used in atopic eczema: pimecrolimus permeates less through skin than corticosteroids and tacrolimus. Int J Pharm 2004; 269(1): 29–35.

73. Billich A et al. Novel cyclosporin derivatives featuring enhanced skin penetration despite increased molecular weight. Bioorg Med Chem 2005; 13(9): 3157–67.

74. Korting HC et al. Different skin thinning potential of equipotent medium-strength glucocorticoids. Skin Pharmacol Appl Skin Physiol 2002; 15(2): 85–91.

75. Isogai M et al. Binding affinities of mometasone furoate and related compounds including its metabolites for the glucocorticoid receptor of rat skin tissue. J Steroid Biochem Mol Biol 1993; 44(2): 141–5.

76. Bonina FP et al. In vitro and in vivo evaluation of polyoxyethylene esters as dermal prodrugs of ketoprofen, naproxen and diclofenac. Eur J Pharm Sci 2001; 14(2): 123–34.

77. Brattsand R, Miller-Larsson A. The role of intracellular esterification in budesonide once-daily dosing and airway selectivity. Clin Ther 2003; 25(Suppl C): C28–41.

78. Lee HJ et al. Prodrug and antedrug: two diametrical approaches in designing safer drugs. Arch Pharm Res 2002; 25(2): 111–36.

79. Gysler A et al. Prednicarbate biotransformation in human foreskin keratinocytes and fibroblasts. Pharm Res 1997; 14(6): 793–7.

80. Jordana M et al. Immune-inflammatory functions of fibroblasts. Eur Respir J 1994; 7(12): 2212–22.

81. Kessler-Becker D, Krieg T, Eckes B. Expression of pro-inflammatory markers by human dermal fibroblasts in a three-dimensional culture model is mediated by an autocrine interleukin-1 loop. Biochem J 2004; 379(Pt 2): 351–8.

82. Levy J et al. Comparison of the effects of calcipotriol, prednicarbate and clobetasol 17–propionate on normal skin assessed by ultrasound measurement of skin thickness. Skin Pharmacol 1994; 7(4): 231–6.

83. Fesq H et al. Improved risk-benefit ratio for topical triamcinolone acetonide in Transfersome in comparison with equipotent cream and ointment: a randomized controlled trial. Br J Dermatol 2003; 149(3): 611–19.

84. Korting HC et al. Liposome encapsulation improves efficacy of betamethasone dipropionate in atopic eczema but not in psoriasis vulgaris. Eur J Clin Pharmacol 1990; 39(4): 349–51.

85. Santos Maia C et al. Drug targeting by solid lipid nanoparticles for dermal use. J Drug Target 2002; 10(6): 489–95.

86. Barnes PJ. Cytokine-directed therapies for asthma. J Allergy Clin Immunol 2001; 108(2 Suppl): S72–6.

87. Schäcke H et al. Dissociation of transactivation from transrepression by a selective glucocorticoid receptor agonist leads to separation of therapeutic effects from side effects. Proc Natl Acad Sci U S A 2004; 101(1): 227–32.

88. Schäcke H et al. SEGRAs: a novel class of anti-inflammatory compounds. Ernst Schering Res Found Workshop 2002; (40): 357–71.

89. Schäcke H, Rehwinkel H. Dissociated glucocorticoid receptor ligands. Curr Opin Investig Drugs 2004; 5(5): 524–8.

90. Buttgereit F, Burmester GR, Lipworth BJ. Optimised glucocorticoid therapy: the sharpening of an old spear. Lancet 2005; 365(9461): 801–3.

91. Zollner TM, Boehncke WH, Kaufmann R (eds). Atopische Dermatitis. Berlin: Blackwell Science, 2002.

15

Clinical aspects of glucocorticoid treatment

Kristian Thestrup-Pedersen

BACKGROUND

The first report on the efficacy of topical steroids became available in 1952, when compound F (i.e. hydrocortisone) was documented to be effective in various dermatoses including the treatment of atopic eczema.[1] Five decades of clinical documentation and the experience of many doctors have proven the usefulness of topical steroids, which together with emollients today still are the 'gold standard' of treatment for atopic eczema. Although hundreds of trials have shown their efficacy, most have been limited to a treatment period of up to 4 weeks, and long-term trials are remarkably few.

BIOCHEMISTRY OF STEROIDS

Any topical steroid needs to have a few basic characteristics of its molecule, which stems from the cholesterol ring (Figure 15.1). The position on the molecule of double bonds and various side chains has a major impact on their biological efficacy. The 'gluco-corticoid effect' versus the 'mineralo-corticoid effect' also depends upon the presence of double bonds and side chains. As an example all topical steroids must have a hydroxyl (-OH) group at position 11 as they are inactive without. A double bond between 1 and 2, fluorination at position 9, and modifications of the side chains in 16,17 position bring increased potency to the molecule. The most recently marketed products all have their side chains at the 16 or 17 position removed at first passage through the liver, therefore – in theory – having less systemic effects than molecules, where the side chains are not removed.

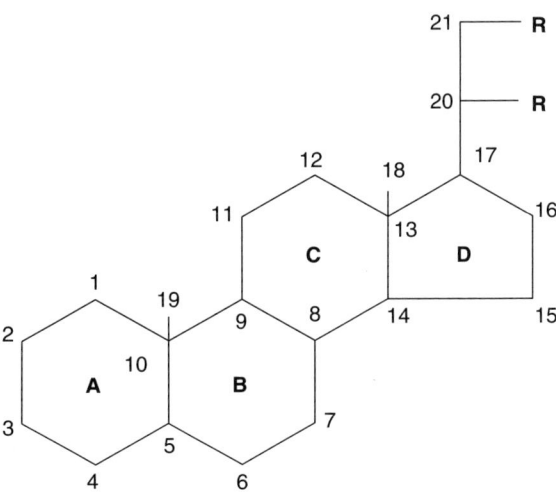

Figure 15.1 The steroid molecule used for topical steroids.

The potency of steroids is based on their vasoconstriction capacity[2] combined with their clinical effect. Topical steroids are listed into 4 groups, ranging from mild potency, i.e. hydrocortisone acetate 1%, through moderate and potent to very potent steroids.[3] A listing of these groups can be found in various pharmacological manuals.

ACTIONS OF TOPICAL STEROIDS

Anti-inflammatory effects

Steroids are effective in eczema, because they have a broad spectrum of activity on the inflammation creating

Table 15.1   A listing of anti-inflammatory effects of topical steroids

- A broad anti-inflammatory effect on T lymphocytes through a blockade of the release of cytokines leading to the almost immediate diminishing of itch, which is probably cytokine mediated
- Blocking of dendritic cells in antigen presentation and their removal from epidermis and dermis
- Blocking and removal of mast cells from the skin
- Down-regulation of chemokine receptors on inflammatory cells
- Down-regulation of adhesion molecules inhibiting cellular emigration to the skin
- Vasoconstriction inhibiting migration of T cells and eosinophils
- Inhibition of other mediator cascades (prostaglandins, leukotrienes)

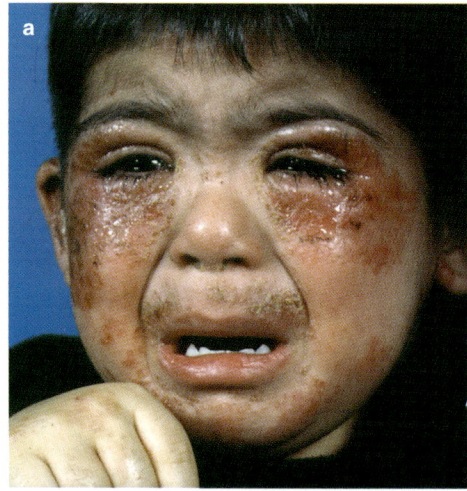

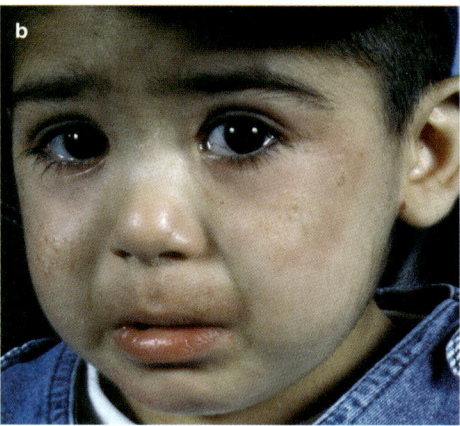

Figure 15.2   A 14-month-old child (a) before and (b) 1 week after treating the eczema with a topical steroid.

eczema. Table 15.1 lists a number of effects which will improve the eczema.

All these effects have a 'shot-gun' effect on the skin inflammation. In addition, the effects come quickly as steroid molecules are easily absorbed into the skin.

Absorption of steroids in different anatomical regions

An important study looked at the absorption of ³H-labelled hydrocortisone acetate in various regions of the body in healthy volunteers.[4] If absorption through the skin on the volar aspect of the forearm was used as 'standard', it was observed that the absorption of steroids on scrotal skin was 42 × higher, on face 6–8 × higher and in palms 0.2 × higher (or 5-fold lower). Thus, absorption varies depending on the anatomical region, something which should be considered when prescribing topical steroids.

Absorption of steroid is increased when the skin barrier is disrupted as it is in patients with atopic eczema. Thus, plasma cortisol levels became increased even after application of hydrocortisone acetate. When the skin barrier is repaired the absorption falls.[5,6]

EFFICACY, DOSING, DURATION, AND AMOUNT OF STEROIDS TO BE USED

Efficacy

Figure 15.2 a,b shows a 14-months-old child before and 1 week after treating his eczema once daily with

mometasone furoate. The pictures illustrate what is known from daily practice: topical steroids clear eczema and they do so fast.

Table 15.2 lists the outcome of a recent study documenting how the majority of patients aged 12–65 years and with atopic eczema can control their eczema using fluticasone propionate and how they, on a long-term basis, can prevent a relapse through twice weekly application of steroid on previously treated areas.

Patients were treated daily for 4 weeks to induce remission, when 9% discontinued because of lack of effect. The remaining patients (91%) were eligible for maintenance treatment. Note how prophylactic treatment keeps

Table 15.2 Atopic eczema control by patients aged 12–65 years old using fluticasone propionate twice weekly

Maintenance treatment	Fluticasone cream 0.05% twice weekly + emollient	Placebo cream daily
Number of patients	70	84
Outcome after 16 weeks		
Relapse	19%	64%
No relapse	81%	36%

81% without eczema for a 4-month period; note too that emollients are able to keep one-third of the patients in remission over a 16-week period.[7]

Dosing

Infants
Infants, at the moment, only have steroids registered as an anti-inflammatory topical treatment for eczema. They work well, and if the eczema is mild to moderate, low potency topical steroids like hydrocortisone acetate or hydrocortisone butyrate will be highly effective in many children. Following remission of eczema, emollients can for a certain time keep the skin normal and the steroid can be applied again for a short course, if symptoms of eczema relapse. However, the quite extensive steroid phobia among parents often leads to a lack of compliance.[8]

Children and adults
Children and adults with severe eczema often need the advantage of the quick effects on symptom relief from potent topical steroids. Following remission less potent steroids can be used or intermittent treatment can be initiated for long-term control.[7] It seems equally effective to use short bursts of a potent topical corticosteroid versus prolonged use of a mild preparation in children with mild to moderate atopic eczema.[9]

Application frequency and duration of treatment

A few studies show that application once daily is as effective as twice daily for the same steroid.[10] This author therefore recommends that emollients are used in the morning as itch is less present in the morning

hours, but when the child becomes tired in the afternoon, bouts of itching occur and steroids should then be applied. Emollients are steroid-sparing,[11] maybe because the stratum corneum acts as a reservoir for steroids and application of emollients induces a steroid release.[12]

A recent survey on topical steroids and their use in atopic eczema underlines that we are lacking comparative studies on different steroids for the various forms of atopic eczema and especially how to use steroids for long-term control.[13]

Amount of steroids to be used for eczema treatment

The 'fingertip unit' was introduced as a practical and instructive way of dosing the amount of steroid which is relevant for the various anatomical regions.[14,15] Table 15.3 shows the recommended maximal use of mild to moderate topical steroid per week according to the age of the child. If potent steroids are used it is recommended to use half the amount only. The amounts are based on how much is needed if all skin was affected by eczema, and the steroid was applied once daily.

Wet dressing

This dosing of steroids is very effective for children with severe, often oozing eczema.[16] The reason is that wet dressings leave a cooling effect on the skin, leading to relief of itch. At the same time steroid absorption is dramatically increased. Wet dressings have a further drawback, as they are a very time-consuming way of applying steroids, often requiring an experienced nurse. They should be restricted for severe cases only and for short-term treatment: i.e. a maximum of 2 weeks.

Dispensary forms

Steroids are easy to dissolve; therefore they can be applied in ointments, which are good for dry skin and lead to improved absorption of the steroid. Creams are better for oozing eczema and where the occlusive effects of ointments are counterproductive for a normal transepidermal water evaporation. Creams are cosmetically much more acceptable for the patient. For hairy body areas, gels or lotions are the best way for an easy application of steroid. The dispensary forms of topical steroids are therefore optimal.

Combinations with antiseptics or antibiotics

There are many products on the market combining a topical steroid with antibacterial and antifungal drugs.

Table 15.3 Recommended weekly cumulative use of steroid according to age								
Age	3 months	6 months	12 months	2 years	3 years	5 years	7 years	10 years	12 years
Grams	28	33	42	47	56	70	86	100	100

The role of *Staphylococcus aureus* and its secretion of superantigens, and the possible role of *Pityrosporoum ovale* for head and neck dermatitis (HNAD) has been considered. There are well-conducted studies showing that addition of Fucidin (fusidic acid) to hydrocortisone led to a significantly quicker remission of atopic eczema during the initial 2 weeks of treatment,[17] but other studies using a different antiseptic are not able to support this finding.[18,19] It is known that topical steroids themselves will reduce the number of *S. aureus* on the skin, when the eczema is cleared.[20] However, addition of a soap with 1.5% triclocarban acting against *S. aureus* led to a significant reduction in eczema activity.[21] Addition of an antifungal compound (ketoconazole) to hydrocortisone cream could however not give a significant beneficial effect in the treatment of HNAD in adults.[22] Systemic antibiotics over a 4-week period did not change the activity of atopic eczema.[23] The Health Assessment Report does therefore not at the moment recommend use of a combinatory treatment with topical steroids and antimicrobials, neither topically nor systemically.[13] However, it is a fact that many of these products are used by doctors. Recent observations from the UK could indicate that using such products should be only initially to avoid the risk of resistance development.[24]

DURATION OF TREATMENT INCLUDING PROPHYLACTIC USE OF TOPICAL STEROIDS

Topical steroids will within a treatment period of 4 weeks either completely clear or significantly reduce the eczema activity.[7,9] Many parents or patients therefore stop treatment as eczema has gone and they are afraid of side effects. On continuing with emollients one-third of patients can stay clear of eczema for up to 4 months,[7] but the 'prophylactic use' of topical steroids has now become established as an efficient and economical way of keeping atopic eczema under control.[7,25,26] There seem to be very few clinical side effects from using potent topical steroid twice weekly except in the face and genital regions, where hydrocortisone is recommended. One study measured skin thickness using ultrasound and observed that 10% of the patients did develop some skin atrophy.[9]

SIDE EFFECTS INCLUDING CONTACT ALLERGY

A list of potential side effects is shown below:

- Skin atrophy through atrophy of epidermis and disruption of collagen and elastic fibres in dermis leading to potential development of striae distensae (Figure 15.3).
- Skin vessel fragility leading to teleangiectasia and bleeding, especially seen in elderly patients, but rarely in children (Figure 15.4).
- Systemic absorption with increase of plasma cortisol and a potential risk of HPA disturbance; especially seen during the initial days of eczema treatment because of disrupted skin barrier.
- Inhibition of melanocyte activity, which in some patients will lead to hypopigmentation.
- Iatrogenic dermatitis caused by excessive use of topical steroid with a relatively too high 'efficacy' e.g. hypertrichosis, steroid acne, perioral dermatitis, tinea incognito, pustular psoriasis.

The side effects can be evident within 1 week of treatment as seen by diminished skin thickness on ultrasound investigation. Side effects are much more common among elderly patients. They rarely occur in children with atopic eczema, when properly used. The reason for side effects is that collagen synthesis is inhibited[27] with a diminished elasticity and increased fragility of the various structures in the skin.

Adrenal function and plasma cortisol levels

All topical steroids are absorbed through the skin and even treatment with hydrocortisone acetate in active atopic eczema will lead to increased plasma cortisol levels.[5,6] However, it has been shown that the adrenal function is normal after topical steroids.[28–30] There was no growth inhibition of children during a 2-week treatment of children with a potent topical steroid; actually the removal of eczema led to catch-up growth, i.e. a significant increase of the growth rate in children after controlling the eczema.[31] Most children relapsed within 2 weeks, indicating the need for long-term treatment strategies.

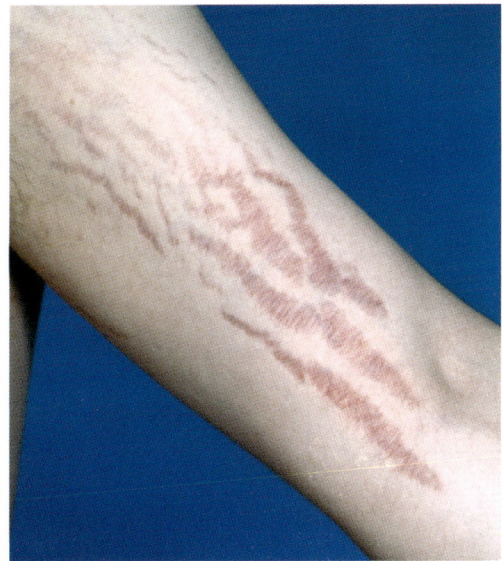

Figure 15.3   Striae distensae following longterm usage of potent topical steroid.

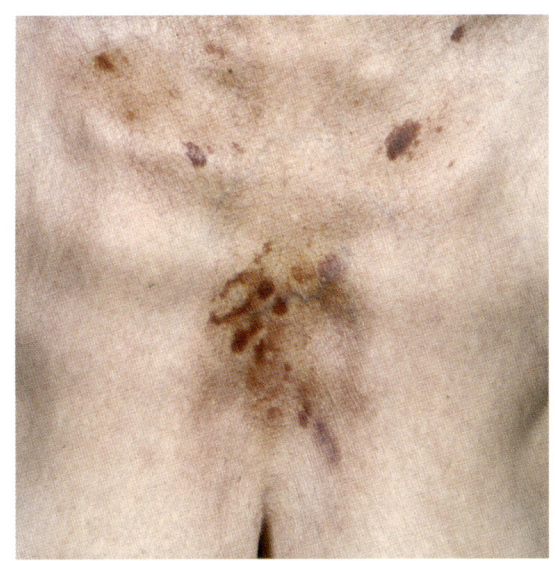

Figure 15.4   Ecchymoses in an elderly lady following longterm usage of potent topical steroid.

The use of topical steroids during pregnancy does not bring risks for the child.[32] This was concluded as pregnant women on systemic steroids because of asthma did not have increased risks regarding their child.

Contact allergy to topical steroids

Contact allergy to topical steroids is by some investigators claimed to occur in up to 4% of all atopic eczema patients.[33] However, in Denmark the prevalence of contact eczema is around 1%.[34] Eczema not responding to topical steroids should be investigated for eventual steroid contact allergy. Reading of the tests should include a 7-day reading.

USE OF SYSTEMIC STEROIDS

There is a surprising lack of use of systemic steroids in atopic eczema.[35] The reason are the side effects including the possibility of osteoporosis. Some parents or patients lack sufficient insight into their disease often accompanied by a relative lack of compliance leading to insufficient eczema control. If so, a low dose of systemic steroids can be used for some months. Likewise, an acute severe flare may be cured with a short-term intensive systemic dose, e.g. 40 mg prednisolone for 1 week, and then a reduction over a couple of weeks.

THE FUTURE OF STEROIDS

Although the new calcineurin inhibitors are now available with their advantages of being effective, specific, and without the side effects of steroids, there surely is a future for topical steroids in atopic eczema. The steroids are here to stay. The future will show how the two different topical compounds are used. This author recommends the use of steroids in the acute phase (see Figure 15.2 a,b), but then switching to topical calcineurin inhibitors for long-term control.

REFERENCES

1. Sultzberger MB, Witten VH. The effect of topically applied compound F in selected dermatoses. J Invest Dermatol 1952; 19: 101–2.
2. Goa KL. Clinical pharmacology and pharmacokinetic properties of topically applied corticosteroids. A review. Drugs 1988; 36 (Suppl 5): 51–61.
3. Poulsen J, Rorsman H. Ranking of glucocorticoid creams and ointments. Acta Derm Venereol 1980; 60: 57–60.
4. Maibach HI. In vivo percutaneous penetration of corticoids in man and unresolved problems in their efficacy. Dermatologica 1976; 152(Suppl 1): 11–25.
5. Turpeinen M, Salo OP, Leisti S. Effect of percutaneous absorption of hydrocortisone on adrenocortical responsiveness in infants with severe skin disease. Br J Dermatol 1986; 115: 475–84.
6. Turpeinen M, Mashkilleyson N, Bjorksten F, Salo OP. Percutaneous absorption of hydrocortisone during exacerbation and remission of atopic dermatitis in adults. Acta Derm Venereol 1988; 68: 331–5.
7. Berth-Jones J, Damstra RJ, Golsch S et al. Twice weekly fluticasone propionate added to emollient maintenance treatment to

reduce risk of relapse in atopic dermatitis: randomised, double blind, parallel group study. Br Med J 2003; 326: 1367–70.

8. Charman CR, Morris AD, Williams HC. Topical corticosteroid phobia in patients with atopic eczema. Br J Dermatol 2000; 142: 931–6.

9. Thomas KS, Armstrong S, Avery A et al. Randomised controlled trial of short bursts of a potent topical corticosteroid versus prolonged use of a mild preparation for children with mild or moderate atopic eczema. BMJ 2002; 321: 1–7.

10. Bleehen SS, Chu AC, Hamann I et al. Fluticasone propionate 0.05% cream in the treatment of atopic eczema: a multicentre study comparing once-daily treatment and once-daily vehicle cream application versus twice-daily treatment. Br J Dermatol 1995; 133: 592–7.

11. Lucky AW, Leach AD, Laskarzewski P, Wenck H. Use of an emollient as a steroid-sparing agent in the treatment of mild to moderate atopic dermatitis in children. Ped Dermatol 1997; 14: 321–4.

12. Turpeinen M. Absorption of hydrocortisone from the skin reservoir in atopic dermatitis. Br J Dermatol 1991; 124: 358–60.

13. Hoare C, Li Wan Po A, Williams H. Systematic review of treatments for atopic eczema. Health Technol Assess 2000; 4(37): 1–191. (www.ncchta.org)

14. Long CC, Finlay AU. The fingertip unit – a new practical measure. Clin Exp Dermatol 1991; 16: 444–7.

15. Long CC, Mills CM, Finlay AY. A practical guide to topical therapy in children. Br J Dermatol 1998; 138: 293–6.

16. Devillers AC, Oranje AP. Efficacy and safety of 'wet-wrap' dressings as an intervention treatment in children with severe and/or refractory atopic dermatitis: a critical review of the literature. Br J Dermatol 2006; 154: 579–85.

17. Ramsay, CA, Savoie JM, Gilbert M et al. The treatment of atopic dermatitis with topical fusidic acid and hydrocortisone acetate. J Eur Acad Dermatol Venereol 1996; 7(Suppl 1): 15–22.

18. Ainley-Walker PF, Patel L, David TJ. Side to side comparison of topical treatment in atopic dermatitis. Arch Dis Child 1998; 79: 149–52.

19. Stalder JF, Fleury M, Sourisse M et al. Comparative effects of two topical antiseptics (chlorhexidine vs KMnO₄) on bacterial skin flora in atopic dermatitis. Acta Derm Venereol (Stockh) 1992; 176(Suppl): 132–4.

20. Nilsson EJ, Henning CG, Magnusson J. Topical corticosteroids and Staphyloccus aureus in atopic dermatitis. J Am Acad Dermatol 1992; 27: 29–34.

21. Breneman DL, Hanifin JM, Berge CA, Keswick BH, Neumann PB. The effect of antibacterial soap with 1.5% triclocarban on Staphylococcus aureus in patients with atopic dermatitis. Cutis 2000; 66: 296–300.

22. Broberg A, Faergemann J. Topical antimycotic treatment of atopic dermatitis in the head/neck area. A double-blind randomised study. Acta Derm Venereol 1995; 75: 46–9.

23. Ewing CI, Ashcroft C, Gibbs AC et al. Flucloxacillin in the treatment of atopic dermatitis. Br J Dermatol 1998; 138: 1022–9.

24. Ravenscroft JC, Layton AM, Eady EA et al. Short-term effects of topical fusidic acid or mupirocin on the prevalence of fusidic acid resistant (FusR) Staphylococcus aureus in atopic eczema. Br J Dermatol 2003; 1010–7.

25. Faergemann J, Christensen O, Sjövall P et al. An open study of efficacy and safety of long-term treatment with mometasone furoate fatty cream in the treatment of adult patients with atopic dermatitis. J Eur Acad Dermatol Venereol 2000; 14: 393–6.

26. van der Meer JB, Glazenburg EJ, Mulder PG, Eggink HF, Coenraads PJ. The management of moderate to severe atopic dermatitis in adults with atopical fluticasone propionate. Br J Dermatol 1999; 140: 1114–21.

27. Haaspasaari K-M, Risteli J, Oikarinen A. Recovery of human skin collagen synthesis after short-term topical corticosteroid treatment and comparison between young and old subjects. Br J Dermatol 1996; 135: 65–9.

28. Patel L, Clayton PE, Addison GM, Prince DA, David TJ. Adrenal function following topical steroid treatment in children with atopic dermatitis. Br J Dermatol 1995; 132: 950–5.

29. Jorizzo J, Levy M, Lucky A et al. Multicenter trial for long-term safety and efficacy comparison of 0.05% desonide and 1% hydrocortisone ointments in the treatment of atopic dermatitis in pediatric patients. J Am Acad Dermatol 1995; 33: 74–7.

30. Friedlander SF, Bebert AA, Allen DB. Safety of fluticasone propionate cream 0.05% for the treatment of severe and extensive atopic dermatitis in children as young as 3 months. J Am Acad Dermatol 2002; 46: 387–93.

31. Heuck C, Wolthers OD. Calculation of knemometric growth rates in group studies of children treated with exogenous glucocorticoids. Ann Human Biol 1997; 24: 411–18.

32. Kieffer M, Weismann K, Hjorth N. Pregnancy and treatment with glucocorticoids. Ugeskr Laeger 1986; 148: 160–2.

33. Reitamo S. Lauerma AI. Forstrom L. Detection of contact hypersensitivity to topical corticosteroids with hydrocortisone-17-butyrate. Contact Dermatitis 1989; 21: 159–65.

34. Vestergaard L, Andersen KE. Contact allergy to local steroids. Contact allergy to corticosteroids among consecutively tested patients with eczema. Ugeskr Laeger 1997; 159: 5662–6.

35. Aylett SE, Atherton DJ, Preece MA. The treatment of difficult atopic dermatitis in childhood with oral beclomethasone dipropionate. Acta Derm Venereol (Stockh) 1992; 176(Suppl): 123–5.

16

Phototherapy of atopic dermatitis

Sonja A Grundmann and Stefan Beissert

INTRODUCTION

Phototherapy of atopic dermatitis (AD) has been largely empirical since the beneficial effect of solar exposure has been appreciated for decades. In the early 1920s it was recognized that sea climate can improve AD and later it was appreciated that AD improved during the summer season. In 1948 the beneficial effects of phototherapy were studied in a systematic way by exposing patients to radiation emitted from carbon arc lamps. From the 1970s on, fluorescent lamps with more or less precisely defined emission spectra were applied, and these types of lamps are still in use. Within recent years new modalities like UVA1 and narrow band UVB were introduced. Although the basis of phototherapy of AD is still empirical today, parts of the new developments are already based on the advances in photoimmunology and molecular biology.

UVB PHOTOTHERAPY

UVB therapy (290–320 nm) has a long tradition in treating AD since UVB is the oldest phototherapeutic regimen available. UVB phototherapy of atopic patients actually started with the exposure of patients to carbon arc lamps. Since the introduction of UVB fluorescent and mercury arc lamps, UVB was the therapeutic regimen of choice for quite a long time.

The efficacy of UVB was documented in a variety of studies.[1–3] In one of the first studies 17 atopic patients were irradiated on one half of the body with broad-band UVB and on the other half with visible light.[1] The UVB exposure was performed with either 0.5 minimal erythema dose (MED) or with 1.0 MED. Therapy over 8 weeks led in 13 patients to a complete healing of the lesions compared to visible light exposed areas.[1] The same group also examined the therapeutic dose response to UVB by irradiating one half of the body with 0.8 MED and one half with 0.4 MED UVB for 8 weeks in a total of 24 patients.[1] However, although both UVB doses were found to be effective, no significant differences were found between the doses applied, arguing for far erythemogenic doses being equally effective to near erythemogenic doses.[1]

In another study 107 atopic patients were treated with UVB once daily for 4–19 days. A beneficial effect was observed in 93% of the cases and led to a reduction in the need for topical corticosteroids which were allowed during the study period.[4] However, looking at the emission spectra of the irradiation device used by the authors it must be stated that the Psorilux® 9050 lamp also emitted to a certain extent in the UVA range. Therefore, it is not clear whether this investigation should be allocated to the pure UVB or to the UVA/B studies.

The most frequent indication for UVB therapy was and still is psoriasis. Comparison of the therapeutic spectra indicated the highest antipsoriatic efficacy in the range of around 313 nm.[5] This was confirmed by Parrish et al, who demonstrated that 304 and 313 nm were optimally effective even at suberythemogenic doses.[6] To optimally meet these requirements for antipsoriatic activity the Philips TL01 fluorescent lamp emitting narrow-band UVB (311–313 nm) was introduced.[7] Due to the omission of the short wave part of the UVB range, narrow-band UVB is much less erythemogenic. Whether narrow-band UVB is less carcinogenic than broad-band UVB is still a matter of debate,[8] because data investigating the carcinogenic risks of narrow-band UVB and broad-band UVB are limited in humans. In 2004 the first retrospective study was published concerning the skin cancer risk in 195 psoriasis patients treated with broad-band or narrow-band UVB phototherapy. The main endpoint was the development of skin tumours during an observation period of 10 years. The 10-year observation period did not provide evidence for a significant increased skin cancer risk in these patients. To differentiate the risk of both phototherapies and to distinguish the overall risk, prospective longitudinal studies with prolonged follow-up periods are required.[9] No increased incidence of squamous cell carcinoma or melanoma was obtained from the data of 1908 patients with a median number of 23 treatments and a median follow-up duration of 4 (0.04–13) years, though the risk of basal cell carcinoma was increased twofold. However, to determine the true carcinogenic risk, longer follow-up is essential as well.[10]

A recently published study estimates that based on the human carcinogenesis action spectrum, the risk of narrow-band UVB lamps is 50% more carcinogenic for equal erythemal doses than selected broad-band lamps. Epidemiologic evidence of this provoking theory is still pending.[11] In line with this hypothesis is the finding that narrow-band UVB irradiation produced more malignant skin tumours in Ogg1 knockout mice compared to controls.[12]

Nevertheless, narrow-band UVB has turned out to be more effective in treating psoriasis and fewer treatments are needed to achieve remission. Hence, one can anticipate that because of the fewer exposures necessary the risk may be lower. Because of its superiority, narrow-band UVB has almost entirely replaced broad-band UVB. Consequently, narrow-band UVB has been also tried in a variety of other indications including AD.[13–18]

Patients sometimes complain about the worsening of itch and sweating during phototherapy, which especially occurred during UVA/UVA1 application. Therefore, in an open study, 21 severely affected AD patients were treated with air-conditioned narrow-band UVB phototherapy 3 times weekly for 12 weeks. This treatment regimen resulted in a 68% reduction in AD severity scores and a concomitant 88% reduction in topical corticosteriod use.[13] After a follow-up period of 6 months, 6 patients had relapsed and the remaining 15 continued to derive long-term benefit.[8] These data clearly demonstrate the effectiveness of narrow-band UVB for treatment of AD and furthermore show that long-term benefit can be achieved by phototherapy. The efficacy of narrow-band UVB for atopic eczema therapy has been confirmed by others. In this report UVB 311 nm notably reduced AD after 3 weeks of irradiation.[18] During this time a cumulative dose of 9 J/cm^2 was delivered. The therapeutic efficacy of narrow-band UVB has also been evaluated in children. The response was good to excellent in 80% of the 40 children (mean age 11 years). The most frequent adverse effects reported were facial and truncal erythema as well as xerosis.[16,17] A recent study from Jury et al observed 25 children with AD who were treated with narrow-band UVB. It was reported that 68% of children achieved minimal residual diseases after treatment. However, the report did not comment on the eczema severity, length of remission, or whether topical treatment was continued during treatment with narrow-band UVB.[19] A 6-year (1999–2005) retrospective study of 50 patients represents the largest study of narrow-band UVB phototherapy for children with AD. In 40% of these patients with severe enzema, clearance or minimal residual activity was achieved with narrow-band UVB, and the median length of remission was 3 months.[20] Because these patients were permitted to use topical steroids during phototherapy it is, however, difficult to draw any conclusions on the actual therapeutic efficacy of narrow-band UVB alone. These findings show that UVB 311 nm can be successfully used for the phototherapy of children with AD. Nevertheless, based on the potential long-term adverse events it should be not regarded as a first-line treatment.[21]

Since different forms of phototherapy have been reported to be of therapeutic benefit for atopic patients it is important to compare their efficacy. To this end, narrow-band UVB was applied on one half of the body and compared to 8-methoxypsoralen bath-PUVA [psoralen plus UVA (PUVA)] on the other half in 12 patients with severe AD. Treatment was performed 3 times weekly for 6 weeks. After cessation of phototherapy, a decrease in the mean baseline Scoring Atopic Dermatitis (SCORAD) score by 66% by bath PUVA and by 64% by UVB 311 nm treatment was observed.[13] No severe adverse effects were reported to either of the two forms of phototherapy. Hence, both regimens appear to be equally effective for the therapy of AD. In a more recent randomized controlled trial, narrow-band UVB, broad-band UVA, and visible light phototherapy were compared for treating AD. Irradiation was performed with narrow-band UVB in 26 patients, 24 received UVA, and 23 visible light twice weekly for 12 weeks.[15] Narrow-band UVB was very effective in moderate-to-severe adult AD.[15] Furthermore, the data failed to support the benefit of broad-band UVA phototherapy for AD since only moderate effects were noted. Remission was maintained in the narrow-band UVB-treated group over a follow-up period of 3 months. However, this investigation failed to demonstrate a significant topical corticosteroid-sparing effect by either irradiation regimens as has been reported before.[13] Combination of narrow-band UVB phototherapy with cyclosporin A has been reported to be effective in the treatment of AD. Patients with severe AD were treated with oral short-term cyclosporin A for 4 weeks. Subsequently, cyclosporin A was washed out for 4–6 weeks followed by narrow-band UVB phototherapy applied 3 times a week for up to 2 months. This regimen resulted in good clinical response. However, the study did not investigate long-term effects of this protocol, and this combination has to be viewed very critically, especially regarding its carcinogenic potential.[22]

A more recent investigation conducted by Legat et al confirmed the advantages of narrow-band UVB for treating chronic AD. This relatively small trial compared narrow-band UVB to medium-dose UVA1 via half-side comparison in 9 patients with chronic AD. Treatment with narrow-band UVB reduced the clinical severity score (Costa score) by 40% while treatment with UVA1 did not achieve any statistically significant disease reduction. Furthermore, patients reported notably more improvement in disease severity with narrow-band UVB and a better reduction of pruritus.[23] A recent systemic review concluded that in view of its efficacy, benefit–risk profile and costs, narrow-band UVB should be considered as the first-line phototherapeutic option for moderately severe AD.[24] Clearly, more clinical trials are needed to investigate important issues such as carcinogenity and effectiveness in skin diseases other than psoriasis. Taken together, narrow-band UVB is a very effective treatment alternative for atopic patients, which will lead to reduction in disease activity, extent of disease, and pruritus.

While the role of long-term PUVA treatment in the induction of skin tumours is undisputed, in humans the role of UVB phototherapy in skin carcinogenesis is less clear. Macve et al observed in a murine study that tumour outgrowth is enhanced by broad-band UVB but not by narrow-band UVB and UVA1.[25] In another study performed in mutant mice, UVB but not UVA was observed to be responsible for the induction of mammalian cutaneous malignant melanoma.[26] The long-term skin cancer risk of narrow-band UVB is thought to be less than that of PUVA photochemotherapy.[27] However, no data are at present available to quantify the long-term risk of developing skin cancer in children undergoing narrow-band UVB. The mechanisms underlying the beneficial therapeutic effects of UVB are still not entirely clear. For a long time it was believed that UVB can only act in the epidermis due to its lower penetration in comparison to UVA. However, there is recent evidence that UVB can also reach the upper parts of the dermis. UVB is known to induce apoptosis via induction of nuclear DNA damage but also via direct activation of death receptors.[28] Accordingly, it was shown that the therapeutic effect of narrow-band UVB is associated with the induction of apoptosis of T lymphocytes in the psoriatic lesions.[29] Although not experimentally proven, the same effect may apply for AD. In addition, UVB causes immunosuppression by inhibiting antigen presentation and inducing the release of immunosuppressive cytokines, such as interleukin (IL)-10. UVB preferentially inhibits Th1 immune responses and is even able to skew immune reactions towards a Th2 type. At first glance, this would argue against a beneficial effect of UVB in AD, since atopy in general is regarded as a Th2-driven disease. This, however,

may only apply for the early stage of AD, if at all, while in the chronic stage there is a shift towards a Th1 reaction with high levels of interferon-gamma which also explains why chronic AD resembles much more a delayed-type hypersensitivity response. In this case, the immunosuppressive properties of UVB should be of benefit. This may also explain why chronic atopic lesions usually respond better to UVB than acute lesions.

Additionally, narrow-band UVB has a significant influence on antimicrobial peptides, bacterial colonization of the skin surface, and bacterial superantigenes. The skin of patients with AD expresses altered levels of antimicrobial peptides, like hBD1 (human beta defensin 1) or cathelicidines like LL-37, compared with healthy or psoriatic skin. The observed altered expression of these factors might be caused by the need to deal with a modified bacterial skin flora. This pathological antimicrobial response could explain the disposition for bacterial infections in atopic skin. Phototherapy can significantly alter the mRNA levels of antimicrobial peptides in atopic eczema.[30] Furthermore, the narrow-band UVB therapy reduces skin surface bacteria and their superantigen production. Both factors have been shown to trigger AD disease activity.[31]

UVA/B PHOTOTHERAPY

Combination phototherapy consisting of UVA and UVB irradiations has quite a long tradition in the phototherapy of atopic eczema.[3,32,33] UVA/B therapy can be applied by using lamps, the emission spectrum of which includes both ranges (e.g. Metec Helarium), or by combining the exposure to UVA and UVB lamps. The latter can be done depending on the technical equipment in a simultaneous or a subsequent manner. UVA/B therapy was preferentially used since comparison studies revealed UVA/B superior to conventional broad-band UVB for AD.[32] In this study irradiation was given 5 times per week. The average number of treatments was 18 in the UVA/B and 20 in the UVB group. Altogether 48% complete remission was achieved in 23 patients with UVA/B phototherapy compared to complete remission in only 27% of the 33 patients treated with UVB. These results were confirmed by a later report by Jekler et al.[3] Thirty patients with AD underwent phototherapy with a combination of UVA and UVB on one side of the body and UVB on the other. Irradiation was performed 3 times per week for a total of 8 weeks. In this clinical evaluation significant differences in favour of UVA/B treatment were reported for overall scores as well as for the pruritus score.[3] However, when the effect of the two therapies on the extent of the dermatitis was compared, no statistically significant differences were noted.

A disadvantage of the lamps, which emit both UVA and UVB, is dosimetry since it is impossible to dose UVA and UVB separately. In devices which are equipped with UVA and UVB lamps, both spectra can be dosed individually. UVA/B therapy was preferentially used in former times because it turned out to be superior to broad-band UVB. Since the introduction of narrow-band UVB and UVA1, UVA/B therapy has lost some of its importance but is still in use. A combination of narrow-band UVB and UVA for AD in children resulted in a more or equal than 90% reduction of the SCORAD index in 45.5% and a 70–90% reduction in another 22.7% of patients.[34] A recent inverstigation of adult patients with AD demonstrated that continuing topical therapy with corticosteroids during UVA/UVB treatment resulted in significant clinical improvement. In addition, topical corticosteroids reduced the total UVB dose and duration of treatment without any overall difference on remission or the frequency of side effects compared with UVA/UVB monotherapy.[35]

UVA(1) PHOTOTHERAPY

In contrast to the very frequently used combination of UVA and UVB, pure UVA therapy is applied rather rarely. This may be due to the fact that the conventional UVA fluorescent bulbs have only a limited output and thus require extremely long, almost intolerable, exposure times to achieve biologically effective doses. UVA therapy got a new input by the introduction of the UVA1 devices. UVA1 comprises the long wavelength range from 340 to 400 nm.[36–41] The rationale for using UVA1 was the assumption of reducing the adverse effects by omitting the UVA2 part (320–340 nm), which is closely related to the UVB range. The major advantage of the UVA1 devices, however, was the capacity to emit rather high doses in a reasonable amount of time. Initially, these high-power UVA1 lamps were primarily used to perform photoprovocations in patients suffering from polymorphic light eruption and lupus erythematosus.

Since with these devices high doses of UVA1 could be applied without inducing sunburn reaction, these lamps were also used for therapeutic purposes. UVA1 has been reported to be beneficial for patients with acute atopic eczema.[36,37] In addition, UVA1 penetrates deeper into the skin than UVB and UVA2; therefore higher doses should reach the dermis and the deeper blood vessel plexus and cause biological effects.[42,43]

In the first pilot study to assess the effectiveness of UVA1 irradiation for the treatment of AD a single dose of 130 J/cm^2 UVA1 was given for 15 consecutive days.[37] This treatment regimen was compared to UVA/B irradiation (starting doses 30 mJ/cm^2 UVB and 7 J/cm^2

UVA, respectively). UVA1 irradiation was significantly more effective in reducing the clinical scores compared to UVA/B therapy. The clinical effectiveness of UVA1 was paralleled by the down-regulation of eosinophilic cationic protein levels, which were markedly reduced after UVA1, but not UVA/B application.[44] It was quite surprising and unexpected that all patients responded completely to UVA1 therapy and that a beneficial effect was already observed after only 6 exposures.[36] These remarkable observations resulted in the prediction that UVA1 high-dose therapy may be the treatment of choice for AD for the future and will open the corticosteroid-free era of AD.

Unfortunately, it took several years until a follow up study was performed, which included more patients and was performed in a multicentre setting.[45] This study compared UVA1 high-dose therapy with topical corticosteroids and UVA/B therapy. The study revealed that the UVA1 regimen was superior in comparison to the other two arms. However, it could not be reproduced that all patients responded and that only a few exposures were needed for clearance.[41,45] Thus one can conclude that UVA1 high-dose therapy is a valuable therapeutic option for the treatment of acute severe AD but is by far not the gold standard as it was advertised based on the initial pilot study.

The disadvantage of the high-power UVA1 devices is the development of heat when applying such high doses, since many atopic patients do not tolerate such temperatures. This was the rationale for the development of UVA1 lamps filtering the infrared part which is responsible for most of the heat. Hence, this spectrum was termed UVA1 cold light. The efficacy of this regimen was shown in a variety of studies. In the study by von Kobyletzki et al 50 patients with atopic eczema were treated for 15 days with 50 J/cm^2/day. During treatment SCORAD score and plasma levels of soluble IL-2 as well as IL-4 receptors were measured. It was found that medium UVA1 cold light irradiation induced a significant reduction of the SCORAD score and cytokine receptor levels after termination of therapy.[38] In the investigation published by Abeck et al 32 atopic patients were treated in the same fashion as described above with medium-dose UVA1 irradiation.[39] Medium-dose UVA1 also induced in these patients a significant lowering of the SCORAD score. This therapeutic effect was still present after a 1-month follow-up. However, after a 3-month follow-up period signs of recurrence of symptoms could be noted.[39]

The different regimens gave rise to quite controversial opinions about the optimal dose. This discussion was also driven by concerns about the safety of such extremely high doses and by the fact that a medium-dose UVA1 regimen was also shown to be of therapeutic benefit.[38,39] Subsequently, a comparative analysis of high-dose versus medium-dose UVA1 irradiation for the treatment of atopic eczema was initiated by several institutions. In the study by Tzaneva et al 10 atopic patients were treated on one half of the body with 130 J/cm^2 and on the other half with 65 J/cm^2 UVA1 each day for 15 days. High-dose UVA1 irradiation led to a 35%, and medium-dose UVA1 to a 28% decrease in the SCORAD score.[40] In another investigation 34 atopic patients were randomized to receive either low-dose (20 J/cm^2), medium-dose (65 J/cm^2) or high-dose (130 J/cm^2) UVA1 treatment once per day for 15 days.[41] It was found that the medium-dose and high-dose treatment regimens were significantly superior compared to the low-dose UVA1-treated group of patients. However, there were no significant beneficial differences between the high-dose and the medium-dose groups with the exception that the tolerability was higher in the medium-dose group. Together, these study results support the concept that medium-dose UVA1 is comparatively as effective as exposure to high doses of UVA1 for the treatment of patients with severe generalized AD. Polderman et al compared in an open prospective study the effect retrospectively of 4-week UVA1 phototherapy to the effect of 3-week treatment in 61 patients who had AD. In that report a medium-dose UVA1 cold light irradiation device was used (45 J/cm^2 5 times weekly). Patients who were treated for 4 weeks showed prolonged therapeutical effects concerning disease activity and quality of life.[46]

Although urgently needed, no randomized study exists which compares the efficacy and safety of the different UVA1 regimens in a sufficiently large number of patients. Accordingly, no state-of-the-art regimen could be designed relating to the optimal dose and the duration and frequency of the treatment. As long as no data concerning the long-term safety in particular of the high-dose therapy are available, preference should be given to the medium-dose regimen.

Localized defined areas of AD can also be treated with partial body UVA1 phototherapy. This has been successfully applied in particular for the treatment of dyshidrotic eczema of the palms and soles. Medium-dose UVA1 phototherapy induced healing of the lesions in 10 out of 12 patients after 15 irradiation cycles.[47] No relapse was noted during a follow-up period for 3 months. Therefore, local UVA1 treatment appears to be an alternative option for the treatment of chronic dermatitis; however, comparative studies against other forms of phototherapy including photochemotherapy are not available.[48]

The major mechanism of action of UVA1 appears to be the induction of apoptosis of T lymphocytes. In-vitro studies have demonstrated that UVA1 irradiation is able to induce apoptosis in T-helper cells obtained from AD patients.[43] UVA1-induced programmed cell death was mediated via singlet oxygen,

since electron quenchers (sodium azide) protected T cells from apoptosis. In turn, deuterium oxide, which induces singlet oxygen, induced T-cell death.[43] This effect appears to be mediated via upregulation of the death ligand CD95L, which subsequently triggers its cognate death receptor CD95 and ultimately initiates the apoptosis programme. The therapeutic effect of UVA1 is attributed to this phenomenon since CD4+ T cells are found in atopic lesions and these T cells undergo apoptosis upon UVA1 exposure, as demonstrated in-situ.[43] The appearance of apoptotic T cells was followed by their depletion from cutaneous lesions, a reduction in the in-situ expression of IFN-gamma by T cells and clearing of the atopic inflammation. Breuckmann et al demonstrated by immunohistological analysis of irradiated atopic skin that UVA1 is also able to modulate the balance between the antiapoptotic integral membrane protein bcl-2 and the p53 protein as potent regulators of T-cell apoptosis.[49,50]

Taken together, UVA1 irradiation acts symptomatically by elimination of the inflammatory lymphocytic infiltrate via induction of apoptosis in these cells. Due to the fact that UVA1 induces apoptosis in T lymphocytes so effectively, this regimen is currently used in an experimental fashion for the treatment of cutaneous T-cell lymphoma.[51]

PHOTOCHEMOTHERAPY

Photochemotherapy combines the application of psoralens with UVA irradiation (PUVA).[52] Mostly 8-methoxypsoralen is used; in some countries (Austria, France) 5-methoxypsoralen is available. Psoralens can be given orally (systemic PUVA) or applied topically. There are two types of topical application, either by bath (bath PUVA) or by cream (cream PUVA). Systemic PUVA has been used successfully for the management of severe atopic eczema.[53–59] Although improvement was observed in the majority of the treated patients, relatively large numbers of exposures had to be given. In addition, several patients who did not continue topical application of corticosteroids developed a rebound after the end of the PUVA therapy. This resulted in the introduction of maintenance treatment which, however, is not ideal because of the long-term adverse effects of chronic PUVA therapy. Since systemic PUVA has been used in dermatology for over 30 years, long-term safety data are now available. Long-term systemic PUVA is certainly associated with the increased risk of developing skin malignancies.[60–62] Thus, a cohort study has shown that substantial exposure to PUVA therapy dramatically increases the risk of non-melanoma skin cancer. After 25 years, more than half of the patients with more than 400 treatments developed at least one squamous cell carcinoma. Almost one third of the patients exposed to more than 200 treatments developed at least one basal cell carcinoma.[60]

PUVA therapy is also known to increase the risk of malignant melanoma, particularly in long-term therapy (>250 treatments).[63–65] On the other hand, the risk of melanoma, squamous cell carcinoma, and to a lesser extent basal cell carcinoma in PUVA must be weighed against the potency of other therapies. Early detection through careful long-term follow-up of patients exposed to repeated PUVA is essential in reducing the long-term morbidity and mortality associated with this therapy. Taken together, performance of long-term PUVA of atopic patients is strongly discouraged.

Acute side effects of systemic PUVA include nausea and vomiting, although this problem is much less common when applying 5-methoxypsoralen instead of 8-methoxypsoralen; theoretically, 5-methoxypsoralen should be given priority over 8-methoxypsoralen. Unfortunatley, 5-methoxypsoralen is not approved in most countries. Other disadvantages of systemic PUVA are the relatively long photosensitivity since psoralens are eliminated not before 8 hours after ingestion, and by the necessity of eye protection by UVA-opaque on the days of psoralen ingestion.

These actions are not required when applying psoralens topically.[58,66] For bath PUVA, patients are bathing in warm water that contains approximately 0.5–1.0 mg psoralen per litre for 20–30 minutes. UVA exposure has to be performed immediately after bathing. An alternative is the topical application of a psoralen cream (cream PUVA). Usually a water-in-oil ointment containing 0.0006% 8-methoxypsoralen is applied to a defined area of lesional skin 1 hour before irradiation. Cream PUVA has been shown to be very effective in treating patients with chronic hand and foot dermatitis.[66] Since many atopic patients suffer from dyshidrotic eczema, cream PUVA represents a favourite therapeutic option for these patients. In 70% of the treated patients complete remission has been reported by using cream PUVA. A study comparing cream PUVA with bath PUVA in chronic dermatitis revealed cream PUVA to be superior to the bath route in clearing the lesions.[58] The 'PUVA cream' may additionally moisturize the skin, an effect which may contribute to the beneficial effect. Furthermore, cream PUVA is easier to handle and thus cheaper.

The mechanisms underlying the therapeutic effects of PUVA are much less understood compared to UVA or UVB treatment. Since PUVA is most effective in psoriasis, which is a hyperproliferative skin disease, it is believed that UVA-induced DNA-psoralen photoadducts inhibit cell proliferation, leading to inhibition of cell activation and effector function(s).[67] In fact, inhibition of cell proliferation is observed at psoralen concentrations and UVA doses, respectively, which do not affect cell viability.[68] However, higher doses cause irreversible cell damage, resulting in both apoptosis and necrosis.[68,69] Induction of cell death of lymphocytes by PUVA may be responsible for the anti-inflammatory effects of PUVA and for the beneficial therapeutic effects of PUVA on lymphoproliferative diseases, like cutaneous T-cell lymphoma. Therefore, the rationale of PUVA is to induce remissions of skin diseases by repeated, controlled phototoxic reactions. All theoretical and practical aspects taken together, PUVA will be reserved only for very severe and resistant atopic patients; in most cases, preference will be given to other phototherapeutic regimens.

EXTRACORPOREAL PHOTOPHERESIS

During extracorporeal photopheresis peripheral blood mononuclear cells are obtained from patients and exposed to UVA in the presence of psoralens (8-methoxypsoralen) in an extracorporeal irradiation device.[70] Instead of adding the photosensitizer to the blood, 8-methoxypsoralen may be ingested orally by the patient before treatment. Subsequently, the autologous blood components are reinfused. Extracorporeal photopheresis was initially developed for the treatment of cutaneous T-cell lymphoma, in particular Sézary syndrome. However, it turned out that photopheresis is also effective in (auto)immune mediated diseases, like pemphigus, organ transplant rejection, and graft-versus-host disease.[71–74] Accordingly, some immunosuppressive/modulatory capacity is attributed to this kind of therapy. Therefore, photopheresis was applied experimentally in selected patients with AD that was refractory to conventional therapy. Based on these case reports, the first small trials were conducted and extracorporeal photopheresis turned out to be effective in this indication and in these cases, respectively.[75] This treatment was performed at 4-week intervals and led to the induction of clinical improvement and a reduction of serum IgE levels. However, extracorporeal photopheresis was combined with topical corticosteroids, because by itself this phototherapy regimen was unable to control disease activity. In another report extracorporeal photopheresis was given at 2-week intervals, which led to significant improvement of the lesions.[76] During the treatment-free interval dermatitis began to wax; however, after continuation of extracorporeal photopheresis at 2-week intervals, a decrease in the overall skin score as well as serum ECP (eosinophilic cationic protein) concentrations could be noted. To this end, Radenhausen et al observed in an open clinical trial that, after short-term extracorporeal photephoresis, AD responds with a downregulation of several key inflammatory mediators (ECP, sE-selectin, sIL-2R) accompanying the improved skin conditions. High levels of total IgE turned out to be a predictor of negative outcome in extracorporeal photopheresis treatment.[77] Extracorporeal photopheresis can have a significant therapeutic effect on the quality of life improvement in patients who are refractory to conventional forms of therapy.[78]

In summary, these findings suggest that extracorporeal photopheresis is effective in the treatment of AD in selected patients with severe disease, refractory to conventional therapies. However, extracorporeal photopheresis is expensive and time-consuming and controlled randomized studies with sufficient numbers of patients are still not available. The best efficacy data were derived from the few prospective case studies presented here. Hence, this therapy will be reserved for special atopic cases only.

PERSPECTIVES

Phototherapy is still one of the major therapeutic options for the treatment of AD and this will certainly also apply for the future. New developments, like UV-free phototherapy including infrared irradiation devices, might broaden the indication for phototherapy in inflammatory skin diseases. However, much more research is needed to confirm any efficacy regarding many of the potential indications and in determining when and how this upcoming therapeutic regimen should be used. While the development of phototherapeutic regimens was mostly empirical in the past, recent developments are based on the increase of our knowledge in the pathogenesis of AD as well as in the molecular mechanisms mediating the biological effects of UV radiation.[79–81] Despite these advances, one has to admit that, compared for example to psoriasis, AD responds less reliably to phototherapy in general. There are still a reasonable number of patients who do not respond or even get worse under phototherapy, although they suffer from the same diseases as their fellow patients. This may be due to the fact that AD is a highly complex disease in which numerous factors determine the clinical outcome and the therapeutic response. Therefore it will be of primary importance for the future to identify criteria and parameters, respectively, which will determine whether the patients will respond to phototherapy and in particular to which type of treatment. This will ultimately lead to an individually customized phototherapeutic regimen for each patient.

ACKNOWLEDGMENTS

This work was supported by grants from the German Research Association (DFG SFB 293 B8) and the German Cancer Association (Krebshilfe 1077891) as well as the Interdisciplinary Clinical Research Center Münster (IZKF Münster, Lo2/017/07).

REFERENCES

1. Jekler J, Larkö O. UVB phototherapy of atopic dermatitis. Br J Dermatol 1988; 119: 697–705.
2. Jekler J, Larkö O. UVA solarium versus UVB phototherapy of atopic dermatitis: a paired-comparison study. Br J Dermatol 1991; 125: 569–72.
3. Jekler J, Larkö O. Combined UVA-UVB versus UVB phototherapy for atopic dermatitis: a paired-comparison study. J Am Acad Dermatol 1990; 22: 49–53.
4. Hannuksela M, Karvonen J, Husa M et al. Ultraviolet light therapy in atopic dermatitis. Acta Derm Venereol Suppl (Stockh) 1985; 114: 137–9.
5. Fisher T. UV light treatment of psoriasis. Acta Derm Venereol 1976; 56: 473–9.
6. Parrish JA, Jaenicke KF. Action spectrum for phototherapy of psoriasis. J Invest Dermatol 1981; 76: 359–62.
7. van Weelden H, De La Faille HB, Young E, van der Leun JC. A new development in UVB phototherapy of psoriasis. Br J Dermatol 1988; 119: 11–19.
8. Gibbs NK, Traynor NJ, MacKie RM et al. The phototumorigenic potential of broad-band (270–350 nm) and narrow-band (311–313 nm) phototherapy sources cannot be predicted by their edematogenic potential in hairless mouse skin. J Invest Dermatol 1995; 104: 359–63.
9. Weischer M, Blum A, Eberhard F, Röcken M, Berneburg M. No evidence for increased skin cancer risk in psoriasis patients treated with broadband or narrowband UVB phototherapy: a first retrospective study. Acta Derm Venereol 2004; 84: 370–4.
10. Man I, Crombie IK, Dawe RS, Ibbotson SH, Ferguson J. The photocarcinogenic risk of narrowband UVB (TL-01) phototherapy: early follow-up data. Br J Dermatol 2005; 152: 755–7.
11. Kirke SM, Lowder S, Lloyd JJ et al. A randomized comparison of selective broadband UVB and narrowband UVB in the treatment of psoriasis. J Invest Dermatol 2007; 127: 1641–6.
12. Kunisada M, Kumimoto H, Ishizaki K et al. Narrow-band UVB induces more carcinogenic skin tumors than broad-band UVB through the formation of cyclobutane pyrimidine dimer. J Invest Dermatol 2007; 127: 2865–71.
13. George SA, Bilsland DJ, Johnson BE, Ferguson J. Narrow-band (TL-01) UVB air-conditioned phototherapy for chronic severe adult atopic dermatitis. Br J Dermatol 1993; 128: 49–56.
14. Der-Petrossian M, Seeber A, Hönigsmann H, Tanew A. Half-side comparison study on the efficacy of 8-methoxypsoralen bath-PUVA versus narrow-band ultraviolet B phototherapy in patients with severe chronic atopic dermatitis. Br J Dermatol 2000; 142: 39–43.
15. Reynolds NJ, Franklin V, Gray JC, Diffey BL, Farr PM. Narrow-band ultraviolet B and broad-band ultraviolet A phototherapy in

adult atopic eczema: a randomised controlled trial. Lancet 2001; 357: 2012–16.

16. Collins P, Ferguson J. Narrow-band UVB (TL-01) phototherapy: an effective preventative treatment for the photodermatoses. Br J Dermatol 1995; 132: 956–63.

17. Collins P, Ferguson J. Narrowband (TL-01) UVB air-conditioned phototherapy for atopic eczema in children. Br J Dermatol 1995; 133: 653–5.

18. Grundmann-Kollmann M, Behrens S, Podda M et al. Phototherapy for atopic eczema with narrow-band UVB. J Am Acad Dermatol 1999; 40: 995–7.

19. Jury CS, McHenry P, Burden AD, Lever R, Bilsland D. Narrowband ultraviolet B (UVB) phototherapy in children. Clin Exp Dermatol 2006; 31: 196–9.

20. Clayton TH, Clark SM, Turner D, Goulden V. The treatment of severe atopic dermatitis in childhood with narrowband ultraviolet B phototherapy. Clin Exp Dermatol 2007; 32: 28–33.

21 Hanifin JM, Cooper KD, Ho VC et al. Guidelines of care for atopic dermatitis, developed in accordance with the American Academy of Dermatology (AAD)/American Academy of Dermatology Association 'Administrative Regulations for Evidence-Based Clinical Practice Guidelines'. J Am Acad Dermatol 2004; 50: 391–404.

22. Brazzelli V, Prestinari F, Chiesa MG et al. Sequential treatment of severe atopic dermatitis with cyclosporin A and low-dose narrow-band UV-B phototherapy. Dermatology 2000; 204: 252–4.

23. Legat FJ, Hofewr A, Brabek E et al. Narrowband UVB vs medium-dose UV-A1 phototherapy in chronic atopic dermatitis. Arch Dermatol 2003; 139: 223–4.

24. Gambichler T, Breuckmann F, Boms S, Altmeyer P, Kreuter A. Narrowband UVB phototherapy in skin conditions beyond psoriasis. J Am Acad Dermatol 2005; 52: 660–70.

25. Macve JC, Norval M. Ther effects of UV waveband and cis-urocanic acid on tumour outgrowth in mice. Photochem Photobiol Sci 2002; 1: 1006–11.

26. De Fabo EC, Noonan FP, Fears T, Merlino G. Ultraviolet B but not ultraviolet A radiation initiates melanoma. Cancer Res 2004; 15: 6372–6.

27. Lee E, Koo J, Berger T. UVB phototherapy and skin cancer risk: a review of the literature. Int J Dermatol 2005; 44: 355–60.

28. Kulms D, Pöppelmann B, Yarosh D et al. Nuclear and cell membrane effects contribute independently to the induction of apoptosis in human cells exposed to UVB radiation. Proc Natl Acad Sci U S A 1999; 96: 7974–9.

29. Ozawa M, Ferenczi K, Kikuchi T et al. 312-nanometer ultraviolet B light (narrow-band UVB) induces apoptosis of T cells within psoriatic lesions. J Exp Med 1999; 189: 711–18.

30. Gambichler T, Skrygan M, Tomi NS, Altmeyer P, Kreuter A. Changes of antimicrobial peptide mRNA expression in atopic eczema following phototherapy. Br J Dermatol 2006; 155: 1275–8.

31. Silva SH, Guedes AC, Gontijo B et al. Influence of narrow-band UVB phototherapy on cutaneous mictobiota of children with atopic dermatitis. J Eur Acad Dermatol Venereol 2006; 20: 1114–20.

32. Midelfart K, Sternvold SE, Volden G. Combined UVB and UVA phototherapy of atopic eczema. Dermatologica 1985; 171: 95–8.

33. Jekler J, Larkö O. Phototherapy for atopic dermatitis with ultraviolet A (UVA), low-dose UVB and combined UVA and UVB: two paired-comparison studies. Photodermatol Photoimmunol Photomed 1991; 8: 151–6.

34. Pasić A, Ceović R, Lipozencić J et al. Phototherapy in pediatric patients. Pediatr Dermatol 2003; 20: 71–7.

35. Valkova S, Velkova A. UVA/UVB phototherapy for atopic dermatitis revisited. J Dermatology Treat 2004; 15: 239–44.

36. Krutmann J, Schöpf E. High-dose-UVA1 phototherapy: a novel and highly effective approach for the treatment of acute exacerbation of atopic dermatitis. Acta Derm Venereol Suppl (Stockh) 1992; 176: 120–2.

37. Krutmann J, Czech W, Diepgen T et al. High-dose UVA1 therapy in the treatment of patients with atopic dermatitis. J Am Acad Dermatol 1992; 26: 225–30.

38. von Kobyletzki G, Pieck C, Hoffmann K, Frietag M, Altmeyer P. Medium-dose UVA1 cold-light phototherapy in the treatment of severe atopic dermatitis. J Am Acad Dermatol 1999; 41: 931–7.

39. Abeck D, Schmidt T, Fesq H et al. Long-term efficacy of medium-dose UVA1 phototherapy in atopic dermatitis. J Am Acad Dermatol 2000; 42: 254–7.

40. Tzaneva S, Seeber A, Schwaiger M, Hönigsmann H, Tanew A. High-dose versus medium-dose UVA1 phototherapy for patients with severe generalized atopic dermatitis. J Am Acad Dermatol 2001; 45: 503–7.

41. Dittmar HC, Pflieger D, Schöpf E, Simon JC. UVA1 phototherapy. Pilot study of dose finding in acute exacerbated atopic dermatitis. Hautarzt 2001; 52: 423–7.

42. Breuckmann F, von Kobyletzki G, Avermaete A et al. Mononuclear cells in atopic dermatitis in vivo: immunomodulation of the cutaneous infiltrate by medium-dose UVA1 phototherapy. Eur J Med Res 2002; 7: 315–22.

43. Morita A, Werfel T, Stege H et al. Evidence that singlet oxygen-induced human T helper cell apoptosis is the basic mechanism of ultraviolet-A radiation phototherapy. J Exp Med 1997; 186: 1763–8.

44. von Kobyletzki G, Pieck C, Hoxtermann S, Freitag M, Altmeyer P. Circulating activation markers of severe atopic dermatitis following ultraviolet A1 cold light phototherapy: eosinophil cationic protein, soluble interleukin-2 receptor and soluble interleukin-4 receptor. Br J Dermatol 1999; 140: 966–8.

45. Krutmann J, Diepgen TL, Luger TA et al. High-dose UVA1 therapy for atopic dermatitis: results of a multicenter trial. J Am Acad Dermatol 1998; 38: 589–93.

46. Polderman MC, Wintzen M, le Cessie S, Pavel S. UVA1 cold light therapy in the treatment of atopic dermatitis: 61 patients treated in the Leiden University Medical Center. Photodermatol Photoimmunol Photomed 2005; 21: 93–6.

47. Schmidt T, Abeck D, Boeck K, Mempel M, Ring J. UVA1 irradiation is effective in treatment of chronic vesicular dyshidrotic hand eczema. Acta Derm Venereol 1998; 78: 318–19.

48. Tuchinda C, Kerr HA, Taylor CR et al. UVA1 phototherapy for cutaneous diseases: an experience of 92 cases in the United States. Photodermatol Photoimmunol Photomed 2006; 22: 247–53.

49. Breuckmann F, von Kobyletzki G, Avermaete A, Altmeyes P, Kreuter A. Efficacy of ultraviolet A1 phototherapy on the expression of bcl-2 in atopic dermatitis and cutaneous T-cell lymphoma in vivo: a comparison study. Photodermatol Photoimmunol Photomed 2002; 18: 217–22.

50. Breuckmann F, Pieck C, Kreuter A et al. Opposing effects of UVA1 phototherapy on the expression of bcl-2 and p53 in atopic dermatitis. Arch Dermatol Res 2001; 293: 178–83.

51. Plettenberg H, Stege H, Megahed M et al. Ultraviolet A1 (340–400 nm) phototherapy for cutaneous T-cell lymphoma. J Am Acad Dermatol 1999; 41: 47–50.

52. Fitzpatrick TB, Pathak MA. Research and development of oral psoralen and longwave radiation photochemotherapy: 2000 B.C.-1982 A.D. Natl Cancer Inst Monogr 1984; 66: 165–73.

53. Atherton DJ, Carabott F, Glover MT, Hawk JL. The role of psoralen photochemotherapy (PUVA) in the treatment of severe atopic eczema in adolescents. Br J Dermatol 1988; 118: 791–5.

54. Binet O, Aron-Brunetiere R, Cuneo M, Cesaro MJ. Photochemotherapy via oral route and atopic dermatitis. Ann Dermatol Venereol 1982; 109: 589–90.

55. Morison WL, Parrish J, Fitzpatrick TB. Oral psoralen photochemotherapy of atopic eczema. Br J Dermatol 1978; 98: 25–30.

56. Salo O, Lassus A, Juvakoski T, Kanerva L, Lauharanta J. Treatment of atopic dermatitis and seborrheic dermatitis with

selective UV-phototherapy and PUVA. A comparative study. Dermatol Monatsschr 1983; 169: 371–5.

57. Sannwald C, Ortonne JP, Thivolet J. Oral photochemotherapy in atopic eczema. Dermatologica 1979; 159: 71–7.

58. Grundmann-Kollmann M, Behrens S, Peter RU, Kerscher M. Treatment of severe recalcitrant dermatoses of the palms and soles with PUVA-bath versus PUVA-cream therapy. Photodermatol Photoimmunol Photomed 1999; 15: 87–9.

59. Uetsu N, Horio T. Treatment of persistent severe atopic dermatitis in 113 Japanese patients with oral psoralen photo-chemotherapy. J Dermatol 2003; 30: 450–7.

60. Nijsten TE, Stern RS. The increased risk of skin cancer is persistent after discontinuation of psoralen+ultraviolet A: a cohort study. J Invest Dermatol 2003; 121: 252–8.

61. Stern RS, Liebman EJ, Vakeva L. Oral psoralen and ultraviolet-A light (PUVA) treatment of psoriasis and persistent risk of non-melanoma skin cancer. PUVA Follow-up Study. J Natl Cancer Inst 1998; 90: 1278–84.

62. Lim JL, Stern RS. High levels of ultraviolet B exposure increase the risk of non-melanoma skin cancer in psoralen and ultraviolet A-treated patients. J Invest Dermatol 2005; 124: 505–13.

63. Stern RS; PUVA Follow up Study. The risk of melanoma in association with long-term exposure to PUVA. J Am Acad Dermatol 2001; 44: 755–61.

64. Stern RS, Nichols KT, Väkevä LH. Malignant melanoma in patients treated for psoriasis with methoxsalen (psoralen) and ultraviolet A radiation (PUVA). The PUVA Follow-Up Study. N Engl J Med 1997; 336: 1041–5.

65. Wolff K. Should PUVA be abandoned? N Engl J Med 1997; 336: 1090–1.

66. Stege H, Berneburg M, Ruzicka T, Krutmann J. Cream PUVA photochemotherapy. Hautarzt 1997; 48: 89–93.

67. Lüftl M, Röcken M, Plewig G, Degitz K. PUVA inhibits DNA replication, but not gene transcription at nonlethal dosages. J Invest Dermatol 1998; 111: 399–405.

68. Marks DI, Fox RM. Mechanisms of photochemotherapy-induced apoptotic cell death in lymphoid cells. Biochem Cell Biol 1991; 69: 754–60.

69. Johnson R, Staiano-Coico L, Austin L et al. PUVA treatment selectively induces a cell cycle block and subsequent apoptosis in human T-lymphocytes. Photochem Photobiol 1996; 63: 566–71.

70. Knobler R. Extracorporeal photo-immunotherapy. Hautarzt 1999; 50: 764–5.

71. Greinix HT, Volc-Platzer B, Knobler RM. Extracorporeal photochemotherapy in the treatment of severe graft-versus-host disease. Leuk Lymphoma 2000; 36: 425–34.

72. Greinix HT, Volc-Platzer B, Rabitsch W et al. Successful use of extracorporeal photochemotherapy in the treatment of severe acute and chronic graft-versus-host disease. Blood 1998; 92: 3098–104.

73. Stevens SR, Bowen GM, Duvic M et al. Effectiveness of photopheresis in Sezary syndrome. Arch Dermatol 1999; 135: 995–7.

74. Greinix HT, Volc-Platzer B, Kalhs P et al. Extracorporeal photochemotherapy in the treatment of severe steroid-refractory acute graft-versus-host disease: a pilot study. Blood 2000; 96: 2426–31.

75. Prinz B, Michelsen S, Pfeiffer C, Plewig G. Long-term application of extracorporeal photochemotherapy in severe atopic dermatitis. J Am Acad Dermatol 1999; 40: 577–82.

76. Richter HI, Billmann-Eberwein C, Grewe M et al. Successful monotherapy of severe and intractable atopic dermatitis by photopheresis. J Am Acad Dermatol 1998; 38: 585–8.

77. Radenhausen M, Micheisen S, Plewig G et al. Bicentre experience in the treatment of severe generalised atopic dermatitis with extracorporeal photochemotherapy. J Dermatol 2004; 31: 961–70.

78. Sand M, Bechara FG, Sand D et al. Extracorporeal photopheresis as a treatment for patients with severe, refractory atopic detmatitis. Dermatology 2007; 215: 134–8.

79. Beissert S, Granstein RD. UV-induced cutaneous photobiology. Crit Rev Biochem Mol Biol 1996; 31: 381–404.

80. Beissert S, Schwarz T. Role of immunomodulation in diseases responsive to phototherapy. Methods 2002; 28: 138–44.

81. Beissert S, Schwarz T. Mechanisms involved in ultraviolet light-induced immunosuppression. J Investig Dermatol Symp Proc 1999; 4: 61–4.

17

Antihistamines in atopic dermatitis

Marcus Maurer, Margitta Worm, and Torsten Zuberbier

INTRODUCTION

Pruritus (itching) is one of the most prominent and distressing features of atopic dermatitis (AD). Patient scratching adds to the epidermal damage, thereby increasing transepidermal water loss and drying, possibly leading to secondary infection and inflammation. This in turn results in more itching and more scratching. Antihistamines have traditionally been part of the standard therapy regimen for AD, but a clear understanding of their differences, their effects, and their precise indications is essential if any benefits are actually to be gained from their use.

The role of antihistamines in AD is adjunctive. The primary therapy relies on reducing inflammation with topical corticosteroids and/or calcineurin inhibitors, as well as reducing skin dryness with emollients, as presented in previous chapters of this book. It has often been erroneously assumed that antihistamines possess general antipruritic effects and therefore that almost any antihistamine should be helpful in alleviating the vicious itch-scratch cycle of AD. Although histamine does appear to play a major role in AD pruritus, clinical studies do not support prescribing antihistamines in a generalized indiscriminate pattern. Antihistamines have a variety of pharmacokinetic profiles and properties, which are differentially suited to subpopulations of AD patients with varying clinical presentations. Used under the right indications, specific antihistamines can benefit certain AD patients.

This chapter will begin with an overview of the biology of histamine receptors and the effects they mediate. Next it will present the antihistamines which are most often used for AD. Then this chapter will review the findings of clinical studies on the efficacy of antihistamines for AD patients. Finally it will present differential indications for the selection of appropriate antihistamines for AD patients.

BIOLOGY OF HISTAMINE RECEPTORS

Histamine

Histamine is a naturally occurring, low-molecular-weight amine, synthesized from L-histidine by the enzyme histidine decarboxylase. It is expressed throughout the body and has many important roles in human health.[1] Histamine is the 'quintessential mediator' of early cutaneous inflammation.[2] In the skin, it is released almost exclusively from mast cells. It induces cutaneous vasodilation, oedema, and pruritus.[3]

General overview of histamine receptors

Histamine generates its effects by binding to receptors in the tissues. There are 4 known subtypes of histamine receptors, which have different expression patterns, signalling mechanisms, and functions. They have all been cloned and characterized.[1,4,5] All histamine receptors are transmembrane molecules that transduce extracellular signals via coupled G-protein receptors to intracellular messenger systems. Histamine receptors exist in a state of equilibrium between activated and inactivated forms.[4] They can be tipped in either direction by substances binding to them.[6] Several isoforms exist for each receptor subtype, but their functional differences are largely unknown.[1,4,5] The H_1 and H_2 receptor subtypes are more common, and much more is known about them than the H_3 and H_4 subtypes. Histamine-mediated dermatological effects occur mainly through the H_1 receptor.[3] Furthermore, all available antihistamines used for AD target H_1 receptors.

H_1 receptors

The H_1 receptor is widely expressed in nerve cells, airway and vascular smooth muscles, hepatocytes, endothelial

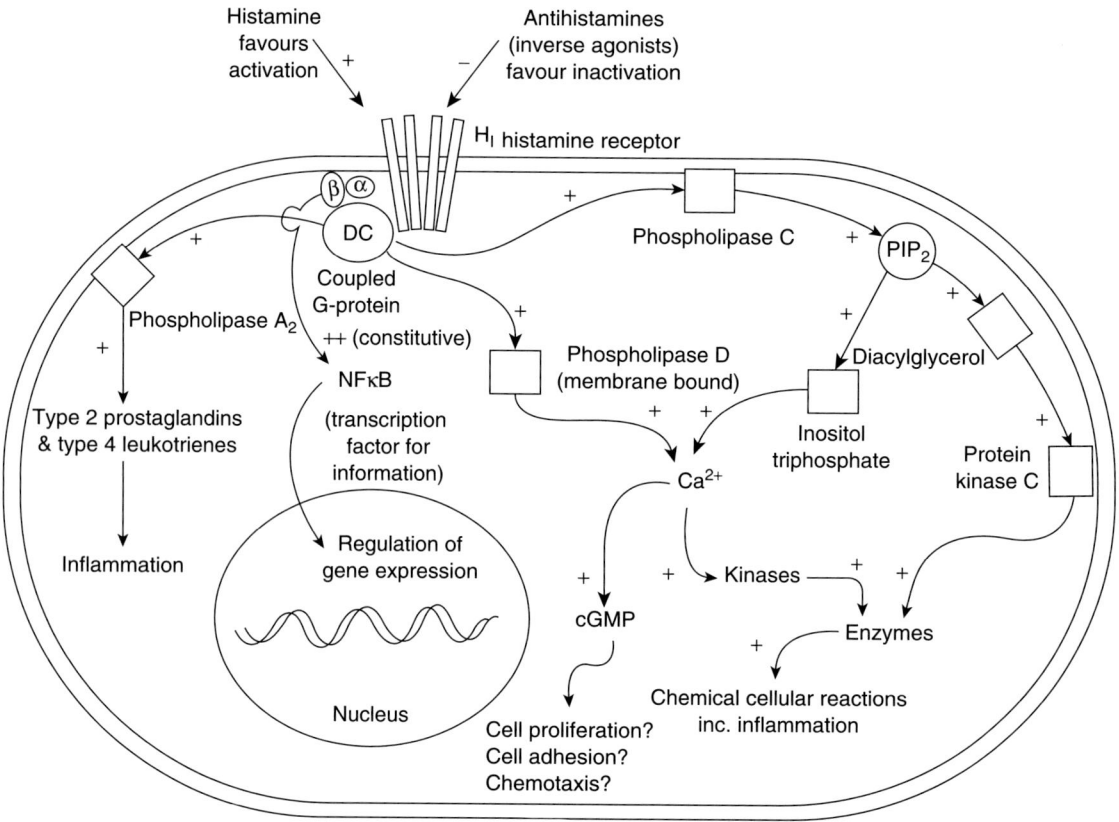

Figure 17.1 Intracellular signalling cascades resulting from stimulation of the H_1 histamine receptor. *Top:* The H_1 receptor is a transmembrane protein, with a constitutive activity in its natural equilibrium state. The binding of histamine (or other agonists) favours the receptor's active conformation, whereas the binding of antihistamines (inverse agonists) favours the receptor's inactive conformation. The H_1 receptor is coupled to a G-protein, $G_{q/11}$, which has three subunits (α, β, γ). Conformation changes in the H_1 receptor activate and deactivate the coupled G protein. The figure shows 3 of the better-known signalling cascades. *Right:* histamine activates phospholipase C, which leads to increased production of kinases and enzymes involved in cellular reactions. It also leads via increased Ca^{2+} to an increase of cGMP, which is considered to play a role in the pathogenesis of AD, perhaps through cellular proliferation, chemotaxis, and/or immune modulation. *Left:* histamine activates phospholipase A_2, which leads to inflammation. *Centre:* directly and/or via phospholipase D, the H_1 receptor regulates NFκB, which then serves as a transcription factor for inflammation. Further effects of histamine on intracellular processes are still being actively investigated, and not all pathways are completely understood.

cells, epithelial cells, neutrophils, eosinophils, monocytes, T cells, and B cells.[4] Via the coupled $G_{q/11}$ protein, it modulates intracellular signals of Ca^{2+}, cGMP, phospholipase D, phospholipase A_2, and NFκB.[4] Figure 17.1 presents the known intracellular signalling cascades resulting from stimulation of an H_1 histamine receptor. Binding of histamine to H_1 receptors mediates a wide range of general effects, including vasodilation, vascular permeability, pain, hypotension, flushing, headache, tachycardia, bronchoconstriction, stimulation of cough receptors, and pruritus.[4] H_1 receptors also have several

roles in allergic and immune reactions, including increasing the release of histamine and other mediators, increasing the expression of cellular adhesion molecules, promoting chemotaxis of eosinophils and neutrophils, increasing antigen-presenting cell capacity and cellular immunity and autoimmunity, and decreasing humoral immunity and IgE production.[4] Binding of histamine to H_1 receptors has a proinflammatory effect.[1] It is not yet known though which of these H_1-receptor-mediated effects may play a role in AD generally and its pruritus specifically.

H_2, H_3, and H_4 receptors

There are 3 other histamine receptors, but they do not currently play any practical role in the treatment of AD. The H_2 receptor has a similar expression pattern as the H_1 receptor. Histamine effects on the H_2 receptor are limited mainly to inhibiting typical cell functioning, mainly by cAMP formation.[4] The binding affinity for histamine to H_3 and H_4 receptors is 3 orders of magnitude lower than to H_1 and H_2 receptors.[4] There is little to no evidence that H_3 receptors exist in the skin,[7] and they are not widely expressed elsewhere. Currently there are no clinically available H_3 antihistamines,[4] and the couple of substances being researched are aimed at disorders involving the central nervous system (CNS), not dermatological problems.[5] The H_4 receptor is rather homologous to the H_3 receptor[5] but has a quite different expression pattern and set of functions.[4] There are initial results to indicate that the H_4 receptor is involved in histamine-induced itch and that novel H_4-receptor inverse agonists might potentially have some positive effects on pruritus that does not respond to H_1-receptor inverse agonists, as is often the case in AD.[5]

The role of histamine in atopic dermatitis

The underlying pathogenesis of AD is not entirely understood, and it is not clearly established whether histamine plays a significant role in the pruritus of AD.[7,8] Earlier studies did find elevated levels of histamine and dermal mast cells in AD patients,[7,8] so it was suggested that AD pruritus was at least partially due to histamine. More recent evidence has not supported the role of histamine in AD.[9] Other possible mediators of AD itch include neuropeptides such as substance P or certain cytokines.[8] Some authors have speculated that pruritus in AD may be due more to central rather than peripheral histamine receptors.[7,8] Stimulation of the H_1 receptor also leads to increased levels of Ca^{2+}, cGMP, NFκB, kinases, and enzymes, among other substances, so histamine may play a variety of other roles in AD, such as promoting inflammation.[4]

The role of histamine in AD is not clearly established but it probably contributes to the itching that characterizes this disorder[7] and it clearly contributes to the urticarial dermographism which is often found in AD patients. Itching is transmitted by distinct C-type nerves, and histamine causes long-lasting stimulation of these C-type nerves, leading to the perception of itching and the motor need to scratch.[3] Scratching aggravates the skin, leading to a vicious cycle of itching and scratching.[8,10,11] Treating AD centrally requires relieving pruritus, and antihistamines have traditionally been one route to pursue this goal.

PHARMACOLOGY OF COMMON ANTIHISTAMINES

Overview

Antihistamines have been widely used for several decades and new ones are continually being researched and developed. All available antihistamines are properly considered 'inverse agonists', meaning that instead of blocking the binding site for receptor activation (as with classical antagonists), their binding stabilizes the receptor in the inactive form, thus reducing the moderate histamine receptor signalling that occurs in the absence of bound substances, or counterbalancing the stimulatory effect of bound histamine.[1,4,7] Effectively all antihistamines for AD are H_1-receptor inverse agonists, and there are over 40 of them available.[4] There are only four available H_2 inverse agonists,[4] and they are almost never discussed in the literature on AD, probably mainly because the affinity of histamine itself for H_2 receptors is 10 times lower than for H_1 receptors.[3] Two small trials have tested the H_2 antihistamine cimetidine, alone or in combination with H_1 antihistamines, yet they found no significant effects. There are presently no clinically available H_3 or H_4 antihistamines,[4] though initial research on H_4 antihistamines is hopeful for AD.[5,12]

H_1 antihistamines are classified as either 'first generation' or 'second generation'. The generally repeated criteria for considering an antihistamine 'second generation' are:

1. It became commercially available after 1980
2. It has a high specificity for the H_1 receptor
3. It has a poor ability to penetrate the CNS, and most characteristically
4. It is non-sedative, though some second-generation antihistamines are sedatives, especially at higher doses.[1,3,8,13]

Although there has sometimes been talk of 'third-generation' antihistamines,[8] this term is now not considered appropriate for any currently existing substance.[1,14] In this section we present information on the antihistamines which are most commonly discussed in the literature on AD. Table 17.1 presents the pharmacokinetic properties of some common antihistamines.

First-generation antihistamines

First-generation antihistamines are the original antihistamines and they have been used for several decades in dermatology. They bind effectively to H_1 receptors but may also block other neurotransmitters.[3] Also, due to their low molecular weight and lipophilicity, they are

Table 17.1 Pharmacokinetics of some commonly used antihistamines

Antihistamine	Recommended dose	Time to peak plasma (h)	Elimination half-life (h)	Action duration (h)	Sedation
Diphenhydramine	variable	2	4–9	12	yes
Chlorpheniramine	4 mg 4–6/d	3	28	4–6	yes
Promethazine	25–60 mg	2–3	11–14	4–6	yes
Cyproheptadine	4 mg 3/d	unknown	unknown	unknown	yes
Hydroxyzine	25–50 mg 3–4/d	2	20.0±4.1	24	moderate
Cetirizine	10 mg 1/d	1	7–10	24	low
Loratadine	10 mg 1/d	1–3	8–15	18–24	none
Desloratadine	5 mg 1/d	1–3	27	24	none
Fexofenadine	120/180 mg 1/d	1–3	14.4	24	none

able to penetrate the blood-brain barrier.[1] Thus first-generation antihistamines often present a range of side–effects, most notably sedation. The term 'sedation' is used to describe various clinical phenomena, ranging from impaired daytime cognitive and motor performance, through feelings of drowsiness and promotion of sleep, to 'hangover' states and reduced morning alertness. Although first-generation antihistamines have been widely used for decades, most of them have never been rigorously evaluated and regulated for their safety.[1]

Diphenhydramine was the first antihistamine ever used, in 1947.[7] Whereas most modern antihistamines have a 24 h duration of action, which enables once daily dosing,[1] diphenhydramine only has 12 h action. It has been reported that diphenhydramine impairs driving performance more than alcohol[1,15] Diphenhydramine has been shown to be ineffective for AD as compared to hydroxyzine.[8]

Chlorpheniramine is another traditional antihistamine, which reaches peak plasma concentration comparatively slowly (3 h) and has a very short action duration (4–6 h). Although a single-patient double-blind trial found it effective, a large double-blind trial and another small double-blind trial both found no benefit for AD.[8]

Promethazine is another representative first-generation antihistamine, which has pronounced sedative effects. The one available study did not find any significant advantage in the treatment of AD.[8]

Cyproheptadine is both a histamine and a serotonin antagonist with clear sedative activity. Two studies have suggested that it reduces pruritus in AD patients; however, both studies found that hydroxyzine was even more effective.[8]

Hydroxyzine is a potent antihistamine with calming properties. All 4 published studies on hydroxyzine in AD have suggested that it is effective, though most of them lacked placebo controls and/or sufficient statistical power to draw solid conclusions.[8,16] One of these studies found that a low dose was as effective as a high dose, while being less sedative.

Second-generation antihistamines

Second-generation antihistamines were first introduced in the early 1980s and are distinguished by their relative non-sedativeness. They have a low penetration of the CNS, because they are lipophobic, do not easily cross the blood–brain barrier, and have lower affinity for central rather than peripheral receptors.[1,3,8] Consequently, they are comparatively non-sedative and lack other side effects often seen in first-generation antihistamines. For these reasons, they are normally preferred over first-generation antihistamines, though in the treatment of pruritus in AD specifically, they have not been shown to be more effective than first-generation antihistamines.[16] It must also be noted that some second-generation antihistamines including cetirizine and levocetirizine are not entirely non-sedative, especially if taken at increased dosages;[7] in fact, only 3 are permitted for use among pilots by the US Federal Aviation Administration: loratadine, fexofenadine, and desloratadine.[1]

Most important in the discussion of the value of modern non-sedating antihistamines in the treatment of atopic eczema are the non-histamine receptor related anti-inflammatory properties of these substances. For example, cetirizine inhibits eosinophil chemotaxis in vitro and in vivo, and reduces LTB_4 release as well as the expression of endothelial adhesion molecules.[17]

Loratadine and desloratadine modulate cytokine release, especially IL-6 and IL-8, from human mast cells and basophils[18] and reduce the expression of endothelial adhesion molecules.[19] Fexofenadine has also been shown to reduce the expression of cellular adhesion molecules and it inhibits the eosinophil-induced release of IL-8, GMCSF, and soluble ICAM-1 from human nasal epithelial cells.[20]

One of the major characteristics of atopic eczema is the high influx of inflammatory cells for which the up-regulation of endothelial adhesion molecules is a prerequisite. Boone and co-workers recently demonstrated that endothelial adhesion molecules, especially ICAM-1 and VCAM-1, are constantly up-regulated in AD.[21] The same authors also showed that cetirizine, at a dosage of 20 mg (twice the recommended dosage for allergic rhinitis), significantly reduces the expression of VCAM-1 as compared to placebo, whereas ICAM-1 was not affected.

Cetirizine is a metabolite of hydroxyzine and a potent antihistamine. One of the few available good-quality randomized controlled trials (RCTs) evaluated cetirizine for 4 weeks in adults with AD at various dosages. Cetirizine was found to be significantly effective compared to placebo but only at the high 40 mg dose level which was sedative as a side effect. Another long-term study has reported that cetirizine was safe and useful in significantly reducing the amount of moderate-to-strong topical corticosteroids used in infants with severe AD.[11] Two other lower quality studies have also supported the use of cetirizine.[16]

Levocetirizine is the active enantiomer of cetirizine and a potent second-generation antihistamine without cardiotoxicity, but so far no trials in AD have been reported.

Terfenadine was one of the first second-generation antihistamines. Because it is relatively free of sedating side effects, it was readily prescribed, often in off-label dosages.[7] Two good-quality studies refuted its effectiveness in AD.[16] Moreover, terfenadine was later found to cause arrhythmias and delays of the QT interval, and is no longer recommended.[1,7] Although cardiotoxicity is not a class effect of antihistamines,[1,7] the rise and fall of terfenadine serves as a cautionary reminder against prescribing antihistamines with inadequate safety testing, especially off-label.

Fexofenadine is the active metabolite of terfenadine, yet has no cardiotoxicity[7] and is non-sedative. In a recent study, Kawashima et al found that twice daily 60 mg fexofenadine in young adults with AD resulted in a rapid improvement in both diurnal and nocturnal pruritus, at a high level of significance compared to placebo, though the effect size was small.[10] The incidence of adverse effects was equal to placebo. Fexofenadine is not metabolized by the liver, and thus the likelihood of drug–drug interactions in patients on other medications is low.[3]

Loratadine is a commonly discussed, long-acting, potent, non-sedative antihistamine with no cardiotoxicity. Although 1 study did not find it effective for AD patients, 2 other small studies have supported its usefulness.[8,16]

Desloratadine is the active metabolite of loratadine; it is also non-sedative and much more potent than loratadine. It has the highest H_1 receptor affinity and is very long-lasting. It is well tolerated, and there is no cardiotoxicity even at 9× the licensed dosage.[7] There do not appear to be any studies yet on its efficacy specifically in AD though.

CLINICAL STUDIES OF ANTIHISTAMINES IN ATOPIC DERMATITIS

Although there may be good biological reasons to hope that antihistamines are effective in AD, only well-designed clinical trials can establish how effective they actually are. To date, the available evidence that antihistamines are effective in treating the pruritus of AD is limited.[22] There do seem to be some benefits for some antihistamines, but most have not yet proven their efficacy for AD patients in prospective placebo-controlled clinical trials.

Quality of available evidence

In a frequently cited paper, Klein et al reviewed the literature on antihistamine treatment of AD.[16] Although antihistamines have been in existence for several decades, they found no large, double-blind, placebo-controlled, randomized clinical trials (RCT) of their efficacy. They found only 3 small RCTs with ambiguous results, and 13 flawed or very small trials and other study designs, the value of which are quite limited. Since that time (1999), only 3 additional good-quality studies (and a few low-quality studies) of antihistamine treatment of AD have appeared. In sum, there is a shortage of solid evidence on the efficacy of antihistamines in treating AD, and more large RCTs are needed. Table 17.2 summarizes the available published clinical evidence on the use of antihistamines for AD.

Review of the efficacy of antihistamines in atopic dermatitis

From the currently available literature, there is no strong evidence that antihistamines on the whole are effective in relieving pruritus or other symptoms in AD patients.[7,16,22] Moreover, it often seems that the effectiveness of some antihistamines is primarily due indirectly to the sedative effect. Klein et al reviewed the 3 available small double-blind RCTs on antihistamines

Table 17.2   Evaluation of antihistamines in AD patients

Antihistamine	Dosage	Duration	Study	Year	Grade	Patients	Efficacious	Remarks
Diphenhydramine	various	2 weeks	Sladek	1989	D	14	No	abstract only
Chlorpheniramine	4 mg qhs	4 weeks	Frosch	1984	C	16	No	w/ & w/o cimetidine
Chlorpheniramine	8 mg bid	6 weeks	Nuovo	1992	C	1	Yes	single-patient study
Chlorpheniramine	12 mg bid	2 weeks	Nuovo	1992	C	1	Yes	single-patient study
Chlorpheniramine	1 or 2 mg OD	4 weeks	Munday	2002	B/A	155	No	sedative
Clemastine	2 mg bid	3 days	Wahlgren	1990	B	25	No	sedative
Clemastine	various	4 weeks	Yoshida	1989	C	123	unclear	unblinded, no placebo control
Promethazine	25 mg qid	6 weeks	Foulds	1981	C	20	No	w/ and w/o cimetidine
Cyproheptadine	0.25 mg/kg	1 week	Klein	1980	C	10	claimed	no placebo control
Cyproheptadine	4 mg tid	7 days	Baraf	1976	C	12	Yes	study 30 years old
Hydroxyzine	25 mg tid	7 days	Baraf	1976	C	12	Yes	study 30 years old
Hydroxyzine	25 mg tid	1 week	Monroe	1992	C	14	claimed	not significant vs placebo
Hydroxyzine	0.7 mg/kg	2 weeks	Simons	1984	C	12	claimed	no placebo control
Hydroxyzine	1.4 mg/kg	2 weeks	Simons	1984	C	12	claimed	no placebo control
Hydroxyzine	1.25 mg/kg	1 week	Klein	1980	C	10	claimed	no placebo control
Hydroxyzine	various	2 weeks	Sladek	1989	D	14	No	abstract only
Trimeprazine	20 mg	3 days	Savin	1979	C	12	Yes	sedative
Trimeprazine	10 mg tid	2 days	Krause	1983	C	7	Yes	sedative
Astemizole	10 mg	19–40 days	Krause	1983	C	6	No	no longer available
Astemizole	10 mg OD	4 weeks	Nuovo	1992	C	1	No	no longer available
Cetirizine	10 mg OD	4 weeks	Hannuksela	1993	B	26	No	non-sedative
Cetirizine	20 mg OD	4 weeks	Hannuksela	1993	B	34	No	non-sedative
Cetirizine	40 mg OD	4 weeks	Hannuksela	1993	B	35	Yes	sedative

(Continued)

Table 17.2 *(Continued)*

Antihistamine	Dosage	Duration	Study	Year	Grade	Patients	Efficacious	Remarks
Cetirizine	various	8 weeks	LaRosa	1994	C	12	Yes	non-sedative
Cetirizine	0.25 mg/kg bid	18 months	Diepgen	2002	–	350	unevaluated	>10% drop-out
Cetirizine	10 mg	12 weeks	Guzik	2002	D	34	claimed	article in Polish
Cetirizine	10 mg bid	4 weeks	Behrendt	1990	C	not stated	claimed	no placebo control
Terfenadine	60 mg bid	4 weeks	Behrendt	1990	C	not stated	claimed	no longer available
Terfenadine	60 mg bid	3 days	Wahlgren	1990	B	25	No	no longer available
Terfenadine	120 mg bid	1 week	Berth-Jones	1989	B	24	No	no longer available
Terfenadine	60 mg tid	2 days	Krause	1983	C	6	No	no longer available
Terfenadine	120 mg bid	2 weeks	Nuovo	1992	C	1	No	no longer available
Terfenadine	60 mg tid	10 days	Doherty	1989	C	16	Yes	no longer available
Acrivastine	8 mg tid	10 days	Doherty	1989	C	13	Yes	>15% drop-out
LN2974	15 mg bid	3 days	Savin	1986	C	10	No	unavailable
Loratadine	various	2 weeks	Chunharas	2002	C	48	No	
Loratadine	10 mg OD	3 x 2 weeks	Langeland	1994	C	16	Yes	
Loratadine	10 mg OD	1 week	Monroe	1992	C	14	Yes	
Fexofenadine	60 mg bid	1 week	Kawashima	2003	A	201	Yes	highly significant
Olopatadine	10 mg OD	4 weeks	Furukawa	2004	C	15	claimed	no placebo group
Oxatomide or Epinastine	30 mg bid 20 mg OD	2 weeks	Imaizumi	2003	C	32	claimed	poorly designed study
Cimetidine (H₂)	400 mg qid	6 weeks	Foulds	1981	C	20	No	w/ and w/o promethazine
Cimetidine (H₂)	400 mg qid	4 weeks	Frosch	1984	C	16	No	w/ chlorpheniramine

OD = on demand, qid = once daily, qhs = once daily at night time, bid = twice daily, tid = three times a day. Clinical trials quality grading: Grade A: Well-designed, randomized, controlled trial; Grade B: Randomized, controlled trial with minor limitations; Grade C: Observational study, flawed or very small trial; Grade D: Expert opinion, case report.

used in the treatment of AD, and they found that 2 refuted their use, while 1 supported them, but all had some limitations to their conclusions:

1. Berth-Jones et al conducted a small RCT of 120 mg of terfenadine twice daily for 1 week.[23] They concluded that terfenadine was not effective in relieving pruritus, but due to the small sample size and the imprecision of the clinical measurements, a possible treatment effect could not be definitively ruled out.[16]
2. Wahlgren et al performed a small cross-over RCT on 25 adults receiving 60 mg terfenadine twice daily, 2 mg clemastine fumarate twice daily, or placebo, for 3 days.[24] They found no significant differences in clinical outcomes between the three treatment conditions.
3. Hannuksela et al conducted a parallel-group RCT of cetirizine at 10 mg, 20 mg, and 40 mg, and placebo for 4 weeks on 178 adults, 51 of whom had to be excluded from the final analysis.[25] They found that the pruritus scores of all 4 patient groups improved significantly compared to baseline, but only the 40 mg group improved significantly more than the placebo group. They reported that 40 mg cetirizine (which is 4 times the recommended normal dose),[10] was sedative and conceded that the improvement was due to this effect.

Since Klein et al completed their 1999 review, only 3 other good-quality antihistamine trials have appeared in the literature:

1. Diepgen reported on an 18-month long, multi-country RCT of 0.25 mg/kg cetirizine versus placebo on 795 infants with AD and a family history of AD, of whom 99 dropped out (nearly equally from both conditions).[11] The value of the study is limited though because concomitant use of any other medications was allowed if reported, and because asthma onset, not pruritus, was the clinical outcome of interest. The authors did find though that among the subgroup of infants with severe AD, cetirizine led to a reduction of the amount and duration of moderate-to-strong topical corticosteroids used.
2. Munday et al reported on a multicentre, double-blind, placebo-controlled trial of chlorpheniramine in 155 children with AD.[26] They found chlorpheniramine no more effective than placebo in alleviating symptoms, and that it did not reduce the amount of topical treatment used. They took this as evidence against the view that antihistamines are effective due to sedation.

3. Kawashima et al investigated the efficacy of twice daily 60 mg fexofenadine for 1 week in reducing pruritus in young adult AD patients.[10] Their study was a large, double-blind, randomized, placebo-controlled trial, which was methodologically well-designed and well-reported. They found that fexofenadine rapidly improved both diurnal and nocturnal pruritus, at a high level of significance compared to placebo. The incidence of adverse effects was equal to placebo. It should be noted though that the mean effect size difference was small (additional improvement over placebo was 0.25 on a 0–8 compound scale). The evidence for the efficacy of antihistamines in AD from these more recent studies, along with all the studies reviewed by Klein et al, was characterized in a recent narrative review article as 'not convincing'.[1]

Positive findings for antihistamines in atopic dermatitis

Although altogether these studies have not provided sufficient evidence for the general efficacy of antihistamines in the treatment of AD,[1,3,7,8,16,22,27] they have provided an interesting insight into why some antihistamines may be helpful for some patients in managing AD. It has often been remarked that improvements in the clinical condition and patient quality of life (QoL) may be due primarily to the promotion of restful sleep, rather than to a direct reduction of symptoms.[3,8,22] Klein et al likewise underscore that Hannuksela et al only found a significantly greater improvement from cetirizine versus placebo when it was administered at sedating levels.[16] Although sedation as an unintended side effect might at first be seen as undesirable, it would seem that this is why some antihistamines are effective in reducing itching for some patients. O'Donoghue et al suggest that 'a good night's rest' improves the patient's (and possibly parents') 'overall demeanor' and therefore tolerance of the disease.[3] Another further possible explanation is based on an earlier study by Savin et al.[28] The sedative effect of trimeprazine tartrate and of trimipramine maleate (and perhaps of many other sedating antihistamines as well), reduces the amount of time during the night that the patient spends waking up or in shallow stage 1 sleep, and increases the amount of time in sleep stages 2–4 and REM, where he or she has much less deliberate motor activity. In Savin's study, those 2 antihistamines did not reduce the probability that a patient would itch in any given stage of sleep. As a result of this antihistamine-induced shift from broken/shallow to deeper sleep, patients would spend less time during the night scratching themselves and thereby exacerbating their condition. Since the management of itching is one of the more important principles of treatment of AD,[11] this particular sedative effect should not be discounted. Nonetheless, not all antihistamines are effective simply because they are sedative. Promethazine,[8] chlorpheniramine,[26] and clemastine,[16] for example, have all been found ineffective in clinical trials, despite being clearly sedative. The effectiveness of some other sedative antihistamines therefore cannot be due solely to an indirect general effect of sedation.

INDICATIONS FOR ANTIHISTAMINE USE IN ATOPIC DERMATITIS

Historical prescribing pattern

Antihistamines have been widely prescribed for AD during the past few decades, perhaps too widely.[8] One reason for this is the erroneous belief that antihistamines have non-specific antipruritic properties which will stop itching in any skin disease.[7] Also, because they are often effective in other allergic conditions and because it has been assumed that histamine plays a major role in the pruritus of AD, it has been widely assumed and hoped that antihistamines are effective also in AD.[8,16] The available evidence does not support such a widespread and indiscriminate prescribing pattern for antihistamines.[1,8,16,22] On the other hand though, it would be overly restrictive to summarily dismiss the whole class of antihistamines, as some authors seem implicitly to do,[27] especially considering the challenging long-term course of AD and the shortage of other effective options available for controlling itching.[8,22] A careful and discriminatory reading of the literature provides several indications about which antihistamines may be beneficial for which patients. A differential and targeted prescription of antihistamines may yield more satisfying clinical results than what is found in the existing studies which randomly prescribe a given antihistamine to an all-inclusive collective of AD patients.

Differentially targeted Indications

There is a general acknowledgement that sedative antihistamines often provide benefit for patients whose pruritus is primarily nocturnal and/or who are experiencing sleep disturbances.[3,8,16,22] Hydroxyzine, which is both sedative and calming, has often been found to be beneficial when prescribed for night time use, and it may represent a good option for patients complaining of sleep disturbances due to pruritus. For patients with milder pruritus yet pronounced sleeping troubles, cyproheptadine

may be better suited. The second-generation hydroxyzine metabolite cetirizine has shown itself to be effective when sedative and able to reduce topical corticosteroid use among patients with severe AD. Thus it also seems well suited for patients with severe AD that is more nocturnal, if prescribed at a high dosage. For these and other sedative antihistamines, it is important to note that the patients themselves may not always recognize these sedative effects.[1] Thus, clear patient education is essential for safety, and sedative antihistamines are more or less counterindicated for patients who are elderly, have pre-existing cognitive impairment, or who must remain alert (e.g. to operate a vehicle).[1,7]

Low-sedative and non-sedative antihistamines may be helpful for patients whose AD is more diurnal and who have other histamine-based comorbidities, such as allergic rhinitis, chronic urticaria, dermographism, or allergen-induced asthma.[8,13,16,22] Loratadine, or alternatively its more potent metabolite desloratadine, may be the first option of antihistamine for this subpopulation of AD patients. Aside from these, non-sedative antihistamines do not yet appear beneficial for AD patients, except for fexofenadine.

Fexofenadine has been shown to be more effective than placebo for both diurnal and nocturnal AD pruritus,[10] without sedation or other side effects. For patients without comorbidities or pronounced sleep disruption, fexofenadine seems to be the most useful antihistamine currently available and tested. The mean effect size above placebo is small though (0.25 on a 0–4 × 2 point scale),[10] so patients (and their physicians) should not expect fexofenadine to be a 'magic bullet' cure for AD pruritus. But some relief is better than no relief and, given its safety and lack of side effects, there does not seem to be any reason not to try it with AD patients.

Safety of antihistamines

Antihistamines are generally considered to be safe and not associated with significant side effects.[22] Although the earlier antihistamines have never been rigorously tested for safety, they have been widely used for decades.[1,29] The main concern is their sedative effect. Second-generation antihistamines are relatively free of sedative and other side effects. They have either been shown to be relatively free of cardiotoxicity or have been removed from the market.[1,7] No H_1 antihistamine currently available in the USA is considered to have carcinogenic or tumour-promoting effects.[1] H_1 antihistamines are not associated with foetal risk in pregnancy, though the US FDA at best classifies them as category B in this regard.[1,7] Thus there are generally no strong reasons against prescribing H_1 antihistamines to AD patients on a trial basis along with appropriate patient education.

CONCLUSIONS

Antihistamines have been widely prescribed for decades for the goal of alleviating the pruritus of AD. Clinical studies on the efficacy of antihistamines for AD patients do not support this kind of indiscriminate usage. Many antihistamines are simply ineffective compared to placebo for AD patients or present no advantages compared to other antihistamine options. However, certain antihistamines are recommendable for certain subgroups of AD patients, and most antihistamines are considered safe. Sedative antihistamines, such as hydroxyzine, cyproheptadine, and cetirizine, appear beneficial for night time use in patients whose pruritus is more nocturnal or who are suffering from associated sleep disturbances. Second-generation antihistamines, such as loratadine and desloratadine, appear beneficial for patients with comorbid conditions such as allergic rhinitis, chronic urticaria, dermographism, or allergen-induced asthma. Fexofenadine has demonstrated a small but highly significant reduction of pruritus in AD, so it should be somewhat helpful for many AD patients. Currently it seems to be the first option of antihistamine for all AD patients who do not fall into the previous two subgroups. There is a distant hope that 'third-generation' antihistamines (designed by molecular techniques) or H_4-receptor inverse agonists will eventually provide stronger, more general alleviation of pruritus in AD patients sometime in the future. In the meanwhile, discriminate review of the individual patient history and a differential approach to prescription may often enable antihistamines to be beneficial adjuncts in the overall treatment regimen.

REFERENCES

1. Simons FER. Advances in $H_{(1)}$-Antihistamine. N Engl J Med 2004; 351: 2203–17.
2. Greaves MW, Sabroe RA. Histamine: the quintessential mediator. J Dermatol 1996; 23: 739–40.
3. O'Donoghue M, Tharp MD. Antihistamines and their role as antipruritics. Dermatol Ther 2005; 18: 333–40.
4. Akdis CA, Simons FER. Histamine receptors are hot in immunopharmacology. Eur J Pharmacol 2006; 533: 69–76.
5. de Esch IJP, Thurmond RL, Jongejan A, Leurs R. The H_4 receptor as a new therapeutic target for inflammation. Trends Pharmacol Sci 2005; 26: 462–9.
6. Leurs R, Church MK, Taglialatela M. H_1-antihistamines: inverse agonism, anti-inflammatory actions and cardiac effects. Clin Exp Allergy 2002; 32: 489–98.
7. Greaves MW. Antihistamines in dermatology. Skin Pharmacol Physiol 2005; 18: 220–9.
8. Herman SM, Vender RB. Antihistamines in the treatment of atopic dermatitis. J Cutan Med Surg 2003; 7: 467–73.
9. Reitamo S, Ansel JC, Luger TA. Itch in atopic dermatitis. J Am Acad Dermatol 2001; 45: 55–6.
10. Kawashima M, Tango T, Noguchi T, Inagi M, Nakagawa H et al. Addition of fexofenadine to a topical corticosteroid reduces the pruritus associated with atopic dermatitis in a 1-week randomized, multicentre, double-blind, placebo-controlled, parallel-group study. Br J Dermatol 2003; 148: 1212–21.
11. Diepgen TL. Long-term treatment with cetirizine of infants with atopic dermatitis: a multi-country, double-blind, randomized, placebo-controlled (the ETAC™ trial) over 18 months. Pediatr Allergy Immunol 2002; 13: 278–86.
12. Fung-Leung WP, Thurmond RL, Ling P, Karlsson L. Histamine H_4 receptor antagonists: the new antihistamines? Curr Opin Investig Drugs 2004; 5: 1174–83.
13. Slater JW, Zechnich AD, Haxby DG. Second-generation antihistamines. Drugs 1999; 57: 31–47.
14. Holgate ST, Canonica GW, Simons FER et al. Consensus Group on New-Generation Antihistamines (CONGA): present status and recommendations. Clin Exp Allergy 2003; 33: 1305–24.
15. Weiler JM, Bloomfield JR, Woodworth GG et al. Effects of fexofenadine, diphenhydramine, and alcohol on driving performance: a randomized, placebo-controlled trial in the Iowa Driving Simulator. Ann Intern Med 2000; 132: 354–63.
16. Klein PA, Clark RA. An evidence-based review of the efficacy of antihistamines in relieving pruritus in atopic dermatitis. Arch Dermatol 1999; 135: 1522–5.
17. Zuberbier T, Henz BM. Use of cetirizine in dermatologic disorders. Ann Allergy Asthma Immunol 1999; 83: 476–80.
18. Lippert U, Kruger-Krasagakes S, Moller A, Kiessling U, Czarnetzki BM. Pharmacological modulation of IL-6 and IL-8 secretion by the H1-antagonist decarboethoxy-loratadine and dexamethasone by human mast and basophilic cell lines. Exp Dermatol 1995; 4: 272–6.
19. Molet S, Gosset P, Lassalle P, Czarlewski W, Tonnel AB. Inhibitory activity of loratadine and descarboxyethoxyloratadine on histamine-induced activation of endothelial cells. Clin Exp Allergy 1997; 27: 1167–74.
20. Abdelaziz MM, Devalia JL, Khair OA, Bayram H, Prior AJ, Davies RJ. Effect of fexofenadine on eosinophil-induced changes in epithelial permeability and cytokine release from nasal epithelial cells of patients with seasonal allergic rhinitis. J Allergy Clin Immunol 1998; 101: 410–20.
21. Boone M, Lespagnard L, Renard N, Song M, Rihoux JP. Adhesion molecule profiles in atopic dermatitis vs. allergic contact dermatitis: pharmacological modulation by cetirizine. J Eur Acad Dermatol Venereol 2000; 14: 263–66.
22. Hanifin JM, Cooper KD, Ho VC et al. Guidelines of care for atopic dermatitis. J Am Acad Dermatol 2004; 50: 391–404.
23. Berth-Jones J, Graham-Brown RAC. Failure of terfenadine in relieving the pruritus of atopic dermatitis. Br J Dermatol 1989; 121: 635–7.
24. Wahlgren CF, Hägermark Ö, Bergström R. The antipruritic effect of a sedative and a non-sedative antihistamine in atopic dermatitis. Br J Dermatol 1990; 122: 545–51.
25. Hannuksela M, Kalimo K, Lammintausta K et al. Dose ranging study: cetirizine in the treatment of atopic dermatitis in adults. Ann Allergy 1993; 70: 127–33.
26. Munday J, Bloomfield R, Goldman M, Robey H, Kitowska GJ et al. Chlorpheniramine is no more effective than placebo in relieving the symptoms of childhood atopic dermatitis with a nocturnal itching and scratching component. Dermatology 2002; 205: 40–5.
27. Williams HC. Atopic dermatitis. N Engl J Med 2005; 352: 2314–24.
28. Savin JA, Paterson WD, Adam K et al. Effects of trimeprazine and trimipramine on nocturnal scratching in patients with atopic eczema. Arch Dermatol 1979; 115: 313–15.
29. Kaufman DW, Kelly JP, Rosenberg L et al. Recent patterns of medication use in the ambulatory adult population in the United States: the Slone Survey. JAMA 2002; 287: 337–44.

18

Systemic immunomodulation

John Berth-Jones

INTRODUCTION

Most patients with atopic dermatitis (AD) are able to achieve very adequate control of their disease using the range of topical treatments described in other chapters of this book. There are, however, a relatively small number of sufferers at the extreme end of the spectrum of severity for whom the eczema simply cannot be controlled with these first line treatments Figure 18.1 illustrates severe atopic dermatitis.

The impact of the disease on the quality of life (QoL) for these patients can be devastating.[1] These patients rarely enjoy a good nights sleep as they are constantly disturbed by the pruritus. Adult patients experience difficulties with work whilst children may be repeatedly absent from school. Many of these patients experience difficulty establishing and maintaining satisfactory relationships. In some cases repeated admissions to hospital are required, each being followed by a prompt relapse after discharge.

It is in these severe cases that systemic treatment with the immunosuppressant drugs described in this chapter becomes necessary. When they are effective the improvement in QoL for such patients is often dramatic. There are hazards associated with these systemic treatments but with adequate supervision and careful monitoring the risks are justified by the benefit.

AZATHIOPRINE

Azathioprine is a synthetic purine analogue used as a cytotoxic immunosuppressant and corticosteroid sparing agent in a wide variety of inflammatory and autoimmune diseases. Even within dermatology this drug has found a wide range of applications but dermatologists are most familiar with its use in immunobullous dermatoses such as bullous pemphigoid and pemphigus vulgaris. The structural formula is shown in Figure 18.2.

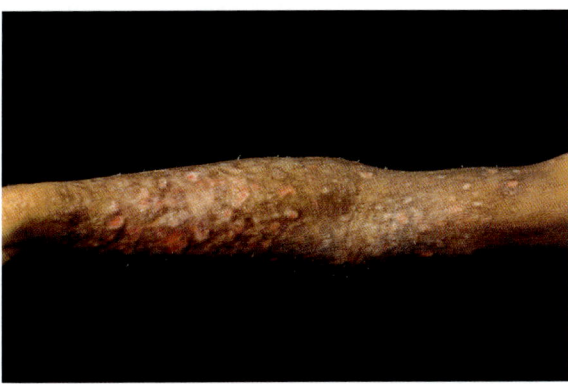

Figure 18.1   Severe atopic dermatitis.

Azathioprine

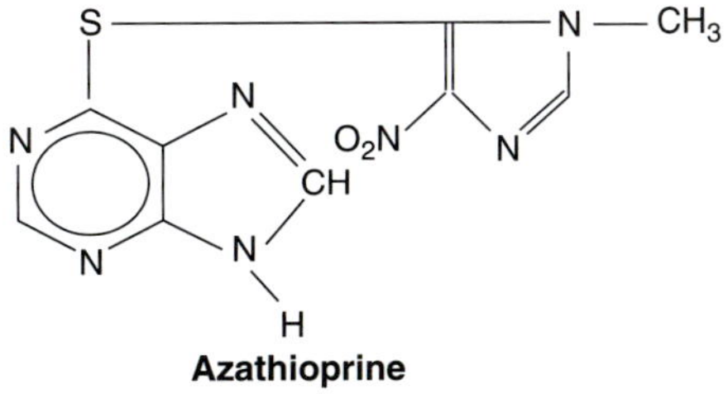

Figure 18.2   Structure of azathioprine – a purine analogue.

Mechanism of action

The active metabolites of azathioprine are also purine analogues of which the most important is 6-thioguanine. These inhibit purine synthesis and metabolism and consequently synthesis of DNA and RNA. Incorporation of these analogues into DNA and RNA in place of adenine and guanine may result in formation of brittle strands subject to breaks and point mutations. Azathioprine demonstrates pronounced antiproliferative and immunosuppressant effects. Both T-cell and B-cell mechanisms, as well as antigen presenting cell function have been shown to be suppressed by azathioprine.[2-5]

Treatment regimen

Doses employed have generally ranged from 50–300 mg daily or up to 2.5 mg/kg/day. In patients receiving allopurinol the dose should be reduced by 75%. Lower doses should be used for patients with moderate or low levels of thiopurine methyltransferase and it is advisable to avoid the use of this drug altogether in patients with very low levels of this enzyme (see below). Low doses should be used, at least initially, in patients with hepatic impairment as metabolism may be reduced. Azathioprine is usually given as a single daily dose but it is sometimes useful to split this if nausea or other mild side effects occur.

Metabolism

Azathioprine is rapidly metabolized to 6-mercaptopurine (6-MP) which is subsequently acted upon by 3 enzymatic pathways:

1. Hypoxanthine guanine phosphoribosyl transferase (HGPRT) converts 6-MP to its active metabolites, including 6-thioguanine.
2. Thiopurine methyltransferase (TPMT) metabolizes 6-MP to inactive metabolites. Genetic polymorphisms in this enzyme are known to be a major cause of the marked variability in efficacy and toxicity of azathioprine. Although several different mutations have been found in the TPMT gene, the population can be broadly divided into three phenotypes demonstrating high, moderate or low levels of TPMT activity (corresponding, respectively, to normal genotype, heterozygosity and homozygosity for non-functional genes). In the white Caucasian population approximately 1 in 300 are homozygous for a low activity mutation which can result in pancytopenia when these patients are treated with ordinary doses of azathioprine.[6] Eleven per cent demonstrate intermediate activity and the majority show high levels of TPMT activity. The latter group probably require relatively high doses of azathioprine to achieve optimal efficacy.
3. Xanthine oxidase also metabolizes 6-MP to inactive metabolites. This enzyme is not so prone to genetic variability but can be inhibited pharmacologically by allopurinol and related drugs. This may produce a dangerous interaction between azathioprine and these drugs with the risk of pancytopenia.

Toxicity and side-effect profile

Azathioprine is generally regarded as a relatively safe cytotoxic immunosuppressant but side effects are not uncommon. The greatest concern is bone marrow suppression and this is the main constraint on the dose that can be used. Most often, marrow suppression manifests as lymphopenia but any or all cell lines may be affected.[7-10] Anaemia is usually macrocytic but macrocytosis may or may not progress to anaemia.[8,9] Thrombocytosis has also been observed, and may precede thrombocytopenia.[9] As discussed above, an estimated 1 in 300 individuals is unable to metabolize azathioprine normally and is prone to development of profound pancytopenia when conventional doses are administered.

Abnormalities of liver enzymes may result from azathioprine therapy and may be more common in the atopic population (see below). Other hypersensitivity phenomena include various exanthemata, gastrointestinal disturbances, pneumonitis, myopathy,[11] pyrexia, arthralgia and renal dysfunction.[12] In occasional severe cases anaphylactic reactions and hypotension can occur.[13]

As with all immunosuppressive drugs there are risks which result from the immunosuppression. Under some circumstances there is an increased risk of malignancy, particularly lymphoreticular malignancy, associated with the use of azathioprine.[14,15] This has been most prominent in patients profoundly immunosuppressed following organ transplantation.[16] In other groups of patients, such as those with inflammatory bowel disease[17] or multiple sclerosis,[18] no increased risk has been established. This would suggest that it is the intensity and duration of immunosuppression, rather than treatment with azathioprine specifically, that is responsible for the increase in malignancy.

Unlike many cytotoxic drugs, azathioprine probably does not usually affect fertility and neither is it generally considered teratogenic.[7] However, it is certainly advisable to avoid the use of this drug, whenever possible, in women of childbearing age, and especially those at risk of pregnancy.

Monitoring

Prior to treatment with azathioprine patients should be screened for any contraindication to immunosuppression. It is recommended that patients should have a full blood count, including platelet count and differential white cell count, before starting, and at weekly intervals for at least 6 weeks after starting azathioprine. Subsequently, the intervals between haematological assessments may be gradually extended, provided there is no cause for concern. The maximum interval should not exceed 3 months. Liver function tests and serum

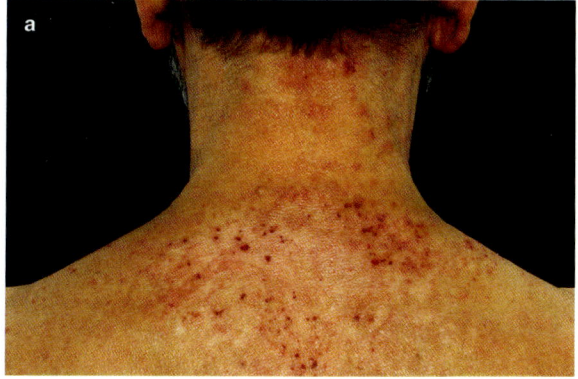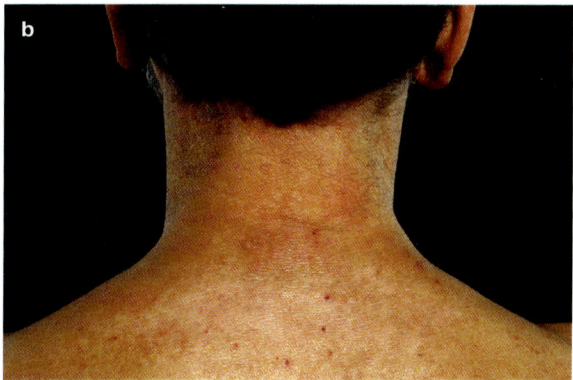

Figure 18.3   Severe atopic dermatitis (a) before and (b) after 3 months of treatment with azathioprine 2.5 mg/kg/day (a patient participating in the clinical trial illustrated in Figure 18.4).

creatinine should also be monitored. It is also recommended that patients should be examined at 6-month intervals for evidence of cutaneous or lymphoreticular malignancy. Patients should be advised to comply fully with screening programmes for malignancies such as breast or cervical cancers.

The hazard of developing marrow suppression during treatment with azathioprine can now be predicted in many cases by the assay of TPMT. Where available, and when time permits, it is recommended that this assay should be performed prior to commencing treatment. When normal levels of TPMT have been demonstrated, haematological monitoring need not be quite so frequent, although this is still required.

Drug interactions

There are relatively few drug interactions with azathioprine. Most important is the interaction with allopurinol discussed above. This drug inhibits azathioprine metabolism, increasing the potential for toxicity. Captopril may increase the risk of marrow suppression. Neuromuscular blocking agents may be increased (succinylcholine) or reduced (tubocurarine) in efficacy. The action of warfarin may be reduced by azathioprine.

Clinical experience of azathioprine in atopic dermatitis

Azathioprine does not seem to suit every patient with severe AD but it can certainly be highly effective when it is well tolerated (Figure 18.3). The efficacy of azathioprine in AD is evidenced by the frequency with which it is used. A survey of UK dermatologists indicated that 75% used azathioprine for this disease.[19] The published experience is still quite limited and, until recently, this has been entirely uncontrolled. With the exception of one early description of 3 cases,[20] all the

published reports have indicated that the majority of patients with severe AD respond well.

In small case series, Morrison et al[21] reported a good response in 2 and Younger et al[22] in 3 cases of severe adult AD.

August[23] treated 25 patients suffering from various types of eczema with azathioprine at 2.5 mg/kg/day and reported that the patients suffering from AD responded less well than those with other types of eczema.

Lear et al,[24] in a retrospective review, reported their results from treatment of 35 patients, ranging in age from 5–70, with severe longstanding AD. Azathioprine was used at an initial dose of 50 mg bd in most cases and the median duration of treatment was 7 months. Patients were asked to grade the efficacy of the drug on a scale of 0 (no effect) to 10 (100% improvement) and the average score was 6.9.

Buckley et al[25] published data on 10 adult patients with severe AD treated with azathioprine for at least 12 months. Eight improved considerably although 3 seemed to become refractory to the drug.

Scerri reported a good or excellent response in 6 of 10 adults with severe AD using doses ranging from 50–150 mg daily.[26]

Chu[27] reported the results of treating one 6-year-old and 26 adult patients suffering from severe AD with azathioprine at the dose of 2.5 mg/kg/day for periods of 4 weeks to 27 months. The drug was well tolerated by all the patients. Three adults failed to respond, leading to withdrawal of treatment at 3 months. The rest demonstrated 70–100% improvement, generally over the first 2 months.

Murphy et al reported results from treatment of 48 children with severe atopic eczema aged 6–16 years.[28] Initial doses ranged from 2–3.5 mg/kg/day. The response was considered good or excellent in 41 cases. The improvement was usually observed after 2–6 weeks. Adverse events included a single episode of eczema

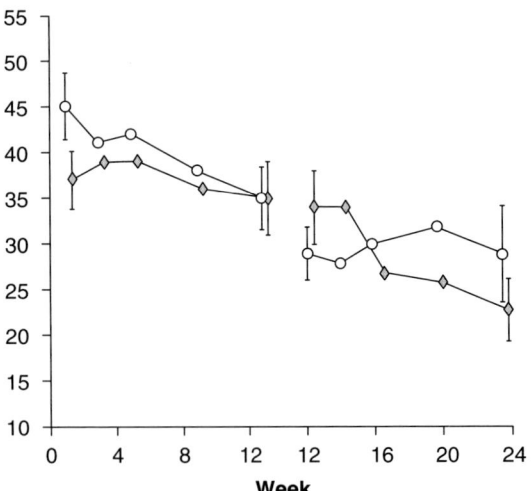

SASSAD

○ Subjects receiving azathioprine 2.5 mg/kg/day (n = 18) followed by placebo (n = 11)

◊ Subjects receiving placebo (n = 17) followed by azathioprine (n = 15)

Figure 18.4 Mean SASSAD scores during treatment for 3 months with azathioprine and placebo in a crossover trial. Error bars show standard errors (SEM).

herpeticum. Nausea, vomiting, and diarrhoea occurred in 1 child and another developed a hypersensitivity reaction comprising urticaria and vomiting. Mild, transient changes in liver enzymes were observed in 5 cases. The assay of TPMT activity was considered helpful in improving the safety of the treatment.

Meggitt et al reported results from treatment of 12 adult cases of AD in an open study using the TPMT to determine the dose used, which ranged from 0.5–2.5 mg/kg/day.[29] An objective sign score was used to monitor disease activity. There was a mean reduction of 26% in the sign score after a treatment duration ranging from 4–16 weeks.

In a retrospective case study Kuanprasert et al[30] reported that AD was well-controlled in 30 out 38 cases treated with maintenance doses of azathioprine ranging from 25–200 mg per day. Four of their patients were unable to tolerate the drug, 1 of whom developed pancytopenia.

Berth-Jones et al conducted a trial of double-blind, placebo-controlled, crossover design to investigate the efficacy of azathioprine in adult patients with severe AD and the tolerability of the drug in this population.[31] Azathioprine was used at the dose of 2.5 mg/kg/day and each treatment period was of 3 months' duration. Disease activity was monitored using the six area, six sign, atopic dermatitis (SASSAD) score. Of 37 subjects enrolled, 16

were withdrawn, 12 during azathioprine treatment and 4 during placebo treatment. The SASSAD score fell by 26% during treatment with azathioprine versus 3% on placebo (P<0.01) (Figure 18.4). Pruritus, sleep disturbance, and disruption of work and daytime activity also improved significantly on azathioprine but not on placebo. This response of the sign score can be compared to the response to ciclosporin (see Figure 18.6 below) which has been assessed in a trial of similar design. The response to azathioprine is less rapid and less complete than the response to ciclosporin. However, the dermatitis was still improving after 3 months on azathioprine so a greater improvement seems likely to be achievable with continued treatment.

The adverse events experienced by the subjects in this trial were significant. Gastrointestinal disturbances were reported by 14 patients during azathioprine treatment and 4 were withdrawn as a result of severe nausea and vomiting. Leukopenia was observed in 2 patients and deranged liver enzymes in 8 patients during treatment with azathioprine.

Meggitt et al have reported a further double-blind, randomized, placebo-controlled trial,[32] which was of parallel-group design. Sixty-three adult patients were randomized. TPMT enzyme activity was used to establish azathioprine dose. There was again a significant improvement in SASSAD score on azathioprine, 37% versus 20% in the placebo group. In contrast to the previous study, there was a marked placebo effect. Pruritus and the physician's global assessment also improved significantly better in the azathioprine group. Six patients withdrew from azathioprine treatment due to nausea or hypersensitivity.

Conclusions

Azathioprine appears to be an effective and useful drug in both adults and children with severe AD. In comparison to ciclosporin it is probably less effective and certainly slower acting but it has an entirely different side-effect profile. Unfortunately azathioprine is not consistently well tolerated and susceptible individuals can develop marrow suppression, hypersensitivity reactions, or hepatitis. Haematological and biochemical monitoring (especially of liver enzymes) are essential. The advent of the TPMT assay will make this treatment safer by helping to predict which patients are most liable to develop profound marrow suppression.

CICLOSPORIN

Ciclosporin is a non-cytotoxic immunosuppressant. This was the first of an important class of drugs now known as calcineurin inhibitors. It is rather paradoxical that ciclosporin was used initially in psoriasis, which had not previously been considered an autoimmune disease, well before it was used in AD, which has always been regarded as a disorder involving the immune system.

Ciclosporin is a cyclic peptide containing 11 amino acids with molecular weight 1203 and the structural formula shown in Figure 18.5.

Mechanism of action

Ciclosporin inhibits lymphocyte activation. This is effected by blocking transduction of the signal from the lymphocyte receptor to induce lymphokine transcription. The drug requires a cyclophilin for activity and is only active when bound to a member of this family of enzymes which are cis-trans isomerases abundant in the cytoplasm of most types of cell. The ciclosporin/cyclophilin complex binds to and inhibits a cytoplasmic enzyme – calcineurin phosphatase. Calcineurin is a calcium-calmodulin dependent serine-threonine phosphatase. Among the substrates of this enzyme is the transcription activating factor NFAT (nuclear factor of activated T cells). After removal of a phosphate group, NFAT is able to enter the nucleus and 'activate' the lymphocyte by promoting transcription of lymphokines such as IL-2, γ–interferon, GMCSF, IL-3, IL-4, TNFα and others. Activation of T4 lymphocytes with both Th1 and Th2 lymphokine profiles can therefore be prevented by inhibiting calcineurin.

In vitro studies have demonstrated numerous other properties of ciclosporin including an ability to inhibit the function of antigen presenting cells, inhibition of the release of mast cell mediators including histamine and leukotrienes, and actions on keratinocytes including the inhibition of proliferation and cytokine secretion. However, at least in vitro, much higher concentrations of the drug are usually required to produce these effects than are required to inhibit lymphocyte activation.

Treatment regimen

Doses used for treatment of AD have generally ranged from 2.5–5 mg/kg/day. The maximum dose should not usually be exceeded as toxicity is dose related. Measuring dose according to body weight in this way can result in relative overdose of obese subjects. Conversely, children tend to be relatively underdosed but this results in a useful extra safety margin and in the author's experience young patients often respond surprisingly well to lower doses.

The author recommends advising patients at the outset that a short course of treatment is planned. In those patients who tolerate the drug well treatment can then be extended if necessary. A short course of 2 or 3 months[9] duration appears remarkably safe but long-term therapy carries significant risks (see below).

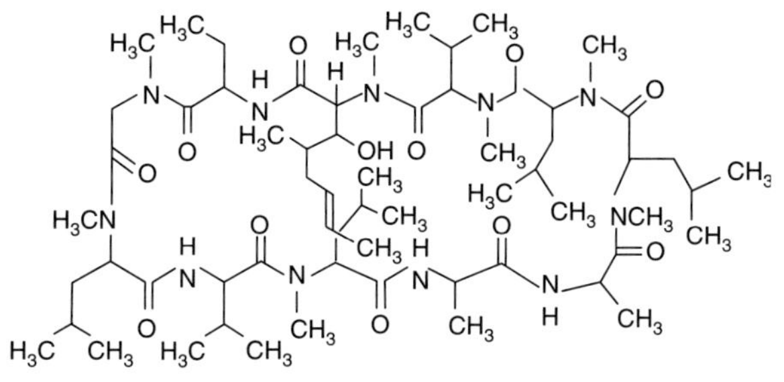

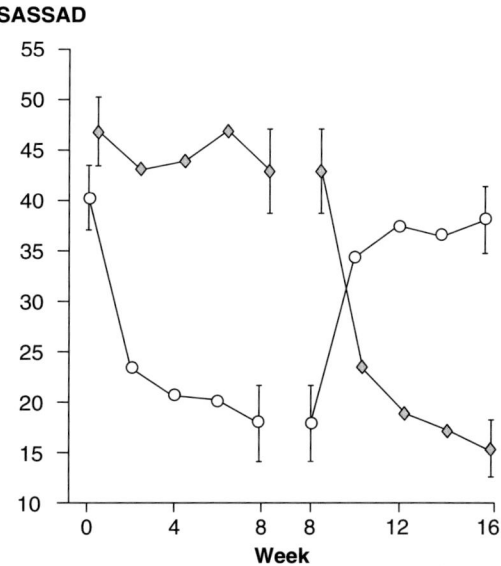

Ciclosporin

Figure 18.5 Structural formula of ciclosporin, a cyclic undecapeptide.

SASSAD

○ Subjects receiving ciclosporin 5 mg/kg/day (n = 17) followed by placebo (n = 17)

◇ Subjects receiving placebo (n = 16) followed by ciclosporin (n = 16)

Figure 18.6 Mean SASSAD scores during treatment for 8 weeks with ciclosporin and placebo in a crossover trial. Error bars show standard errors (SEM).

The speed of response is dose related. Most patients with severe AD greatly appreciate prompt relief from the pruritus. Since toxicity is not usually a problem in the short term there seems little advantage in starting at the lower end of the dose range.

Treatment should be tailed off gradually over at least 4 weeks, not abruptly discontinued, as AD may relapse very promptly and the sudden return of severe pruritus can be distressing, especially to children.

Metabolism

Ciclosporin undergoes metabolism to inactive products by cytochrome P450 type 3A isoenzymes (especially isoenzyme 3A4). It is therefore subject to numerous metabolic interactions with other drugs which can significantly alter blood levels of ciclosporin and/or the interacting drug.

Toxicity and side-effect profile

The most frequent problem requiring withdrawal of ciclosporin is renal impairment which is related to dose and duration of treatment.[33] Even short courses of treatment at the dose of 5 mg/kg/day may produce a measurable effect on renal function.[34] This appears to be reversible provided that the recommended dose rate of 5 mg/kg/day is not exceeded and that the dose is reduced, and treatment stopped if required, to prevent the serum creatinine rising to more than 130% of baseline. However, even when these guidelines are followed it cannot be stated that renal impairment is 100% reversible. In a series of 8 patients with psoriasis treated by Korstanje et al for an average of 12 months, glomerular filtration rate (GFR) had fallen by 17.8% and remained 9.8% below baseline even 4 months after stopping ciclosporin.[35] Zachariae et al have reported histological changes in the kidney in a group of 30 psoriasis patients treated with doses of up to 6 mg/kg/day for 6 months to 8 years.[36] Changes became pronounced after 2 years and the authors considered that after 2 years, if ciclosporin therapy was to be continued, estimations of GFR and renal biopsies should be performed. Powles et al reported on the renal function of 29 patients with psoriasis treated with ciclosporin for between 5 and 11 years and monitored using a combination of serum creatinine, isotope GFR estimations, and renal biopsies.[37] In the worst case, histology revealed 25% glomerular obsolescence after 10 years of treatment. The higher the dose and the longer the duration of treatment the less reversible the renal changes are likely to be but, most importantly, renal function generally recovers at least partially and does not seem to become progressive after treatment is discontinued.[37]

Additional manifestations of nephrotoxicity are the increases in serum potassium and urate consistently observed during treatment. Although these are rarely severe enough to require dose adjustment it is advisable to monitor serum potassium and urate.

Treatment with ciclosporin results in an increase in blood pressure which can be detected even in the short term. Significant hypertension may develop at any time during treatment and this is probably a dose-dependent effect. Hypertension resulting from ciclosporin therapy can either be treated along conventional lines or the dose of ciclosporin can be reduced. Nifedipine appears to have a protective effect on renal function during ciclosporin treatment. This is therefore a particularly useful drug if it is considered necessary to treat hypertension.

An increase in serum bilirubin is often observed during ciclosporin treatment. In the author's experience the largest rises have occurred in subjects who already had an elevated bilirubin prior to treatment (Gilbert's syndrome). Isolated increases in serum bilirubin do not usually require dose adjustment. Rises in transaminases appear to be relatively rare and should prompt screening for occult viral hepatitis.

Other side effects include arthralgia, gastrointestinal disorders (nausea, abdominal pain, diarrhoea), gingival hyperplasia, headache, hypertrichosis, paraesthesiae, and tremor. Nausea is most frequently encountered after the first few doses and usually resolves. Gum hypertrophy is a side effect which may be slightly more common in children than adults. This may respond to improved dental hygiene or a reduction in dose. Hypertrichosis is often seen to some degree and may be a particular problem in female patients with dark hair. Ciclosporin is known to raise serum cholesterol and triglyceride levels.

Infections, including herpes simplex, have not been a prominent problem during treatment of AD. However ciclosporin is hazardous in patients who have suffered from hepatitis B or C.

The risk of malignancy developing as a result of immunosuppression is difficult to quantify at present but appears to be small. Although there is no doubt that the risk of diverse malignancies, including cutaneous tumours and lymphomas, is increased in transplant patients, this group undergoes immunosuppression of a different order of magnitude to dermatological patients. Cutaneous malignancy is a particular hazard in patients who have received significant doses of therapeutic ultraviolet irradiation.[38]

Monitoring

Before starting ciclosporin it is important to assess the suitability of the patients by carefully checking for contraindications. These include renal disease; uncontrolled hypertension; hyperlipidaemia; active chronic infection or evidence of previous infection with hepatitis B or C; or a history of malignancy. Ciclosporin is not known to be teratogenic but should be avoided in pregnancy if not essential. In the elderly, the usefulness of ciclosporin tends to be restricted by a lower renal reserve.

Blood pressure should be recorded and examination performed for malignancy or infection. Lymphadenopathy should be documented at baseline. Patients should be encouraged to comply with any available routine screening for neoplasia.

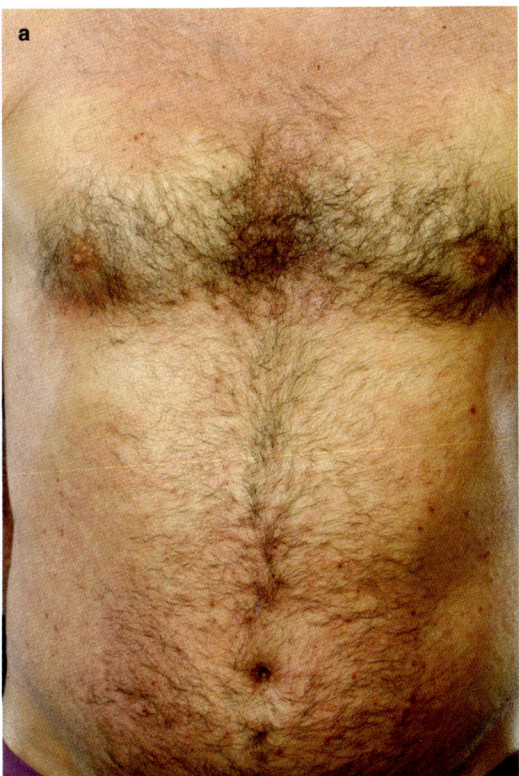 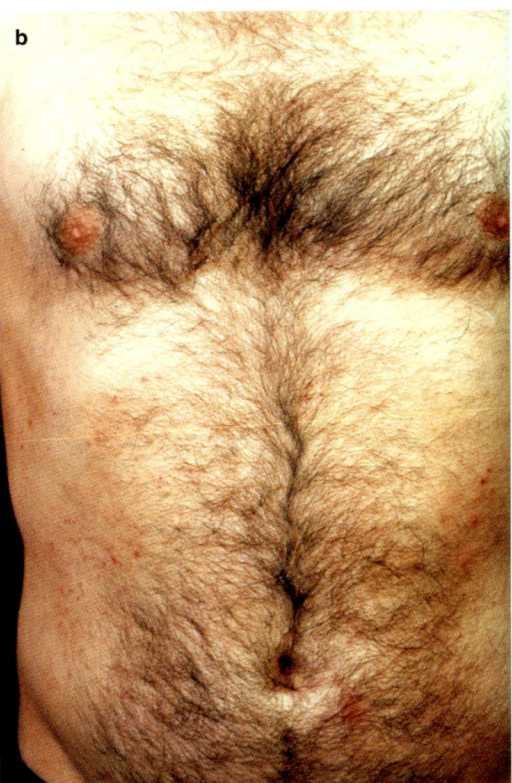

Figure 18.7   Severe atopic dermatitis on the abdomen (a) before and (b) after 8 weeks of treatment with ciclosporin 5 mg/kg/day (in a patient participating in the clinical trial illustrated in Figure 18.6).

Serum creatinine should be measured to establish a baseline. It is often surprising how much this varies from day to day, so whenever possible the author usually obtains 3 estimations at intervals of a few days, and uses the mean as the baseline value. Other useful investigations at baseline are serum electrolytes, urate liver function tests and lipids, and urinalysis to detect proteinuria or haematuria which may be indicative of pre-existing renal disease.

Patients should be reviewed after 2 and 4 weeks on ciclosporin and then monthly, or fortnightly if there is any cause for concern. During long-term maintenance therapy, if the treatment has been well tolerated for 6 months, it is possible to extend the review interval to 6 or 8 weeks in some patients.

Serum creatinine should be checked at each visit. Small reductions in GFR in the normal kidney are not detected by monitoring serum creatinine because tubular secretion of creatinine increases to compensate. However, in subjects in whom renal function is already impaired, the creatinine rises much more promptly with small changes in the GFR. This investigation is therefore most sensitive in the circumstances where

it is most important. As discussed above, published experience suggests that changes in renal function are, for practical purposes, reversible after stopping treatment provided that the dose is reduced as required to prevent a sustained rise in serum creatinine of more than 30%.

Blood pressure should also be monitored at each review. If hypertension develops this can either be treated or the dose of ciclosporin can be reduced.

Blood levels of ciclosporin have not proved a useful means of predicting the risk of nephrotoxicity during the treatment of skin disease.

Drug interactions

Ciclosporin is a drug with a narrow therapeutic index. Relatively small changes in blood levels can markedly influence efficacy and toxicity. Drug interactions are therefore an important consideration. Numerous drugs affect the hepatic metabolism of ciclosporin. Important examples of drugs inhibiting ciclosporin metabolism are erythromycin, itraconazole, diltiazem and verapamil. Drugs which may accelerate ciclosporin metabolism include phenytoin, rifampicin and carbamazepine. New drug interactions are frequently reported and it is essential to consult an up-to-date reference list of drug interactions whenever other drugs are prescribed for patients taking ciclosporin.

It is best to avoid ciclosporin, if possible, in patients requiring any other potentially nephrotoxic drugs, including non-steroidal anti-inflammatory agents.

Ciclosporin is also generally best avoided in patients taking additional immunosuppressant or carcinogenic therapies. Concomitant (or intercurrent) phototherapy is therefore undesirable since this is both carcinogenic and immunosuppressive.

Clinical experience with ciclosporin in treating atopic dermatitis

A sizable volume of research has now been published on the use of ciclosporin in this indication. This began with a series of uncontrolled observations[39] which were followed by controlled trials of crossover[40–42] and parallel-group design[43] to confirm the efficacy and tolerability of the drug. Subsequent research has examined long-term treatment, compared different treatment regimens and, perhaps most importantly, examined the efficacy and tolerability of ciclosporin in childhood AD.

Figures 18.6 and 18.7 illustrate the results of a crossover trial of ciclosporin in atopic dermatitis. There can be no doubt that ciclosporin is highly effective in AD. The pruritus can be improved within 24 hours of starting treatment. Not only the signs and symptoms of the disease but also the QoL for patients[44] have all been shown to improve during treatment. The requirement for topical steroids is also reduced by this treatment and this can be useful in circumstances where the use of large quantities of topical corticosteroids is causing concern.

Children respond well and seem to tolerate ciclosporin at least as well as adults.[45,46] Changes in renal function and blood pressure have been less than those seen in adults when children are treated with doses of up to 5 mg/kg/day although it is possible that this simply reflects a relatively lower dose, as children metabolize the drug more rapidly.

Long-term studies of up to 12 months' duration indicate that the response can be maintained without tachyphylaxis and that the drug is well tolerated over this period of time.[47,48] Initial anxiety that herpes simplex and other infections might be increased has proved largely unfounded. In some individuals treatment has apparently induced prolonged remissions after treatment was discontinued[49] but it is difficult to be certain whether this merely represents the natural history of the disease.

As stated above, dose reduction should be gradual rather than abrupt as the dermatitis may relapse very promptly. This can be achieved either by reducing the daily dose or by giving the drug once daily and then gradually increasing the number of days between doses. An interesting study by Munro et al[42] compared a reducing dosage (1 mg/kg/day steps) and a reducing frequency of treatment (1 day decrements). Dose or frequency was reduced every 2 weeks. Improvement was maintained by both regimens; however, ciclosporin 5 mg/kg once every 5 days was more effective than 1 mg/kg/day.

Intermittent short courses of ciclosporin are probably more difficult to use in AD than in psoriasis due to the greater speed of relapse in AD. This approach has been investigated both in adults[50] and in children[51] and may be somewhat better tolerated by adults. Even short courses of treatment should be tailed off and not stopped abruptly.

The dose required is usually about 3 mg/kg day and even severe cases usually respond well to this dose. A more rapid improvement is seen if treatment is started at a higher dose and then reduced, but a lower cumulative exposure can be achieved by starting with a lower dose and increasing this until control is achieved.

Conclusions

Ciclosporin is a rapidly acting and highly effective treatment for AD in adults and children. In the short term, this treatment is generally very well tolerated, especially in children, but careful monitoring is required. Nephrotoxicity is cumulative and becomes a real concern in the longer term. There are also some real (and some theoretical) concerns over the hazards of immunosuppression.

METHOTREXATE

Methotrexate is a cytotoxic immunosuppressant drug very familiar to dermatologists as it is used so extensively for treating psoriasis. It is an analogue of folic acid (Figure 18.8). Although it is sometimes used in AD there is surprisingly little published on the use of methotrexate for this indication.

Mechanism of action

There are probably several different mechanisms by which methotrexate exerts immunosuppressive and antiproliferative effects most of which are related to folate antagonism. As discussed below, intracellular methotrexate activity is mainly due to the polyglutaminated intracellular form of the drug. This inhibits dihydrofolate reductase, the enzyme responsible for conversion of folic acid to tetrahydrofolate. The latter is required for transfer of single carbon moieties used in many metabolic pathways, notably synthesis of pyrimidine (thymidylate) and purine nucleotides required for synthesis of DNA and RNA.

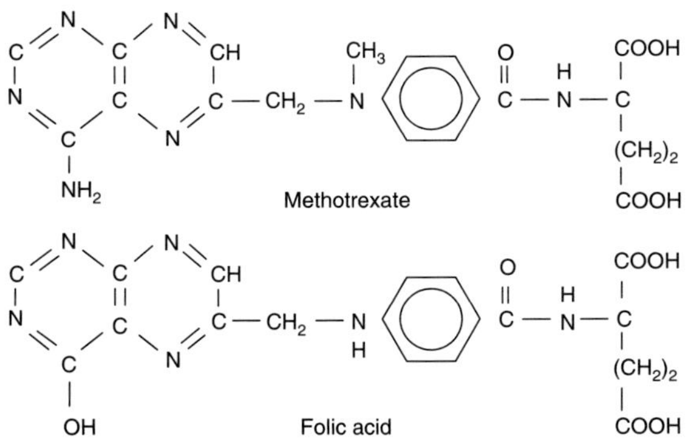

Figure 18.8   Methotrexate is an analogue of folic acid.

In addition, methotrexate polyglutamate directly inhibits other enzymes involved in the single carbon transfer pathways required for purine and pyrimidine synthesis. These include thymidylate synthetase and aminoimidazole carboxamide ribosyl (AICAR) transformylase. Inhibition of thymidylate synthetase reduces production of the pyrimidine base thymidylate required for DNA synthesis.[52] Inhibition of the transformylase may result in accumulation of its substrate and consequently increased levels of extracellular adenosine.[53] Interaction of adenosine with specific receptors, particularly the A2A receptor, inhibits leucocyte chemotaxis and production of inflammatory cytokines such as TNFα.[54–56] Methotrexate has been shown to selectively induce apoptosis in activated peripheral blood T lymphocytes.[57] Only a small part of this activity appeared to be related to adenosine release. The ability of methotrexate to inhibit nucleotide synthesis may play a more important role.[58]

Treatment regimen

No regimen has been developed specifically for use in AD. Methotrexate is therefore generally employed in a similar way as in other autoimmune and inflammatory disease. In the treatment of psoriasis doses are usually given once weekly and range from 2.5–30 mg.[59] The lower end of this range is useful mainly in elderly patients with impaired renal clearance, more usual doses lying in the range 10–20 mg weekly. In cases where absorption or compliance is questionable, methotrexate can be given by intramuscular injection. This can also be helpful when gastrointestinal intolerance occurs.

A regimen which proved successful in a prospective series of 12 patients with AD is described below.

Metabolism

Methotrexate is rapidly absorbed following oral administration.[60] The bioavailability varies considerably between individuals whilst remaining relatively consistent within individuals.[61] Bioavailability after oral administration tends to diminish somewhat as the dose is increased, possibly due to saturation of the transport mechanism.[62] The area under the plasma concentration/time curve is lower in children, suggesting that bioavailability may vary with age.[63] Methotrexate is more rapidly and probably more completely absorbed if taken while fasting than on a full stomach.[60,64] In plasma, methotrexate is largely (50–70%) bound to albumin.[65] The drug is actively transported into cells. It then undergoes polyglutamylation which has the effect of 'trapping' methotrexate within the intracellular compartment. It is this intracellular reservoir which is metabolically active and this is the reason why methotrexate need only be administered once weekly.

Methotrexate is partially metabolized in the liver to 7-hydroxymethotrexate. Most of the drug is excreted in the urine within 24 hours of oral or intramuscular administration, 80% as unchanged drug and 3% as the hydroxylated metabolite.[66] The elimination half-life is estimated at 7.5 hours.[60] The rate of clearance is related to creatinine clearance which at least partly explains the reduced clearance rate with increasing age.[60] Clearance increases with increasing body weight. The clearance rate is some 17% lower in females than males, indicating that females are at higher risk of toxicity.[60] In addition to filtration by the glomeruli, methotrexate is actively secreted in the renal tubule.[67] Significant amounts of methotrexate are excreted in bile.[68] Enterohepatic circulation takes place so that only a small proportion is eliminated via the gastrointestinal tract.

Toxicity and side-effect profile

Common side effects during methotrexate therapy include nausea and other gastrointestinal disturbances. Splitting the dose over 2 or 3 days, taking food with the drug, use of antiemetics, parenteral administration, or addition of folic acid supplements may ameliorate these effects.

Bone marrow suppression is a real hazard with methotrexate therapy. Macrocytosis may be the first indication of this. Anaemia, leukopenia, thrombocytopenia or pancytopenia may develop. When such a disaster occurs, folinic acid can be used as a rescue therapy to counteract these effects.

Hepatotoxicity is a major constraint on methotrexate therapy and requires careful monitoring (see below).

Pulmonary toxicity may manifest as an acute pneumonitis or as gradual development of fibrosis. The latter seems to occur more often in the rheumatology population than in dermatological patients. Methotrexate increases plasma homocysteine. Hyperhomo-cysteinaemia is associated with increased risk of vascular disease, so this raises the possibility that methotrexate may also increase risk of vascular disease.

Monitoring

Prior to starting treatment with methotrexate, screening is required to exclude hepatic and renal disease. Haematological monitoring is recommended at weekly intervals for 4 weeks after initiation of treatment and after any dose increment.

Monitoring liver enzymes is recommended and often gives warning of hepatitis but cannot be relied upon in the long term as on occasions serious degrees of fibrosis may develop without changes in transaminases. Whilst many authorities continue to recommend liver biopsy as the only reliable method of detecting hepatic fibrosis[69] the need for this to be performed on a strictly routine basis has recently been increasingly questioned.[70] Measurement of procollagen type III amino terminal peptide (PIIINP) seems likely to prove reliable as an indicator of fibrosis.[71,72] The study of hepatic blood flow by dynamic hepatic scintigraphy has also been proposed as a non-invasive method to detect liver fibrosis induced by methotrexate.[73,74] This technique detects the changes in hepatic portal blood flow which accompany fibrosis.

Drug interactions

There are a wide range of drugs that interact with methotrexate and increase the toxicity of this drug so an up-to-date source of reference on drug interactions should always be consulted when other drugs are prescribed concurrently.

Nephrotoxic drugs are likely to impair methotrexate excretion, increasing toxicity. The same effect may result when drugs are given which inhibit the renal elimination of methotrexate such as probenecid and penicillins. Nonsteroidal anti-inflammatory drugs, including salicylates, interact by both these mechanisms.

Concomitant use of hepatotoxic drugs, notably ethanol (and probably also retinoids), is likely to result in additive hepatotoxicity.

Folate antagonists such as trimethoprim and cotrimoxazole can dangerously potentiate the action of methotrexate. Other sulphonamides, pyrimethamine (used in antimalarials), dapsone, and phenytoin also have this effect.

Displacement of methotrexate from plasma protein binding is an often cited but less firmly established mechanism of interaction.[75]

Clinical experience with methotrexate in treatment of atopic dermatitis

Methotrexate is used for AD and is considered to be effective, although there is relatively little published evidence relating to its efficacy.[76]

Methotrexate has been reported to be helpful in the management of pompholyx in adults.[77] Doses ranging from 12.5–22.5 mg weekly led to significant improvement or clearing in 5 severe cases within 1–2 months. In all these patients oral corticosteroid therapy was substantially reduced or eliminated.

Shaffrali et al[78] described the use of methotrexate in a group of 5 elderly patients with severe eczematous eruptions, one of whom had a lifelong history of AD. Four of these cases responded well.

Balasubramaniam et al reported successful use of methotrexate to treat severe and refractory AD in a 50-year-old woman.[79]

Goujon et al reported a retrospective series of 20 adult patients suffering from moderate to severe AD, treated with methotrexate for 3 months to 2.5 years, with weekly doses ranging from 7.5–25 mg.[80] At 3 months of treatment 15 patients had improved and in 13 the improvement was estimated at greater than 70%. Tolerability was reported as generally good, although 2 patients discontinued the treatment due to nausea and elevation of liver enzymes.

Recently a prospective series of 12 adult patients treated with methotrexate for moderate to severe AD was reported by Weatherhead et al[81] Methotrexate was first administered as a 5 mg test dose, increasing to 10 mg weekly from weeks 2–4, and then increased further by 2.5 mg every fourth week up to a maximum of 22.5 mg weekly. The mean SASSAD score fell by 52% from 35 to 16 over 24 weeks. Most improvement occurred during the first 12 weeks. Dermatology Life Quality Index (DLQI) also improved. These data would suggest that methotrexate may be comparable in efficacy to ciclosporin and, at 12 weeks of treatment, possibly more effective than azathioprine.

Bateman et al recently followed disease progress in a patient undergoing progressive reduction in the dose of methotrexate for AD. Association was demonstrated between levels of allergen specific T cells (reactive to Fel d 1, a cat allergen) and disease activity (monitored using the SASSAD), as the disease deteriorated during reduction of the methotrexate dose. The authors proposed that methotrexate acts by reducing effector T cells as well as memory cells retaining the capacity to proliferate in vitro.

It is interesting to observe that methotrexate is not infrequently used for treating children with other indications. It is reported to be helpful in the treatment of severe childhood asthma,[82] arthritis,[83] and inflammatory bowel disease.[84] Methotrexate has also been used for severe childhood psoriasis.[85]

Conclusions

Methotrexate is considered to be effective as a treatment for AD although further data are needed to confirm this. This drug has the advantage of being very familiar to dermatologists. Careful monitoring of bone marrow and liver function are required and physicians must remain alert to the numerous potential interactions with other drugs. There is considerable published experience of using methotrexate in children for various indications, although not in atopic dermatitis.

MYCOPHENOLATE MOFETIL

Mycophenolate mofetil is an ester of mycophenolic acid, a fungal metabolite with cytotoxic properties (Figure 18.9). It has been developed mainly as an immunosuppressant for use in renal transplantation but has found several additional applications, notably in rheumatoid disease.[86] Mycophenolate is occasionally used by dermatologists for treatment of AD (see below). Other potential indications include psoriasis,[87] pompholyx,[88] and immunobullous disease.[89]

Mechanism of action

Mycophenolic acid, the active metabolite of mycophenolate mofetil, inhibits inosine monophosphate dehydrogenase (IMPDH), especially the type II isoform expressed in B and T lymphocytes. This enzyme is required for de novo synthesis of guanosine nucleotides for incorporation into DNA and RNA. The relatively high activity in inhibiting the type II isoform of IMPDH found in lymphocytes, combined with the relative importance of de novo synthesis of guanine in lymphocytes, which lack the alternative salvage pathway active in most other cells, result in a high degree of specificity for inhibition of lymphocyte function.[90,91] Both T and B lymphocyte function are suppressed by this drug.[91] The activity of antigen presenting cells may also be suppressed.[92]

Treatment regimen

Mycophenolate mofetil is most often used at doses ranging from 500 mg to 1 g twice daily. Higher doses (e.g. 1.5 g twice daily) are also sometimes used but require careful monitoring to avoid inadvertent marrow suppression.

Metabolism

Mycophenolate mofetil is the morpholino ester of mycophenolic acid (Figure 18.9). This ester is rapidly absorbed with 90% bioavailability. It is a prodrug, and is immediately hydrolysed by esterases in the gut to mycophenolic acid, the active compound. Mycophenolic acid undergoes glucuronidation in the liver. It is excreted in bile and significant enterohepatic circulation takes place. The main route of elimination is in the urine, as the glucuronide.

Toxicity and side-effect profile

Mycophenolate mofetil is a well-tolerated drug. The most frequent side effects are gastrointestinal disturbances including nausea, vomiting, abdominal pain,

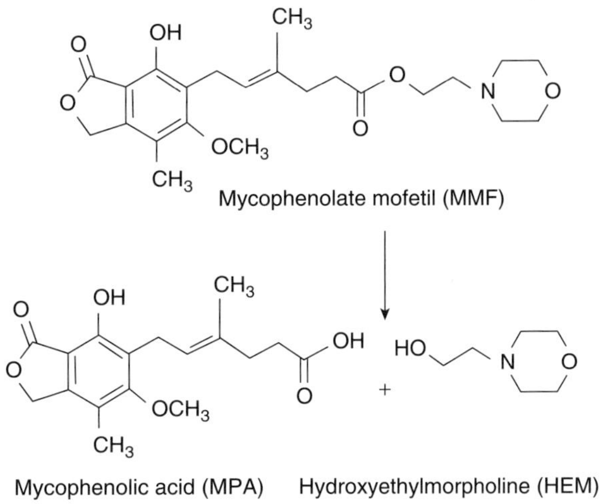

Figure 18.9 Mycophenolate mofetil is a morpholino ester of mycophenolic acid and is rapidly hydrolysed during transport through the gut wall.

and diarrhoea. Marrow suppression can occur but is uncommon at standard doses. There are, of course, risks associated with immunosuppression and both malignancies and infections have been reported. Mycophenolate has proved teratogenic in animal studies and should be avoided in pregnancy whenever possible. Neurological events reported during treatment with mycophenolate have included dizziness, weakness, insomnia, and tremor. Elevation of liver enzymes has been reported in 2 patients treated for AD but is not generally regarded as a frequent event.[93]

Monitoring

Haematological monitoring should be performed on a weekly basis for 4 weeks, then on alternate weeks for 3 months and monthly thereafter.

Drug interactions

Aciclovir, ganciclovir and probenecid compete with mycophenolic acid glucuronide for tubular secretion. Antacids containing magnesium and aluminium hydroxides reduce absorption of mycophenolate. Bile acid binding resins such as cholestyramine interrupt the enterohepatic circulation of mycophenolate and reduce blood levels.

Simultaneous administration of azathioprine is not recommended as both drugs inhibit inosine monophosphate dehydrogenase.

Clinical experience in treatment of atopic dermatitis

The efficacy of mycophenolate mofetil in AD remains somewhat controversial. There are several reports of cases responding but success has not been universal and may depend on the severity of the disease. No controlled studies are yet available. Mycophenolate is also sometimes used in combination with other immunosuppressants such as ciclosporin with the aim of obtaining a dose-sparing effect on these more toxic drugs. All but one of the published reports of treatment of AD with mycophenolate have involved treatment of adults, although there is considerable experience with the use of this drug in children from other disciplines, especially in the field of transplantation.

The first report of AD responding to mycophenolate mofetil was published by Grundmann-Kollman et al in 1999.[94] Two cases responded to daily doses of 2 g. Satchell et al then raised concern by reporting a patient in whom initial marked improvement in the eczema was followed, during treatment at the dose of 2 g daily, by development of staphylococcal septicaemia and endocarditis.[95]

In a prospective study, 10 adult patients with severe eczema were treated with 1 g daily for a week, then 2 g daily for 11 weeks.[96] The mycophenolate was well tolerated. Insomnia necessitated a dose reduction in 1 case. The eczema improved and serum IgE levels also fell. Circulating levels of IL-10 were also reduced whilst levels of interferon-γ increased.

Benez et al reported responses which were maintained during long-term treatment in 3 cases using doses of 1–2 g daily for 12–29 months.[97]

Grundmann-Kollmann et al then reported an additional 10 patients, treated with 1 g twice daily for 4 weeks, followed by 500 mg bd for 4 weeks. Seven patients responded well, 2 improved then relapsed and 1 was withdrawn after initial improvement due to herpetic retinitis.[98]

In a Korean study, 7 patients with moderate to severe disease were treated with mycophenolate mofetil 2 g daily for 6 weeks and followed up for another 6 weeks. Six of the 7 patients finished the treatment courses. Symptoms and signs were significantly improved and no severe side effects were observed. During the follow-up period, patients were treated with topical steroids and oral antihistamine and no flares occurred.[99]

In an American report, Murray et al retrospectively reviewed a series of 20 adults treated for AD with mycophenolate mofetil using doses from 1–3 g/day. Treatment duration extended from 4–200 weeks. Seventeen were reported to improve within 4 weeks. Most patients tolerated the treatment well although 4 developed episodes of herpes zoster and others reported gastrointestinal side effects, fatigue, anorexia, and headache.

In the first report of the use of mycophenolate mofetil in childhood AD, Heller et al described the results in a retrospective series of 14 patients aged 2–16. Initial doses ranged from 12–40 mg/kg/day,

divided into 2 doses. Doses were titrated upward until patients achieved remission or reached a dose of 75 mg/kg/day (with a 3 g daily maximum). Four achieved complete clearance, 4 had more than 90% improvement whilst only 1 failed to respond at all. The treatment was well tolerated in all cases.

In contrast to these reports, Hansen et al reported 5 severe cases which failed to respond to mycophenolate mofetil 1–1.25 g twice daily after 4–12 weeks.[100]

It has been suggested that the failure of these patients to respond may have been related to exceptional disease severity.[101]

The author has not found mycophenolate mofetil very helpful in very severe adult cases of AD at doses of 2–3 g daily. However, the drug has been very well tolerated. Gastrointestinal disturbances, especially diarrhoea, have occasionally been troublesome.

Conclusions

The place of mycophenolate in the treatment of AD remains to be established. Efficacy may be limited but mycophenolate is generally well tolerated and is probably the least toxic of the drugs described in this chapter.

REFERENCES

1. Long CC, Funnell CM, Collard R, Finlay AY. What do members of the National Eczema Society really want? Clin Exp Dermatol 1993; 18: 516–22.
2. Levin RH, Landy M, Frie E. The effects of 6-MP on immune responses in man. N Engl J Med 1964; 271: 16–22.
3. Levy J, Barnett EV, MacDonald NS et al. The effect of azathioprine on gammaglobulin synthesis in man. J Clin Invest 1972; 51: 2233–8.
4. Younger IR, Harris DWS, Colver GB. Azathioprine in dermatology. J Am Acad Dermatol 1991; 25: 281–8.
5. Liu H, Wong C. In vitro immunosuppressive effects of methotrexate and azathioprine on Langerhans cells. Arch Dermatol Res 1997; 289: 94–7.
6. Anstey A, Lennard L, Mayou SC, Kirby JD. Pancytopenia related to azathioprine – an enzyme deficiency caused by a common genetic polymorphism: a review. J Roy Soc Med 1992; 85: 752–6.
7. Lawson DH, Lovatt GE, Gurton CS, Hennings RC. Adverse effects of azathioprine. Adverse Drug React Acute Poisoning Rev 1984; 3: 161–71.
8. Du Vivier A, Munro DD, Verbov J. Treatment of psoriasis with azathioprine. Br Med J 1974; 1(5897): 49–51.
9. Hewitt J, Escande JP, Leibowitch M, Francheschini P. Trial therapy of psoriasis with azathioprine. Bull Soc Fr Dermatol Syphiligr 1970; 77: 392–6.
10. Pinals RS. Azathioprine in the treatment of chronic polyarthritis: longterm results and adverse effects in 25 patients. J Rheumatol 1976; 3: 140–4.
11. Clayton R. Azathioprine in psoriasis. Br Med J 1974; 2: 443.
12. McHenry PM, Allan JG, Rodger RS, Lever RS. Nephrotoxicity due to azathioprine. Br J Dermatol 1993; 128: 106.
13. Jones JJ, Ashworth J. Azathioprine-induced shock in dermatology patients. J Am Acad Dermatol 1993; 29: 795–6.

14. Gruber SA, Skjei KL, Sothern RB et al. Cancer development in renal allograft recipients treated with conventional and cyclosporine immunosuppression. Transplant Proc 1991; 23: 1104–5.

15. Tennis P, Andrews E, Bombardier C et al. Record linkage to conduct an epidemiologic study on the association of rheumatoid arthritis and lymphoma in the province of Saskatchewan, Canada. J Clin Epidemiol 1993; 46: 685–95.

16. Kinlen LJ, Shiel AGR, Peto J, Doll R. Collaborative United Kingdom – Australian study of cancer in patients treated with immunosuppressive drugs. Br Med J 1979; 2: 1461–6.

17. Connell WR, Kamm MA, Dickson M et al. Long-term neoplasia risk after treatment in inflammatory bowel disease. Lancet 1994; 343: 1249–52.

18. Armato MP, Pracucci G, Ponziani G et al. Long term safety of azathioprine therapy in multiple sclerosis. Neurology 1993; 43: 831–3.

19. Tan BB, Lear JT, Gawkrodger DJ, English JSC. Azathioprine in dermatology: a survey of current practice in the U.K. Br J Dermatol 1997; 136: 351–5.

20. Gunnar S, Johansson O, Juhlin L. Immunoglobulin E in "healed" atopic dermatitis and after treatment with corticosteroids and azathioprine. Br J Dermatol 1970; 82: 10–13.

21. Morrison JGL, Schulz EJ. Treatment of eczema with cyclophosphamide and azathioprine. Br J Dermatol 1978; 98: 203–7.

22. Younger IR, Harris DW, Colver GB. Azathioprine in dermatology. J Am Acad Dermatol 1991; 25: 281–6.

23. August PJ. Azathioprine in the treatment of eczema and actinic reticuloid. Br J Dermatol 1982; 107(suppl 22): 23.

24. Lear JT, English JSC, Jones P, Smith AG. Retrospective review of the use of azathioprine in severe atopic dermatitis. J Am Acad Dermatol 1996; 35: 642–3.

25. Buckley DA, Baldwin P, Rogers S. The use of azathioprine in severe adult atopic eczema. J Eur Acad Dermatol 1998; 11: 137–40.

26. Scerri L. Azathioprine in dermatological practice. An overview with special emphasis on its use in non-bullous inflammatory dermatoses. Adv Exp Med Biol 1999; 455: 343–8.

27. Chu AC. The role of systemic therapy in atopic eczema. CME Bulletin Dermatology. London: Rila Publications Ltd, 1999; 2: 23–8.

28. Murphy LA. Atherton D. A retrospective evaluation of azathioprine in severe childhood atopic eczema, using thiopurine methyltransferase levels to exclude patients at high risk of myelosuppression. Br J Dermatol 2002; 147: 308–15.

29. Meggitt SJ, Reynolds NJ. Azathioprine for atopic dermatitis. Clin Exp Dermatol 2001; 26: 369–75.

30. Kuanprasert N, Herbert O, Barnetson RS. Clinical improvement and significant reduction of total serum IgE in patients suffering from severe atopic dermatitis treated with oral azathioprine. Australas J Dermatol 2002; 43: 125–7.

31. Berth-Jones J, Takwale A, Tan E et al. Azathioprine in severe adult atopic dermatitis: a double-blind, placebo-controlled, crossover trial. Br J Dermatol 2002; 147: 324–30.

32. Meggitt SJ, Gray JC, Reynolds NJ. Azathioprine dosed by thiopurine methyltransferase activity for moderate-to-severe atopic eczema: a double-blind, randomised controlled trial. Lancet 2006; 367(9513): 839–46.

33. Young EW, Ellis CN, Messana SM et al. A prospective study of renal structure and function in psoriasis patients treated with cyclosporin. Kidney Int 1994; 46: 1216–22.

34. Berth-Jones J, Sowden JM, Feehally J, Graham-Brown RAC. Treatment of severe refractory atopic dermatitis with cyclosporin. Lancet 1991; 338: 643.

35. Korstanje MJ, Bilo HJ, Stoof TJ. Sustained renal function loss in psoriasis patients after withdrawal of low-dose cyclosporin therapy. Br J Dermatol 1992; 127: 501–4.

36. Zachariae H, Kragballe K, Hansen HE et al. Renal biopsy findings in long-term cyclosporin treatment of psoriasis. Br J Dermatol 1997; 136: 531–5.

37. Powles AV, Hardman CM, Porter WM et al. Renal function after 10 years' treatment with cyclosporin for psoriasis. Br J Dermatol 1998: 138; 443–9.

38. Marcil I, Stern RS. Squamous-cell cancer of the skin in patients given PUVA and ciclosporin: nested cohort crossover study. Lancet 2001; 358(9887): 1042–5.

39. Van Joost T, Stolz E, Heule F. Efficacy of low-dose cyclosporine in severe atopic skin disease. Arch Dermatol 1987; 123: 166–7.

40. Sowden JM, Berth-Jones J, Ross JS et al. Double-blind, controlled, crossover study of cyclosporin in adults with severe refractory atopic dermatitis. Lancet 1991; 338: 137–40.

41. Wahlgren CF, Scheynius A, Hagermark O. Antipruritic effect of oral ciclosporin in atopic dermatitis. Acta Derm Venereol (Stockh) 1990; 70: 323–9.

42. Munro CS, Levell N, Friedmann P, Shuster S. Low dose or intermittent cyclosporin maintains remission in atopic eczema. Br J Dermatol 1992; 127(Suppl 40): 13–14.

43. Van Joost T, Heule F, Korstanje M et al. Cyclosporin in atopic dermatitis: a multicentre placebo-controlled study. Br J Dermatol 1994; 130: 634–40.

44. Salek MS, Finlay AY, Luscombe DK et al. Cyclosporin greatly improves the quality of life of adults with severe atopic dermatitis. A randomized, double-blind, placebo-controlled trial. Br J Dermatol 1993; 129: 422–30.

45. Berth-Jones J, Finlay AY, Zaki I et al. Cyclosporin in severe childhood atopic dermatitis: a multicenter study. J Am Acad Dermatol 1996; 34: 1016–21.

46. Zaki I, Emerson R, Allen BR. Treatment of severe atopic dermatitis in childhood with cyclosporin. Br J Dermatol 1996; 135(Suppl 48): 21–4.

47. Berth-Jones J, Graham-Brown RAC, Marks R et al. Long-term efficacy and safety of cyclosporin in severe adult atopic dermatitis. Br J Dermatol 1997; 136: 76–81.

48. Zonneveld IM, De Rie MA, Beljaards RC et al. The long term safety and efficacy of cyclosporin in severe refractory atopic dermatitis: a comparison of two dosage regimens. Br J Dermatol 1996; 135(suppl 48): 15–20.

49. Sepp N, Fritsch PO. Can cyclosporin A induce permanent remission of atopic dermatitis? Br J Dermatol 1993; 128: 213–16.

50. Granlund H, Erkko P, Sinisalo M, Reitamo S. Cyclosporin in atopic dermatitis: time to relapse and effect of intermittent therapy. Br J Dermatol 1995; 132: 106–12.

51. Ahmed I, Berth-Jones J, Friedmann PS et al. Short course versus continuous therapy with cyclosporin in severe childhood atopic dermatitis. Br J Dermatol 1998; 139 (suppl 51): 22.

52. Baggott JE, Morgan SL, Ha TS et al. Antifolates in rheumatoid arthritis: a hypothetical mechanism of action. Clin Exp Rheumatol 1993; 11 (suppl 8): S101–5.

53. Cronstein BN, Naime D, Ostad E. The antiinflammatory mechanism of methotrexate. Increased adenosine release at inflamed sites diminishes leukocyte accumulation in an in vivo model of inflammation. J Clin Invest 1993; 92: 2675–82.

54. Montesinos MC, Desai A, Delano D et al. Adenosine A2A or A3 receptors are required for inhibition of inflammation by methotrexate and its analog MX-68. Arthritis Rheum 2003; 48: 240–7.

55. Chan ES, Cronstein BN. Molecular action of methotrexate in inflammatory diseases. Arthritis Res 2002; 4: 266–73.

56. Ohta A, Sitkovsky M. Role of G-protein-coupled adenosine receptors in downregulation of inflammation and protection from tissue damage. Nature 2001; 414(6866): 916–20.

57. Genestier L, Paillot R, Fournel S et al. Immunosuppressive properties of methotrexate: apoptosis and clonal deletion of activated peripheral T cells. J Clin Invest 1998; 102: 322–8.

58. Quemeneur L, Gerland LM, Flacher M et al. Differential control of cell cycle, proliferation, and survival of primary T lymphocytes by purine and pyrimidine nucleotides. J Immunol 2003; 170: 4986–95.

59. Griffiths CEM, Camp RDR, Barker JNWN. Psoriasis. In: Burns T, Breathnach S, Cox N, Griffiths C, eds. Rook's Textbook of Dermatology, 7th edn., Oxford: Blackwell Science, 2004; 35: 37–40.

60. Godfrey C, Sweeney K, Miller R et al. The population pharmacokinetics of long-term methotrexate in rheumatoid patients. Br J Clin Pharmacol 1998; 46: 369–76.

61. Lebbe C, Beyeler C, Gerber NJ, Reichen J. Intraindividual variability of the bioavailability of low dose methotrexate after oral administration in rheumatoid arthritis. Ann Rheum Dis 1994; 53: 475–7.

62. Hamilton RA, Kremer JM. Why intramuscular methotrexate may be more efficacious than oral dosing in patients with rheumatoid arthritis. Br J Rheumatol 1997; 36: 86–90.

63. Albertioni F, Flato B, Seideman P et al. Methotrexate in juvenile rheumatoid arthritis. Evidence of age dependent pharmacokinetics. Eur J Clin Pharmacol 1995; 47: 507–11.

64. Dupuis LL, Koren G, Silverman ED, Laxer RM. Influence of food on the bioavailability of oral methotrexate in children. J Rheumatol 1995; 22: 1570–3.

65. Bleyer WA. The clinical pharmacology of methotrexate: new applications of an old drug. Cancer 1978; 41: 36–51.

66. Seideman P, Beck O, Eksborg S, Wennberg M. The pharmacokinetics of methotrexate and its 7-hydroxy metabolite in patients with rheumatoid arthritis. Br J Clin Pharmacol 1993; 35: 409–12.

67. Masereeuw R, Russel FG, Miller DS. Multiple pathways of organic anion secretion in renal proximal tubule revealed by confocal microscopy. Am J Physiol 1996; 271: 1173–82.

68. Hendel J, Brodthagen H. Entero-hepatic cycling of methotrexate estimated by use of the D-isomer as a reference marker. Eur J Clin Pharmacol 1984; 26: 103–7.

69. Roenigk HH Jr, Auerbach R, Maibach H et al. Methotrexate in psoriasis: consensus conference. J Am Acad Dermatol 1998; 38: 478–85.

70. Zachariae H. Liver biopsies and methotrexate: a time for reconsideration? J Am Acad Dermatol 2000; 42: 531–4.

71. Zachariae H, Heickendorff L, Sogaard H. The value of aminoterminal propeptide of type III procollagen in routine screening for methotrexate-induced liver fibrosis: a 10-year follow-up. Br J Dermatol 2001; 144: 100–3.

72. Boffa MJ, Smith A, Chalmers RJ et al. Serum type III procollagen aminopeptide for assessing liver damage in methotrexate-treated psoriatic patients. Br J Dermatol 1996; 135: 538–44.

73. McHenry PM, Bingham EA, Callender ME et al. Dynamic hepatic scintigraphy in the screening of psoriatic patients for methotrexate-induced hepatotoxicity. Br J Dermatol 1992; 127: 122–5.

74. VanDooren-Greebe RJ, Kuijpers AL, Buijs WC et al. The value of dynamic hepatic scintigraphy and serum aminoterminal propeptide of type III procollagen for early detection of methotrexate-induced hepatic damage in psoriasis patients. Br J Dermatol 1996; 134: 481–7.

75. Furst DE. Practical clinical pharmacology and drug interactions of low-dose methotrexate therapy in rheumatoid arthritis. Br J Rheumatol 1995; 34(Suppl 2): 20–5.

76. Sidbury R, Hanifin JM. Systemic therapy of atopic dermatitis. Clin Exp Dermatol 2000; 25: 559–66.

77. Egan CA, Rallis TM, Meadows KP, Krueger GG. Low-dose oral methotrexate treatment for recalcitrant palmoplantar pompholyx. J Am Acad Dermatol 1999; 40: 612–14.

78. Shaffrali FC, Colver GB, Messenger AG, Gawkrodger DJ. Experience with low-dose methotrexate for the treatment of eczema in the elderly. J Am Acad Dermatol 2003; 48: 417–19.

79. Balasubramaniam P, Ilchyshyn A. Successful treatment of severe atopic dermatitis with methotrexate. Clin Exp Dermatol 2005; 30: 436–7.

80. Goujon C, Berard F, Dahel K et al. Methotrexate for the treatment of adult atopic dermatitis. Eur J Dermatol 2006; 16: 155–8.

81. Weatherhead SC, Wahie S, Reynolds NJ, Meggitt SJ. An open-label, dose-ranging study of methotrexate for moderate-to-severe adult atopic eczema. Br J Dermatol 2007; 156: 346–51.

82. Guss S, Portnoy J. Methotrexate treatment of severe asthma in children. Pediatrics 1992; 89: 635–9.

83. Cron RQ. Current treatment for chronic arthritis in childhood. Curr Opin Pediatr 2002; 14: 684–7.

84. Gremse DA, Crissinger KD. Ulcerative colitis in children: medical management. Paediatr Drugs 2002; 4: 807–15.

85. Kumar B, Dhar S, Handa S, Kaur I. Methotrexate in childhood psoriasis. Pediatr Dermatol 1994; 11: 271–3.

86. Goldblum R. Therapy of rheumatoid arthritis with mycophenolate mofetil. Clin Exp Rheumatol 1993; 11(suppl 8): 117–19.

87. Spatz S, Rudnicka A, McDonald CJ. Mycophenolic acid in psoriasis. Br J Dermatol 1978; 98: 429–35.

88. Pickenacker A, Luger TA, Schwarz T. Dyshidrotic eczema treated with mycophenolate mofetil. Arch Dermatol 1998; 134: 378–9.

89. Bohm M, Beissert S, Schwarz T et al. Bullous pemphigoid treated with mycophenolate mofetil. Lancet 1997; 349(9051): 541.

90. Allison AC, Eugui EM. Mycophenolate mofetil and its mechanisms of action. Immunopharmacology 2000; 47: 85–118.

91. Eugui EM, Mirkovich A, Allison AC. Lymphocyte-selective antiproliferative and immunosuppressive effects of mycophenolic acid in mice. Scand J Immunol 1991; 33: 175–83.

92. Mehling A, Grabbe S, Voskort M et al. Mycophenolate mofetil impairs the maturation and function of murine dendritic cells. J Immunol 2000; 165: 2374–81.

93. Hantash B, Fiorentino D. Liver enzyme abnormalities in patients with atopic dermatitis treated with mycophenolate mofetil. Arch Dermatol 2006; 142: 109–10.

94. Grundmann-Kollmann M, Korting HC, Behrens S et al. Successful treatment of severe refractory atopic dermatitis with mycophenolate mofetil. Br J Dermatol 1999; 141: 175–6.

95. Satchell AC, Barnetson RS. Staphylococcal septicaemia complicating treatment of atopic dermatitis with mycophenolate. Br J Dermatol 2000;143: 202–3.

96. Neuber K, Schwartz I, Itschert G, Dieck AT. Treatment of atopic eczema with oral mycophenolate mofetil. Br J Dermatol 2000; 143: 385–91.

97. Benez A, Fierlbeck G. Successful long-term treatment of severe atopic dermatitis with mycophenolate mofetil. Br J Dermatol 2001; 144: 638–9.

98. Grundmann-Kollmann M, Podda M, Ochsendorf F et al. Mycophenolate mofetil is effective in the treatment of atopic dermatitis. Arch Dermatol 2001; 137: 870–3.

99. Lee SW, Park YM, Kim HO, Kim CW. Therapeutic efficacy of mycophenolate mofetil in atopic dermatitis. Korean J Dermatol 2002; 40: 908–13.

100. Hansen ER, Buus S, Deleuran M, Andersen KE. Treatment of atopic dermatitis with mycophenolate mofetil. Br J Dermatol 2000; 143: 1324–6.

101. Grundmann-Kollmann M, Kaufmann R, Zollner TM. Treatment of atopic dermatitis with mycophenolate mofetil. Br J Dermatol 2001; 145: 351–2

19

Topical calcineurin inhibitors

Thomas A Luger, Martin Steinhoff, Anita Remitz, and Sakari Reitamo

INTRODUCTION

Two topical calcineurin inhibitors (TCIs), tacrolimus, and the ascomycin derivative pimecrolimus, have been developed for the treatment of atopic dermatitis (AD). Tacrolimus ointment (0.03%, 0.1%) and pimecrolimus cream (1%) are now commonly regarded as effective therapies for AD, and both compounds have been approved by the authorities of many countries for the treatment of this disease. Tacrolimus ointment is marketed with the tradename Protopic®, and pimecrolimus cream mainly with the tradename Elidel®. Other tradenames for topical pimecrolimus include Aregen®, Isaplic®, Rizan®, Ombex®, and Velov®. The indication for both tacrolimus ointment and pimecrolimus cream is treatment of AD not responsive to first-line treatment with corticosteroids, or when corticosteroids are contraindicated. In most countries the indication of tacrolimus ointment is for moderate to severe AD from the age of 2 years on, and for pimecrolimus cream for mild to moderate AD, also from the age of 2 years on. The indication for the use of these compounds in AD is until clearance of the lesion, and restarting the treatment when new symptoms occur.

In the present chapter we will focus on the preclinical and clinical data on tacrolimus ointment and pimecrolimus cream. While the data on short-term management of AD are abundant, optimal long-term management of AD with the TCIs is still under study. Therefore, strategies for the long-term use of these compounds will be discussed. In addition, we will discuss the use of TCIs in skin diseases other than AD.

ORIGIN OF CALCINEURIN INHIBITORS

Ciclosporin was the first calcineurin inhibitor to be used in AD. Oral treatment was effective in placebo-controlled trials, although the treatment was usually

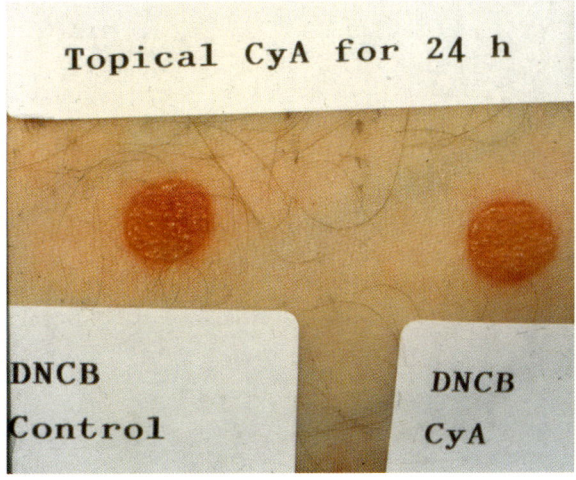

Key:

AP1, activator protein-1 transcription factor;
CanB, calmodulin B; *DAG*, diacylglycerol;
Ca^{2+}, ionic calcium;
FKBP12, tacrolimus/pimecrolimus-binding protein 12;
IL-2, interleukin-2; IP3, inositol triphosphate;
mRNA, messenger ribonucleic acid;
NFAT, nuclear factor of activated T cells; P, phosphate group; PKC, phosphokinase C; PLCγ1, phospholipase Cγ1;
TCR-complex, T-cell receptor complex.

Figure 19.1 Ciclosporin (CyA) does not supress a dinitrochlotobenzene (DNCB) challenge reaction in an individual presensitized with DNCB.

combined with topical corticosteroids.[1,2] Early attempts to develop a topical formulation with ciclosporin showed promise in animal models of allergic contact dermatitis, whereas no efficacy was noted in suppression of human allergic contact dermatitis (Figure 19.1).[3] However, a topical 10% ciclosporin gel showed weak efficacy in AD.[4,5] Today, topical ciclosporin formulations are used for atopic eye disease.[6]

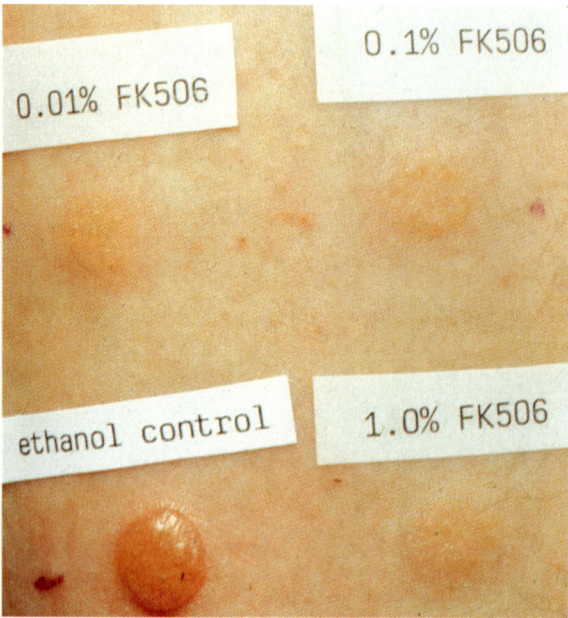

Figure 19.2 Topical tacrolimus (FK506) suppresses DNCB challenge reaction in an individual presensitized with DNCB. Photo by Antti Lauerma.

In contrast to ciclosporin, topical tacrolimus was effective in an identical model of suppression of human, allergic contact dermatitis as used earlier for ciclosporin[7] (Figure 19.2). Topical tacrolimus ointment also proved to be effective in AD.[8,9] Compared to ciclosporin, tacrolimus has a lower molecular weight and a higher specific activity both in vitro and in vivo.[10] Both ciclosporin and

tacrolimus are natural products. Ciclosporin was isolated from a fungus, whereas tacrolimus was isolated from the fungus-like bacteria *Streptomyces tsukubaensis*.[11] Ascomycin is an antifungal compound isolated from *S. hygroscopicus* var. *ascomyceticus*.[12] It shows a close relationship to tacrolimus. Pimecrolimus is a semisynthetic derivative of ascomycin[13] (Figure 19.3). In addition to the topical form, oral pimecrolimus has shown promise in the treatment of AD in a clinical study.[14] In addition to pimecrolimus, several other ascomycin derivatives have been tried in animal models.[15] So far none of them have been developed for treatment of human disease.

MODE OF ACTION OF TOPICAL CALCINEURIN INHIBITORS

Tacrolimus and pimecrolimus both bind with a different affinity to the same cytosolic immunophilin receptor (FK binding protein-12 or macrophilin-12).[16] In contrast, ciclosporin recognizes a different cytosolic receptor named cyclophilin.[17] The macrophilin complex formed either with tacrolimus or pimecrolimus inhibits a calcium-dependent serine-threonine phosphatase defined as calcineurin (Figure 19.4). Thereby, dephosphorylation, and nuclear translocation of a cytosolic transcription factor, the nuclear factor of activated T-cell protein (NFATp), is inhibited.[18] As a consequence, the production of cytokines such as interleukin-2 (IL-2), IL-4, IL-8, tumor necrosis factor alpha (TNFα), interferon gamma (IFNγ), and granulocyte-macrophage colony-stimulating factor (GM-CSF) is blocked resulting in the inhibition of TH1-lymphocyte as well as TH2-lymphocyte activation.

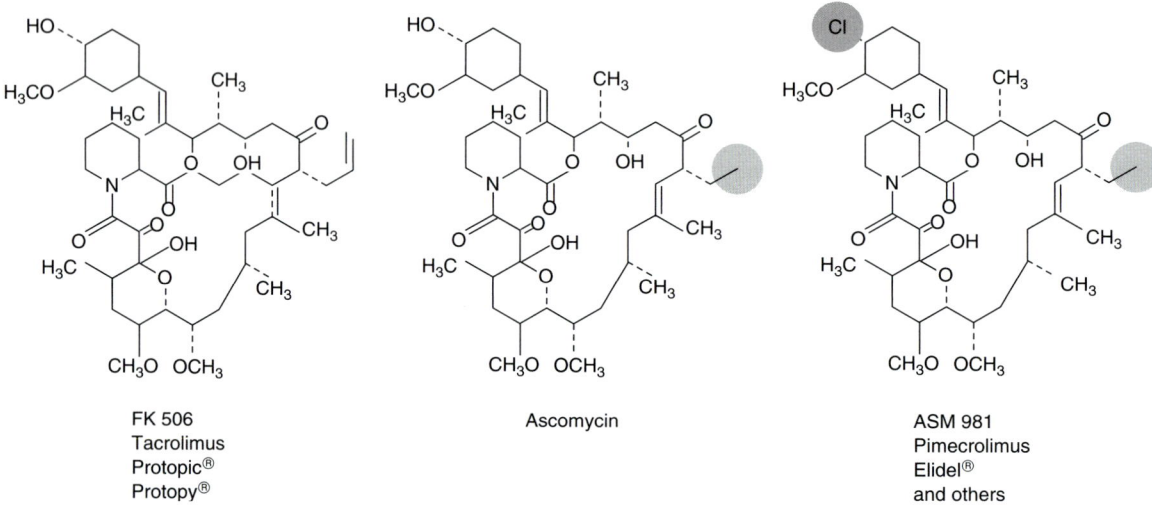

Figure 19.3 Molecular structures of tacrolimus, ascomycin and pimecrolimus.

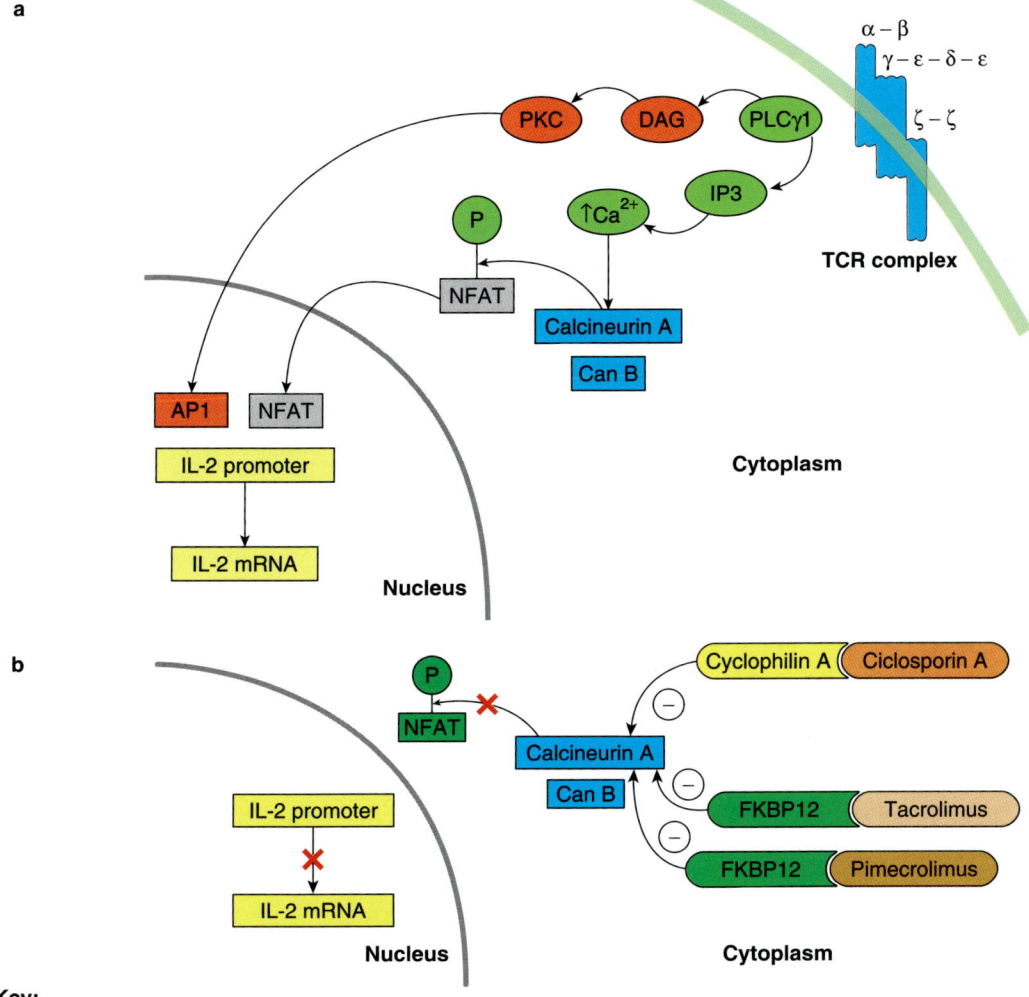

Key:

AP1, activator protein-1 transcription factor; *CanB*, calmodulin B; *DAG*, diacylglycerol; Ca²⁺, ionic calcium; *FKBP12*, tacrolimus/pimecrolimus-binding protein 12; *IL-2*, interleukin-2; IP3, inositol triphosphate; mRNA, messenger ribonucleic acid; NFAT, nuclear factor of activated T cells; P, phosphate group; PKC, phosphokinase C; PLCγ1, phospholipase Cγ1; TCR-complex, T-cell receptor complex.

Figure 19.4   T-cell activation (a) and inhibition of calcineurin activation (b). Inhibition of calcineurin activation prevents translocation of NFAT within the nucleus.

Moreover, topical pimecrolimus produces anti-inflammatory effects by downregulating IL-5, IL-10, and IL-13 both in CD4+ and CD8+ T cells.[19] Pimecrolimus also diminishes the number of CD1+ inflammatory epidermal dendritic cells from the epidermis.[19,20] Both topical tacrolimus and pimecrolimus induce apoptosis in cutaneous T lymphocytes but not in Langerhans cells.[20,21] In addition, the release of mast cell mediators such as histamine is also inhibited by tacrolimus and pimecrolimus.[22,23] Pimecrolimus, as known so far, is unable to alter the function of dendritic cells such as costimulatory molecule expression or the capacity to stimulate T-lymphocyte proliferation.[24] In contrast to corticosteroids, topical application of pimecrolimus does not affect the density of epidermal Langerhans cells.[25] Tacrolimus inhibits cytokine production from eosinophils, mast cells, and basophils, and reduces the capacity of Langerhans cells to activate T cells (reviewed in Alomer et al[26]). Tacrolimus was found to alter certain functions of Langerhans cells, and inflammatory dendritic epidermal cells (IDEC), such as the expression of the high-affinity receptor for IgE (FcεRI).[27] On the inflammatory epidermal and dermal cells of the skin, tacrolimus shows opposing effects to corticosteroids. In Langerhans cells, in vitro, tacrolimus downregulates the expression of FcεRI; in contrast, betamethasone upregulates its expression.[28] The downregulation of FcεRI is of potential clinical significance in the therapy of AD. It is not known whether the action of tacrolimus on FcεRI depends on NFATp. In an in vivo intervention study of AD with topical tacrolimus, an increased proportion of CD1a+ cells in the epidermis of AD lesions decreased to normal during clinical improvement with tacrolimus ointment.[29] The CD1a+ population consisted of Langerhans cells and IDEC. The decrease in CD1a+ cells was mainly due to a decrease in IDEC, and not Langerhans cells, suggesting a normalization in the function of dendritic cells by tacrolimus treatment.

The in vivo anti-inflammatory capacity of tacrolimus and pimecrolimus has also been investigated in animal models of contact dermatitis. Both compounds were able to block the elicitation phase of allergic contact dermatitis. In vivo animal studies have shown that pimecrolimus, in contrast to tacrolimus, had no effect on the sensitization phase of allergic contact dermatitis, and thus apparently does not impair the primary immune response. This has been further supported by a variety of other animal models of immune-mediated diseases. Using a localized rat model of 'graft-versus-host disease' (GvhD), pimecrolimus was significantly less effective than tacrolimus. In another rat model of kidney transplantation, pimecrolimus again was less effective in preventing graft rejection when compared to tacrolimus or ciclosporin. Moreover, upon investigation of the effect on T-helper cell assisted B-cell activation in rats, pimecrolimus turned out to be significantly weaker when compared to tacrolimus.[26,29] The atopy patch test (APT) is regarded as a human model of induction of eczema in patients with AD. Environmental antigens cause a T-cell mediated response visible as an eczematous reaction. In this model, pre-treatment with both tacrolimus and pimecrolimus failed to suppress the APT.[30,31]

Potentially the greatest advantage of the TCIs in the treatment of AD is their lack of atrophogenicity, which makes long-term treatment possible when needed. In contrast to glucocorticosteroids TCIs do not suppress collagen synthesis by fibroblasts.[32,33]

POTENTIAL SYSTEMIC EXPOSURE BY TOPICAL CALCINEURIN INHIBITORS

The question of potential systemic exposure is one major concern in any case of the development of a novel compound for topical application. Therefore, the capacity of pimecrolimus to penetrate into, and to permeate through, the skin was investigated in vitro using human cadaver skin, compared to corticosteroids or tacrolimus. Accordingly, the amount of pimecrolimus penetrating into the skin was similar to that of corticosteroids or tacrolimus. However, pimecrolimus was observed to permeate significantly less through skin compared to corticosteroids or tacrolimus.[34] Therefore, one may suggest that following the topical application of pimecrolimus, the risk of systemic exposure, and the ultimate possibility of systemic side effects, are most unlikely. This has been supported by several pharmacokinetic studies which proved that after topical use of pimecrolimus in patients with AD, serum concentrations were equally low regardless of the age, severity of disease, and body area treated. In 99% of the samples tested, concentrations were below 2 ng/ml, which is far below the level of 10–15 ng/ml required for a systemic anti-inflammatory activity.[35] Serum concentrations of pimecrolimus in this range did not cause toxic adverse events as has been shown in several clinical trials.[36] Although the metabolism of pimecrolimus in the skin has not yet been carefully, investigated, it might be assumed that it is removed by desquamation. In contrast, serum tacrolimus levels after topical application were detected more frequently following topical application in patients with AD. However, usually these levels were low and transient because circulating tacrolimus was no longer detectable upon improvement of skin barrier function after short-term treatment.[9,37] The reason for the observed differences between tacrolimus and pimecrolimus, however, is not completely understood. Possible explanations may be the different structure, and differences in lipophilicity, as well as content of lipophilic groups of these compounds. Taken together the potential of systemic exposure by TCIs is low with the exception of some patients with severe genetic barrier defects in their skin, namely patients with Netherton syndrome.[38]

CLINICAL STUDIES OF ATOPIC DERMATITIS WITH TOPICAL CALCINEURIN INHIBITORS

Both tacrolimus and pimecrolimus have been developed for the topical treatment of AD and approved for this indication in many countries around the world. Tacrolimus is available as 0.03% and 0.1% ointment whereas pimecrolimus currently is available as 1% cream. In most counties tacrolimus is approved for the treatment of moderate and severe cases of AD in adults, and children < 2 years old. In Europe and the United States, pimecrolimus has been approved for the treatment of mild and moderate cases of AD in adults, and children under 2 years of age. However, in some other countries pimecrolimus is approved for the therapy of AD regardless of age and severity of the disease. Many clinical studies have been performed demonstrating that both compounds are highly effective in the treatment of AD. We now briefly summarize the available experience of tacrolimus and pimecrolimus in the short-term as well as long-term management of infants, children, and adults suffering from AD.

Short-term studies with tacrolimus ointment

Placebo-controlled studies

The first placebo-controlled clinical study in 13–60-year-old patients with AD has clearly shown that after 3 weeks of treatment with tacrolimus ointment in 3 different concentrations (0.03%, 0.1%, and 0.3%) a significant improvement of pruritus and eczematous lesions has been noted.[9] These findings were confirmed by several subsequent studies using 3–12-week treatment protocols for patients with moderate and severe disease. Accordingly, ~70% of the patients experienced at least a 75% improvement of their symptoms (reviewed in Quelle-Roussel et al[33]). Compared to placebo, both 0.03% and 0.1% tacrolimus were more effective.

Tacrolimus versus topical corticosteroids

Tacrolimus ointment has been compared to topical corticosteroids in several short-term controlled studies of a few weeks. In adult patients with moderate to severe AD, 0.1% tacrolimus ointment was as effective as hydrocortisone butyrate 0.1% ointment, whereas 0.03% tacrolimus were less effective.[39] In a similar study in children of 2–15 years of age, both 0.1% and 0.03% tacrolimus were more effective than 1% hydrocortisone acetate ointment.[40] In all previously mentioned studies tacrolimus ointment was used twice daily. In one study in children once-daily to twice-daily treatments of 0.03% tacrolimus ointment were compared. In addition one patient group had 1% hydrocortisone acetate twice daily. Both tacrolimus groups showed better efficacy than the hydrocortisone group.[41] Patients with moderate disease had similar results with once- or twice-daily treatment. In contrast patients with severe disease showed better efficacy with twice-daily treatment.[41] In recent studies tacrolimus ointment has been compared in adults and in children to 0.005% fluticasone pivalate ointment, and in children with severe AD having an acute flare to 0.1% methyl prednisolone aceponate ointment. In these studies 0.1% tacrolimus ointment was superior to 0.005% fluticasone ointment in adults, whereas 0.03% ointment was similar to fluticasone pivalate ointment in children.[42,43] Mometasone furoate 0.1% ointment was superior to tacrolimus ointment 0.03% for clinical score, itch, and adverse events, although the success rate of treatment was similar with the two treatments.[44]

Tacrolimus ointment versus pimecrolimus cream

In a multicentre, randomized, investigator-blinded, 6-week study (n = 1065), the efficacy and safety of tacrolimus ointment (0.1%) was compared to pimecrolimus 1% cream in adult and paediatric patients. Tacrolimus was more effective than pimecrolimus in adults and children with moderate/severe AD, and at week 1 with mild AD. Tacrolimus was also superior with respect to itch scores and onset of action, while no differences were observed concerning unexpected side events.[45,46] Taken together, these studies have provided convincing evidence that the application of tacrolimus ointment for the treatment of AD in adults as well as children after a short time of 3–7 days results in a significant improvement of any disease-specific signs and symptoms such as pruritus as well as eczema.

Long-term studies with tacrolimus ointment

Safety and efficacy

The impressive efficacy of short-term treatment was the rationale for performing long-term studies to confirm the efficacy and safety of tacrolimus ointment for the long-term management of AD. In a multicentre, open-label non-comparative trial, a total of 316 patients aged 18 years and older with moderate to severe AD, 200 patients (for 6 months) and 116 (for 12 months) were enrolled. Patients were instructed to apply 0.1% tacrolimus ointment twice daily on all affected skin areas (5–60%) until 1 week after complete clearance. The additional use of emollients without any active compound was allowed.[47] Efficacy end points included a combined score based on a modified Eczema Area and Severity Index (EASI) as well as an investigator's global assessment.[47] Safety assessments included monitoring of adverse events, clinical laboratory values, and tacrolimus blood concentrations. The study was completed by 77.5% of the patients and within the first week of treatment most of them experienced a significant amelioration of the symptoms. A further increasing improvement was noted until month 3 after treatment, which in most cases lasted until the end of the study. The mean EASI score was 23.7 at the beginning of the study, which decreased to 13.5 at week 1, and finally was 6.1 after 6 months or 12 months, respectively. After 12 months excellent improvement (≥ 90%) or clearance of the symptoms was reported in 68.2% of those patients. An improvement (≥ 50%) was noted in 90.9% of the cases. Laboratory parameters did not change significantly during the study period. Systemic exposure was low and the maximal blood concentrations of tacrolimus remained below 1 ng/ml in 76% of patients. Local adverse events such as burning sensation (47%) were common but usually only upon initiation of the treatment.

In a more recent 6-month study of 972 adults with moderate to severe AD, tacrolimus 0.1% ointment was compared to corticosteroid treatment, 1% hydrocortisone acetate for the face, and 0.1% hydrocortisone butyrate for other areas.[48] The corticosteroid treatment arm was regarded as the conventional type of treatment for AD. In this study tacrolimus ointment was superior in efficacy throughout the treatment time. Safety results were also similar in that the number of viral and bacterial infections diminished during the treatment. During the first months however, there were more herpes simplex and bacterial infections in the tacrolimus arm. After month 4 both infections were uncommon. These patients were further studied in a 2-year follow-up study.[49] The number of herpes simplex infections went down further. There are now several 4-year safety studies with tacrolimus ointment which all suggest good long-term tolerability both in adults and in children.[50,51] Several safety studies in children with duration from 6 months to 4 years suggest that the safety is equally good both when 0.03% and 0.1% ointment are used.[50–53]

In contrast to topical corticosteroids during long-term treatment with tacrolimus ointment no tachyphylaxis has been observed. The excellent long-term efficacy of tacrolimus ointment for the treatment of AD in children as well as adults has been supported by a variety of other clinical studies. Moreover, several have proven that the long-term application of tacrolimus ointment in infants, children and adults with AD results in a significant improvement of their quality of life.[54]

Pharmacokinetics of topical tacrolimus

It is well known that following the systemic application of tacrolimus severe side effects such as nephrotoxicity and hypertension may occur at plasma levels ≥ 5 ng/ml. Therefore, tacrolimus plasma levels in patients treated with tacrolimus ointment have been monitored very carefully in many clinical trials. The results from different studies, involving a total number of 1057 patients, demonstrate that in 67.1% of the patients tacrolimus plasma levels remained below the level of quantification of 0.5 ng/ml. Low levels were detected in 19.7% (0.5–1 ng/ml) and 9.2% (1–2 ng/ml) of the treated atopic patients. High levels were found in 3.7% (2–5 ng/ml) and 0.4% (≥ 5 ng/ml).[33] In selected patients with a barrier dysfunction, as in Netherton syndrome for example, extremely high blood concentrations (up to 20 ng/ml), which are known to possibly cause systemic adverse events, have been reported.[37] Despite these rare cases, systemic exposure after topical application of tacrolimus is very low. Usually, it is no longer detectable as soon as the eczema vanishes, and when the epidermal barrier function has improved. Moreover, there is no evidence for systemic accumulation resulting in adverse side effects following the long-term treatment with tacrolimus ointment.[40]

Adverse events after tacrolimus treatment

The safety and tolerability of tacrolimus ointment has been investigated carefully in many children and adults with AD. Usually the treatment was reported to be well tolerated. The most common local adverse event was a sensation of burning, which occurred in 29.9% of the children and 46.8% of the adults. Transient itching was noted in some children (23.1%) and adults (25.8%). In the majority of these cases, local adverse events were only noted during the first few days of treatment. Generally, they were mild to moderate.[33] It was also noted in long-term studies that the risk of developing folliculitis or acne may be increased in some young adults.[33] An increased rate of bacterial skin infections could only be observed in one long-term study during the first months of treatment.[51] In the subsequent months the incidence of bacterial infections was reduced. Interestingly, a decreased colonization with Staphylococcus aureus in the eczematous skin lesions was observed.[55] This decrease was already detectable within the first week of treatment and lasted throughout the time period of 1 year. Since tacrolimus exerts direct antimicrobial activity only on selected fungi, e.g. Malassezia furfur,[56] this effect could be due to a normalization of the innate immunity in the skin. Accordingly, it has recently been shown that skin lesions of patients with AD have an impaired capacity to produce antimicrobial peptides such as defensins and cathelicidins.[57–63] This downregulation appears to be due to a predominant TH2 immune response in atopic individuals, since TH2 cytokines such as IL-4 and IL-13 were found to inhibit the production of antimicrobial peptides. Therefore, tacrolimus, by inhibiting TH2 cytokines, may upregulate the production of antimicrobial peptides, which ultimately leads to a decreased colonization of microbial agents. A long-term study on recall antigen reaction showed that treatment of AD with tacrolimus ointment results in restoration of recall antigen reactions, which can be interpreted as a restoration of TH1-type immunity and hence control of TH2 cytokines.[64]

Restoration of collagen synthesis by tacrolimus monotherapy

The limiting factor of long-term treatment with topical corticosteroids is skin atrophy. Many investigations have been performed to evaluate the effect of tacrolimus on fibroblast collagen formation, among them a randomized, double-blind study in 14 patients with AD and 12 healthy volunteers. Tacrolimus (0.03% and 0.1%), betamethasone valerate, and a vehicle control were applied to the abdominal skin under occlusion. After 1 week, skin thickness was evaluated, and the content of procollagen peptides was measured in suction blister fluids. Betamethasone valerate-treated areas showed a decrease of carboxy-terminal propeptides of procollagen I (17%), amino-terminal propeptides of procollagen I (17.6%), amino-terminal propeptides of procollagen III (39.5%), and a reduction in skin thickness. In contrast, tacrolimus had no effect on procollagen propeptide production, and caused no reduction of skin thickness.[32]

The absence of skin atrophy is a major advantage of tacrolimus and has been confirmed also in long-term studies.[65] Long-term monotherapy of 12 months with tacrolimus ointment restored collagen synthesis and thus reversed skin atrophy. Interestingly, patients with AD and bronchial asthma requiring treatment with inhaled corticosteroids had very low collagen synthesis at baseline. However, treatment with tacrolimus monotherapy restored their collagen synthesis, although these patients continued their treatment with inhaled corticosteroids throughout the study, suggesting a protective effect of tacrolimus on the skin.

Tacrolimus ointment and skin cancer

The use of systemic immunosuppressants is associated with an increased incidence of UV-induced skin cancer.[66,67] Therefore, it was crucial to evaluate the potential risk of developing skin cancer following the topical application of tacrolimus. According to several pieces of evidence, the potential of tacrolimus ointment to cause skin cancer appears to be rather low. This is also supported by the observation that no commentary of skin cancer has been reported associated with the application of tacrolimus ointment after more than 5 years of clinical experience.[68] In animal studies it was demonstrated that tacrolimus is capable of inhibiting the development of phorbol ester-induced skin tumours.[69] Tacrolimus was also found to inhibit the activation of the tumour growth factor beta-1 receptor (TGFβ1R) which plays an important role in wound healing and tumour formation.[70] Recently, it has been shown that tacrolimus as well as pimecrolimus are able to inhibit the UV-induced thymidin-dimer formation, and thus prevent DNA damage.[71] There is also evidence for tacrolimus being able to prevent keratinocyte apoptosis. However, the question of tumour formation following long-term treatment with topical tacrolimus cannot be answered beyond doubt at present.

Therefore, concomitant UV therapy should be avoided and the patients should be instructed to take UV-protective measure.[72]

Short-term studies with pimecrolimus cream

Pimecrolimus versus placebo

The efficacy of pimecrolimus 1% cream for the treatment of AD in adults, children, and infants has been proven in several clinical studies.[73–75] In a proof of concept study in adults with moderate AD, pimecrolimus 1% cream was applied in comparison to vehicle once or twice daily for a period of 3 weeks. The twice-daily application resulted in a 71.9% improvement of the eczematous lesions, whereas an improvement rate of only 37.7% was observed in lesions which were treated once daily. In areas treated with vehicle, the mean improvement was 10.3% or 6.2%, respectively.[73]

Since no significant drug-related side effects were observed in this study, pimecrolimus cream was applied twice daily in any of the following studies.

Pimecrolimus versus corticosteroids

In a randomized, double-blind, multicentre study, 260 patients with AD were treated for 3 weeks with pimecrolimus cream at different concentrations (0.05%, 0.2%, 0.6%, and 1.0%), vehicle cream, or 0.1% betamethasone 17-valerate cream for dose-finding. According to this study, pimecrolimus 1% cream was most effective with a median EASI decrease of 47%. Betamethasone valerate treatment resulted in a median percent change from baseline of 78%. Furthermore, pruritus was shown to be effectively controlled by pimecrolimus within 1 week of treatment. Of note, no serious adverse events were obtained in any of the treatment groups, and a transient burning or a feeling of warmth in the treated areas was the most commonly reported side effect.[74]

To further evaluate the efficacy and safety of a twice-daily application of pimecrolimus 1% cream in children (2–17 years) and infants (3–23 months) with mild, moderate, or even severe AD, several multicentre clinical trials have been performed (reviewed in Breur et al[75]). A total of 403 children and 186 infants were included in these studies. After 6 weeks of treatment in a double-blind phase, patients were continued on an open-labelled 20-week extension phase. Both in children and infants, pimecrolimus 1% cream in comparison to vehicle proved to be highly effective in improving eczema as well as pruritus after only 8 days of treatment. Treatment was well tolerated and no increased incidence of side effects, including viral or bacterial infections, was reported.[76] Therapeutic effects were independent of ethnic origin and disease severity.[77] These results were confirmed in a recent double-blind study. During a 4-week period of treatment, pimecrolimus cream reduced the mean eczema area and severity index by 71.5% as compared to an increase by 19.4% in the vehicle control group. The eczema reduction was statistically significant at day 4. At this time, significant improvements of sleep loss and pruritus were observed.[78] A significant improvement of pimecrolimus on sleep disturbances was also observed by others.[79] Another study in infants (n=250) and children (n=711) clearly supports the observation of pimecrolimus 1% cream being a safe and effective therapeutic option in children and infants. Of note, significantly more patients in the pimecrolimus group were maintained without glucocorticoid therapy.[80]

Long-term studies with pimecrolimus cream

The efficacy of pimecrolimus in the topical long-term management of AD has been investigated in several studies with a 6- or 12-month follow-up.[76] In several multicentre, randomized, double-blind studies 192 adults,[81] 713 children (2–17 years of age),[82] and 250 infants (3–23 months of age)[83] were enrolled. Patients were randomized to apply twice-daily pimecrolimus cream or vehicle cream (conventional therapy) upon the first signs of a flare (itching, erythema). In the case of uncontrolled flare, patients of both groups were allowed to use moderately potent topical corticosteroids until clearing. After 6 as well as 12 months, of treatment, significantly fewer infants in the pimecrolimus group (67.6%) developed a severe flare requiring corticosteroids, as compared to the conventional therapy group (30.4%).

The efficacy of the pimecrolimus treatment in infants was also reflected by a significant EASI reduction of 61.8% after 6 weeks and >80% after 12 months.[82] Similar results were obtained with children, since after 6 months of treatment with pimecrolimus significantly more children remained without any flare (61%) in comparison to the control group (34.2%).[81] In a recent study, the long-term control of AD with pimecrolimus cream was further investigated in infants and young children for 1 year (n=91) or 2 years (n=76). While no patients had to discontinue therapy because of side effects, treatment was safe and well tolerated. Interestingly, the incidence of systemic and skin infections including eczema herpeticatum (n=2) was not statistically significant.[84,85] Among adults, 45% of the pimecrolimus-treated patients but only 18.8% in the vehicle group experienced no flare during the treatment period of 6 months.[76] The mean time until the first flare was 144 days in the pimecrolimus group, while it was 26 days in the vehicle group, and thus 5 times faster.[81]

In any of these long-term studies a significant improvement of pruritus was observed as early as after 2–4 days of pimecrolimus application.[82] Moreover, several studies have shown that pimecrolimus treatment has a significantly greater beneficial effect on the quality of life in patients with AD.[81] These studies provide evidence that pimecrolimus 1% cream is effective for the treatment of mild, moderate, and severe AD in adults as well as children and infants. Moreover, there is clear evidence that lesions in the face and neck — which are often difficult to treat — respond even better to pimecrolimus treatment than eczematous lesions in other areas of the body.[77] Pimecrolimus was safe and well tolerated during the entire study period, no clinically relevant drug-related systemic events occurred and no significant difference between treatment groups in terms of infections and application site reactions were observed. In addition, there was no evidence of systemic immunosuppression according to a comparable response to recall antigens. Thus, treatment with pimecrolimus 1% cream is safe and effective in the topical long-term management of AD (Figure 19.5).

Pharmacokinetics of pimecrolimus cream

Accordingly, in adults and children as well as infants, pimecrolimus blood concentrations after topical application were usually below the level of verification (>0.5 ng/ml or >0.1 ng/ml). Pharmacokinetic studies have further been performed in 52 adults and 58 paediatric patients aged from 3 months to 14 years with moderate to severe AD.[73,86] The body surface area (BSA) affected ranged from 10 to 92% and in most patients ≥40% BSA was affected at baseline. In this study, pimecrolimus 1% cream was applied twice daily for 3 weeks or 1 year, respectively, and pimecrolimus blood concentrations were evaluated at different time points. In all patients, blood concentrations were consistently low (99% <2 ng/ml) regardless of the age, severity, extent of the skin area treated, and the duration of therapy.[73] In adults, blood concentrations ranged from <0.5 to 1.4 ng/ml and in children from <0.1 to 2.6 ng/ml. During the 1-year extension period, no accumulation was observed and only a minimal increase was detected with rising BSA during treatment. In children, the highest concentration measured was 2.6 ng/ml.[73,86] This is significantly below the blood levels of ≥15 ng/ml which are required for systemic immunomodulation in patients with psoriasis or AD. Moreover, these blood concentrations did not cause any detectable toxicity during the study period of 12 weeks.[88]

Recently, the low risk of systemic exposure after topical treatment with pimecrolimus was confirmed by case reports demonstrating very low blood levels in

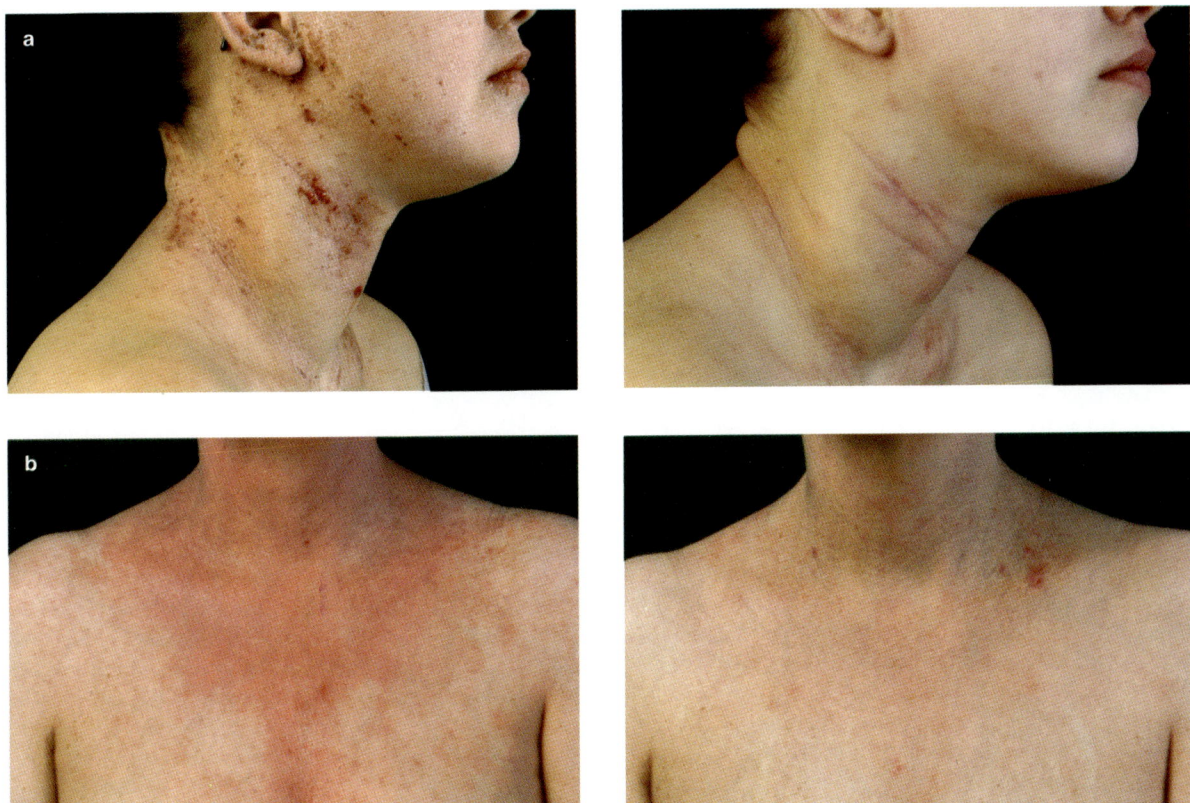

Figure 19.5   (a) AD before (left), and 10 days after treatment with pimecrolimus 1% cream twice daily (right). (b) AD before (left) and after treatment with tacrolimus 0.1% cream twice daily (right).

children with Netherton syndrome. Treatment of the total body surface area with pimecrolimus 1% cream resulted in a significant improvement of the eczematous skin lesions within a few days. However, in contrast to tacrolimus, blood levels in these patients remained low, between 1.5 and 2 ng/ml, and no accumulation was detected even after 3 months of daily application.[87,89,90] These findings indicate that the risk of systemic adverse events due to systemic exposure is negligible. This has been supported by the data of different long-term studies indicating no signs of systemic toxicity, immunosuppression, local or systemic infections.[81–83] In summary these studies showed that pimecrolimus has an excellent safety profile and was well tolerated locally and systemically.

Adverse events with pimecrolimus cream

The most frequently observed local adverse events following the topical application of pimecrolimus cream are burning and a feeling of warmth. In most cases these sensations were regarded as mild and transient, lasting only 1–3 days. The incidence of these local

effects also seemed to be dependent on the age of the patients, as burning occurred in 2.5% of the infants, 10.5% of the children, and 14.6% of the adults during the first days of pimecrolimus application.[81–83] In addition the severity of disease plays a role in the incidence of these adverse events. According to recent data the burning sensation following the topical application of TCIs appears to be due to the release of preformed neuromediators from primary afferent nerve endings. Accordingly, a depletion of substance P, which is known to cause burning, was observed in cutaneous nerves following the application of both tacrolimus and pimecrolimus.[91–93] Alcohol intake also may show erythema and a burning sensation of the skin both after pimecrolimus and tacrolimus treatment.

Pimecrolimus and cancer

In several clinical studies the potential risk of an increased incidence of skin infections following the topical application of pimecrolimus has been carefully investigated. As a result of these investigations long-term application of pimecrolimus 1% cream is not associated with a significantly increased risk for the development of fungal bacterial or viral skin infections.[81–83] Although treatment with pimecrolimus as well as tacrolimus was associated with a slight but not significant increase of local viral infections – mainly herpes simplex infections of the skin – in none of these cases have serious complications been reported, and they responded well to the conventional antiviral treatment.[5] However, the current recommendation is to stop treatment with TCIs until total clearance of the viral infection. Surprisingly the incidence of bacterial infections was found to be decreased during the application of pimecrolimus or tacrolimus, respectively. Since neither of these two compounds has a direct antibacterial activity, this effect most likely is due to a normalization of the innate defence which is known to be impaired in atopic individuals. This is supported by a recent report indicating that due to the increased production of TH2 cytokines such as IL-4 and IL-13, the production of antimicrobial peptides is downregulated. Thus, topical anti-inflammatory treatment causing a downregulation of TH2 cytokine production results in an upregulation of antimicrobial peptide production and subsequently to decreased microbial colonization of the skin.[48]

There is concern that topical treatment with calcineurin inhibitors may impair the outcome of vaccination in infants and children. However, there is also evidence that the capacity to respond to vaccination with an appropriate antibody production is not affected upon treatment with pimecrolimus. Accordingly, pimecrolimus does not affect the function and migration of antigen-presenting dendritic cells and thus will not impair the primary immune response. This is supported by the finding in an animal model that – in contrast to ciclosporin A or tacrolimus – the systemic application of pimecrolimus after immunization did not diminish the production of specific IgM or IgG.[92] In order to further support this assumption, clinical trials are currently under investigation.[84]

In contrast to corticosteroids, neither tacrolimus nor pimecrolimus affects collagen synthesis, and therefore in animal models as well as in humans they do not cause skin atrophy even after long-term application. Accordingly, in 16 healthy volunteers the atrophogenic potential of pimecrolimus was compared to that of betamethasone 17-valerate 0.1%, triamcinolone acetonide, and the corresponding vehicles. After 4 weeks, the twice-daily application of pimecrolimus cream did not reveal any signs of skin atrophy. In contrast, corticosteroids caused a significant reduction in skin thickness from day 8 onwards as shown by sonographic evaluation as well as histological analysis.[33]

The use of systemic immunosuppressants such as ciclosporin A is well known to be associated with an increased risk for the development of UV-induced skin cancer. The long-lasting experience with topical corticosteroids indicates that this might not be applicable for the local treatment with immunomodulators. This was further supported by a report from an animal study demonstrating that the topical application of pimecrolimus cream and additional UV irradiation in comparison to the vehicle control after 12 months was not associated with an increased incidence of skin tumours.[93] In addition, it has recently been shown that the topical treatment with both tacrolimus and pimecrolimus prevents the UV-mediated formation of dimethyl-thymidin dimers, suggesting a rather protective effect of these compounds. However, there is still need for more thorough investigations in the future. Therefore, the current recommendation is still not to combine pimecrolimus with concurrent UV therapy and to recommend the use of appropriate sun screens.[71,93,94]

Oral pimecrolimus for atopic dermatitis

Oral treatment with pimecrolimus may be an effective option for the treatment of therapy-resistant moderate to severe AD. Therefore, a randomized, double-blind, placebo-controlled dose-finding study of 2 parallel groups (n = 103) was performed. Patients were treated with either placebo or pimecrolimus (10, 20, 30 mg twice daily) and observed for a 12-week treatment phase and a 12-week post-treatment phase. Hydrocortisone acetate 1% was allowed as concomitant topical medication. The authors observed a significant dose-dependent improvement in the eczema area and severity index of 66.6% at week 7 in the group treated with 30 mg twice daily. Of note, the treatment was well tolerated, especially with respect to nephrotoxicity and hypertension.[14] Thus, systemic pimecrolimus appears to be a promising therapeutic drug for treatment of recalcitrant AD that cannot be topically controlled.

DO TOPICAL IMMUNOMODULATORS HAVE AN EFFECT ON THE NATURAL HISTORY OF ATOPIC DERMATITIS?

Before TCIs, monotherapy of AD was performed only with topical corticosteroids, as UV treatments and oral immune suppressive agents are usually combined with topical corticosteroid treatment. Topical corticosteroids are indicated for short-term use. In clinical practice they tend to be used intermittently long term, especially in patients with more severe forms of AD. TCIs have made monotherapy of AD possible without corticosteroids. Monotherapy with TCIs long term makes it possible to study the effects of inhibition of early T-cell activation in AD without simultaneous effects on connective tissue cells, which is always the

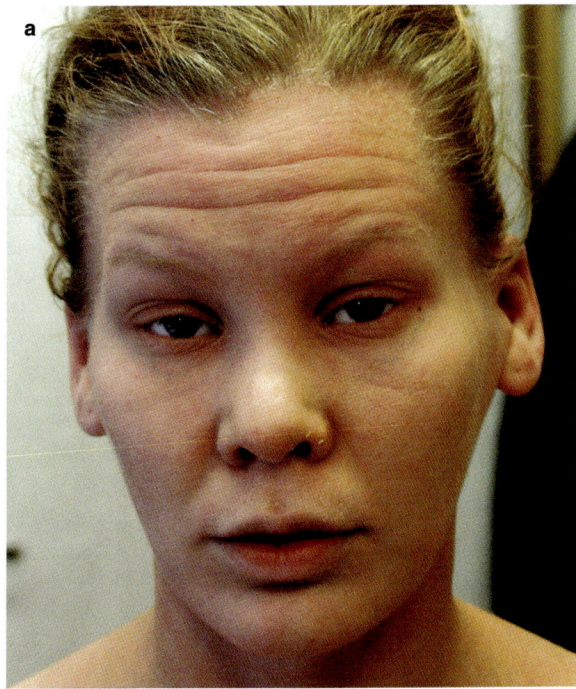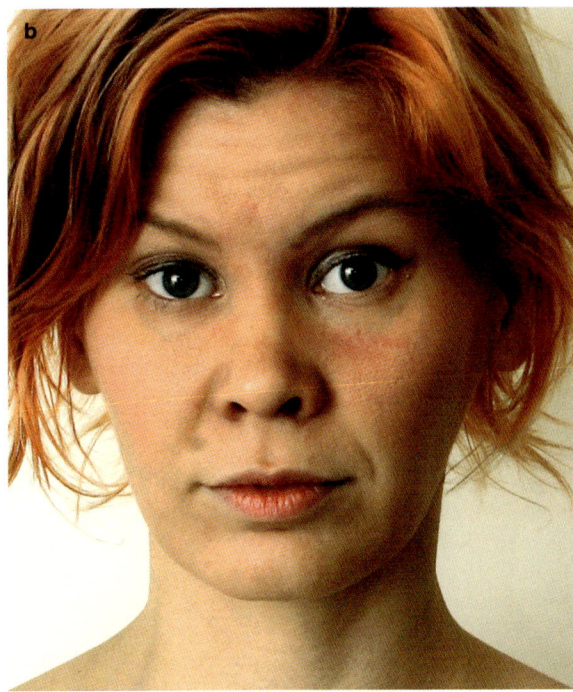

Figure 19.6   A patient previously treated with topical corticosteroids and oral ciclosporin A. (a) At baseline prior to intermittent monotherapy with tacrolimus ointment. (b) After 6 years

case with corticosteroid treatment. If T-cell activation plays an important role in the pathogenesis and clinical symptoms of AD it should be interesting to see the long-term effects of TCIs in AD. TCIs differ from topical corticosteroids in that they can be used as long as needed, as they do not possess any atrophogenic potential. Therefore both adults and children with AD show long-term results, which are characterized not only by clinical improvement but also by a decreased use of tacrolimus ointment over time[47] (Figure 19.6).

Long-term studies of monotherapy with TCIs have shown a constant improvement of AD. In contrast, when the face has been treated with tacrolimus ointment and the rest of the body with a corticosteroid, only a short-term improvement in the facial AD was seen.[95] This suggests that monotherapy with TCIs should be used whenever possible. In clinical practice, hand eczema in AD is often resistant to TCI treatment. Similarly, the hairy scalp is difficult to treat with the current formulations. Therefore, a limited role for corticosteroids during TCI treatment has to be accepted. Topical treatments have been traditionally used for an intensive period with a following treatment break of 1 to several weeks. This has been used mainly to reduce the skin thinning activity of corticosteroids. With TCIs it has been possible to treat until all symptoms of active disease vanish, including the itch. Recent studies suggest that, after initial treatment of

AD, the long-term outcome of AD can be improved by using twice-weekly tacrolimus ointment for all body regions previously affected. This treatment has resulted in less disease flares compared to previous treatment modes.[96,97] At the present we have patients who have used TCI monotherapy for over 10 years. Typical for such patients is a good clinical condition, diminished need for treatment, diminished occurrence of viral infections, normal results with vaccinations, and improvement of atopic airway symptoms. No increase in malignancies have been observed.[98]

CONCLUSIONS AND FUTURE PERSPECTIVES

For the first time since the introduction of topical corticosteroids more than 50 years ago, topical calcineurin inhibitors such as pimecrolimus and tacrolimus have established a novel, effective, and safe treatment modality for most patients suffering from AD. In contrast to these 2 compounds, any of the currently used treatments for mild and moderate AD is associated with a higher risk of developing adverse events. Therefore, the long-term use of therapeutic modalities such as corticosteroids or phototherapy is limited. Topical calcineurin inhibitors are the first compounds which are suited for a long-term treatment of inflammatory skin diseases such as AD.[99,100]

The extremely good results of both pimecrolimus and tacrolimus for the treatment of AD have subsequently stimulated many investigators to test their efficacy in other inflammatory skin diseases. In case reports or small uncontrolled clinical trials, the successful use of both compounds for the treatment of psoriasis in the face and intertrigenous areas have been reported.[101,102] Moreover, pimecrolimus and tacrolimus have been successfully applied to treat seborrhoeic eczema,[103] steroid-induced perioral dermatitis, steroid-induced rosacea,[104] erythroteleangiectatic as well as papulopustular and oedematous rosacea,[105] perianal dermatitis, chronic actinic dermatitis,[106] disseminated granuloma annulare,[107,108] lichen planus,[109] and some forms of hand eczema. Mucous lesions of lichen planus[110] and lichen sclerosus et atrophicans also have been shown to respond well to treatment with TCIs.[111,112] The therapy of vitiligo with calcineurin inhibitors also appears to be promising,[113] although UV light may be additionally mandatory.[114,115] Successful treatment of cutaneous chronic GvhD with topical pimecrolimus cream has also been described.[116,117] This observation may be of specific importance in those patients with highly atrophic skin. In contrast to animal models, the treatment of alopecia areata in humans with these new compounds was not effective.[118] There is also evidence for an efficacy of pimecrolimus and tacrolimus for the treatment of pyoderma gangraenosum, skin lesions of systemic lupus erythematosus or dermatomyositis, bullous autoimmune diseases, lichen amyloidosus, lichen aureus, and chronic actinic dermatitis. It is also very important to analyse economical aspects of a – at a first glance – very expensive novel therapeutic development against AD. Recently, the economics of TCIs for the treatment of AD were investigated. In certain patients, topical immunomodulators are cost-effective and show an acceptable incremental cost utility,[119] although involving higher costs as compared to glucocorticosteroids.[119] Thus, considering the extremely high expenses of drug development, and the uncertainty of long-term efficacy, a fair calculation may often be difficult. Moreover, between topical immunomodulators, comparative head-to-head data are only limited. Another problem is the frequently performed comparison with historical data which in each case were collected under not identical conditions, and in different collectives of patients. In summary, a recent study concluded that the costs, especially non-drug-related costs, of long-term treatment with the novel TCIs appears to be comparable or even cheaper than current comparable therapies.[120] However, none of these studies have yet considered any socioeconomic aspects.

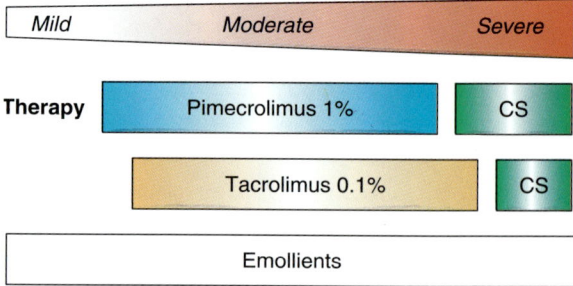

Figure 19.7   A new paradigm for the treatment of AD. CS, topical corticosteroids.

The introduction of this new group of topical compounds has allowed the establishment of a novel paradigm for the treatment of AD, and a reduction of the need for other therapies often associated with severe side effects. Upon the first symptoms of AD, patients should start using calcineurin inhibitors. Only in cases where the disease cannot be controlled may the intermittent use of other anti-inflammatory compounds such as glucocorticosteroids be recommended. Although a cure of AD is still not possible, novel compounds such as tacrolimus and pimecrolimus may provide an effective, safe, and perhaps even prophylactic treatment. Therefore the use of systemic immunosuppressants with sometimes severe side effects may in the future be limited to very severe forms of AD which cannot be controlled by these newly introduced compounds.

The future position of these novel compounds in the treatment of AD and other inflammatory skin diseases will be dependent on further clinical studies. However, already today, TCIs have changed our attitude towards the treatment of patients with acute as well as chronic AD (Figure 19.7).

REFERENCES

1. Sowden JM, Berth-Jones J, Ross JS et al. Double-blind, controlled, crossover study of cyclosporin in adults with severe refractory atopic dermatitis. Lancet 1991; 338: 137–40.
2. Camp RD, Reitamo S, Friedmann PS et al. Cyclosporin A in severe, therapy-resistant atopic dermatitis: report of an international workshop, April 1993. Br J Dermatol 1993; 129: 217–20.
3. Reitamo S, Käyhkö K, Lauerma AI et al. Topical cyclosporine and contact dermatitis in guinea pig and man. Arch Dermatol 1989; 125: 568.
4. de Prost Y, Bodemer C, Teillac D. Randomized double-blind placebo-controlled trial of local cyclosporin in atopic dermatitis. Acta Derm Venereol Suppl (Stockholm) 1989; 144: 136–8.
5. de Rie MA, Meinardi MM, Bos JD. Lack of efficacy of topical cyclosporin A in atopic dermatitis and allergic contact dermatitis. Acta Derm Venereol 1991; 71: 452–4.
6. Hingorani M, Calder VL, Buckley RJ et al. The immunomodulatory effect of topical cyclosporin A in atopic keratoconjunctivitis. Invest Ophthalmol Vis Sci 1999; 40: 392–9.

7. Lauerma AI, Maibach HI, Granlund H et al. Inhibition of contact allergy reactions by topical FK506. Lancet 1992; 340: 556.

8. Nakagawa H, Etoh T, Ishibasi Y et al. Tacrolimus ointment for atopic dermatitis. Lancet 1994; 344: 883.

9. Ruzicka T, Bieber T, Schöpf E et al. A short-term trial of tacrolimus ointment in atopic dermatitis. N Engl J Med 1997; 337: 816–21.

10. Puzik A, Schultz C, Iblher P et al. Effects of cyclosporin A, tacrolimus and sirolimus on cytokine production in neonatal immune cells. Acta Pediatr 2007; 96: 1483–9.

11. Goto T, Kino T, Hatanaka H et al. Discovery of FK-506, a novel immunosuppressant isolated from Streptomyces tsukubaensis. Transplant Proc 1987; 19 (5 Suppl 6): 4–8.

12. Arai T, Koyama Y, Suenaga T et al. Ascomycin, an antifungal antibiotic. J Antibiot Ser A 1962; 15: 231–2.

13. Grassberger M, Baumruker T, Enz A et al. A novel anti-inflammatory drug, SDZ ASM 981, for the treatment of skin diseases: in vitro pharmacology. Br J Dermatol 1999; 141: 264–73.

14. Wolff K, Fleming C, Hanifin J et al. Efficacy and tolerability of three different doses of oral pimecrolimus in the treatment of moderate to severe AD: a randomized controlled trial. Br J Dermatol 2005; 152: 1296–303.

15. Mollison KW, Fey TA, Gauvin DM et al. Discovery of ascomycin analogs with potent topical but weak systemic activity for treatment of inflammatory skin diseases. Curr Pharm Des 1998; 4: 367–79.

16. Bochelen D, Rudin M, Sauter. Calcineurin inhibitors FK506 and SDZ ASM 981 alleviate the outcome of focal cerebral ischaemic/reperfusion injury. J Pharmacol Exp Ther 1999; 288: 653–9.

17. Mrowietz U. Macrolide immunosuppressants. Eur J Dermatol 1999; 9:346–51.

18. Reitamo S. Tacrolimus. A new topical immunomodulatory therapy for atopic dermatitis. J Allergy Clin Immunol 2001; 107: 445–8.

19. Simon D, Vassina E, Yousefi S, Braathen LR, Simon HU. Inflammatory cell numbers and cytokine expression in AD after topical pimecrolimus treatment. Allergy 2005; 60: 944–51.

20. Hoetzenecker W, Ecker R, Kopp T et al. Pimecrolimus leads to an apoptosis-induced depletion of T cells but not Langerhans cells in patients with atopic dermatitis. J Allergy Clin Immunol 2005; 115: 1276–83.

21. Schuller E, Oppel T, Bornhövd E et al. Tacrolimus ointment causes inflammatory dendritic epidermal cell depletion but no Langerhans cell apoptosis in patients with atopic dermatitis. J Allergy Clin Immunol 2004; 114: 137–43.

22. Hatfield SM, Mynderse JS, Roehm NW. Rapamycin and FK506 differentially inhibit mast cell cytokine production and cytokine-induced reciprocal antagonists. J Pharmacol Exp Ther 1992; 261: 970–6.

23. Zuberbier T, Chong SU, Grunow K et al. The ascomycin macrolactam pimecrolimus (Elidel, SDZ ASM 981) is a potent inhibitor of mediator release from human dermal mast cells and peripheral blood basophils. J Allergy Clin Immunol 2001; 108: 275–80.

24. Kalthoff FS, Chung J, Musser P, Stuetz A. Pimecrolimus does not affect the differentiation, maturation and function of human monocyte-derived dendritic cells, in contrast to corticosteroids. Clin Exp Immunol 2003; 133: 350–9.

25. Meingassner JG, Kowalsky E, Schwendinger H, Elbe-Burger A, Stutz A. Pimecrolimus does not affect Langerhans cells in murine epidermis. Br J Dermatol 2003; 149: 853–7.

26. Alomar A, Berth-Jones J, Bos JD et al. The role of topical calcineurin inhibitors in atopic dermatitis. Br J Dermatol 2004; 151 (Suppl 70): 3–27.

27. Wollenberg A, Sharma S, von Bubnoff D et al. Topical tacrolimus (FK506) leads to profound phenotypic and functional alterations of epidermal antigen presenting dendritic cells in atopic dermatitis. J Allergy Clin Immunol 2001; 107: 519–25.

28. Panhans-Gross A, Novak N, Kraft S et al. Human epidermal Langerhans cells are targets of the immunosuppressive macrolide tacrolimus (FK506). J Allergy Clin Immunol 2001; 107: 345–52.

29. Stuetz A, Grassberger M, Meingassner JG. Pimecrolimus (Elidel, SDZ ASM 981) – preclinical pharmacologic profile and skin selectivity. Semin Cutan Med Surg 2001; 20: 233–41.

30. Oldhoff JM, Knol EF, Laaper-Ertmann M. Modulation of the atopy patch test: tacrolimus 0.1% compared with triamcinolone acetonide 0.1%. Allergy 2006; 61: 622–8.

31. Weissenbacher S, Traidl-Hoffmann C, Eyerich K et al. Modulation of atopy patch test and skin prick test with 1% pimecrolimus cream. Int Arch Allergy Immunol 2006; 140: 239–44.

32. Reitamo S, Rissanen J, Remitz A et al. Tacrolimus ointment does not affect collagen synthesis: results of a single-center randomized trial. J Invest Dermatol 1998; 111: 396–8.

33. Quelle-Roussel C, Paul C, Duteil L et al. The new topical ascomycin derivative SDZ ASM 981 doers not induce skin atrophy when applied to normal skin for four weeks: a randomised, double-blind controlled study. Br J Dermatol 2001; 44: 507–13.

34. Billich A, Aschauer H, Aszodi A, Stuetz A. Percutaneous absorption of drugs used in atopic eczema: pimecrolimus permeates less through skin than corticosteroids and tacrolimus. Int J Pharm 2004; 269: 29–35.

35. Van Leent EJ, Ebelin ME, Burtin P et al. Low systemic exposure after repeated topical application of pimecrolimus (Elidel), SD Z ASM 981) in patients with atopic dermatitis. Dermatology 2002; 204: 63–8.

36. Marsland AM, Griffiths CE. The macrolide immunosuppressants in dermatology: mechanisms of action. Eur J Dermatol 2002; 12: 618–22.

37. Kawashima M, Nakagawa H, Ohtsuki M, Tamaki K, Ishibashi Y. Tacrolimus concentrations in blood during topical treatment of atopic dermatitis. Lancet 1996; 348: 1240–1.

38. Allen A, Siegfried E, Silverman R et al. Significant absorption of topical tacrolimus in 3 patients with Netherton syndrome. Arch Dermatol 2001; 137: 747–50.

39. Reitamo S, Rustin M, Ruzicka T et al. Efficacy and safety of tacrolimus ointment compared with that of hydrocortisone butyrate ointment in adult patients with atopic dermatitis. J Allergy Clin Immunol 2002; 109: 547–55.

40. Reitamo S, Van Leent EJ, Ho V et al. Efficacy and safety of tacrolimus ointment compared with that of hydrocortisone acetate ointment in children with atopic dermatitis. J Allergy Clin Immunol 2002; 109: 539–46.

41. Reitamo S, Harper J, Bos J et al. 0.03% tacrolimus ointment applied once or twice daily is more efficacious than 1% hydrocortisone acetate in children with moderate to severe atopic dermatitis. Br J Dermatol 2004; 150: 554–62.

42. Doss N, Reitamo S, Dubertret L et al. Efficacy and safety of 0.1% tacrolimus ointment (Protopic) versus a potent corticosteroid ointment as second-line treatment in adults with moderate to severe atopic dermatitis of the face. European Academy of Dermatology and Venereology, Annual meeting, Vienna 2007. Abstract. Poster 53

43. Doss N, Kamoun MR, Dubertret L et al. Efficacy of tacrolimus 0.03% ointment as second-line treatment for children with moderate to severe atopic dermatitis: evidence from a randomised, double-blind noninferiority trial vs fluticasone 0.005% ointment. Submitted.

44. Bieber T, Vick K, Folster-Holst R et al. Efficacy and safety of methylprednisolone aceponate ointment 0.1% compared to tacrolimus 0.03% in children and adolescents with an acute flare of severe atopic dermatitis. Allergy 2007; 62: 184–9.

45. Ashcroft DM, Dimmock P, Garside R et al. Efficacy and tolerability of topical pimecrolimus and tacrolimus in the treatment of

atopic dermatitis: meta-analysis of randomised controlled trials. BMJ 2005; 330: 516.

46. Paller AS, Lebwohl M, Fleischer AB Jr et al. Tacrolimus ointment is more effective than pimecrolimus cream with a similar safety profile in the treatment of atopic dermatitis: results from 3 randomized, comparative studies. J Am Acad Dermatol 2005; 52: 810–22.

47. Reitamo S, Wollenberg A, Schopf E et al. Safety and efficacy of 1 year of tacrolimus ointment monotherapy in adults with atopic dermatitis. The European Tacrolimus Ointment Study Group. Arch Dermatol 2000; 136: 999–1006.

48. Reitamo S, Ortonne JP, Sand C et al. A multicentre, randomized, double-blind, controlled study of long-term treatment with 0.1% tacrolimus ointment in adults with moderate to severe atopic dermatitis. Br J Dermatol 2005; 152: 1282–9.

49. Reitamo S, Ortonne JP, Sand C et al. Long-term treatment with 0.1% tacrolimus ointment in adults with atopic dermatitis: results of a two-year, multicentre, noncomparative study. Acta Derm Venereol 2007; 87: 406–12.

50. Hanifin JM, Paller AS, Eichenfield L et al. Efficacy and safety of tacrolimus ointment for up to 4 years in patients with atopic dermatitis. J Am Acad Dermatol 2005; 53(2 Suppl 2): S186–94.

51. Reitamo S, Rustin M, Harper J et al. A 4-year follow-up study of atopic dermatitis therapy with 0.1% tacrolimus ointment in children and adult patients. Br J Dermatol, submitted.

52. Remitz A, Harper J, Rustin M et al. Long-term safety and efficacy of tacrolimus ointment for the treatment of atopic dermatitis in children. Acta Derm Venereol 2007; 87: 54–61.

53. Kang S, Lucky AW, Pariser D, Lawrence I, Hanifin JM. Long-term safety and efficacy of tacrolimus ointment for the treatment of atopic dermatitis in children. J Am Acad Dermatol 2001; 44: S58–64.

54. Drake L, Prendergast M, Maher R et al. The impact of tacrolimus ointment on health-related quality of life of adult and pediatric patients with atopic dermatitis. J Am Acad Dermatol 2001; 44: S65–72.

55. Remitz A, Kyllonen H, Granlund H et al. Tacrolimus ointment reduces staphylococcal colonization of atopic dermatitis lesions. J Allergy Clin Immunol 2001; 107:196–7.

56. Nakagawa H, Etoh T, Yokota Y et al. Tacrolimus has antifungal activities against Malassezia furfur isolated from healthy adults and patients with atopic dermatitis. Clin Drug Investig Suppl (Stockholm) 1996; 12: 244–50.

57. Agerberth B, Buentke E, Bergman P et al. Malassezia sympodialis differently affects the expression of LL–37 in dendritic cells from atopic eczema patients and healthy individuals. Allergy 2006; 61: 422–30.

58. Fellermann K, Wehkamp J, Stange EF. Antimicrobial peptides in the skin. N Engl J Med 2003; 348: 361–3.

59. Harrison JM, Ramshaw IA. Cytokines, skin, and smallpox – a new link to an antimicrobial peptide. Immunity 2006; 24: 245–7.

60. Howell MD, Gallo RL, Boguniewicz M et al. Cytokine milieu of atopic dermatitis skin subverts the innate immune response to vaccinia virus. Immunity 2006; 24: 341–8.

61. Howell MD, Novak N, Bieber T et al. Interleukin–10 downregulates anti-microbial peptide expression in atopic dermatitis. J Invest Dermatol 2005; 125: 738–45.

62. Howell MD, Wollenberg A, Gallo RL et al. Cathelicidin deficiency predisposes to eczema herpeticum. J Allergy Clin Immunol 2006; 117: 836–41.

63. Ong PY, Ohtake T, Brandt C et al. Endogenous antimicrobial peptides and skin infections in atopic dermatitis. N Engl J Med 2002; 347: 1151–60.

64. Mandelin J, Remitz A, Virtanen H et al. Recall antigen reactions in patients with atopic dermatitis treated with tacrolimus ointment for one year. J Allergy Clin Immunol in press.

65. Kyllönen H, Remitz A, Mandelin JM, Elg P, Reitamo S. Effects of 1-year intermittent treatment with topical tacrolimus monotherapy on skin collagen synthesis in patients with atopic dermatitis. Br J Dermatol 2004; 150: 1174–81.

66. Parrish JA. Immunosuppression, skin cancer, and ultraviolet A radiation. N Engl J Med 2005; 353: 2712–13.

67. Yarosh DB, Pena AV, Nay SL, Canning MT, Brown DA. Calcineurin inhibitors decrease DNA repair and apoptosis in human keratinocytes following ultraviolet B irradiation. J Invest Dermatol 2005; 125:1020–5.

68. Soter NA, Fleischer AB Jr, Webster GF, Monroe E, Lawrence I. Tacrolimus ointment for the treatment of atopic dermatitis in adult patients: part II, safety. J Am Acad Dermatol 2001; 44: S39–46.

69. Jiang H, Yamamoto S, Nishikawa K, Kato R. Anti-tumor-promoting action of FK506, a potent immunosuppressive agent. Carcinogenesis 1993; 14: 67–71.

70. Yao D, Dore JJ Jr, Leof EB. FKBP12 is a negative regulator of transforming growth factor-beta receptor internalization. J Biol Chem 2000; 275: 13149–54.

71. Tran C, Lübbe J, Antille C et al. Calcineurin inhibitors and skin cancer. J Invest Dermatol 2003; 121: 1072A.

72. Trautmann A, Akdis M, Schmid-Grendelmeier P et al. Targeting keratinocyte apoptosis in the treatment of atopic dermatitis and allergic contact dermatitis. J Allergy Clin Immunol 2001; 108: 839–46.

73. Van Leent EJ, Graber M, Thurston M et al. Effectiveness of the ascomycin macrolactam SDZ ASM 981 in the topical treatment of atopic dermatitis. Arch Dermatol 1998; 134: 805–9.

74. Luger T, Van Leent EJ, Graeber M et al. SDZ ASM 981: an emerging safe and effective treatment for atopic dermatitis. Br J Dermatol 2001; 144: 788–94.

75. Breuer K, Werfel T, Kapp A. Safety and efficacy of topical calcineurin inhibitors in the treatment of childhood atopic dermatitis. Am J Clin Dermatol 2005; 6: 65–77.

76. Eichenfield LF, Lucky AW, Boguniewicz M et al. Safety and efficacy of pimecrolimus (ASM 981) cream 1% in the treatment of mild and moderate atopic dermatitis in children and adolescents. J Am Acad Dermatol 2002; 46: 495–504.

77. Eichenfield LF, Lucky AW, Langley RG et al. Use of pimecrolimus cream 1% (Elidel) in the treatment of atopic dermatitis in infants and children: the effects of ethnic origin and baseline disease severity on treatment outcome. Int J Dermatol 2005; 44: 70–5.

78. Kaufmann R, Folster-Holst R, Hoger P et al. Onset of action of pimecrolimus cream 1% in the treatment of atopic dermatitis. J Allergy Clin Immunol 2004; 114: 1183–8.

79. Leo HL, Bender BG, Leung SB et al. Effect of pimecrolimus cream 1% on skin condition and sleep disturbance in children with atopic dermatitis. J Allergy Clin Immunol 2004; 114: 691–3.

80. Papp K, Staab D, Harper J et al. Effect of pimecrolimus cream 1% on the long-term course of pediatric atopic dermatitis. Int J Dermatol 2004; 43: 978–83.

81. Meurer M, Folster-Holst R, Wozel G et al. Pimecrolimus cream in the long-term management of atopic dermatitis in adults: a six-month study. Dermatology 2002; 205: 271–7.

82. Wahn U, Bos JD, Goodfield M et al. Efficacy and safety of pimecrolimus cream in the long-term management of atopic dermatitis in children. Pediatrics 2002; 110: e2.

83. Kapp A, Papp K, Bingham A et al. Long-term management of atopic dermatitis in infants with topical pimecrolimus, a non-steroid anti-inflammatory drug. J Allergy Clin Immunol 2002; 110: 277–84.

84. Papp KA, Breuer K, Meurer M et al. Long-term treatment of atopic dermatitis with pimecrolimus cream 1% in infants does not interfere with the development of protective antibodies after vaccination. J Am Acad Dermatol 2005; 52: 247–53.

85. Papp KA, Werfel T, Folster-Holst R et al. Long-term control of atopic dermatitis with pimecrolimus cream 1% in infants and young children: a two-year study. J Am Acad Dermatol 2005; 52: 240–6.

86. Harper J, Green A, Scott G et al. First experience of topical SDZ ASM 981 in children with atopic dermatitis. Br J Dermatol 2001; 144: 781–7.

87. Rappersberger K, Komar M, Ebelin ME et al. Pimecrolimus identifies a common genomic anti-inflammatory profile, is clinically highly effective in psoriasis and is well tolerated. J Invest Dermatol 2002; 119: 876–87.

88. Wolff K, Caro I, Murell D et al. Safety profile of oral pimecrolimus in atopic eczema and psoriasis: a pooled analysis from two dose-finding studies. J Invest Dermatol 2003; 121: 1245A.

89. Oji V, Beljan G, Beier K et al. Topical pimecrolimus: a novel therapeutic option for Netherton syndrome. Br J Dermatol 2005; 153: 1067–8.

90. Henno A, Choffray A, De La Brassinne M. [Improvement of Netherton syndrome associated erythroderma in two adult sisters through use of topical pimecrolimus]. Ann Dermatol Venereol 2006; 133: 71–2.

91. Stander S, Steinhoff M, Stander H et al. Morphological evidence of neuropeptide release and mast cell degranulation in tacrolimus and pimecrolimus treated murine skin. J Invest Dermatol 2003; 121: 912A.

92. Stander S, Stander H, Seeliger S, Luger TA, Steinhoff M. Topical pimecrolimus (SDZ ASM 981) and tacrolimus (FK 506) transiently induces neuropeptide release and mast cell degranulation in murine skin. Br J Dermatol 2007; 156: 1020–6.

93. Mahl A, Roman D, Court M, Vit P, Ulrich P. Pimecrolimus shows, in contrast to tacrolimus and cyclosporine, only marginal effects on immunization by oral administration in a rat model. J Invest Dermatol 2003; 121: 1226A.

94. Ring J, Barker J, Behrendt H et al. Review of the potential cocarcinogenicity of topical calcineurin inhibitors: position statement of the European Dermatology Forum. J Eur Acad Dermatol Venereol 2005; 19: 663–71.

95. Wooltorton E. Eczema drugs tacrolimus (Protopic) and pimecrolimus (Elidel): cancer concerns. CMAJ 2005; 172: 1179–80.

96. Sugiura H, Uehara M, Hoshino N et al. Long-term efficacy of tacrolimus ointment for recalcitrant facial erythema resistant to topical corticosteroids. Arch Dermatol 2000; 136: 1062–3.

97. Wollenberg A, Reitamo S, Girolomoni G et al. A novel approach to disease control with 0.1% tacrolimus ointment in adults with atopic dermatitis: results of a randomised, multicentre, comparative study. Allergy in press.

98. Thaci D, Reitamo S, Gonzalez Ensenat MA et al. Proactive disease management with 0.03% tacrolimus ointment in children with atopic dermatitis: results of a randomised, multicentre, comparative study. Br J Dermatol in press.

99. Arellano FM, Wentworth CE, Arana A et al. Risk of lymphoma following exposure to calcineurin inhibitors and topical steroids in patients with atopic dermatitis. J Invest Dermatol 2007; 127: 808–16.

100. Nghiem P, Pearson G, Langley RG. Tacrolimus and pimecrolimus: from clever prokaryotes to inhibiting calcineurin and treating atopic dermatitis. J Am Acad Dermatol 2002; 46: 228–41.

101. Bieber T, Cork M, Ellis C et al. Consensus statement on the safety profile of topical calcineurin inhibitors. Dermatology 2005; 211: 77–8.

102. Mansouri P, Farshi S. Pimecrolimus 1 percent cream in the treatment of psoriasis in a child. Dermatol Online J 2006; 12: 7.

103. Martin Ezquerra G, Sanchez Regana M et al. Topical tacrolimus for the treatment of psoriasis on the face, genitalia, intertriginous areas and corporal plaques. J Drugs Dermatol 2006; 5: 334–6.

104. Rallis E, Nasiopoulou A, Kouskoukis C et al. Pimecrolimus cream 1% can be an effective treatment for seborrheic dermatitis of the face and trunk. Drugs Exp Clin Res 2004; 30: 191–5.

105. Chu CY. The use of 1% pimecrolimus cream for the treatment of steroid-induced rosacea. Br J Dermatol 2005; 152: 396–9.

106. Crawford KM, Russ B, Bostrom P. Pimecrolimus for treatment of acne rosacea. Skinmed 2005; 4: 147–50.

107. de Almeida HL Jr, de Oliveira Filho UL. Topical pimecrolimus is an effective treatment for balanitis circinata erosiva. Int J Dermatol 2005; 44: 888–9.

108. Rigopoulos D, Prantsidis A, Christofidou E et al. Pimecrolimus 1% cream in the treatment of disseminated granuloma annulare. Br J Dermatol 2005; 152: 1364–5.

109. Cyr PR. Diagnosis and management of granuloma annulare. Am Fam Physician 2006; 74: 1729–34.

110. Scheer M, Kawari-Mahmoodi N, Neugebauer J et al. [Pimecrolimus (Elidel) for therapy of lichen ruber mucosae.] Mund Kiefer Gesichtschir 2006; 10: 403–7.

111. Swift JC, Rees TD, Plemons JM et al. The effectiveness of 1% pimecrolimus cream in the treatment of oral erosive lichen planus. J Periodontol 2005; 76: 627–35.

112. Luesley DM, Downey GP. Topical tacrolimus in the management of lichen sclerosus. BJOG 2006; 113: 832–4.

113. Wollina U, Hansel G, Koch A. Topical pimecrolimus for skin disease other than AD. Expert Opin Pharmacother 2006; 7: 1967–75.

114. Coskun B, Saral Y, Turgut D. Topical 0.05% clobetasol propionate versus 1% pimecrolimus ointment in vitiligo. Eur J Dermatol 2005; 15: 88–91.

115. Mehrabi D, Pandya AG. A randomized, placebo-controlled, double-blind trial comparing narrowband UV-B plus 0.1% tacrolimus ointment with narrowband UV-B plus placebo in the treatment of generalized vitiligo. Arch Dermatol 2006; 142: 927–9.

116. Ostovari N, Passeron T, Lacour JP et al. Lack of efficacy of tacrolimus in the treatment of vitiligo in the absence of UV-B exposure. Arch Dermatol 2006; 142: 252–3.

117. Conrotto D, Carrozzo M, Ubertalli AV et al. Dramatic increase of tacrolimus plasma concentration during topical treatment for oral graft-versus-host disease. Transplantation 2006; 82: 1113–5.

118. Schmook T, Kraft J, Benninghoff B et al. Treatment of cutaneous chronic graft-versus-host disease with topical pimecrolimus. Bone Marrow Transplant 2005; 36: 87–8.

119. Pitt M, Garside R, Stein K. A cost-utility analysis of pimecrolimus vs. topical corticosteroids and emollients for the treatment of mild and moderate atopic eczema. Br J Dermatol 2006; 154: 1137–46.

120. Ellis CN, Drake LA, Prendergast MM et al. Cost-effectiveness analysis of tacrolimus ointment versus high-potency topical corticosteroids in adults with moderate to severe atopic dermatitis. J Am Acad Dermatol 2003; 48: 553–63.

121. Ellis C, Luger T, Abeck D et al. International Consensus Conference on atopic dermatitis II (ICCAD II): clinical update and current treatment strategies. Br J Dermatol 2003; 148 (Suppl 63): 3–10.

20

Possible clinical associations of atopic dermatitis with bronchial asthma

Sakari Reitamo, Maili Lehto, Hannele Virtanen, Rita Haapakoski, Harri Alenius, Anita Remitz, and Antti Lauerma

INTRODUCTION

Atopic dermatitis (AD) is often accompanied by atopic airway disease, i.e. allergic rhinitis and/or bronchial asthma. In children the first symptoms of AD usually precede the airway symptoms. This phenomenon is often called the atopic march. Epidemiological studies suggest a relationship between the severity of AD, and the degree of atopic sensitization, and bronchial asthma. Patients with established AD often show bronchial hyperresponsiveness, respiratory symptoms, and eosinophilic airway inflammation. Recent findings of impaired barrier function of the skin induced by mutations of the filaggrin and other epidermal genes which lead to an increased risk for bronchial asthma further emphasize the key role of the epidermal barrier in both AD and atopic airway disease. Murine models of AD and asthma further suggest that the skin is the primary organ in the sensitization to aeroallergens leading to asthma-like reactions in the airways. Taken together these findings suggest an association of AD and bronchial asthma. Although it is tempting to speculate that effective treatment of AD at an early age might intervene with airway symptoms, only a few studies have addressed this issue. In the present chapter we discuss current knowledge on the relationship of AD and asthma and intervention studies in AD with atopic airway disease.

Atopic dermatitis is a T-cell-mediated inflammation exacerbated by an impaired barrier function of the skin

Environmental allergens can enter the body through skin, airways, and gastrointestinal tract and in sensitized individuals they evoke a variety of allergic manifestations.[1,2] In healthy human skin the upper layer of the epidermis plays a key role in the prevention of penetration of environmental allergens to the organism. In healthy normal skin peptides with a molecular mass of more than 500 D scarcely penetrate the skin.[3] In AD environmental allergens of up to 20 kD are capable of penetrating the skin. Effective treatment of the skin inflammation with topical calcineurin inhibitors has been shown to normalize the barrier function of the skin resulting in decrease of transepidermal water loss, suggesting a normalization of the barrier function. The barrier function is not only dependent on inflammatory response of the skin, as recent studies have shown that a high percentage of patients with AD have mutations of epidermal proteins leading to impaired barrier function of the skin. Mutations of the filaggrin genes are among those studied in depth. Interestingly a recent study showed that loss-of-function mutations of the filaggrin gene not only increases the risk for AD but also for bronchial asthma.[4]

Atopy is regarded as a disease which shows a lack of balance between T helper 1 and T helper 2 types of cells. Th1 cells are responsible for cell-mediated immunity and Th2 cells for antibody-mediated immunity. Impaired Th1 functions are typical for atopy in general, which clinically is shown as microbial infections and lack of reactions to environmental microbial antigens. In contrast, the Th2 functions are increased, which is shown for example in the increased levels of IgE. However, in the AD skin, Th2-type dominance is only seen in the acute phase of the disease, as Th2-type cytokines IL-4, IL-5 and IL-13 characterize the inflammatory response in the inflamed skin. In the chronic phase of the disease, however, Th1-type cytokines, IL-12 and IFN-γ, are highly expressed and predominate over Th2 cytokines. Interestingly, long-term treatment with either topical corticosteroids or topical calcineurin inhibitor such as tacrolimus, restores Th1-type immunity in patients with AD, as shown in the normalization of recall antigen responses.[5]

Since approximately 70–80% of patients with AD have elevated levels of serum IgE and specific IgE antibodies to environmental allergens, this points to an important role for environmental allergens in AD. It has been hypothesized that aeroallergens, such as house-dust mite and pollen allergens, may penetrate into the skin in sensitized atopic subjects, bind to high affinity IgE receptors on the Langerhans and other antigen-presenting cells, and then cause T-cell-mediated inflammatory responses leading to the eczema reaction.[6] In support of this theory, house-dust mite specific T cells have been found in the inflamed and non-inflamed skin of AD patients sensitized to this mite.[7] This IgE is vital for the presentation of the environmental allergens to the antigen-presenting cells of the epidermis which then process the environmental antigens to T cells. A further activation of the T cells is caused by bacterial enterotoxins. To conclude, environmental antigens such as aeroallergens are capable of penetrating the epidermis in AD skin, and can, together with bacterial enterotoxins, cause a specific and non-specific activation of T cells which leads to clinical symptoms of AD. The activation pathway can be blocked with corticosteroids or topical calcineurin inhibitors. However, of these only topical calcineurin inhibitors can effectively suppress the enterotokin induced T-cell response.[8]

CLINICAL FORMS OF ATOPIC AIRWAY DISEASE

Airways are continuously exposed to inhaled particles, microbes, and harmless antigens to which either immunity or tolerance is induced. Allergic rhinitis and allergic asthma are two important allergic disorders, which affect the upper and lower parts of the respiratory tract, respectively. Similar inflammatory features are found in these diseases, such as vasodilation and local infiltration of mast cells, macrophages, eosinophils, dendritic cells, and T cells. However, the importance of affected structures differs: smooth muscles are essential components in lower airways and blood vessels in upper airways. In addition, the surface of the epithelium plays an important role in the development of asthma.[9]

Asthma is commonly divided into IgE-mediated allergic asthma and non-IgE-mediated asthma (non-allergic asthma).[10,11] Eighty per cent of childhood asthma and over 50% of adult asthma has been reported to be allergic in this manner. The mechanisms which initiate non-allergic asthma are not well-defined. Asthma is a phenotypically heterogeneous disorder that results from complex interactions between environmental and genetic factors. Allergic asthma is triggered by allergen-induced activation of submucosal mast cells in the lower airways.[12] This leads to immediate bronchial constriction and amplified secretion of fluid and mucus, causing respiratory distress. A central aspect of asthma is chronic airway inflammation which is characterized by the continuous presence of Th2 lymphocytes, and eosinophilic, neutrophilic, and other leukocytes. These cells act together to cause improper remodelling of the airways, accompanied by augmented mucus production. Th2 cytokines such as IL-13 may directly affect airway epithelial cells and cause the induction of goblet-cell metaplasia and the secretion of mucus.[13] Bronchial epithelial cells express the chemokine receptor CCR3 and also produce at least two of the ligands for this receptor – CCL5 (RANTES) and CCL11 (eotaxin 1). These chemokines attract more Th2 cells and eosinophils to the damaged lungs which can increase the Th2 response. Additionally, recent studies indicate that CCL11 has a profibrogenic effect on human airway epithelial cells and fibroblasts through the chemokine receptor CCR3.[14,15] Th2 cytokines and chemokines also have a direct effect on airway smooth muscle cells and lung fibroblasts leading to airway remodelling. Remodelling comprises thickening of the airway walls by hyperplasia and hypertrophy of the smooth muscle layer and mucous glands, with the final development of fibrosis.

Initially, allergic asthma is driven by a response to a specific allergen, but chronic inflammation seems to continue unabated even in the absence of allergen exposure. The airways become hyperreactive, and factors other than re-exposure to antigen can trigger asthma symptoms. For instance, environmental irritants, such as cigarette smoke, typically induce airway hyperreactivity. In addition, viral or bacterial respiratory infections can exacerbate asthma by inducing a Th2-dominated local response.[16,17]

MOUSE MODELS FOR ALLERGIC DISEASES

Mouse models have been largely used for study of allergic disorders due to the availability of immunological tools, such as transgenic and knockout mouse strains and antibodies. Mouse models of AD can be roughly categorized into the following groups:

1. Mouse models (NC/Nga) with spontaneous development of AD[18]
2. Genetically modified mice, transgenic or knockout, e.g. with regard to IL-4 and IL-18[19,20]
3. AD-like skin lesions after epicutaneous ovalbumin sensitization[21,22]
4. Humanized mouse models of AD such as the SCID. mutant mice (severe combined immunodeficiency)[23]

For the time being, the limited availability and the lack of standardized mice housing conditions make the use of NC/Nga mice inconvenient. Humanized SCID and genetically modified mice are important tools when examining specific mechanisms of diseases. On the other hand, a mouse model making use of repeated epicutaneous protein exposure[24] imitates reasonably well naturally occurring cutaneous sensitization. In this model, tape stripping is an important feature provoking the development of general skin injury characteristic of AD.

Allergic asthma is a complex condition characterized by increased amounts of systemic IgE, elevated allergen-specific Th2 cells and their products, airway hyperreactivity (AHR), and structural changes in the lung.[25] Animal models of both acute and chronic allergic airway responses have been described, although none of these models encompasses all aspects of human asthma.[26–30] Moreover, considerable differences in the airway reactivity between different mice strains exist.[31,32] The most widely used mouse model of acute asthma involves intraperitoneal injections with ovalbumin combined with alum, followed by repeated ovalbumin challenges intratracheally, intranasally, or by inhalation. This evokes a marked eosinophilic inflammation and AHR, which is independent of IgE, B cells, or mast cells, but dependent on CD4 + T cells.[33] The presence of effector T cells is essential and sufficient to provide the necessary Th2 cytokines to evoke both histological changes and induced AHR.[29] Chronic asthma models with remodelling of lung tissue have been reported but these models are difficult to standardize.[30,34,35]

A few studies have used mouse models to examine the pathological mechanisms involved in natural rubber latex (NRL) allergy.[36,37] BALB/c mice have been the most commonly investigated mice strain, but in two studies C57BL/6 and B6C3F1 mice were also used.[38,39] Crude NRL has been the allergen used in almost all studies[38–41] but recombinant Hev b 5 has also been administered in two studies.[42,43] One group has been interested in the effects of NRL in the lungs which they have investigated by using intranasal and intraperitoneal sensitization.[38,40,41] They found increased levels of total IgE, IL-4, IL-5 and eosinophils in the blood.[38] Eosinophils were detected in the lungs and AHR occurred after methacholine (MCh) challenge.[40,41] Experiments in IL-4 knockout BALB/c mice showed no eosinophils or IgE antibodies, confirming the importance of this cytokine in the initiation of this response.[41] It is, however, of interest that IL-4 knockout mice exhibited a weak AHR to MCh.[40,41]

Woolhiser et al[39] studied the effects of intranasal (IN), subcutaneous and epicutaneous exposure by using crude NRL as allergen. They found increased total IgE levels by all exposure routes and detected the presence of several IgE bands with cutaneous exposure. However, the results of different exposure routes are not comparable because NRL dosage and exposure times were different. Slater and co-workers[42,43] used recombinant Hev b 5 with maltose binding protein to sensitize BALB/c mice by the IN route. Hev b 5 specific IgG1 or IgE antibodies were found in the blood. A significant lymphoid cell infiltration, but no mucus secretion, was seen in the lungs when the allergen was given together with lipopolysaccharide (LPS). These mouse model studies indicate that IgE antibodies appear after cutaneous, intranasal and intraperitoneal exposure to NRL. It seems evident that IN exposure to NRL can evoke eosinophilic lung inflammation and AHR in the sensitized mice.

EFFECT OF EXPOSURE ROUTES ON LUNG INFLAMMATION AND AIRWAY HYPERREACTIVITY

The role of different exposure routes in the induction of lung inflammation and airway hyperreactivity in a murine model of allergic asthma was studied. We used natural rubber latex (NRL) as a model allergen as it contains the major NRL allergen Hev b 6.02 (hevein), which is well-characterized. In addition, hevein with reduced allergenicity has been constructed for possible use in immunotherapy studies.[44] We used the intracutaneous (IC) route for skin exposure, IN (intranasal) route for airway exposure, and intraperitoneal (IP) route for systemic exposure. IC and IN immunizations were done without adjuvants, reflecting more the real-life sensitization route in people suffering from allergic symptoms. Sensitization protocols are shown in Figure 20.1. The study showed overwhelmingly that the skin is the most efficient route of sensitization, whilst sensitization through airways exposure fails to induce allergic asthma.[45]

IC and IP exposure caused perivascular and peribronchial inflammation of lung tissues after airway allergen challenge, whereas after IN exposure, only a slight, mostly perivascular inflammation was detected (Fig 20.2a). The number of eosinophils increased dramatically after IC treatment, but not after IP or IN exposure in lung tissues (Figure 20.2a), whereas significant amounts of eosinophils and lymphocytes were seen in BAL fluid samples of IC and IP allergen-exposed mice (Figure 20.2b). In line with the histological results, eosinophils were virtually absent and only a few lymphocytes were present in the BAL of intranasally exposed mice.[45]

Airway hyperreactivity (AHR) to inhaled methacholine (MCh) increased vigorously in response to IC and IP allergen exposure followed by NRL airway challenge (Figure 20.3a). In contrast, IN allergen exposure did not induce AHR and the control mice group exhibited a slightly elevated but statistically non-significant response to inhaled MCh. PAS staining of lung sections

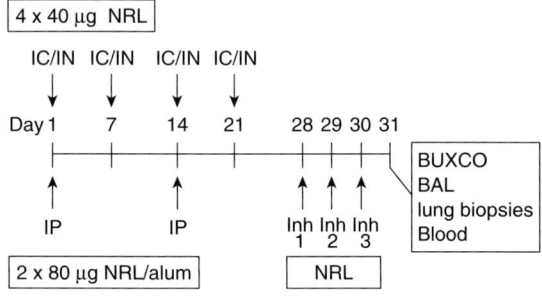

Figure 20.1 Intracutaneous (IC), intraperitoneal (IP) and intranasal (IN) exposure schedules. Mice were exposed for 4 weeks before airway challenge. In saline (SAL) groups exposures were made with phosphate-buffered saline and with natural rubber latex (NRL) in NRL groups. Airway challenges were made by NRL. Airway hyperreactivity to methacholine was measured 24 hours after airway challenges and different samples were taken for subsequent analysis.

showed that animals treated intracutaneously or intraperitoneally with NRL displayed a significant increase in mucus production, as seen in the high amount of goblet cells around the bronchiolar lumen (Fig 20.3b). Intranasal NRL exposure induced only a slight and insignificant enhancement of mucus production in the airways.[45]

Expression of mRNA of several CC chemokines, which attract eosinophils (CCL3, CCL8, CCL11, and CCL24) or Th2 (CCL1 and CCL17) cells was measured. It was noted that IC, IP, and IN exposure and airway challenge significantly elevated mRNA expression of CCL1, CCL8, CCL11, CCL17, and CCL24 relative to the PBS-treated control mice. Expression of CCL3 mRNA significantly increased after IC and IP NRL exposure, but not after IN exposure. In general, expression of most chemokines was significantly higher after IC NRL exposure (CCL1, CCL3, CCL8, CCL17, and CCL24) or IP exposure (CCL1, CCL3, CCL8, CCL17, and CCL24) compared to IN treatment. Expression of

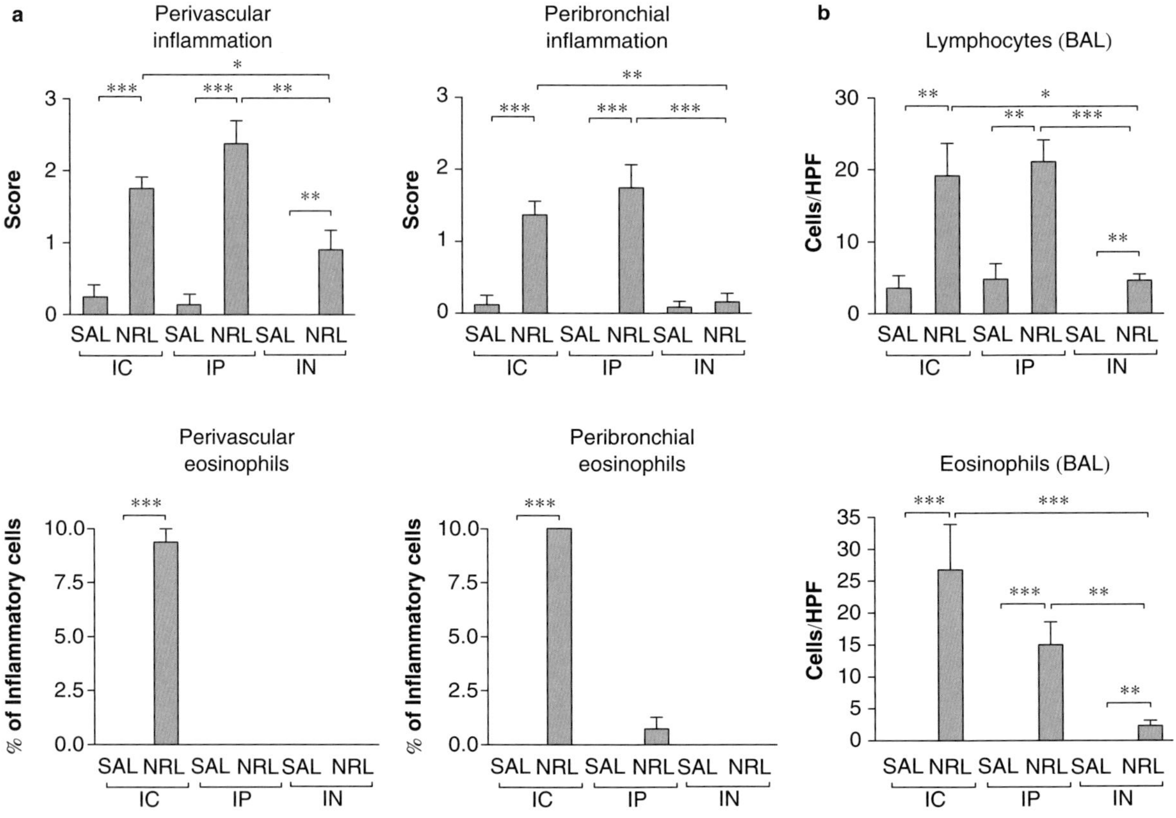

Figure 20.2 Lung inflammation (a) Inflammation was expressed as score values and eosinophils as percentages of inflammatory cells (n = 7–12 mice per group). (b) Lymphocytes and eosinophils in bronchoalveolar lavage (BAL) fluids were counted per high-power field (HPF) (n = 12–16 mice per group). The columns and error bars represent mean ± SEM; *p < 0.05, **p < 0.01, ***p < 0.001.

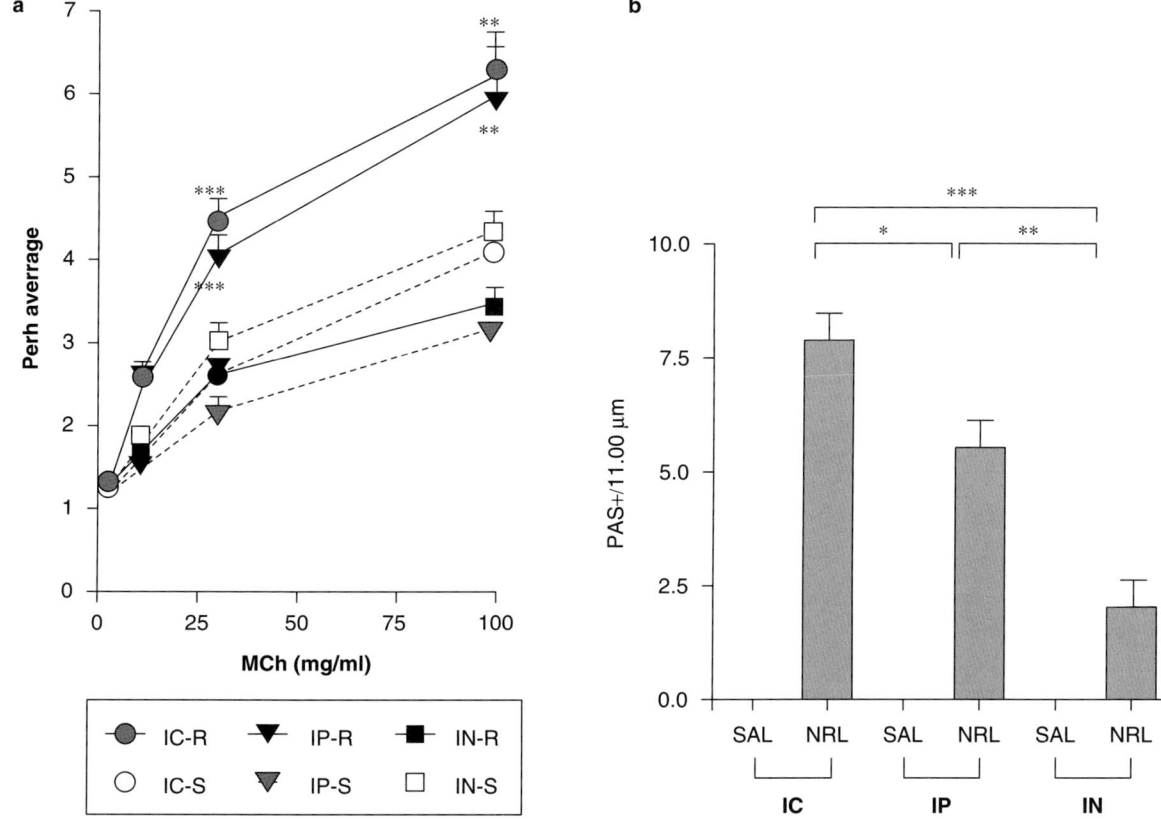

Figure 20.3   Airway hyperresponsiveness and lung mucus production (a) Airway hyperreactivity was expressed by average enhanced pause (Penh) values in relation to increasing doses (1–100 mg/ml) of aerosolized methacholine (MCh). Data represent mean ± SEM. (b) The number of mucus-producing cells was represented as periodic acid-Schiff (PAS) positive cells. The columns and error bars represent mean ± SEM; ns = non-significant, *p < 0.05, **p < 0.01, ***p < 0.001; n = 12–16 mice per group.

chemokine receptors (CCR1, CCR3, CCR4, and CCR8), which bind these CC ligands, was also analysed. All exposure routes significantly increased mRNA expression of these chemokine receptors. Expression of CCR1 and CCR8 mRNAs was significantly higher after IC and IP sensitization compared to intranasally treated mice. A markedly higher level of CCR3 mRNA was seen in intracutaneously sensitized mice compared to the corresponding intranasally sensitized group.[45]

The cytokine expression profile at the mRNA level revealed differences between different exposure routes. IC and IP exposure to NRL increased the expression levels of IL-4 and IL-13 mRNA, but only IC exposure significantly increased the expression of IL-5 mRNA in lung compared to PBS-treated controls (Figure 20.4a). In addition, the IL-13 mRNA level was elevated (8-fold) in the intranasally NRL exposed mice in comparison

with the controls. IC exposure elicited significantly higher expression of IL-4, IL-5, and IL-13 mRNA compared to the IN group. The mRNA levels of regulatory cytokine IL-10 were enhanced significantly in all NRL exposed groups, especially in intranasally treated mice (Figure 20.4b). On the other hand, a significant elevation in the levels of TGF-β1 mRNA was observed after IN and IP NRL exposure but not after IC exposure. In addition, the TGF-β1 mRNA levels were significantly higher in IN and IP exposed mice than in IC exposed mice (Figure 20.4b). Forkhead box 3 (Foxp3) transcription factor mRNA expression also increased significantly after IP and IN NRL administration but not after IC exposure (Figure 20.4b) with the elevation in expression being most marked after IN NRL exposure.[45]

Total and Hev b 6.01-specific IgE antibodies were strongly elevated after IC and IP exposure, but not after IN exposure to NRL.[45] In the murine study described

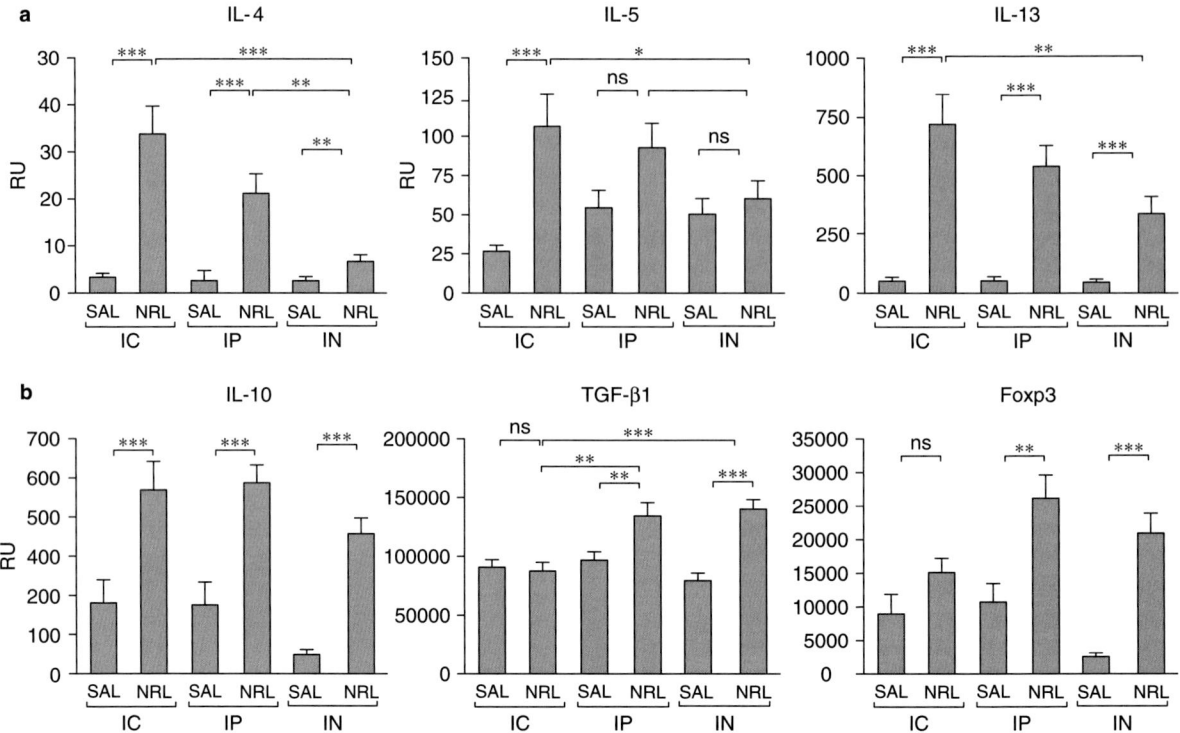

Figure 20.4 Expression levels of cytokines and Foxp3 mRNAs. T-helper type 2 cytokine mRNA (a) and regulatory cytokine and forkhead box 3 (Foxp3) mRNA (b) expression in lung samples after exposures to vehicle (saline (SAL)) or natural rubber latex (NRL). The columns and error bars represent mean ± SEM; ns = non-significant, *p < 0.05, **p < 0.01, ***p < 0.001; n = 12–15 mice per group.

above,[45] IC and IN exposures were performed with the same total amount (160 µg) of NRL without adjuvants. When the airways were challenged with NRL in IC exposed mice, a more intense lung eosinophilia was found than in IN and IP exposed mice. IC and IP exposures, but not IN exposure, induced significant mucus production and AHR to inhaled MCh. In agreement with these findings, a previous study revealed that topical NRL exposure to tape stripped skin also increased AHR to inhaled MCh, whereas intratracheal exposure of NRL had no influence on the airway response.[46,47] These results in mice clearly indicate that repeated cutaneous NRL exposure can efficiently sensitize the lungs, and therefore predispose this tissue to NRL-allergic asthma.

Th2 cytokines IL-4 and IL-13 are most important regulators of IgE class switching[48] and IL-13 also participates in AHR and mucus production.[13] In the present experiments, all 3 (IC, IP, and IN) NRL exposure routes were able to upregulate IL-4 and IL-13 mRNA in the lungs of the mice. The increase was, however, highest after IC exposure and lowest after IN exposure. It is known that IL-5 is especially involved in the

recruitment and survival of eosinophils.[49] In the present study, IL-5 mRNA expression was increased significantly after IC but not after IP or IN exposure. One effect of IL-5 could then be the influx of eosinophils into the lungs, a finding which was especially marked in IC exposed mice. In line with the present findings, a previous study documented that IP sensitization with NRL glove extract or Hev b 5 can induce IL-5 protein into the BAL fluid.[50] It is of interest that mRNA expression of eosinophil-attracting chemokines (CCL3, CCL8, CCL11, CCL24) and their receptors (CCR1, CCR3) was significantly higher in the lungs of IC exposed mice compared to the lungs of IN exposed mice. CCL1 and CCL17 chemokines are known to attract Th2 cells.[51] Expression of these chemokine mRNAs was also higher after IC and IP exposure compared to IN exposure in mice, and the same was true for Th2 associated chemokine receptor CCR8. In summary, these findings indicate that repeated cutaneous NRL allergen exposure also effectively sensitizes the lungs. Thereafter, NRL airway challenge is able to upregulate different inflammatory chemokines and chemokine receptors. The next step seems to be the influx of eosinophils and Th2 lymphocytes into the lung tissue, the cells which are important in allergic airway inflammation.

Airway inflammation, mucus production, and AHR were substantially lower in IN exposed mice compared to intracutaneously exposed mice. Therefore we measured the mRNA levels of regulatory cytokines IL-10 and TGF-β1.[51–53] Interestingly, expression of IL-10 was higher after IN exposure than after IC and IP exposure in mice. In addition, both TGF-β1 and Foxp3, which is a marker for CD4 + CD25+ T regulatory cells,[54,55] were significantly upregulated after IN exposure. These findings in mice suggest that an allergen exposure to the airways, but not to the skin, could also activate regulatory mechanisms for the inflammation and in this process IL-10 and TGF-β1 as well as Foxp3 + regulatory T cells could be the key players. This suggestion is in line with the concept that the mucosal immune system is programmed to induce tolerance to ingested or inhaled allergens.[56–59] A recent mouse study with NRL provided further evidence for the fact that tolerance can take place when allergen exposure initially occurs in the nasal mucosa.[60] These investigators observed that IN exposure, when performed before IP exposure, prevented antibody responses to Hev b 1 and Hev b 3. A similar induction of tolerance has also been observed in mice after IN administration of the birch pollen allergen Bet v 1.[61,62] The IN administration suppressed both the allergic immune responses and airway inflammation and the induction of tolerance seemed to be due to Foxp3+ CD4 + T cells.[62]

HUMAN STUDIES ON PREVENTION OR REVERSAL OF THE ATOPIC MARCH

The only studies performed so far to prevent asthma have been with oral H_1 receptor antagonists, i.e antihistamines. The most widely studied antihistamine for the prevention of the atopic march has been cetirizine. Cetirizine was compared to placebo for 18 months in infants 1–2 years of age with AD. After 18 months, follow-up was continued for a further 18 months. There was no difference in the cumulative prevalence of asthma between active and placebo treatment in the intention-to-treat population. Those infants with an evidence of sensitivity to house dust mite, grass pollen, or both, who were treated with cetirizine, were significantly less likely to have asthma compared with those treated with placebo over 18 months of treatment. This effect was sustained for the grass-pollen sensitized infants throughout the study period. In the house dust mite sensitized group there was a gradual narrowing of the difference between active and placebo treatment in

terms of cumulative prevalence of asthma at the end of 36 months but no evidence of rebound immediately after the treatment was stopped. In the placebo population there was a slightly increased risk of sensitization to egg, house dust mite, grass pollen, and cat.[63]

The lack of a significant effect on the prevention of the atopic march with oral cetirizine may be due to the fact that it is not an effective treatment of asthma. As previously noted in mice the main sensitization route is via the epidermis. In the cetirizine study patients could use topical corticosteroids, but the details of use are not clear. As previously noted in mice, the main sensitization route is via the epidermis. Currently there are no studies with topical long-term treatment of infants with AD to prevent the progression to atopic airway disease.

Effect of topical calcineurin inhibitor in patients with AD and atopic airway disease

We earlier noted that many patients with moderate-to-severe AD who achieved control of the AD with long-term use of tacrolimus ointment had a subjective relief of symptoms of asthma. Therefore, we prospectively assessed the effects of topical-intermittent long-term treatment with tacrolimus ointment in 64 patients aged 13–56 years who had moderate to severe AD. Treatment in this uncontrolled study was for 4 years.[64] Bronchial histamine challenge for hyperresponsiveness was done at baseline and after 1 year of treatment, and total serum IgE and respiratory symptoms were determined at baseline and after 1 and 4 years of treatment. The body surface area of AD cleared significantly, and bronchial hyperresponsiveness, as well as asthma and rhinitis symptoms, all showed significant improvement. Patients whose AD improved most also showed a decreasing trend in serum IgE levels. This study suggests that effective long-term topical treatment may improve not only AD but also reverse atopic airway disease. Controlled studies should be performed to confirm these findings. A study with a protocol similar to the cetirizine study for infants with AD prior to established asthma would also be needed. Topical calcineurin inhibitors would be ideal for such a study, as they, in contrast to corticosteroids, do not impair the integrity of the skin.

REFERENCES

1. Kay AB. Allergy and allergic diseases. First of two parts. N Engl J Med 2001; 344: 30–7.
2. Kay AB. Allergy and allergic diseases. Second of two parts. N Engl J Med 2001; 344: 109–13.
3. Bos JD, Meinardi MM. The 500 Dalton rule for the skin penetration of chemical compounds and drugs. Exp Dermatol 2000; 9: 165–9.

4. Marenholz I, Nickel R, Ruschendorf F, Schullz F, Esparza-Gordillo J et al. Filagrin loss-of-function mutations predispose to phenotypes involved in the atopic march. J Allergy Clin Immunol 2006; 118: 866–71.

5. Mandelin et al, Remitz A, Virtamen H, Reitamo S. Recall-antigen reactions in patient with atopic dermatitis treated with tacrolimus ointment for one year. Submitted.

6. Bruijnzeel-Koomen CA, Fokkens WJ, Mudde GC, Bruijnzeel PL. Role of Langerhans cells in atopic disease. Int Arch Allergy Appl Immunol 1989; 90(Suppl 1): 51–6.

7. Bohle B, Schwihla H, Hu HZ, Friedl-Hajek R, Sowka S et al. Long-lived Th2 clones specific for seasonal and perennial allergens can be detected in blood and skin by their TCR-hypervariable regions. J Immunol 1998; 160: 2022–7.

8. Leung DY, Bieber T. Atopic dermatitis. Lancet 2003; 361: 151–60.

9. Cookson W. The immunogenetics of asthma and eczema: a new focus on the epithelium. Nat Rev Immunol 2004; 4: 978–88.

10. Humbert M, Menz G, Ying S, Corrigan CJ, Robinson DS et al. The immunopathology of extrinsic (atopic) and intrinsic (non-atopic) asthma: more similarities than differences. Immunol Today 1999; 20: 528–33.

11. Johansson SG, Bieber T, Dahl R, Friedmann PS, Lanier BQ et al. Revised nomenclature for allergy for global use: Report of the Nomenclature Review Committee of the World Allergy Organization, October 2003. J Allergy Clin Immunol 2004; 113: 832–6.

12. Bousquet J, Jeffery PK, Busse WW, Johnson M, Vignola AM. Asthma. From bronchoconstriction to airways inflammation and remodeling. Am J Respir Crit Care Med 2000; 161: 1720–45.

13. Kuperman DA, Huang X, Koth LL, Chang GH, Dolganov GM et al. Direct effects of interleukin-13 on epithelial cells cause airway hyperreactivity and mucus overproduction in asthma. Nat Med 2002; 8: 885–9.

14. Beck LA, Tancowny B, Brummet ME, Asaki SY, Curry SL et al. Functional analysis of the chemokine receptor CCR3 on airway epithelial cells. J Immunol 2006; 177: 3344–54.

15. Puxeddu I, Bader R, Piliponsky AM, Reich R, Levi-Schaffer F et al. The CC chemokine eotaxin/CCL11 has a selective profibrogenic effect on human lung fibroblasts. J Allergy Clin Immunol 2006; 117: 103–10.

16. Friedlander SL, Busse WW. The role of rhinovirus in asthma exacerbations. J Allergy Clin Immunol 2005; 116: 267–73.

17. Lemanske RF, Jr. Busse WW. 6. Asthma: Factors underlying inception, exacerbation, and disease progression. J Allergy Clin Immunol 2006; 117: S456–61.

18. Matsuda H, Watanabe N, Geba GP, Sperl J, Tsudzuki M et al. Development of atopic dermatitis-like skin lesion with IgE hyperproduction in NC/Nga mice. Int Immunol 1997; 9: 461–6.

19. Chan LS, Robinson N, Xu L. Expression of interleukin-4 in the epidermis of transgenic mice results in a pruritic inflammatory skin disease: an experimental animal model to study atopic dermatitis. J Invest Dermatol 2001; 117: 977–83.

20. Konishi H, Tsutsui H, Murakami T, Yumikura-Futatsugi S, Yamanaka K et al. IL-18 contributes to the spontaneous development of atopic dermatitis-like inflammatory skin lesion independently of IgE/stat6 under specific pathogen-free conditions. Proc Natl Acad Sci U S A 2002; 99: 11340–5.

21. Wang LF, Lin JY, Hsieh KH, Lin RH. Epicutaneous exposure of protein antigen induces a predominant Th2-like response with high IgE production in mice. J Immunol 1996; 156: 4077–82.

22. Spergel JM, Paller AS. Atopic dermatitis and the atopic march. J Allergy Clin Immunol 2003; 112: S118–27.

23. Carballido JM, Biedermann T, Schwarzler C, de Vries JE. The SCID-hu Skin mouse as a model to investigate selective chemokine mediated homing of human T-lymphocytes to the skin in vivo. J Immunol Methods 2003; 273: 125–35.

24. Spergel JM, Mizoguchi E, Brewer JP, Martin TR, Bhan AK et al. Epicutaneous sensitization with protein antigen induces localized allergic dermatitis and hyperresponsiveness to methacholine after single exposure to aerosolized antigen in mice. J Clin Invest 1998; 101: 1614–22.

25. Cohn L, Elias JA, Chupp GL. Asthma: mechanisms of disease persistence and progression. Annu Rev Immunol 2004; 22: 789–815.

26. Kips JC, Anderson GP, Fredberg JJ, Herz U, Inman MD et al. Murine models of asthma. Eur Respir J 2003; 22: 374–82.

27. Epstein MM. Do mouse models of allergic asthma mimic clinical disease? Int Arch Allergy Immunol 2004; 133: 84–100.

28. Taube C, Dakhama A, Gelfand EW. Insights into the pathogenesis of asthma utilizing murine models. Int Arch Allergy Immunol 2004; 135: 173–86.

29. Boyce JA, Austen KF. No audible wheezing: nuggets and conundrums from mouse asthma models. J Exp Med 2005; 201: 1869–73.

30. Fulkerson PC, Rothenberg ME, Hogan SP. Building a better mouse model: experimental models of chronic asthma. Clin Exp Allergy 2005; 35: 1251–3.

31. Takeda K, Haczku A, Lee JJ, Irvin CG, Gelfand EW. Strain dependence of airway hyperresponsiveness reflects differences in eosinophil localization in the lung. Am J Physiol Lung Cell Mol Physiol 2001; 281: L394–402.

32. Whitehead GS, Walker JK, Berman KG, Foster WM, Schwartz DA. Allergen-induced airway disease is mouse strain dependent. Am J Physiol Lung Cell Mol Physiol 2003; 285: L32–42.

33. Corry DB, Grunig G, Hadeiba H, Kurup VP, Warnock ML et al. Requirements for allergen-induced airway hyperreactivity in T and B cell-deficient mice. Mol Med 1998; 4: 344–55.

34. McMillan SJ, Lloyd CM. Prolonged allergen challenge in mice leads to persistent airway remodelling. Clin Exp Allergy 2004; 34: 497–507.

35. Wegmann M, Fehrenbach H, Fehrenbach A, Held T, Schramm C et al. Involvement of distal airways in a chronic model of experimental asthma. Clin Exp Allergy 2005; 35: 1263–71.

36. Meade BJ, Woolhiser M. Murine models for natural rubber latex allergy assessment. Methods 2002; 27: 63–8.

37. Herz U, Renz H, Wiedermann U. Animal models of type I allergy using recombinant allergens. Methods 2004; 32: 271–80.

38. Kurup VP, Kumar A, Choi H, Murali PS, Resnick A et al. Latex antigens induce IgE and eosinophils in mice. Int Arch Allergy Immunol 1994; 103: 370–7.

39. Woolhiser MR, Munson AE, Meade BJ. Role of sensitization routes in the development of type I hypersensitivity to natural rubber latex in mice. Am J Ind Med Suppl 1999; 1: 139–41.

40. Thakker JC, Xia JQ, Rickaby DA, Krenz GS, Kelly KJ et al. A murine model of latex allergy-induced airway hyperreactivity. Lung 1999; 177: 89–100.

41. Xia JQ, Rickaby DA, Kelly KJ, Choi H, Dawson CA et al. Immune response and airway reactivity in wild and IL-4 knock-out mice exposed to latex allergens. Int Arch Allergy Immunol 1999; 118: 23–9.

42. Slater JE, Paupore EJ, Elwell MR, Truscott W. Lipopolysaccharide augments IgG and IgE responses of mice to the latex allergen Hev b 5. J Allergy Clin Immunol 1998; 102: 977–83.

43. Slater JE, Paupore EJ, O'Hehir RE. Murine B-cell and T-cell epitopes of the allergen Hev b 5 from natural rubber latex. Mol Immunol 1999; 36: 135–43.

44. Karisola P, Mikkola J, Kalkkinen N, Airenne KJ, Laitinen OH et al. Construction of hevein (Hev b 6.02) with reduced allergenicity for immunotherapy of latex allergy by comutation of six amino acid residues on the conformational IgE epitopes. J Immunol 2004; 172: 2621–8.

45. Lehto M, Haapakoski R, Wolff H, Majuri ML, Mäkelä MJ et al. Cutaneous, but not airway, latex exposure induces allergic lung inflammation and airway hyperreactivity in mice. J Invest Dermatol 2005; 125: 962–8.

46. Howell MD, Weissmann DN and Jean Meae B. Latex sensitization by dermal exposure can lead to airway hyperreactivity. Int Arch Allergy Immunol 2002; 128: 204–11.

47. Howell MD, Tomazic VS, Leakakos T, Truscott W et al. Immunomodulatory effect of endotoxin on the development of latex allergy. 2004. Journal of Allergy Clin Immunol. 113: 916–24.

48. Geha RS, Jabara HH, Brodeur SR, The regulation of immunoglobulin E class-switch recombination. 2003. Nat Rev Immunol 2003; 3: 721–32.

49. Hamelmann E, Gelfand BW. IL-5-induced airway eosinophilia one key to asthama? Immunol Rev. 179: 182–191.

50. Hardy CL, Kenins L, Drew AC, Rolland JM, O'Hehir RE. Characterization of a mouse model of allergy to a major occupational latex glove allergen Hev b 5. Am J Respir Crit Care Med 2003; 167: 1393–9.

51. Panina-Bordignon P, Papi A, Mariani M, Di Lucia P, Casoni G et al. The C-C chemokine receptors CCR4 and CCR8 identify airway T cells of allergen-challenged atopic asthmatics. J Clin Invest 2001; 107: 1357–64.

52. Akbari O, Stock P, DeKruyff RH, Umetsu DT. Role of regulatory T cells in allergy and asthma. Curr Opin Immunol 2003; 15: 627–33.

52. Terui T, Sano K, Shirota H, Kunikata N, Ozawa M et al. TGF-beta-producing CD4+ mediastinal lymph node cells obtained from mice tracheally tolerized to ovalbumin (OVA) suppress both Th1- and Th2-induced cutaneous inflammatory responses to OVA by different mechanisms. J Immunol 2001; 167: 3661–7.

53. Nagler-Anderson C, Bhan AK, Podolsky DK, Terhorst C. Control freaks: immune regulatory cells. Nat Immunol 2004; 5: 119–22.

54. Fontenot JD, Gavin MA, Rudensky AY. Foxp3 programs the development and function of CD4+CD25+ regulatory T cells. Nat Immunol 2003; 4: 330–6.

55. Khattri R, Cox T, Yasayko SA, Ramsdell F. An essential role for Scurfin in CD4+CD25+ T regulatory cells. Nat Immunol 2003; 4: 337–42.

56. Macaubas C, DeKruyff RH, Umetsu DT. Respiratory tolerance in the protection against asthma. Curr Drug Targets Inflamm Allergy 2003; 2: 175–86.

57. Mayer L, Shao L. Therapeutic potential of oral tolerance. Nat Rev Immunol 2004; 4: 407–19.

58. Holmgren J, Czerkinsky C. Mucosal immunity and vaccines. Nat Med 2005; 11: S45–53.

59. Lefrancois L, Puddington L. Intestinal and pulmonary mucosal T cells: local heroes fight to maintain the status quo. Annu Rev Immunol 2006; 24: 681–704.

60. Hufnagl K, Wagner B, Winkler B et al. Induction of mucosal tolerance with recombinant Hev b3 for prevention of latex allergy in BALB/c mice. Clin Exp Immunol. 133: 170–6.

61. Winkler B, Baier K, Wagner S, Repa A, Eichler HG et al. Mucosal tolerance as therapy of type I allergy: intranasal application of recombinant Bet v 1, the major birch pollen allergen, leads to the suppression of allergic immune responses and airway inflammation in sensitized mice. Clin Exp Allergy 2002; 32: 30–6.

62. Winkler B, Hufnagl K, Spittler A, Ploder M, Kallay E et al. The role of Foxp3+ T cells in long-term efficacy of prophylactic and therapeutic mucosal tolerance induction in mice. Allergy 2006; 61: 173–80.

63. Warner JO, ETAC Study Group, Early treatment of atopic child. A double-blinded, randomized, placebo-controlled trial of cetirizine in preventing the onset of asthma in children with atopic dermatitis: 18 months' treatment and 18 months' posttreatment follow-up. J Allergy Clin Immunol 2001; 108: 929–37.

64. Virtanen H, Remitz A, Malmberg P. Topical tacrolimus in the treatment of atopic dermatitis – Does it benefit the airways? A 4-year open follow-up. J Allergy Clin Immunol 2007; 120: 1464–6.

21

Experimental therapeutic strategies for the treatment of atopic dermatitis

Thomas A Luger and Martin Steinhoff

INTRODUCTION

Colossal progress in the understanding of the cellular and molecular mechanisms involved in inflammatory, allergic as well as autoimmune diseases, and the recent discoveries in biotechnology have led to the development of several novel immunomodulating and anti-inflammatory agents including drugs and specific biologics ('biological response modifiers') such as cytokines, antibodies and fusion proteins which may be helpful for future treatments of atopic dermatitis (AD).[1-3] Consequently, new therapeutic strategies emerged by the use of these immunomodulating drugs (Table 21.1). As a consequence of the improved understanding of the molecular mechanism underlying immune-mediated diseases, several new targets have been identified, leading to the development of even more specific agonists or antagonists. Moreover, new therapies using in vitro modified antigen-presenting cells (APCs) are currently under investigation.[4]

AD is characterized by various immunological abnormalities. Consequently, many molecular structures are targeted in order to combat AD. One major immunological abnormality is driving of Th0 towards a Th2 lymphocyte pattern upon antigenic challenge. Accordingly, increased IgE production, reduced IFN-γ concentrations, and increased IL-4 and IL-5 production appear to be crucial pathways in the pathophysiology of AD which have to be aimed at. This chapter briefly summarizes some of these recent developments in view of their efficacy and safety for the treatment of AD. Novel and experimental drugs for the treatment of pruritus in AD are summarized in Chapter 10.

DRUGS

Many new immunomodulatory drugs such as ciclosporin A (CyA), tacrolimus, pimecrolimus, sirolimus, leflunomide, mycophenolate mofetil, and others have been recently introduced for the treatment of AD. Among these compounds, the development of calcineurin inhibitors (CI) that are either new or for topical application, including tacrolimus, pimecrolimus, and ISA 247, currently appears to be the most promising approach (Table 21.1).[5-9] In a randomized placebo-controlled double-blind study with patients suffering from psoriasis, a 75% reduction was observed within 12 weeks as compared to placebo with ISA247.[10] While serum creatinine increased in patients treated with ISA247, it remained within the normal range. After binding to distinct cytosolic immunophilins CI inhibit the phosphatase calcineurin and thus interrupt the nuclear translocation of the cytoplasmic subunit of the nuclear factor of activated T cells (NF-AT). As a consequence the transcription of immunomodulating and proinflammatory cytokine genes (IL-2, IFN-γ, IL-4, and TNFα) is blocked.[11] Because of their molecular structure and their binding behaviour to different immunophilins, CI may differ significantly in their biological activities as well as in their toxic profile.

Pimecrolimus was the first immunomodulating drug that primarily has been developed for the therapy of AD.[12] Both tacrolimus and pimecrolimus have been recently introduced for the topical treatment of this disease. Although the structure of both compounds is similar, pimecrolimus is significantly more lipophilic which may account for its preferential distribution to epithelial structures and its low affinity for lymphoid

Table 21.1   Novel immunomodulating agents and biologics for the treatment of inflammatory and atopic diseases

Agent	Properties
Drugs	
Mycophenolate mofetil	Pyrimidine synthesis inhibitor
Leflunomide	Purine synthesis inhibitor
Tacrolimus, pimecrolimus, ascrolimus, ISA 247	Macrolactam calcineurin inhibitors
Sirolimus (rapamycin)	S6 kinase inhibitor
Merimempodib	Nucleotide biosynthesis inhibitor
Paldesine	Nucleotide biosynthesis inhibitor
BCX-1777	Nucleotide biosynthesis inhibitor
Imiquimod	Activator of TLR 7
Resiquimod	Activator of TLR 8
Cytosine-P-5 vanine (LP5)	Activator of TLR 9, TH1 switch
Biologics	
Il1R antagonist (Anakinra[N])	IL-1 suppression
Altrahincept	S IL-4R
Nepolizmas	Anti-IL-5Mab
IL-4, IL-10, IL-11	Immunodeviating cytokines
Infliximab	Chimeric anti-TNFα
Adalimumab	Humanized anti-TNFα
Etanercept	TNFα-RII and Fc (IgG$_1$) fusion protein
CDP870	PEGylated Fab of a humanized anti-TNFα
PEG-TNF-RI	PEGylated soluble TNF-RI
ABX IL-8	Humanized anti-IL-8
Efalizumab	Humanized anti-CD11a
Alefacept	LFA3 and Fc (IgG$_1$) fusion protein
Siplizumab	Humanized anti-CD2
Visilizumab	Humanized anti-CD3
HuMax-CD4	Humanized anti-CD4
OKT(R)cdr4a	Humanized anti-CD4
IDEC 114	Humanized anti-CD80
IDEC 131	Humanized anti-CD40
CTLA-4 Ig	CTLA-4 and Fc (IgG$_1$) fusion protein
Basiliximab	Chimeric anti-IL2Rα
Daclizumab	Humanized anti-IL2Rα
Denileukin diftitox	IL-2 and diphtheria toxin (DAB$_{389}$) fusion protein

organs.[13,14] In several animal models, the immunosuppressing potential of pimecrolimus turned out to be significantly less when compared to that of tacrolimus. There is also evidence that the topical application of CI to the skin may not be associated with an increased risk for the development of ultraviolet light mediated skin tumours.[15,16] Accordingly, the potential of CI such as pimecrolimus to impair a primary immune response is very low, and very recently both tacrolimus and pimecrolimus have been shown to protect epidermal cells from UV-induced thymidine dimer formation.[17]

One major advantage of pimecrolimus and tacrolimus in comparison to topically applied glucocorticosteroids is that even after long-term application there is no evidence of skin atrophy. Pimecrolimus – in comparison to tacrolimus – permeates to a lesser degree through the skin, suggesting a lower risk of systemic exposure.[13] Accordingly, only minimal and transient levels of pimecrolimus have been detected in the circulation of patients being treated with pimecrolimus cream regardless of the age, severity, extent of lesions treated, duration of therapy, and time of sampling following the application.[5,18,19] Similarly, after topical application of tacrolimus blood levels were usually low and transient. However, blood concentrations identical to those observed after systemic application with tacrolimus have been reported in patients with severe disease or skin barrier dysfunctions.[6,20] Systemic adverse events following topical treatment with tacrolimus or pimecrolimus have not been reported as of yet.

Consequently, both tacrolimus ointment and pimecrolimus cream proved to be highly effective therapies for AD and have been approved by the authorities of many countries for the treatment of this disease.[19] The most common adverse event was transient skin burning within the first week of treatment.[19,21] However, skin burning caused by pimecrolimus cream was reported to be less intense and less frequent as compared to tacrolimus. The low profile of adverse events for these agents for the first time allows long-term treatment of AD beginning from early childhood as soon as the first symptoms appear. Moreover, continuous and early anti-inflammatory interventions using either tacrolimus or pimecrolimus may prevent the development of chronic eczematous lesions and ultimately result in disease modification. From several reports one may also conclude that both tacrolimus ointment and pimecrolimus cream are efficient for the treatment of many other inflammatory skin diseases including seborrhoeic dermatitis, contact dermatitis, rosacea, as well as autoimmune diseases such as lupus erythematosus and dermatomyositis, for example.[6,19] However, future clinical trials are required to determine the long-term efficacy and safety of these compounds.[22]

Beside the well-established immunosuppressant CyA (3–5 mg/kg b.w.),[23–25] other immunomodulatory small molecule drugs are currently considered as being a useful alternative for the treatment of AD are for example sirolimus (rapamycin), leflunomide, and mycophenolate mofetil (MMF) (Table 21.2).[26–30]

Sirolimus belongs to the group of macrolactam immunomodulators and inhibits the IL-2R mediated signal transduction pathway, but in contrast to others such as CyA, tacrolimus, or pimecrolimus, it does not inhibit calcineurin. In addition to being used successfully in transplantation medicine there is also evidence that sirolimus in combination with a subtherapeutic dose of CyA is effective in the treatment of psoriasis with the advantage of a reduced toxicity.[29] Moreover, topical sirolimus has been demonstrated to be effective and safe for the treatment of psoriasis lesions.[31]

Both MMF and leflunomide inhibit key enzymes in nucleotide biosynthesis, a step that is crucial for T-cell activation and antibody formation. They do not act in the nucleus and thus apparently have an advantageous side-effect profile. Therefore, both agents are now widely used for the treatment of immune-mediated diseases such as rheumatoid arthritis.

There are several case reports on the successful treatment of bullous autoimmune diseases, psoriasis, atopic, and others with MMF.[26,32–36] Of note, the successful treatment of severe refractory AD has been demonstrated with MMF.[37,38] However, side effects such as liver abnormalities and septicaemia were also observed in patients with AD after MMF treatment.[39,40]

Leflunomide is an immunomodulating compound with immunosuppressive properties, targeting primarily T lymphocytes by inhibiting pyrimidine de novo synthesis.[17] Because T-cell activation and Th1/Th2 imbalance is a crucial step in the pathophysiology of AD, leflunomide may be a useful therapeutic target. For leflunomide, a beneficial role for the treatment of severe AD was shown in 2 patients.[41] Moreover, experimental evidence suggests that leflunomide may modulate eotaxin activity in eosinophils independent of its antimetabolite activity.[42] Of note, the clinical severity scores in AD seem to correlate with plasma levels of eosinophil granule proteins (e.g. eosinophil-derived neurotoxin (EDN)) and with the infiltrative capacity of eosinophils to the site of inflammation in AD lesions.[43,44]

However, more controlled clinical studies which are currently being performed are necessary to reveal the safety and efficacy of MMF and leflunomide for the treatment of AD and other skin diseases.

Other recently designed nucleotide biosynthesis inhibitors include compounds such as merimempodib, paldesine, BCX-1777, and others.[45–50] First clinical trials have been performed for the treatment of psoriasis.[51]

TOLL-LIKE RECEPTOR AGONISTS

Toll-like receptors (TLRs) are key molecules involved in microbial recognition by the immune system. At present, 10 members of the TLR family have been identified in mammals.[52] They recognize microbial structures such as bacterial lipopolysaccharides, bacterial DNA, and viral double stranded DNA. There is also evidence that some probiotics which appear to be effective in allergy prevention may function via interaction with TLRs. The number of ligands for these receptors is growing, and it appears that multiple ligands exist for each receptor. TLRs activate common signalling pathways leading to the activation of nuclear kappa B (NFκB) transcription factor and the mitogen activated protein kinases (MAPKs) which results in the production of

Table 21.2 Novel therapeutic approaches for the treatment of atopic dermatitis and other diseases – phases of development (Modified from Homey B, Steinhoff M, Ruzicka T, Leung DY. Cytokines and chemokines orchestrate atopic skin inflammation. J Allergy Clin Immunol 2006; 118: 178–89.)

| Drug description | Name | Therapeutic approach in atopic dermatitis | | Disease | Approval or phase of development |
		Preventative*	Therapeutic**		
CCR1 antagonist	–	x		Inflammation	Preclinical
CCR5 antagonist tauschen CCR4 and -5)	UK-427,857, SCH-C, SCH-D, TAK 449	x		HIV transplantation	Preclinical, Phase I
CXCR4 antagonist	AMD-3100	x		HIV, rheumatoid arthritis, asthma	Preclinical, Phase I
Recombinant human IL-1 receptor antagonist (IL-1RA)	Anakinra	x		Rheumatoid arthritis	yes
Recombinant soluble human TNFα receptor	Etanercept	x	x	Rheumatoid arthritis, Crohn's disease, psoriasis	yes
Pegylated recombinant soluble human TNFα receptor	Pegsunercept	x	x	Rheumatoid arthritis	Phase II
Anti-human TNFα	Infliximab	x	x	Rheumatoid arthritis, Crohn's disease, psoriasis	yes
Anti-human TNFα	Adalimumab	x	x	Rheumatoid arthritis, Crohn's disease	Phase II/III
Anti-human IFN-γ	HuZAF		x	Crohn's disease, psoriasis	Phase I/II
Anti-human IL-4	SB240683, pascolizumab		x	Asthma	PhaseI/II
Soluble human IL-4 receptor	–		x	Asthma	Phase II
Anti-human CD25	Daclizumab		x	Transplantation, asthma	yes, Phase I/II
Anti CD2	Sipilizumab		x	Psoriasis	Phase
Anti-human IL-2 receptor	Basiliximab			Transplantation	yes
Anti-human CD11a	Efalizumab	x		Psoriasis	Phase III
Anti-LFA$_3$	Alefacept	x	x	Psoriasis	yes
Anti-human CD$_3$	Nuvion (Visilizumab)		x	GvHD	Phase I/II
Anti-human CD4	HuMax-CD4®			Psoriasis	Phase __
	OKT(R)cdr4a			Psoriasis	Phase __
Anti-human IgE	Omalizumab	x		Asthma	Yes
	Rnv nab – E25	x		Asthma, rhinitis	Phase X?
NF-AT inhibition	FK506, tacrolimus		x	Atopic dermatitis	yes
NF-AT inhibition	SDZ ASM 981, pimecrolimus	x	x	Atopic dermatitis	yes

*Preventative administration is understood as long-term management of the disease and reduction of the frequency of acute flares.
**Therapeutic administration means treatment of established lesions.

proinflammatory cytokines.[53,54] On the other hand, individual TLRs via their specific signalling systems may induce immune response to a given microbial agent. Thus TLRs are crucial components of both the innate and adaptive immune response.

Imidazoquinolones such as imiquimod and resiquimod bind to TLR7 and TLR8, respectively, which results in the activation of macrophages and other cells and the induction of cytokine production (predominately IFNα, TNFα and IL-12). Subsequently, this cytokine milieu is responsible for an immunodeviation towards Th1 required for cytotoxicity and an effective antiviral and antitumoural activity.[55,56]

Several clinical trials have proved the efficacy of topical immunotherapy with imiquimod in the treatment of anogenital warts resulting in remission rates up to 75%.[52,57] There is also evidence from preliminary studies demonstrating that imiquimod is very effective in the treatment of actinic keratosis, basal cell carcinomas, squamous cell carcinomas, and skin metastases of solid tumours.[55,58] The efficacy of this promising new approach to treat skin tumours and Th2-mediated diseases such as atopic eczema or asthma needs to be evaluated in further clinical trials.[59,60]

Cytosine-phosphate-guanine (CpG) motifs lacking C5 methylation are abundant in all bacterial and some viral genomes. They were found to switch an immune response towards Th1 via NFκB activation and the induction of Th1 cytokines. Moreover, it was recently shown that TLR9 is responsible for CpG oligodeoxynucleotide (ODN)-mediated effects. Therefore, CpG ODN vaccination strategies are currently being investigated for their efficacy in enhancing the immune response against tumours.[61] There is also evidence from animal studies and first clinical trials suggesting that CpG ODN may be effective for the treatment of allergic diseases or as an adjuvant immunotherapy.[62,63] Further clinical studies will ultimately reveal which of the current approaches using CpG ODN is most suited to improve our current strategies for the treatment of tumours and allergic diseases. With respect to AD, the induction of predominantly T helper (Th)1-type cytokine profiles by TLR agonists such as imiquimod might have further benefits by shifting the dominant Th2-type response in AD to a more potent Th1 response.[52]

BIOLOGICS

Biologics are synthetically generated proteins used as immunomodulating agents. So far, recombinant cytokines, monoclonal antibodies, toxin-labelled proteins and fusion proteins have been produced and clinically tested. Biologics are agents with specific cellular targets such as cell surface molecules (adhesion molecules, receptors), or intracellular molecules (e.g. transcription factors), which are designed to imitate or inhibit the actions of naturally occurring proteins. They are derived from living sources such as humans, animals, plants and micro-organisms. Biologics can modulate several immunological disease pathways like lymphocyte (T- or B-cell) activation, antigen-presenting cells (APC)/lymphocyte interactions, endothelial cell activation or adhesion, as well as the release of cytokines, interferons, amines, and chemokines.[1,2]

In the skin, biologics have been used for the treatment of inflammatory skin diseases (AD, psoriasis), B-cell lymphoma, and cutaneous T-cell lymphoma (CTCL). Clinical trials revealed biologics to be highly efficient including short- and long-term remissions. As compared to many immunosuppressants, biologics may have a favourable adverse-effect profile. Treatment with conventional drugs (systematic steroids, ciclosporin, methotrexate, and mycophenolate mofetil) or photochemotherapy may have severe short- or long-term side effects in AD patients. Thus, novel understandings about the pathophysiology of AD led to new strategies for technically produced proteins.

Because generic names of biologics led to confusion, a strict nomenclature has been introduced. Receptor-antibody fusion proteins end with '-cept'. Generic names of chimeric monoclonals end with '-ximab,' humanized monoclonals end with '-zumab,' and human monoclonal antibodies (Mab) end with 'umab'. Table 21.1 lists biologics that are approved for dermatological indications or are at present under investigation for treatment of dermatological conditions including AD.

Advances in the understanding of the complex molecular mechanisms of immune reactions have led to the identification of several new extracellular as well as intracellular targets such as cytokine receptors, adhesion molecules, and transcription factors that may be used for novel anti-inflammatory and immunomodulating strategies. Approaches to block these specific targets are: humanized or fully human antibodies directed against cytokines or their receptors, soluble receptors that bind to secreted cytokines, receptor antagonists, fusion protein constructs targeting cytokines or cell surface molecules and transcription factor inhibitors.[2] A new generation of high affinity cytokine blockers called 'cytokine traps' has recently been developed, although further deep studies on the efficacy in humans are still lacking. However, no evidence currently suggests this way to be beneficial. The 'traps' consist of the extracellular domain of two distinct cytokine receptor components involved in binding the cytokine and the constant region of IgG. These 'traps' have been shown to potently block cytokines in vitro and in vivo and currently are being evaluated in first clinical trials for their efficacy in the therapy of cytokine-driven diseases.[64,65]

However, no further clinical trials have been recently published.

IL-1

In addition, targeting IL-1 represents a further promising approach for the treatment of inflammatory diseases. Accordingly, a recombinant human interleukin-1 receptor antagonist (IL-1RA) (e.g. Anakinra®), which is currently being investigated for its efficacy in patients with rheumatoid arthritis, may also be useful in psoriasis.[66] Recent studies in various diseases and Schniezler's syndrome support the idea that targeting the IL-IR may be a promising way to follow in the future. Studies in AD are currently lacking.

IL-2

DAB$_{389}$IL-2 (denileukin diftitox) was the first IL-2 receptor specific fusion protein in which the receptor binding domain of the diphtheria toxin has been replaced by human IL-2 and the membrane translocating and cytotoxic domains have been retained. Clinical and laboratory investigations have demonstrated a selective destruction of IL-2 receptor expressing T lymphocytes and DAB$_{389}$IL-2 has been used successfully in clinical trials for the treatment of cutaneous T-cell lymphomas and psoriasis. The most common side effects observed were flu-like symptoms with severity increasing at higher doses.[67,68]

Antibodies against the IL-2Rα chain (daclizumab, basiliximab, and inolimomab), antibodies against T-cell markers, and IL-2/toxin fusion proteins are currently being investigated in many T-cell-mediated diseases. According to clinical studies there is some evidence for the efficacy of anti-IL-2 in the treatment of psoriasis.[69–71] Recently, in a patient with severe chronic AD the successful use of basiliximab, a chimeric anti-IL-2 receptor monoclonal antibody, has been reported.[72]

IL-4, IL-5

In animal experiments it has been shown that IL-4 shifts the differentiation of naïve and probably also memory T cells towards a Th2 phenotype in an antigen-specific fashion. Analysis of mite infestation in various knockout mice revealed that IgE production in response to these ectoparasites was dependent on T cells, IL-4, and CD40L.[73] A recently published clinical study indicates that the treatment of psoriasis with rhIL-4 results in a significant improvement of the PASI score (up to 80%) within 6 weeks and seems to be well tolerated.[74] Thus IL-4 appears to have a considerable potential for the treatment of Th1-mediated diseases. In patients with atopic asthma, promising results with soluble IL-4 receptor (altrakincept) and anti-IL-5 Mab (mepolizumab) have

been reported.[75] Thus far, no clinical trials have been published using anti-IL-4-directed therapies in patients with AD. Thus, these biologics appear to be promising therapeutic tools for the treatment of AD.

IL-16

IL-16 is secreted from keratinocytes and Langerhans cells (LCs) and is an important chemokine for the recruitment of CD4+ T cells, monocytes, eosinophils, and LCs in the inflamed skin. Serum and RNA expression of this cytokine positively correlate with the acuity of AD.[76] Its therapeutic potential has been considered to be beneficial for the treatment of AD, as well as asthma and inflammatory bowel disease. For example, IL-16 downregulates antigen-driven T cell activation as well as Th2 cytokine production. So far, no clinical trials have been published using agonists of IL-16.

IL-18 binding protein

Il-18 has been shown to be involved in the pathophysiology both of AD and psoriasis. Of note, transgenic mice overexpressing IL-18 have been shown to form AD-like lesions. Its binding partner, the decoy receptor IL-18 binding protein (IL-18 BP) also suppresses inflammatory responses during contact hypersensitivity. This concept has to await further clarification.[77]

IL-31

An auspicious member of the cytokine family for the treatment of AD is IL-31 (reviewed in[78,79]). Of note, transgenic mice overexpressing IL-31 released by T cells and macrophages showed an AD-like skin disease consisting of a T-cell infiltrate and pruritus, similar to AD in humans. IL-31 activates the IL-31 receptor (IL-31R), a heterodimeric receptor composed of the IL-31 receptor A (IL-31RA) subunit and the oncostatin M receptor (OSMR) subunit. Interestingly, IL-31 is upregulated in pruritic forms of cutanous inflammation.[80,81] These findings were recently confirmed in mice: in NC/Nga mice, the expression of cutaneous IL-31 mRNA with scratching behaviour was significantly higher than that in NC/Nga mice without scratching behaviour. Thus, IL-31 may participate in the cause of itch sensation and promote scratching behaviour.[82,83] IL-31 may be a new link between the immune and neural systems by regulating inflammation as well as itch. Therefore, soluble IL-31 as well as the IL-31R are potential targets for the treatment of AD.

Anti-IgE

In AD, an important therapeutic pathway lies in the IgE-induced blockade of FcεRI receptors on LCs. Strategies to block IgE using a humanized murine neutralizing antibody (omalizumab)[84–87] directed against the high affinity IgE receptor in patients with moderate and severe asthma have demonstrated significant steroid-sparing effects.[81,88] The combination treatment with anti-IgE in addition to specific immunotherapy was found to be effective in polysensitized children and adolescents with seasonal allergic rhinitis.[89] A humanized Mab directed against IgE (rhuMab-E25) also successfully blocked the interaction of free IgE with mast cells and basophiles. Moreover, placebo-controlled studies demonstrated a clinical effect in patients with allergic rhinitis and moderate to severe asthma.[90] Recent reports indicate the efficacy of omalizumab in a certain subgroup of AD patients. Unfortunately, no placebo-controlled double-blind studies exist thus far for AD.[91] However, one may expect that the anti-IgE strategy may be capable of reducing the relapse frequency for AD rather than healing acute lesions in AD patients.[91]

Interferon-γ

As a cytokine, IFN-γ drives the T-cell response into a Th1 direction. It potently inhibits IL-4, IL-5, and IgE synthesis, and suppresses Th2 proliferation. Accordingly, several clinical studies have focused on the therapeutic effects of IFN-γ to combat AD. More than a decade ago, Hanifin et al had already demonstrated that once daily subcutaneous injections of recombinant IFN-γ significantly reduced the eczema over a 12-week period. Moreover, the compound was a safe, well-accepted, and effective drug reducing itching, clinical symptoms, and eosinophilia in severe AD.[92] Clinical as well as experimental examinations revealed that a higher dosage $(1.5 \times 10E6 \, IU/m^2)$ was superior as far as the maintenance of clinical improvement was concerned in comparison to a lower dosage $(0.5 \times 10E6 \, IU/m^2)$. An anti-human IFN-γ antibody (HuZAF) has been tested in phase I/II trials for the treatment of Crohn's disease.[93,94] It has also been used in a placebo-controlled clinical trial for the treatment of moderate to severe AD. Interestingly, approximately 50% of the patients responded to a subcutaneous treatment over 6 weeks with a continuous improvement over 3 months.[95,96] In sum, although IFN-γ appears in principle to be an interesting target, success is hampered from a relatively low efficacy of this drug in AD, as well as adverse effects such as flu-like symptoms and the subcutaneous application.

TNFα

Several different agents that neutralize the proinflammatory cytokine TNFα such as a humanized antibody (infliximab), a full human antibody (adalimumab), and a protein containing the TNFα receptor (TNFαRII) fused with a humanized immunoglobulin fragment (etanercept) are available for the treatment of inflammatory diseases,[2,97,98] with psoriasis or psoriasis arthritis as an approved indication[98–103] in addition to rheumatoid arthritis or Crohn's disease. A pegylated form of a recombinant soluble human TNFα receptor is currently under investigation (Pegsunercept).

Certain, mainly in vitro data indicate a role of TNFα in the acute or chronic phase of AD.[60] In clinical trials, however, a beneficial effect of infliximab was only observed in 2 of 9 patients.[104] In contrast, patients were observed who developed AD lesions after infliximab therapy.[105,106] According to the fact that TNFα does not appear to play an essential role in the pathophysiology of AD or even ameliorate this disease, TNFα blockers do not seem to be beneficial for the treatment of AD.

CD2 (LFA₃)

In a preliminary clinical trial, an antibody binding to CD2 (siplizumab) which is expressed on memory effector T lymphocytes was successfully evaluated in psoriasis.[107] Its counterpart, LFA₃TIP (alefacept), is a human fusion protein where the CD2-binding domain of LFA₃ has been linked to the Fc portion of human IgG₁, leading to functional blockade of the LFA₃/CD2 pathway.[108] Thus alefacept by binding to CD2 inhibits the function of CD4+ and CD8+ T cells and selectively reduces memory-effector CD45RO+ T cells. Treatment with alefacept (12 weeks) significantly improved psoriasis in comparison to placebo, and a second course of alefacept after 12 weeks was found to provide additional benefit. Alefacept has been shown to provide long-lasting periods of remission. It was well tolerated without any serious short-term side effects.[109–111] However, monitoring of CD4+ cells may be required. Alefacept was the first biologic which has been approved in the USA for the treatment of psoriasis. The IL-13 production by peripheral blood T cells from AD patients does not require CD2 costimulation.[112]

Expression of and responses to CD2 and CD3 in 18-month-old children with and without AD. Atopy was associated with a low proportion of CD2+ lymphocytes. Responsiveness to PHA, which activates lymphocytes partly via the sheep erythrocyte receptor, CD2, was reduced in the allergic children. The anti-CD3-induced proliferation declined more rapidly with antibody dilution in the allergic than in the non-allergic children. AD was associated with high levels of anti-CD3-stimulated IL-5 secretion. The IL-4/IL-10 and IL-4/IFN-γ ratios were higher in children with elevated total immunoglobulin E (IgE) levels. Skin prick test (SPT)-negative children with eczema produced higher levels of IL-10 than SPT-positive children. In conclusion, atopic children have a reduced T-cell function. AD is associated with increased IL-5 production, while high total IgE levels are associated with high IL-4/IFN-γ and IL-4/IL-10 ratios.[113]

CD3, CD4

An antibody directed against CD3 (visilizumab), a component of the T-cell receptor complex which is expressed on all T lymphocytes, has been reported to have some therapeutic activity in psoriasis but may not be further developed for this indication.[114] Several antibodies have been constructed against CD4 expressed on Th cells. According to first clinical trials, HuMax-CD4 and OKT(R)cdr4a appear to be effective in the treatment of psoriasis.[51,115]

CD11a (LFA-1)

Another promising approach to treat T-cell-mediated diseases is to develop agents that disrupt antigen presentation and thus T-cell activation. Accordingly, antibodies against costimulatory molecules or fusion molecules consisting of costimulatory molecules and Fc portions of human IgG have been developed. Efalizumab is a humanized antibody that binds to the α chain of LFA-1 (CD11a), blocks T-cell trafficking to the dermis and epidermis and inhibits secondary activation of T cells.[116] Side effects consisted of an increased incidence of flu-like symptoms but no organ toxicity. Phase III clinical trials for the treatment of psoriasis are currently ongoing.[109,117] For AD,[118–120] recent reports[118,120] or studies[119] have demonstrated efficacy.[121–123]

CD20

Several clinical studies are currently being performed using strategies that target pathogenic B lymphocytes or T lymphocytes. One may hypothesize that antibodies may have a beneficial effect on the onset of AD when the production of antibodies such as IgE (in IgE-associated AD) may be beneficial. Treatment of CD20 expressing B-cell lymphomas with anti-CD20 (rituximab), a chimeric monoclonal antibody, appears to be promising according to first clinical studies.[124,125] Moreover, rituximab was recently shown to be effective for the treatment of recalcitrant, life-threatening pemphigus.[126] For AD, no clinical studies exist. The adverse effects observed during the treatment of autoimmune diseases may be limiting for the use of anti-CD20 antibodies in AD.

CD25

A human antibody against CD25 (daclizumab) has already been used for the treatment of asthma and in transplantation medicine. Daclizumab blocks the interaction of IL-2 with its receptor. Daclizumab (Zenapax), the humanized form of this antibody, was first approved by the FDA for the prevention of renal allograft rejection. Daclizumab was also shown to be of value for the treatment of patients with non-infectious uveitis, multiple sclerosis, and a neurological disease, defined as human T-cell lymphotropic virus-I associated myelopathy/tropical spastic paraparesis (HAM/TSP). Therapeutic efficacy with daclizumab was also shown in patients with pure red cell aplasia, aplastic anaemia, and psoriasis. Thus, blocking the IL-2/IL-2 receptor system by daclizumab provides a powerful strategy for the prevention of organ allograft rejection and the treatment of patients with select autoimmune diseases. In AD, no controlled studies have been performed to date.

CD28, CD40, CD80

CTLA-4 Ig is a recombinant fusion protein that contains the extracellular domain of the human CTLA-4 fused to human IgG_1 thereby functioning as a high affinity CD28/CTLA-4 antagonist. CTLA-4 Ig inhibits T-cell activation by binding to B7 on antigen-presenting cells. Preliminary data indicate that treatment with CTLA-4 Ig appears to be an effective therapy for psoriasis and atopic diseases.[127–130]

Antibodies against costimulatory molecules such as CD40 (IDEC-131) or CD80 (IDEC-114) are being investigated and in some first clinical trials were found to be promising, safe and well tolerated for the treatment of psoriasis.[51,131] No controlled clinical studies have been published thus far in patients with AD.

T-cell receptor targeting

Restricted T-cell receptor (TCR) gene use has been reported in populations of activated T cells isolated from autoimmune diseases such as rheumatoid arthritis, multiple sclerosis, and psoriasis. One possible strategy for treating psoriasis was therefore to target the appropriate TCR on autoreactive T cells. Vaccines based upon these TCRs have been developed and their safety has already been demonstrated in first clinical trials using Vβ3 and Vβ13.1 TCR peptides.[28]

Transcription factors, signalling molecules

Inhibition of transcription factors such as NFκB which plays an important role in the regulation of inflammatory signals is of particular interest. Recently, a protein consisting of the amino terminal region of the regulatory protein NEMO (NFκB essential modifier), which is required for the activation of NFκB, has been found to selectively inhibit NFκB and thus may be developed as an anti-inflammatory compound.[33] Moreover, the carboxy terminal tripeptide of α-melanocyte-stimulating hormone (αMSH) was also found to block NFκB activation and to exert anti-iflammatory and immunomodulating activities in vivo.[132] Other interesting targets are MAP kinases which are involved in the expression of proinflammatory genes and chronic inflammation.[133]

The rationale for this therapeutic option is to interrupt the recruitment of inflammatory leukocyte to the site of inflammation. The first selectin antagonist, CY-1503 (Cylexin), a sialyl Lewis(X) mimetic, did not cause significant effects as compared to controls. An anti VLA-4 approach (Tysabri) was also unsuccessful,[134–136] This may be due to redundant molecules or receptors. Thus, the question of whether adhesion molecules may be promising targets for the treatment of AD is still open.[137]

Chemokine inhibitors and chemokine receptor blockers

Chemokine receptor antagonists (CCR1, CCR2, CCR4, CCR5, CCR10, CXCR3, CXCR4) have been discussed as promising therapeutic targets for the treatment of inflammatory skin diseases including AD.[138] This is based on their ability to interfere with leukocytes thereby suppressing their recruitment to the skin. This may prevent acute inflammatory excema and lead to long-term remissions of AD. In particular, small molecule antagonists against CCR4 (AMD-3100),[139–141] CCR5 (UK427, UK857, SCH-C, SCH-D, TAK-449)[142,143] and/or CCR10 represent promising targets to prevent the recruitment of pathologically relevant skin-homing CLA+ memory T cells to the inflammatory cutaneous site.[138,144] However, applied into the lesional skin, chemokine antagonists may fail to show significant effects. One problem is that one of the relevant effector cells, the T lymphocyte, has already entered the skin, and has already been activated by its specific antigen.[138]

αMSH

α-Melanocyte-stimulating hormone (α-MSH) is a tridecapeptide derived from the proopiomelanocortin by post-translational processing. Various studies demonstrated evidence for α-MSH being a potent anti-inflammatory agent. These effects are mediated via centrally expressed melanocortin receptors orchestrating descending neurogenic anti-inflammatory pathways. α-MSH also exerts anti-inflammatory effects on immune cells in the skin, suppresses TNFα production, modulates NFκB activation, expression of adhesion molecules and chemokine receptors, production of proinflammatory cytokines and mediators, IL-10 synthesis, T-cell proliferation and activity, inflammatory cell migration, and apoptosis. The anti-inflammatory capacity has been validated in in vivo studies of experimentally induced fever, irritant and allergic contact dermatitis, cutaneous vasculitis and fibrosis, in ocular, gastrointestinal, brain, and allergic airway inflammation, and arthritis. In contrast to α-MSH, the

C-terminal tripeptide KPV lacks the side effect of pigmentation. KDPT, a derivative of KPV, also exerts potent anti-inflammatory effects. The physiochemical properties and the expected low costs of pharmaceutical production render these agents suitable for the future treatment of immune-mediated inflammatory skin and bowel diseases, allergic asthma, eye disease, and arthritis. In humans, the superpotent α-MSH analogue NDP-MSH was recently applied at doses up to 0.16 mg/kg. Adverse events were minimal and consisted only of occasional gastrointestinal upset and facial flushing.[145] Of note, no pigmentation was observed. α-MSH and KPV also possessed antimicrobial activity against *S. aureus* and *Candida albicans*, two major and representative pathogens.[146] It is speculated that D-enantiomers of KPV are relatively stable against peptidase activity compared with their stereochemical analogues suggesting a promising anti-inflammatory drug for the treatment of inflammatory skin diseases including AD.[147]

Tryptase

Recent findings indicate an important role for mast cell-derived tryptase in the pathophysiology of hypersensitivity, atopy, and pruritus.[148] Tryptase is a serine protease released from mast cells upon stimulation. In the extracellular space, tryptase builds a tetramer stabilized by heparin. It can exert various effects in the extracellular space by binding to matrix proteins.[149] Additionally, tryptase can cleave and activate a G-protein-coupled receptor, defined as proteinase-activated receptor-2 (PAR-2). By this unique mechanism, tryptase can modulate the function of keratinocytes,[150] endothelial cells,[151–153] nerves,[154] and mast cells,[155] probably in an autocrine fashion. Proof-of-principle as well as human studies in patients with pruritus demonstrated tryptase to be involved in the pathophysiology of itching in uraemic and AD patients.[156,157] Thus, inhibitors of tryptase or antagonists of PAR-2 may be beneficial for the treatment of AD, especially with respect to both its inflammatory and pruritic symptoms. Future studies with tryptase inhibitors such as nafomastate or novel, currently developed PAR-2 antagonists will have to show whether this pathway may be beneficial for the treatment of AD.

SUMMARY AND CONCLUSIONS

In the last decade, the spectrum of therapeutic strategies for inflammatory skin diseases has largely emerged. Progress in biotechnology such as the possibility of generating humanized molecules targeting specific cellular structures has enabled the development of novel agents. Many of these biologic compounds are recombinant proteins targeting specific soluble or cellular molecules. They are currently being investigated in clinical trials for their efficacy in the treatment of inflammatory skin diseases. Accordingly, psoriasis which is considered as a Th1-cell- and possibly autoimmune-mediated disease has been chosen to evaluate most of the different immune-targeted therapeutic approaches, therefore being a 'pioneer-disease' for the development of novel therapies of immune-mediated skin diseases. Moreover, psoriasis is a visible autoimmune disease which has certain pathogenic features in common with other autoimmune diseases such as rheumatoid arthritis or inflammatory bowel disease. Accordingly, several new agents such as alefacept, efalizumab, pimecrolimus, and others have primarily been developed for the treatment of psoriasis and subsequently may be introduced for the treatment of other autoimmune diseases.

However, there is still no ideal cure available for AD, a disease with a complex and not completely understood pathomechanism. Therefore, it is not surprising that the application of the new biologics or drugs has only rarely resulted in complete remission, and never in all patients. In the future, the combined use of agents aimed at different pathogenetic 'pathways' of this disease will improve the therapeutic efficacy and allow the identification of novel disease-relevant molecules. Considering our increased understanding about the pathophysiology of AD, and about the multiple promising anti-inflammatory approaches which derive therefrom, we predict improved therapeutic strategies for the treatment of excema lesions and pruritus in AD.

REFERENCES

1. Breedveld FC. Therapeutic monoclonal antibodies. Lancet 2000; 355: 735–40.
2. Smolen JS, Steiner G. Therapeutic strategies for rheumatoid arthritis. Nat Rev Drug Discov 2003; 2: 473–88.
3. Nelson RP, Jr., Ballow M. Immunomodulation and immunotherapy: drugs, cytokines, cytokine receptors, and antibodies. J Allergy Clin Immunol 2003; 111: 720–43.
4. Schuler G, Kampgen E. Vaccine therapy of malignant melanoma. Dermatol Ther 1999; 10: 62–73.
5. Wellington K, Jarvis B. Topical pimecrolimus: a review of its clinical potential in the management of atopic dermatitis. Drugs 2002; 62: 817–40.
6. Gupta AK, Adamiak A, Chow M. Tacrolimus: a review of its use for the management of dermatoses. J Eur Acad Dermatol Venereol 2002; 16: 100–14.
7. Aspeslet L, Freitag D, Trepanier D, Abel M, Naicker S et al. ISA(TX)247: a novel calcineurin inhibitor. Transplant Proc 2001; 33: 1048–51.
8. Mollison KW, Fey TA, Gauvin DM, Kolano RM, Sheets MP et al. A macrolactam inhibitor of T helper type 1 and T helper type 2 cytokine biosynthesis for topical treatment of inflammatory skin diseases. J Invest Dermatol 1999; 112: 729–38.
9. Birsan T, Dambrin C, Freitag DG, Yatscoff RW, Morris RE. The novel calcineurin inhibitor ISA247: a more potent immunosuppressant than cyclosporine in vitro. Transpl Int 2005; 17: 767–71.
10. Bissonnette R, Papp K, Poulin Y, Lauzon G, Aspeslet L et al. A randomized, multicenter, double-blind, placebo-controlled phase 2 trial of ISA247 in patients with chronic plaque psoriasis. J Am Acad Dermatol 2006; 54: 472–8.
11. Cather JC, Abramovits W, Menter A. Cyclosporine and tacrolimus in dermatology. Dermatol Clin 2001; 19: 119–37, ix.
12. Paul C, Graeber M, Stuetz A. Ascomycins: promising agents for the treatment of inflammatory skin diseases. Expert Opin Investig Drugs 2000; 9: 69–77.
13. Stuetz A, Grassberger M, Meingassner JG. Pimecrolimus (Elidel, SDZ ASM 981) – preclinical pharmacologic profile and skin selectivity. Semin Cutan Med Surg 2001; 20: 233–41.
14. Meingassner JG, Kowalsky E, Schwendinger H, Elbe-Burger A, Stutz A. Pimecrolimus does not affect Langerhans cells in murine epidermis. Br J Dermatol 2003; 149: 853–7.
15. Meingassner JG, Fahrngruber H, Bavandi A. Pimecrolimus inhibits the elicitation phase but does not suppress the sensitization phase in murine contact hypersensitivity, in contrast to tacrolimus and cyclosporine A. J Invest Dermatol 2003; 121: 77–80.
16. Stuetz A, Baumann K, Grassberger M, Wolff K, Meingassner JG. Discovery of topical calcineurin inhibitors and pharmacological profile of pimecrolimus. Int Arch Allergy Immunol 2006; 141: 199–212.
17. Tran C, Lubbe J, Sorg O, Doelker L, Carraux P et al. Topical calcineurin inhibitors decrease the production of UVB-induced thymine dimers from hairless mouse epidermis. Dermatology 2005; 211: 341–7.
18. Nghiem P, Pearson G, Langley RG. Tacrolimus and pimecrolimus: from clever prokaryotes to inhibiting calcineurin and treating atopic dermatitis. J Am Acad Dermatol 2002; 46: 228–41.
19. Tomi NS, Luger TA. The treatment of atopic dermatitis with topical immunomodulators. Clin Dermatol 2003; 21: 215–24.
20. Allen A, Siegfried E, Silverman R, Williams ML, Elias PM et al. Significant absorption of topical tacrolimus in 3 patients with Netherton syndrome. Arch Dermatol 2001; 137: 747–50.
21. Allen BR. Tacrolimus ointment: its place in the therapy of atopic dermatitis. J Allergy Clin Immunol 2002; 109: 401–3.
22. Bhardwaj SS, Jaimes JP, Liu A, Warshaw EM. A double-blind randomized placebo-controlled pilot study comparing topical immunomodulating agents and corticosteroids for treatment of experimentally induced nickel contact dermatitis. Dermatitis 2007; 18: 26–31.
23. Bemanian MH, Movahedi M, Farhoudi A, Gharagozlou M, Heidari Seraj M et al. High doses intravenous immunoglobulin versus oral cyclosporine in the treatment of severe atopic dermatitis. Iran J Allergy Asthma Immunol 2005; 4: 139–43.
24. Griffiths CE, Katsambas A, Dijkmans BA, Finlay AY, Ho VC et al. Update on the use of ciclosporin in immune-mediated dermatoses. Br J Dermatol 2006; 155(Suppl 2): 1–16.
25. Steffan J, Favrot C, Mueller R. A systematic review and meta-analysis of the efficacy and safety of cyclosporin for the treatment of atopic dermatitis in dogs. Vet Dermatol 2006; 17: 3–16.
26. Frieling U, Luger TA. Mycophenolate mofetil and leflunomide: promising compounds for the treatment of skin diseases. Clin Exp Dermatol 2002; 27: 562–70.
27. Flores F, Kerdel FA. Other novel immunosuppressants. Dermatol Clin 2000; 18: 475–83, ix.
28. Beissert S, Luger TA. Future developments of antipsoriatic therapy. Dermatol Ther 1999; 11: 104–17.
29. Reitamo S, Spuls P, Sassolas B, Lahfa M, Claudy A et al. Efficacy of sirolimus (rapamycin) administered concomitantly with a subtherapeutic dose of cyclosporin in the treatment of severe

psoriasis: a randomized controlled trial. Br J Dermatol 2001; 145: 438–45.

30. Mrowietz U, Christophers E, Altmeyer P. Treatment of severe psoriasis with fumaric acid esters: scientific background and guidelines for therapeutic use. The German Fumaric Acid Ester Consensus Conference. Br J Dermatol 1999; 141: 424–9.

31. Ormerod AD, Shah SA, Copeland P, Omar G, Winfield A. Treatment of psoriasis with topical sirolimus: preclinical development and a randomized, double-blind trial. Br J Dermatol 2005; 152: 758–64.

32. Nousari HC, Sragovich A, Kimyai-Asadi A, Orlinsky D, Anhalt GJ. Mycophenolate mofetil in autoimmune and inflammatory skin disorders. J Am Acad Dermatol 1999; 40: 265–8.

33. Neuber K, Schwartz I, Itschert G, Dieck AT. Treatment of atopic eczema with oral mycophenolate mofetil. Br J Dermatol 2000; 143: 385–91.

34. Hansen ER, Buus S, Deleuran M, Andersen KE. Treatment of atopic dermatitis with mycophenolate mofetil. Br J Dermatol 2000; 143: 1324–6.

35. Grundmann-Kollmann M, Podda M, Ochsendorf F, Boehncke WH, Kaufmann R et al. Mycophenolate mofetil is effective in the treatment of atopic dermatitis. Arch Dermatol 2001; 137: 870–3.

36. Grundmann-Kollmann M, Kaufmann R, Zollner TM. Treatment of atopic dermatitis with mycophenolate mofetil. Br J Dermatol 2001; 145: 351–2.

37. Grundmann-Kollmann M, Korting HC, Behrens S, Leiter U, Krahn G et al. Successful treatment of severe refractory atopic dermatitis with mycophenolate mofetil. Br J Dermatol 1999; 141: 175–6.

38. Benez A, Fierlbeck G. Successful long-term treatment of severe atopic dermatitis with mycophenolate mofetil. Br J Dermatol 2001; 144: 638–9.

39. Hantash B, Fiorentino D. Liver enzyme abnormalities in patients with atopic dermatitis treated with mycophenolate mofetil. Arch Dermatol 2006; 142: 109–10.

40. Satchell AC, Barnetson RS. Staphylococcal septicaemia complicating treatment of atopic dermatitis with mycophenolate. Br J Dermatol 2000; 143: 202–3.

41. Schmitt J, Wozel G, Pfeiffer C. Leflunomide as a novel treatment option in severe atopic dermatitis. Br J Dermatol 2004; 150: 1182–5.

42. Kehrer K, Blumlein K, Wozel G. Eotaxin release is suppressed by the metabolite A 77 1726 of the novel immunomodulating agent leflunomide. Eur J Allergy Clin Immunol 2001; 56(S68): 144.

43. Amerio P, Frezzolini A, Feliciani C, Verdolini R, Teofoli P et al. Eotaxins and CCR3 receptor in inflammatory and allergic skin diseases: therapeutical implications. Curr Drug Targets Inflamm Allergy 2003; 2: 81–94.

44. Breuer K, Kapp A, Werfel T. Urine eosinophil protein X (EPX) is an in vitro parameter of inflammation in atopic dermatitis of the adult age. Allergy 2001; 56: 780–4.

45. Gandhi V, Kilpatrick JM, Plunkett W, Ayres M, Harman L et al. A proof-of-principle pharmacokinetic, pharmacodynamic, and clinical study with purine nucleoside phosphorylase inhibitor immucillin-H (BCX-1777, forodesine). Blood 2005; 106: 4253–60.

46. Filgueira de Azevedo W, Jr., Canduri F, Marangoni dos Santos D, Pereira JH, Dias MV et al. Structural basis for inhibition of human PNP by immucillin-H. Biochem Biophys Res Commun 2003; 309: 917–22.

47. Banti S, Miller PJ, Parker CD, Ananth SL, Horn LL et al. Comparison of in vivo efficacy of BCX-1777 and cyclosporin in xenogeneic graft-vs.-host disease: the role of dGTP in antiproliferative action of BCX-1777. Int Immunopharmacol 2002; 2: 913–23.

48. Schramm VL. Development of transition state analogues of purine nucleoside phosphorylase as anti-T-cell agents. Biochim Biophys Acta 2002; 1587: 107–17.

49. Kicska GA, Long L, Horig H, Fairchild C, Tyler PC et al. Immucillin H, a powerful transition-state analog inhibitor of purine nucleoside phosphorylase, selectively inhibits human T lymphocytes. Proc Natl Acad Sci U S A 2001; 98: 4593–8.

50. Bantia S, Miller PJ, Parker CD, Ananth SL, Horn LL et al. Purine nucleoside phosphorylase inhibitor BCX-1777 (Immucillin-H) – a novel potent and orally active immunosuppressive agent. Int Immunopharmacol 2001; 1: 1199–210.

51. Gniadecki R, Zachariae C, Calverley M. Trends and developments in the pharmacological treatment of psoriasis. Acta Derm Venereol 2002; 82: 401–10.

52. Schiller M, Metze D, Luger TA, Grabbe S, Gunzer M. Immune response modifiers – mode of action. Exp Dermatol 2006; 15: 331–41.

53. Barton GM, Medzhitov R. Toll-like receptor signaling pathways. Science 2003; 300: 1524–5.

54. Sato S, Nomura F, Kawai T, Takeuchi O, Muhlradt PF et al. Synergy and cross-tolerance between toll-like receptor (TLR) 2- and TLR4-mediated signaling pathways. J Immunol 2000; 165: 7096–101.

55. Skinner RB, Jr. Imiquimod. Dermatol Clin 2003; 21: 291–300.

56. Gupta AK, Browne M, Bluhm R. Imiquimod: a review. J Cutan Med Surg 2002; 6: 554–60.

57. Beutner KR, Spruance SL, Hougham AJ, Fox TL, Owens ML et al. Treatment of genital warts with an immune-response modifier (imiquimod). J Am Acad Dermatol 1998; 38: 230–9.

58. Hengge UR, Benninghoff B, Ruzicka T, Goos M. Topical immunomodulators – progress towards treating inflammation, infection, and cancer. Lancet Infect Dis 2001; 1: 189–98.

59. Xie ZQ, Liu LL, Yang GY, Zhu XJ. Effect of topical tacrolimus ointment on expression of Toll-like receptors 2 and 4 in lesional atopic dermatitis skin. Beijing Da Xue Xue Bao 2006; 38: 420–3.

60. Numerof RP, Asadullah K. Cytokine and anti-cytokine therapies for psoriasis and atopic dermatitis. BioDrugs 2006; 20: 93–103.

61. Weiner GJ. The immunobiology and clinical potential of immunostimulatory CpG oligodeoxynucleotides. J Leukoc Biol 2000; 68: 455–63.

62. Horner AA, Raz E. Immunostimulatory sequence oligodeoxynucleotide-based vaccination and immunomodulation: two unique but complementary strategies for the treatment of allergic diseases. J Allergy Clin Immunol 2002; 110: 706–12.

63. Wild JS, Sur S. CpG oligonucleotide modulation of allergic inflammation. Allergy 2001; 56: 365–76.

64. LaDuca JR, Gaspari AA. Targeting tumor necrosis factor alpha. New drugs used to modulate inflammatory diseases. Dermatol Clin 2001; 19: 617–35.

65. Economides AN, Carpenter LR, Rudge JS, Wong V, Koehler-Stec EM et al. Cytokine traps: multi-component, high-affinity blockers of cytokine action. Nat Med 2003; 9: 47–52.

66. Fleischmann RM, Schechtman J, Bennett R, Handel ML, Burmester GR et al. Anakinra, a recombinant human interleukin-1 receptor antagonist (r-metHuIL-1ra), in patients with rheumatoid arthritis: a large, international, multicenter, placebo-controlled trial. Arthritis Rheum 2003; 48: 927–34.

67. Foss FM. Interleukin-2 fusion toxin: targeted therapy for cutaneous T cell lymphoma. Ann N Y Acad Sci 2001; 941: 166–76.

68. Martin A, Gutierrez E, Muglia J, McDonald CJ, Guzzo C et al. A multicenter dose-escalation trial with denileukin diftitox (ONTAK, DAB(389)IL-2) in patients with severe psoriasis. J Am Acad Dermatol 2001; 45: 871–81.

69. Krueger JG, Walters IB, Miyazawa M, Gilleaudeau P, Hakimi J et al. Successful in vivo blockade of CD25 (high-affinity interleukin 2 receptor) on T cells by administration of humanized anti-Tac antibody to patients with psoriasis. J Am Acad Dermatol 2000; 43: 448–58.

70. Mrowietz U, Zhu K, Christophers E. Treatment of severe psoriasis with anti-CD25 monoclonal antibodies. Arch Dermatol 2000; 136: 675–6.

71. Owen CM, Harrison PV. Successful treatment of severe psoriasis with basiliximab, an interleukin-2 receptor monoclonal antibody. Clin Exp Dermatol 2000; 25: 195–7.

72. Kagi MK, Heyer G. Efficacy of basiliximab, a chimeric anti-interleukin-2 receptor monoclonal antibody, in a patient with severe chronic atopic dermatitis. Br J Dermatol 2001; 145: 350–1.

73. Pochanke V, Hatak S, Hengartner H, Zinkernagel RM, McCoy KD. Induction of IgE and allergic-type responses in fur mite-infested mice. Eur J Immunol 2006; 36: 2434–45.

74. Ghoreschi K, Thomas P, Breit S, Dugas M, Mailhammer R et al. Interleukin-4 therapy of psoriasis induces Th2 responses and improves human autoimmune disease. Nat Med 2003; 9: 40–6.

75. Dripps DJ, Brandhuber BJ, Thompson RC, Eisenberg SP. Interleukin-1 (IL-1) receptor antagonist binds to the 80-kDa IL-1 receptor but does not initiate IL-1 signal transduction. J Biol Chem 1991; 266: 10331–6.

76. Loewe R, Holnthoner W, Groger M, Pillinger M, Gruber F et al. Dimethylfumarate inhibits TNF-induced nuclear entry of NF-kappa B/p65 in human endothelial cells. J Immunol 2002; 168: 4781–7.

77. O'Donovan LH, McMonagle EL, Taylor S, Bain D, Pacitti AM et al. A vector expressing feline mature IL-18 fused to IL-1beta antagonist protein signal sequence is an effective adjuvant to a DNA vaccine for feline leukaemia virus. Vaccine 2005; 23: 3814–23.

78. Steinhoff M, Bienenstock J, Schmelz M, Maurer M, Wei E et al. Neurophysiological, neuroimmunological, and neuroendocrine basis of pruritus. J Invest Dermatol 2006; 126: 1705–18.

79. Steinhoff M, Stander S, Seeliger S, Ansel JC, Schmelz M et al. Modern aspects of cutaneous neurogenic inflammation. Arch Dermatol 2003; 139: 1479–88.

80. Sonkoly E, Muller A, Lauerma AI, Pivarcsi A, Soto H et al. IL-31: a new link between T cells and pruritus in atopic skin inflammation. J Allergy Clin Immunol 2006; 117: 411–17.

81. Bilsborough J, Leung DY, Maurer M, Howell M, Boguniewcz M et al. IL-31 is associated with cutaneous lymphocyte antigen-positive skin homing T cells in patients with atopic dermatitis. J Allergy Clin Immunol 2006; 117: 418–25.

82. Takaoka A, Arai I, Sugimoto M, Yamaguchi A, Tanaka M et al. Expression of IL-31 gene transcripts in NC/Nga mice with atopic dermatitis. Eur J Pharmacol 2005; 516: 180–1.

83. Takaoka A, Arai I, Sugimoto M, Honma Y, Futaki N et al. Involvement of IL-31 on scratching behavior in NC/Nga mice with atopic-like dermatitis. Exp Dermatol 2006; 15: 161–7.

84. DuBuske LM. IgE, allergic diseases, and omalizumab. Curr Pharm Des 2006; 12: 3929–44.

85. Graves JE, Nunley K, Heffernan MP. Off-label uses of biologics in dermatology: rituximab, omalizumab, infliximab, etanercept, adalimumab, efalizumab, and alefacept (part 2 of 2). J Am Acad Dermatol 2007; 56: 55–79.

86. Sarinho E, Cruz AA. Anti-IgE monoclonal antibody for the treatment of the asthma and other manifestations related to allergic diseases. J Pediatr (Rio J) 2006; 82: 127–32.

87. Winchester DE, Jacob A, Murphy T. Omalizumab for asthma. N Engl J Med 2006; 355: 1281–2.

88. Milgrom H, Fick RB, Jr., Su JQ, Reimann JD, Bush RK et al. Treatment of allergic asthma with monoclonal anti-IgE antibody. rhuMAb-E25 Study Group. N Engl J Med 1999; 341: 1966–73.

89. Kuehr J, Brauburger J, Zielen S, Schauer U, Kamin W et al. Efficacy of combination treatment with anti-IgE plus specific immunotherapy in polysensitized children and adolescents with seasonal allergic rhinitis. J Allergy Clin Immunol 2002; 109: 274–80.

90. Finn A, Gross G, van Bavel J, Lee T, Windom H et al. Omalizumab improves asthma-related quality of life in patients with severe allergic asthma. J Allergy Clin Immunol 2003; 111: 278–84.

91. Schmitt J, Schakel K. Omalizumab as a therapeutic option in atopic eczema: current evidence and potential benefit. Hautarzt 2007; 58: 128–32.

92. Steinhoff M, Luger TA. The skin cytokine network. In: Bos J, ed. Skin Immune System (SIS). New York: Marcel Dekker Inc, 2004.

93. Hommes DW, Mikhajlova TL, Stoinov S, Stimac D, Vucelic B et al. Fontolizumab, a humanised anti-interferon gamma antibody, demonstrates safety and clinical activity in patients with moderate to severe Crohn's disease. Gut 2006; 55: 1131–7.

94. Reinisch W, Hommes DW, Van Assche G, Colombel JF, Gendre JP et al. A dose escalating, placebo controlled, double blind, single dose and multidose, safety and tolerability study of fontolizumab, a humanised anti-interferon gamma antibody, in patients with moderate to severe Crohn's disease. Gut 2006; 55: 1138–44.

95. Reinhold U, Kukel S, Brzoska J, Kreysel HW. Systemic interferon gamma treatment in severe atopic dermatitis. J Am Acad Dermatol 1993; 29: 58–63.

96. Schneider LC, Baz Z, Zarcone C, Zurakowski D. Long-term therapy with recombinant interferon-gamma (rIFN-gamma) for atopic dermatitis. Ann Allergy Asthma Immunol 1998; 80: 263–8.

97. Weinberg JM, Saini R. Biologic therapy for psoriasis: the tumor necrosis factor inhibitors infliximab and etanercept. Cutis 2003; 71: 25–9.

98. Braun J, Sieper J. Role of novel biological therapies in psoriatic arthritis: effects on joints and skin. BioDrugs 2003; 17: 187–99.

99. Machold KP, Smolen JS. Adalimumab – a new TNF-alpha antibody for treatment of inflammatory joint disease. Expert Opin Biol Ther 2003; 3: 351–60.

100. Gottlieb AB, Chaudhari U, Mulcahy LD, Li S, Dooley LT et al. Infliximab monotherapy provides rapid and sustained benefit for plaque-type psoriasis. J Am Acad Dermatol 2003; 48: 829–35.

101. Mease PJ, Goffe BS, Metz J, VanderStoep A, Finck B et al. Etanercept in the treatment of psoriatic arthritis and psoriasis: a randomised trial. Lancet 2000; 356: 385–90.

102. Mahadevan U, Sandborn WJ. Infliximab for the treatment of orofacial Crohn's disease. Inflamm Bowel Dis 2001; 7: 38–42.

103. Iyer S, Yamauchi P, Lowe NJ. Etanercept for severe psoriasis and psoriatic arthritis: observations on combination therapy. Br J Dermatol 2002; 146: 118–21.

104. Jacobi A, Antoni C, Manger B, Schuler G, Hertl M. Infliximab in the treatment of moderate to severe atopic dermatitis. J Am Acad Dermatol 2005; 52: 522–6.

105. Cassano N, Loconsole F, Coviello C, Vena GA. Infliximab in recalcitrant severe atopic eczema associated with contact allergy. Int J Immunopathol Pharmacol 2006; 19: 237–40.

106. Chan JL, Davis-Reed L, Kimball AB. Counter-regulatory balance: atopic dermatitis in patients undergoing infliximab infusion therapy. J Drugs Dermatol 2004; 3: 315–18.

107. Bayes M, Rabasseda X, Prous JR. Gateways to clinical trials. Methods Find Exp Clin Pharmacol 2002; 24: 371–91.

108. Bashir SJ, Maibach HI. Alefacept (Biogen). Curr Opin Investig Drugs 2001; 2: 631–4.

109. Weinberg JM, Tutrone WD. Biologic therapy for psoriasis: the T-cell-targeted therapies efalizumab and alefacept. Cutis 2003; 71: 41–5.

110. Krueger GG, Ellis CN. Alefacept therapy produces remission for patients with chronic plaque psoriasis. Br J Dermatol 2003; 148: 784–8.

111. Lebwohl M, Christophers E, Langley R, Ortonne JP, Roberts J et al. An international, randomized, double-blind, placebo-controlled phase 3 trial of intramuscular alefacept in patients with chronic plaque psoriasis. Arch Dermatol 2003; 139: 719–27.

112. Simon D, Von Gunten S, Borelli S, Braathen LR, Simon HU. The interleukin-13 production by peripheral blood T cells from atopic dermatitis patients does not require CD2 costimulation. Int Arch Allergy Immunol 2003; 132: 148–55.

113. Jenmalm MC, Aniansson-Zdolsek H, Holt PG, Bjorksten B. Expression of and responses to CD2 and CD3 in 18-month-old children with and without atopic dermatitis. Pediatr Allergy Immunol 2000; 11: 175–82.

114. Weinshenker BG, Bass BH, Ebers GC, Rice GP. Remission of psoriatic lesions with muromonab-CD3 (orthoclone OKT3) treatment. J Am Acad Dermatol 1989; 20: 1132–3.

115. Bachelez H, Flageul B, Dubertret L, Fraitag S, Grossman R et al. Treatment of recalcitrant plaque psoriasis with a humanized non-depleting antibody to CD4. J Autoimmun 1998; 11: 53–62.

116. Cather JC, Cather JC, Menter A. Modulating T cell responses for the treatment of psoriasis: a focus on efalizumab. Expert Opin Biol Ther 2003; 3: 361–70.

117. Gottlieb AB, Miller B, Lowe N, Shapiro W, Hudson C et al. Subcutaneously administered efalizumab (anti-CD11a) improves signs and symptoms of moderate to severe plaque psoriasis. J Cutan Med Surg 2003; 7: 198–207.

118. Weinberg JM, Siegfried EC. Successful treatment of severe atopic dermatitis in a child and an adult with the T-cell modulator efalizumab. Arch Dermatol 2006; 142: 555–8.

119. Takiguchi R, Tofte S, Simpson B, Harper E, Blauvelt A et al. Efalizumab for severe atopic dermatitis: a pilot study in adults. J Am Acad Dermatol 2007; 56: 222–7.

120. Hassan AS, Kaelin U, Braathen LR, Yawalkar N. Clinical and immunopathologic findings during treatment of recalcitrant atopic eczema with efalizumab. J Am Acad Dermatol 2007; 56: 217–21.

121. Griffiths CE, Railan D, Gallatin WM, Cooper KD. The ICAM-3/LFA-1 interaction is critical for epidermal Langerhans cell alloantigen presentation to CD4+ T cells. Br J Dermatol 1995; 133: 823–9.

122. Jockers JJ, Novak N. Different expression of adhesion molecules and tetraspanins of monocytes of patients with atopic eczema. Allergy 2006; 61: 1419–22.

123. Wedi B, Wieczorek D, Stunkel T, Breuer K, Kapp A. Staphylococcal exotoxins exert proinflammatory effects through inhibition of eosinophil apoptosis, increased surface antigen expression (CD11b, CD45, CD54, and CD69), and enhanced cytokine-activated oxidative burst, thereby triggering allergic inflammatory reactions. J Allergy Clin Immunol 2002; 109: 477–84.

124. Coiffier B, Haioun C, Ketterer N, Engert A, Tilly H et al. Rituximab (anti-CD20 monoclonal antibody) for the treatment of patients with relapsing or refractory aggressive lymphoma: a multicenter phase II study. Blood 1998; 92: 1927–32.

125. Czuczman MS, Grillo-Lopez AJ, White CA, Saleh M, Gordon L et al. Treatment of patients with low-grade B-cell lymphoma with the combination of chimeric anti-CD20 monoclonal antibody and CHOP chemotherapy. J Clin Oncol 1999; 17: 268–76.

126. Salopek TG, Logsetty S, Tredget EE. Anti-CD20 chimeric monoclonal antibody (rituximab) for the treatment of recalcitrant, life-threatening pemphigus vulgaris with implications in the pathogenesis of the disorder. J Am Acad Dermatol 2002; 47: 785–8.

127. Abrams JR, Kelley SL, Hayes E, Kikuchi T, Brown MJ et al. Blockade of T lymphocyte costimulation with cytotoxic T lymphocyte-associated antigen 4-immunoglobulin (CTLA4Ig) reverses the cellular pathology of psoriatic plaques, including the activation of keratinocytes, dendritic cells, and endothelial cells. J Exp Med 2000; 192: 681–94.

128. Davenport CM, McAdams HA, Kou J, Mascioli K, Eichman C et al. Inhibition of pro-inflammatory cytokine generation by CTLA4-Ig in the skin and colon of mice adoptively transplanted with CD45RBhi CD4+ T cells correlates with suppression of psoriasis and colitis. Int Immunopharmacol 2002; 2: 653–72.

129. Choi SY, Sohn MH, Kwon BC, Kim KE. CTLA-4 expression in T cells of patients with atopic dermatitis. Pediatr Allergy Immunol 2005; 16: 422–7.

130. Neuber K, Mahnss B, Hubner C, Gergely H, Weichenthal M. Autoantibodies against CD28 are associated with atopic diseases. Clin Exp Immunol 2006; 146: 262–9.

131. Gottlieb AB, Lebwohl M, Totoritis MC, Abdulghani AA, Shuey SR et al. Clinical and histologic response to single-dose treatment of moderate to severe psoriasis with an anti-CD80 monoclonal antibody. J Am Acad Dermatol 2002; 47: 692–700.

132. Slominski A, Wortsman J, Luger T, Paus R, Solomon S. Corticotropin releasing hormone and proopiomelanocortin involvement in the cutaneous response to stress. Physiol Rev 2000; 80: 979–1020.

133. Karin M. Mitogen-activated protein kinase cascades as regulators of stress responses. Ann N Y Acad Sci 1998; 851: 139–46.

134. Norris V, Choong L, Tran D, Corden Z, Boyce M et al. Effect of IVL745, a VLA-4 antagonist, on allergen-induced bronchoconstriction in patients with asthma. J Allergy Clin Immunol 2005; 116: 761–7.

135. Okigami H, Takeshita K, Tajimi M, Komura H, Albers M et al. Inhibition of eosinophilia in vivo by a small molecule inhibitor of very late antigen (VLA)-4. Eur J Pharmacol 2007; 559: 202–9.

136. Tarkowski M, Pacheco KA, Rosenwasser LJ. The effect of antigen stimulation on alpha(4), beta(1) and beta(7) chain integrin expression and function in CD4+ cells. Int Arch Allergy Immunol 2000; 121: 25–33.

137. Zollner TM, Asadullah K, Schon MP. Targeting leukocyte trafficking to inflamed skin: still an attractive therapeutic approach? Exp Dermatol 2007; 16: 1–12.

138. Homey B, Steinhoff M, Ruzicka T, Leung DY. Cytokines and chemokines orchestrate atopic skin inflammation. J Allergy Clin Immunol 2006; 118: 178–89.

139. Hoffjan S, Parwez Q, Petrasch-Parwez E, Falkenstein D, Nothnagel M et al. Association screen for atopic dermatitis candidate gene regions using microsatellite markers in pooled DNA samples. Int J Immunogenet 2006; 33: 401–9.

140. Purandare AV, Somerville JE. Antagonists of CCR4 as immunomodulatory agents. Curr Top Med Chem 2006; 6: 1335–44.

141. Tsunemi Y, Saeki H, Nakamura K, Nagakubo D, Nakayama T et al. CCL17 transgenic mice show an enhanced Th2-type response to both allergic and non-allergic stimuli. Eur J Immunol 2006; 36: 2116–27.

142. Holse M, Assing K, Poulsen LK. CCR3, CCR5, CCR8 and CXCR3 expression in memory T helper cells from allergic rhinitis patients, asymptomatically sensitized and healthy individuals. Clin Mol Allergy 2006; 4: 6.

143. Kato Y, Pawankar R, Kimura Y, Kawana S. Increased expression of RANTES, CCR3 and CCR5 in the lesional skin of patients with atopic eczema. Int Arch Allergy Immunol 2006; 139: 245–57.

144. Homey B, Alenius H, Muller A, Soto H, Bowman EP et al. CCL27-CCR10 interactions regulate T cell-mediated skin inflammation. Nat Med 2002; 8: 157–65.

145. Ugwu SO, Blanchard J, Dorr RT, Levine N, Brooks C et al. Skin pigmentation and pharmacokinetics of melanotan-I in humans. Biopharm Drug Dispos 1997; 18: 259–69.

146. Cutuli M, Cristiani S, Lipton JM, Catania A. Antimicrobial effects of alpha-MSH peptides. J Leukoc Biol 2000; 67: 233–9.

147. Brzoska T, Luger TA, Maaser C, Abels C, Bohm M. alpha-melanocyte-stimulating hormone and related tripeptides. submitted.

148. Steinhoff M, Buddenkotte J, Shpacovitch V, Rattenholl A, Moormann C et al. Proteinase-activated receptors: transducers of proteinase-mediated signaling in inflammation and immune response. Endocr Rev 2005; 26: 1–43.

149. Ossovskaya VS, Bunnett NW. Protease-activated receptors: contribution to physiology and disease. Physiol Rev 2004; 84: 579–621.

150. Buddenkotte J, Stroh C, Engels IH, Moormann C, Shpacovitch VM et al. Agonists of proteinase-activated receptor-2 stimulate upregulation of intercellular cell adhesion molecule-1 in primary human keratinocytes via activation of NF-κB. J Invest Dermatol 2005; 124: 38–45.

151. Seeliger S, Derian CK, Vergnolle N, Bunnett NW, Nawroth R et al. Proinflammatory role of proteinase-activated receptor-2 in humans and mice during cutaneous inflammation in vivo. FASEB J 2003; 17: 1871–85.

152. Shpacovitch VM, Brzoska T, Buddenkotte J, Stroh C, Sommerhoff CP et al. Agonists of proteinase-activated receptor 2 induce cytokine release and activation of nuclear transcription factor kappaB in human dermal microvascular endothelial cells. J Invest Dermatol 2002; 118: 380–5.

153. Shpacovitch VM, Varga G, Strey A, Gunzer M, Mooren F et al. Agonists of proteinase-activated receptor-2 modulate human neutrophil cytokine secretion, expression of cell adhesion molecules, and migration within 3-D collagen lattices. J Leukoc Biol 2004; 76: 388–98.

154. Steinhoff M, Vergnolle N, Young SH, Tognetto M, Amadesi S et al. Agonists of proteinase-activated receptor 2 induce inflammation by a neurogenic mechanism. Nat Med 2000; 6: 151–8.

155. Moormann C, Artuc M, Pohl E, Varga G, Buddenkotte J et al. Functional characterization and expression analysis of the proteinase-activated receptor-2 in human cutaneous mast cells. J Invest Dermatol 2006; 126: 746–55.

156. Steinhoff M, Neisius U, Ikoma A, Fartasch M, Heyer G et al. Proteinase-activated receptor-2 mediates itch: a novel pathway for pruritus in human skin. J Neurosci 2003; 23: 6176–80.

157. Steinhoff M, Steinhoff A, Homey B, Luger TA, Schneider SW. Role of vasculature in atopic dermatitis. J Allergy Clin Immunol 2006; 118: 190–7.

Index

Note: *AD* is used for atopic dermatitis in subheadings

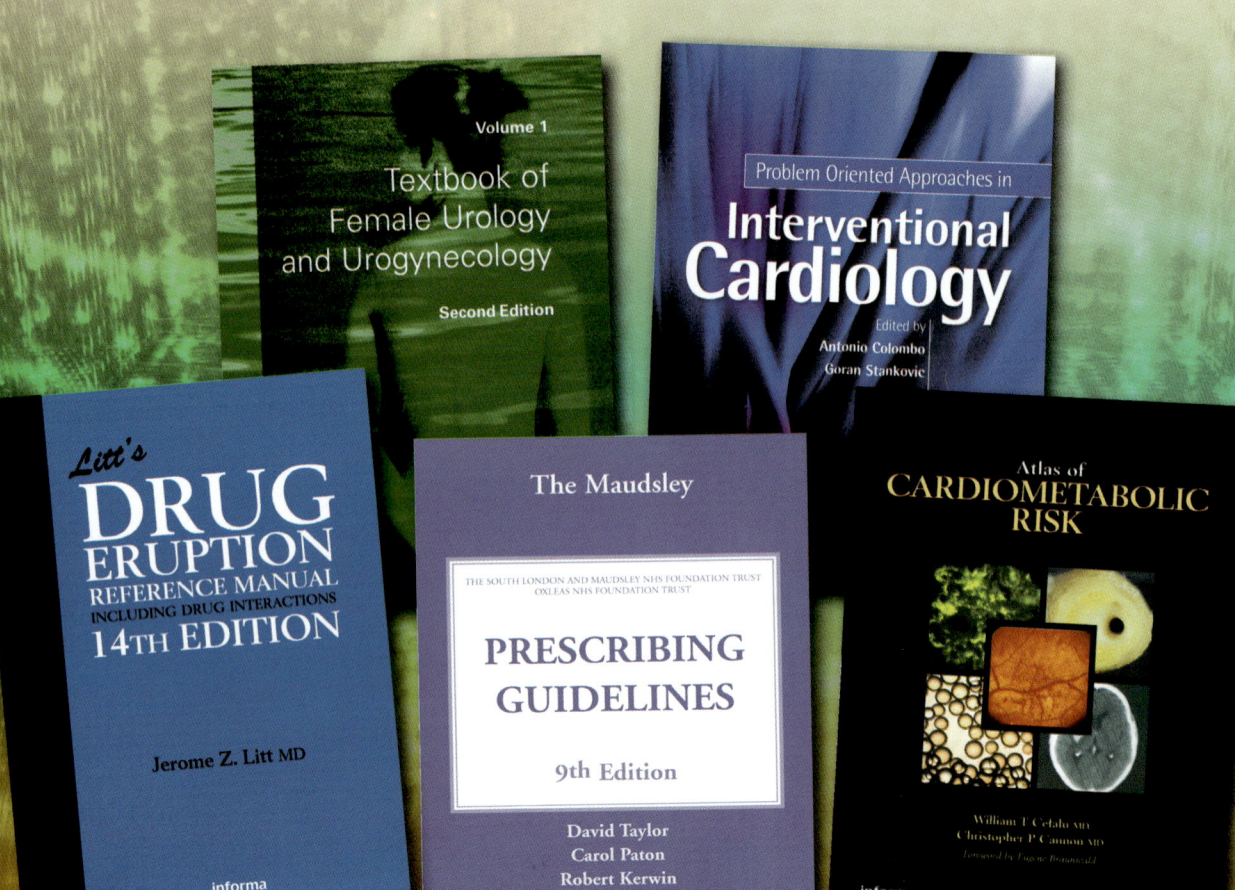

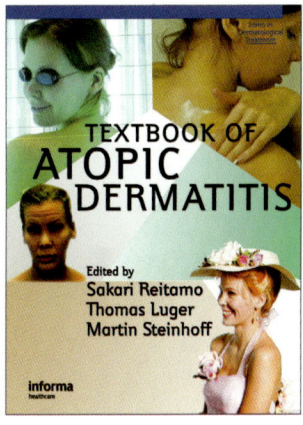